Probiotics: Immunobiotics and Immunogenics

Probiotics: Immunobiotics and Immunogenics

Editor: Simon Bruce

MURPHY & MOORE
www.murphy-moorepublishing.com

www.murphy-moorepublishing.com

MURPHY & MOORE

Cataloging-in-Publication Data

Probiotics : immunobiotics and immunogenics / edited by Simon Bruce.
p. cm.
Includes bibliographical references and index.
ISBN 978-1-63987-461-3
1. Probiotics. 2. Immune system. I. Bruce, Simon.
RM666.P835 P76 2022
615.329--dc23

Murphy & Moore Publishing,
1 Rockefeller Plaza,
New York City, NY 10020, USA

ISBN 978-1-63987-461-3 (Hardback)

Contents

Preface

The live microorganisms which have a beneficial effect on the health of an individual upon their consumption are known as probiotics. The microbial strains which are responsible for the beneficial regulation of the mucosal immune system are collectively known as immunobiotics. They can be used to treat and reduce the severity of numerous diseases and infections in animals and humans. A few of such diseases and infections are allergies, obesity, immunosuppression, intestinal infections and inflammatory bowel disease. Studies have also shown that a few immunobiotic strains are able to regulate the immune-coagulative responses in the respiratory tract and thereby decrease the severity of viral disease. The bioactive compounds present in immunobiotics are termed as immunogenics. This book unravels the recent studies in the field of immunobiotics and immunogenics. Also included herein is a detailed explanation of the various cellular and molecular interactions in immunobiotics. Those in search of information to further their knowledge will be greatly assisted by this book.

Significant researches are present in this book. Intensive efforts have been employed by authors to make this book an outstanding discourse. This book contains the enlightening chapters which have been written on the basis of significant researches done by the experts.

Finally, I would also like to thank all the members involved in this book for being a team and meeting all the deadlines for the submission of their respective works. I would also like to thank my friends and family for being supportive in my efforts.

Editor

1

Unraveling the Differences between Gram-Positive and Gram-Negative Probiotics in Modulating Protective Immunity to Enteric Infections

*Sukumar Kandasamy, Anastasia N. Vlasova, David D. Fischer, Kuldeep S. Chattha[†], Lulu Shao[†], Anand Kumar[†], Stephanie N. Langel, Abdul Rauf, Huang-Chi Huang, Gireesh Rajashekara and Linda J. Saif**

Food Animal Health Research Program (FAHRP), Veterinary Preventive Medicine Department, The Ohio Agricultural Research and Development Center, The Ohio State University, Wooster, OH, USA

Edited by:
Julio Villena,
Reference Centre for Lactobacilli (CERELA-CONICET), Argentina

Reviewed by:
Haruki Kitazawa,
Tohoku University, Japan
Maria Guadalupe Vizoso Pinto,
National University of Tucumán, Argentina

***Correspondence:**
Linda J. Saif
saif.2@osu.edu

The role of intestinal microbiota and probiotics in prevention and treatment of infectious diseases, including diarrheal diseases in children and animal models, is increasingly recognized. Intestinal commensals play a major role in development of the immune system in neonates and in shaping host immune responses to pathogens. Lactobacilli spp. and *Escherichia coli* Nissle 1917 are two probiotics that are commonly used in children to treat various medical conditions including human rotavirus diarrhea and inflammatory bowel disease. Although the health benefits of probiotics have been confirmed, the specific effects of these established Gram-positive (G+) and Gram-negative (G–) probiotics in modulating immunity against pathogens and disease are largely undefined. In this review, we discuss the differences between G+ and G– probiotics/commensals in modulating the dynamics of selected infectious diseases and host immunity. These probiotics modulate the pathogenesis of infectious diseases and protective immunity against pathogens in a species- and strain-specific manner. Collectively, it appears that the selected G– probiotic is more effective than the various tested G+ probiotics in enhancing protective immunity against rotavirus in the gnotobiotic piglet model.

Keywords: rotavirus, probiotics, *Escherichia coli* Nissle, *Lactobacillus*, immunity, children, diarrhea, gnotobiotic piglet disease model

INTRODUCTION

Intestinal commensals constitute more than 1,000 species of bacteria. These commensals are involved in nutrient metabolism, development, and functioning of the gastrointestinal (GI) immune system and protection of the host from pathogens (1–3). Colonization of the GI tract is a gradual process in which *Escherichia coli* and other enterobacteria colonize the intestinal tract early after birth, followed by the subsequent establishment of anaerobes (4). The intestinal microbiota of children only becomes adult-like at 2–3 years of age (5). Perturbation of the intestinal microbiota, or dysbiosis, is associated with various diseases such as inflammatory bowel disease (6) and also affects the efficacy of various vaccines in children (7). Probiotics are widely used to restore gut homeostasis in various medical conditions in humans (8–10) and treat diarrheal diseases in children.

Diarrheal disease is one of the leading cause of deaths in children and it accounts for the death an estimated of 700,000 children annually worldwide (11). Specifically, rotavirus (RV) is a major cause of gastroenteritis in children worldwide. The protective efficacy of available RV vaccines is variable between regions and it is lowest in developing countries such as Southern Asia (50.0%) and sub-Saharan Africa (46.1%) (12). Additionally, lack of access to adequate health-care facilities to manage diarrhea is also associated with higher morbidity and mortality in children in low-income settings. Thus, enhancing vaccine efficacy, along with developing economical approaches to reduce the severity of RV diarrhea are effective strategies to ameliorate severe RV disease. Probiotics and intestinal commensals, crucial interacting partners of the gut immune system (13), are increasingly being considered for treatment of various enteric infections including human retrovirus (HRV) diarrhea (14), human norovirus gastroenteritis (15), antibiotic-associated diarrhea (16), and also to modulate protective antiviral immunity (17).

The beneficial effects of probiotics in reducing the severity of RV diarrhea and modulating viral immunity were observed in randomized clinical studies (18) and experimental studies in animal models (19) (**Table 1**). The Gram-positive (G+) *Lactobacillus* spp. were widely used to treat or prevent RV diarrhea in children. Specifically, prophylactic supplementation of *Lactobacillus rhamnosus* GG (LGG) to children significantly reduced the incidence of HRV disease (20). In our studies, gnotobiotic (Gn) piglets were used to study HRV pathogenesis due to their susceptibility to HRV infection and also the greater anatomic and physiological and immunological similarities between pigs and humans. Dual colonization of Gn piglets with G + LGG and *Bifidobacterium lactis* Bb12 resulted in a significant reduction in both fecal HRV shedding titers and diarrhea severity (21). Further, *Lactobacillus* strains have significant effects in reducing diarrhea severity in children affected by enteric diseases (22).

The effectiveness of probiotics in preventing or treating a disease is dependent on several factors such as class or strains of probiotics, the dosage of probiotics, and heterogeneity of study subjects (40, 41). Several past studies showed strain-specific differences of probiotics in modulating host immune responses (42). Thus, comparative analysis of the health benefits of different classes of probiotics is essential to tailor an effective regimen of probiotic treatment for a disease condition. Specifically variations in microbe-associated molecular patterns between G+ and Gram-negative (G−) bacteria have been attributed to differential induction of innate immunity in a host (43, 44). However, limited studies have been conducted to decipher if differences exist between G+ and G− probiotics in modulating host responses to infectious diseases. In our recent studies (31, 32), we compared the beneficial effects of G+ and G− probiotics in modulating virulent HRV infection as well as host immunity. Specifically, LGG was selected as a G+ probiotic because of its well-documented effects in reducing the severity of RV diarrhea in children (24). For the G− probiotic, we selected *Escherichia coli* Nissle 1917 (EcN) due to its proven effects in attenuating inflammatory disorders and modulating immunity in humans (45). In this review, we focused on the comparisons of the health benefits of G+ and G− probiotics in modulating microbial infections and immunity.

EFFECTS OF G+ VERSUS G− PROBIOTICS ON ENTERIC INFECTIONS AND DIARRHEA

Probiotics have been successfully used to prevent or treat enteric infections in children and animals (**Table 1**). One notable finding is the difference between G+ and G− probiotics in modulating host immunity against microbial diseases. In one study (31), the comparative efficacy of LGG and EcN probiotics in ameliorating HRV disease was assessed in Gn piglets. The EcN colonized piglets had reduced diarrhea severity and also lower mean peak virus shedding titers compared with LGG or uncolonized piglets post-virulent human RV (VirHRV) challenge (31, 32). Both EcN and LGG showed similar colonization patterns as indicated by comparable fecal shedding of each bacterium and also detection of similar levels of each probiotic bacteria in various sections of GI tract. Similarly, EcN supplementation to children with enteric infections resulted in reduced duration of diarrhea (26). Further, supplementation of EcN to infants for the first 5 days immediately after birth resulted in persistence of the probiotic for 6 months as indicated by fecal shedding of EcN (29). Similar to the higher beneficial effects of EcN than LGG on ameliorating HRV infection, higher protective effects against *Salmonella* were observed in EcN compared with *Bifidobacterium choerinum*-supplemented Gn piglets (30). The higher protective effect of EcN against *Salmonella* was associated with increased expression of ZO-1 and occludin in ileal epithelial cells and decreased inflammatory TNF-α cytokine levels in the EcN colonized Gn piglets (30). Consistent with these findings, higher TNF-α levels were induced by G+ commensals as compared with G− commensals using *in vitro* mononuclear cultures (43). EcN supplementation also attenuated lipopolysaccharides (LPS) or trinitrobenzene sulfonic acid-induced inflammatory conditions in a mouse model (46). In summary, the higher ability of G− compared with G+ probiotics in reducing the levels of inflammatory mediators during enteric infections may be major contributing factor in reducing diarrhea severity.

G+ and G− Probiotic Impacts on Modulation of B Cell Responses

Microbial colonization of the GI tract has a significant effect on the maturation of neonatal immune system (47). Consistent with this observation, administration of EcN enhanced serum EcN-specific IgA antibody and polyclonal IgM antibody responses in infants as compared with placebo group (28). Also, mono EcN or dual EcN + LGG colonization significantly increased serum total IgA and IgG responses compared with LGG colonized or uncolonized piglets (31) (**Figure 1**). Similar to systemic immunoglobulin responses, EcN colonization resulted in higher small intestinal total IgA responses compared with LGG colonization in Gn pigs. Thus, EcN had more potent immunostimulatory effects than LGG in terms of inducing mucosal and systemic B cell responses. The underlying mechanism for differential induction of antibody responses by G+ and G− bacteria might be due to variation in IgA inducing factors such as IL-10 cytokine. In fact, G−, but not G+ probiotics, induced higher IL-10 responses in

TABLE 1 | Effects of G+ and G− probiotics on diarrheal diseases and immunity in children and animal models.

Gram-positive probiotic/ commensal bacteria	Gram-negative probiotic/ commensal bacteria	Humans/ animal model/*in vitro* study	Indication	Conclusion(s)	Reference
L. rhamnosus GG (6 × 10^9 CFU/dose)	None	Children	Prophylaxis against diarrheal diseases	Significant reduction in incidence of HRV disease in LGG-supplemented group	(20)
L. rhamnosus GG (10^{10-11} CFU)	None	Children	Effect of LGG on immune responses to HRV in children	LGG significantly enhanced RV-specific IgA antibody responses	(23)
L. rhamnosus GG (10^{10} CFU)	None	Children	Treating diarrhea	Reduced duration of diarrhea	(24)
Lactobacillus paracasei strain ST11 (10^{10} CFU)	None	Children	Treating diarrhea	Reduced severity of non-rotavirus induced diarrhea but no effect on rotavirus diarrhea	(25)
None	*Escherichia coli* Nissle 1917 (EcN) (10^8 CFU)	Children	Treat acute diarrhea in children	Reduced duration of diarrhea by 2.3 days	(26)
None	EcN (3 × 10^8 CFU)	Infants	To assess effects on total IgA responses in infants	Increased serum and stool IgA responses	(27)
None	EcN (10^8 CFU)	Infants	Assess impact on cellular and humoral immunity in infants	Probiotic increased both cellular proliferative and serum total IgA responses	(28)
None	EcN (10^8 CFU)	Infants	Prophylactic administration against bacterial pathogens	Significant reduction in bacterial pathogens in fecal samples	(29)
Bifidobacterium choerinum (5 × 10^8 CFU/ml)	EcN (5 × 10^8 CFU/ ml)	Gn piglets	Protection against *Salmonella enterica* serovar Typhimurium infection	EcN conferred higher protection against disease than *Bifidobacterium choerinum*	(30)
L. rhamnosus GG (10^5 CFU/ml)	EcN (10^5 CFU/ml)	Gn piglets	Compare G+ and G− bacteria effect on HRV infection and immunity	EcN was more effective than LGG in ameliorating HRV disease and enhancing total IgA and NK cell responses	(31, 32)
L. rhamnosus GG (10^5 CFU/ml), *Bifidobacterium lactis* Bb12 (105 CFU/ml)	None	Gn piglets	To study effects on HRV disease	Reduced fecal virus shedding and diarrhea severity in probiotic colonized piglets	(21)
Enterococcus faecium NCIMB 10415 (4.2–4.3 × 10^6/g CFU)	None	Sows and their offspring	Effect on fecal shedding of enteric viruses	Reduced fecal shedding of rotavirus and increased rotavirus specific IgA responses. No effect on hepatitis E virus, encephalomyocarditis virus, and norovirus shedding in feces	(33)
None	EcN (10^{10} CFU/ml)	Pigs	To prevent enterotoxigenic *Escherichia coli* induced diarrhea	Ameliorated clinical signs of diarrhea	(34)
None	EcN (10^8 CFU/ml)	Neonatal calf	Prevention and treatment of diarrhea	Reduction in incidence of diarrheal diseases in prophylactic group. Ameliorated severity of diarrhea in calves with enteric diseases	(35)
Lactobacillus acidophilus A9 (10^8/ ml CFU)	*Escherichia coli* 13-7 (10^6/ml CFU)	Mice	Compare G+ and G− bacteria effect on cytokine responses in mice	*E. coli* 13-7 induced higher IL-12 cytokine compared to *L. acidophilus* A9	(36)
None	EcN (1.5–2 × 10^8 CFU)	Mice	Assess impact on intestinal barrier function in acute dextran sodium sulfate-induced colitis	Strengthened intestinal barrier function	(37)
Lactobacillus casei Shirota	EcN	*In vitro*	Investigate effects on innate immunity	Higher IL-10 and IL-12 induction by EcN than *L. casei* Shirota	(38)
L. plantarum, L. rhamnosus, L. paracasei ssp. paracasei	*Escherichia coli* O6:K13:H1, *Escherichia coli* MS101	*In vitro*	Compare G+ and G− bacteria effect on cytokine responses of monocytes	Lactobacilli-induced higher level of IL-12	(39)

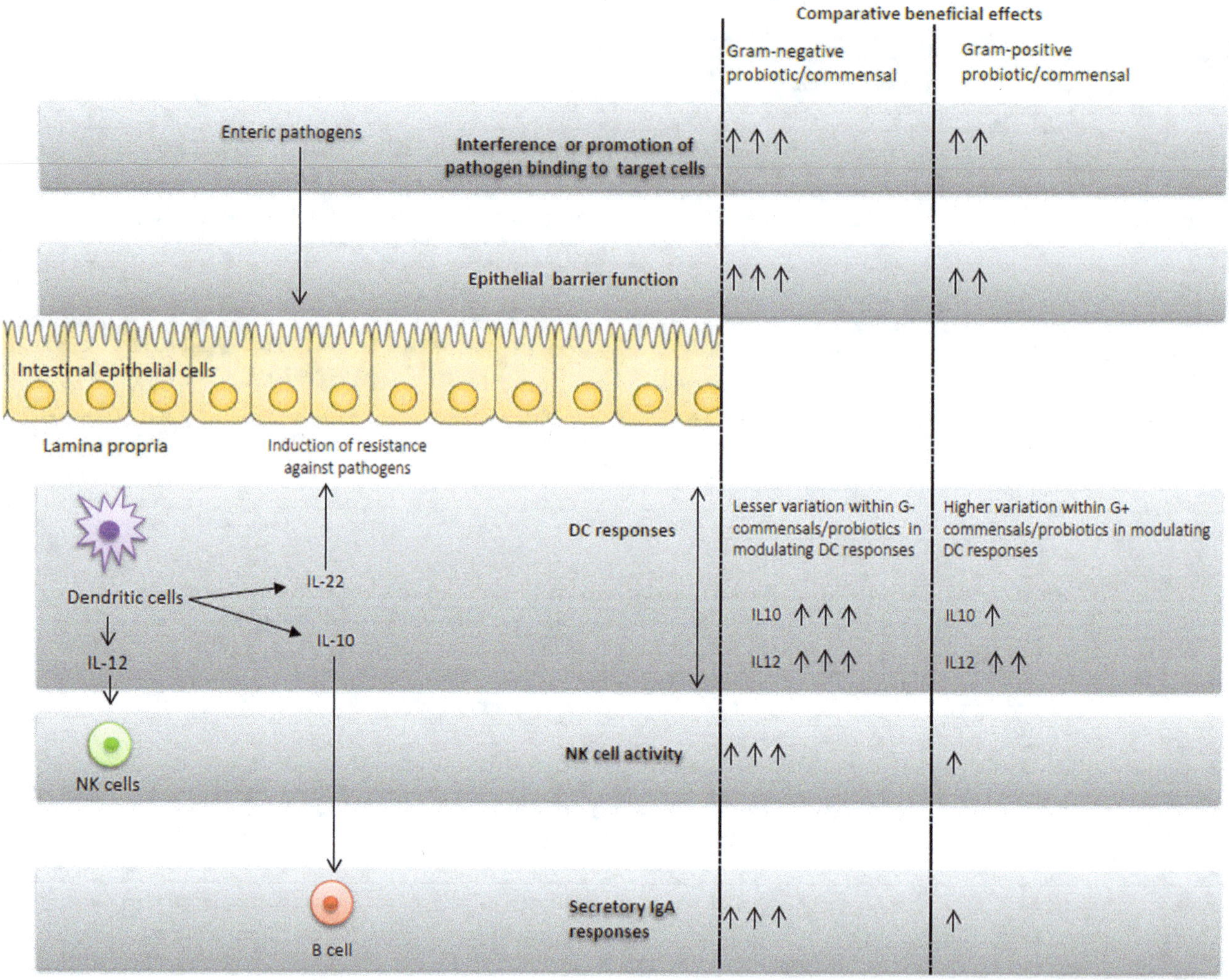

FIGURE 1 | **Schematic representation of the G+ and G− probiotics-induced immunomodulatory effects and proposed potential immune interactions.**

prior studies (31, 48, 49). IL-10 is one of the cytokines that mediates the induction of IgA antibody responses at mucosal sites through enhancing antibody class switching (50). Differences in the microbe-associated molecular patterns between the probiotics might be a potential reason for the differential induction of IL-10 by G+ and G− bacteria. Indeed, both the LPS portion of EcN and whole EcN lysate were identified as potent inducers of IL-10 production in peripheral blood mononuclear cells (51). Further, induction of total IgA responses is at least partially mediated by IL-10 *in vitro* (31). These studies demonstrate that modulation of the cytokine milieu, such as enhanced IL-10 levels, might be a potential mechanism to account for the higher antibody responses observed in G− compared with G+ probiotics groups.

It is also well established that strain-dependent variations in immunomodulatory properties are observed within G+ probiotics (52). Thus, individual probiotic strains within G+ or G− probiotic classes may differ in modulating antibody responses. Consequently, screening of the beneficial effects of individual probiotics is essential to elucidate their impacts on antibody responses.

Impact of Innate Immunity on IgA Responses to G+ versus G− Probiotics

Innate immunity plays an integral role in priming the adaptive immune responses. Thus, probiotics may induce specific changes in innate immunity that may be involved in synergistically enhancing IgA responses. Dual colonization of a G− and G+ probiotic enhanced serum total IgA responses in Gn piglets compared with mono-colonization of the probiotics (31). Thus, G+ and G− bacteria synergistically enhanced the systemic total IgA responses. In fact, combinations of G+ and G− probiotics had additive effects on induction of maturation markers in DCs as well as levels of IL-10 cytokines (53). Thus, considering the known function of DCs in induction of IgA responses (54, 55), the positive effects of combinations of G+ and G− bacteria in modulating DCs may play a role in enhancing IgA responses. Additionally, a previous study (56) also showed that LPS, a TLR4 ligand, synergistically interacted with TLR1/2 ligands which in turn enhanced class-switch recombination in B cells. Thus, synergistic interactions of microbe-associated molecular patterns from G− and G+ probiotics might also play a role in enhancing antibody responses. Apart from DCs, it appears that intestinal epithelial cells also respond differently in terms of producing IgA mediators such as TGF-β and thymic stromal lymphopoietin (TSLP). Specifically, G− commensals induce higher production of TGF-β and TSLP as compared with G+ commensals (57). Further, higher frequencies of splenic $TLR9^+$ mononuclear cells were detected in EcN + LGG colonized compared with the monocolonized EcN or LGG Gn piglets (32). TLR9 recognizes CpG DNA and LGG has a high GC percentage in its genomic DNA (58). Thus, we speculate that higher systemic TLR9 expression in EcN + LGG compared with EcN or LGG monocolonized piglets might be a contributing factor in enhancing immunoglobulin responses as reported in several earlier studies (59, 60).

One unanswered question is the involvement of total IgA levels in modulating immunopathology during microbial infections. Previous studies have shown the involvement of IgA in moderating inflammatory responses through modulating dendritic cells and regulatory T cell functions (61, 62). Further, secretory IgA-commensal complexes were shown to reduce inflammatory responses in intestinal epithelial cells (63). Thus, the role of secretory IgA in mitigating infection-induced inflammatory responses is intriguing and requires further investigation.

Differential Effects of G+ versus G− Probiotics in Modulating Innate Immunity

Probiotics may elicit their beneficial effects against pathogens through modulating innate immunity. A role for innate immunity in mediating host defenses against enteric diseases including RV infection has been elucidated in recent studies (64–67). Specifically, functions of dendritic cells are modulated by various probiotics. It appears that DC populations in the intestine can be modulated by intestinal commensals. This concept is supported by results of an investigation in which depletion of intestinal microbiota resulted in a reduction in DCs numbers in mucosal compartments as well as impaired resistance against influenza virus infection in mice (68). Additionally, G− commensal bacteria have higher immunostimulatory effects on DCs as compared with G+ commensals (69). For example, G− EcN increased frequencies of total plasmacytoid dendritic cells (pDCs) and activated pDCs, more than the G+ LGG probiotic in Gn piglets (32). Also, G− commensals were highly potent in the induction of maturation markers in DCs as compared with G+ commensals (53). Importantly, greater variation was observed among G+ commensals in modulating DC responses, compared with less variation among G− commensals (53). Thus, the distinct ability of G− bacteria such as EcN in modulating frequencies and functions of DCs may have beneficial impacts on induction of protective immunity against pathogens.

In our recently published study (32), we observed higher NK cytotoxic function and increased frequencies of pDCs in EcN colonized compared with LGG colonized or uncolonized piglets. The enhanced NK cell activity coincided with higher serum IL-12 levels *in vivo* in EcN colonized piglets (**Figure 1**) and also DC production of IL-12 *in vitro* (32). Similar to our studies, treatment of murine bone marrow-derived DCs (BMDCs) with EcN resulted in induction of IL-12 and IL-10 cytokines and induction of activation markers in BMDCs (70). In the same study, EcN administration reduced the development of allergen-specific Th2 responses (70). Thus, our results showed that NK cell function can be modulated by probiotics, and more importantly, only G− EcN but not G+ LGG, enhanced NK cell function. These findings were further corroborated by an earlier study in which the germ-free condition impaired the priming of NK cell function by microbial ligands (71). Further, the reduced NK cell function in microbiota-depleted mice was correlated with higher mouse cytomegalovirus titers post-viral challenge (71). A recent study (72) also showed the potential role of the outer membrane vesicles from EcN in induction of IL-22 cytokine responses. IL-22, along with IFN-λ, has been shown to effectively reduce RV replication in a mouse model (66). These results underscore not only the importance of intestinal commensals in regulating innate immunity against viral infections, but also the differential abilities of distinct known G+ or G− probiotics in regulating innate immune cells.

Interactions between Commensals and Viruses That Alter Their Pathogenesis

Direct interactions between viruses and bacteria are being increasingly investigated in recent studies (73–75). Specifically, direct binding of commensal microbiota is associated with either increased or decreased viral infections (76). The ability of mouse mammary tumor virus to bind with LPS was associated with increased virus pathogenicity (77). Similarly, poliovirus stability and viral attachment to target host cells were also enhanced by interaction with bacterial LPS or peptidoglycan (78). Further, EcN binds to HRV *ex vivo* but no such interaction was found between LGG and HRV (31). Also, in this study, prior treatment of epithelial cells with EcN, but not LGG, resulted in a significant reduction in the epithelial attachment of HRV *in vitro*. Further studies are required to elucidate the potential role of physical interactions between EcN and viruses in terms of altering the course of viral infection and pathogenicity. Expression of histo-blood group antigens (HBGA) was observed in some G− intestinal commensal bacteria (79) and certain of those HBGA-expressing bacteria were shown to enhance (73) enteric viral infection. Considering the direct interactions between the commensals and pathogens, any disturbances in microbiota compositions may lead to altered susceptibility or resistance to a particular enteric pathogen. Thus, further studies are required to assess whether any difference exists between G+ and G− bacteria in binding properties with various enteric viruses and the impact on the course of viral pathogenicity.

CONCLUSION

Comparison of the beneficial effects of G+ and G− probiotics and intestinal commensals indicated that the selected G− probiotic had higher beneficial effects in inducing protective immunity against enteric pathogens such as HRV as compared with the selected G+ probiotics in humans and animal models. In our simplified *in vivo* Gn piglet model system, it appears that the induced beneficial effects of G− EcN against HRV disease may be accomplished by the integrated interaction of DCs, NK cells, and immunoglobulins as well as direct binding of EcN to virus (**Figure 1**). Most of the initial studies showed that G− probiotics have higher immunostimulatory effects and better protective effects against HRV as compared with G+ probiotics. It remains to be determined whether these findings can be generalized to all G− commensals. Further, the potential ability of different G+ and G− probiotics to alter the composition as well as functionalities of the intestinal microbiota, and the consequences of these changes on microbial infections and vaccines is unclear. Identification of the essential components of probiotics that induce the beneficial effects against pathogens may also be useful in identifying probiotics or their products as novel adjuvants for vaccines.

AUTHOR CONTRIBUTIONS

All authors listed have made substantial direct contribution to the work.

ACKNOWLEDGMENTS

This work was supported by a grant from the NIAID, NIH (grant # R01 A1099451 to LJS, AV, and GR) and federal funds appropriated to the Ohio Agricultural Research and Development Center (OARDC) of The Ohio State University. The authors thank Dr. J. Hanson, R. Wood, and J. Ogg, J. Chepngeno, and K. Scheuer for their technical assistance.

REFERENCES

1. Nicholson JK, Holmes E, Kinross J, Burcelin R, Gibson G, Jia W, et al. Host-gut microbiota metabolic interactions. *Science* (2012) 336:1262–7. doi:10.1126/science.1223813
2. Kamada N, Chen GY, Inohara N, Nunez G. Control of pathogens and pathobionts by the gut microbiota. *Nat Immunol* (2013) 14:685–90. doi:10.1038/ni.2608
3. Kamada N, Nunez G. Role of the gut microbiota in the development and function of lymphoid cells. *J Immunol* (2013) 190:1389–95. doi:10.4049/jimmunol.1203100
4. Scholtens PA, Oozeer R, Martin R, Amor KB, Knol J. The early settlers: intestinal microbiology in early life. *Annu Rev Food Sci Technol* (2012) 3:425–47. doi:10.1146/annurev-food-022811-101120
5. Yatsunenko T, Rey FE, Manary MJ, Trehan I, Dominguez-Bello MG, Contreras M, et al. Human gut microbiome viewed across age and geography. *Nature* (2012) 486:222–7. doi:10.1038/nature11053
6. Arrieta MC, Stiemsma LT, Amenyogbe N, Brown EM, Finlay B. The intestinal microbiome in early life: health and disease. *Front Immunol* (2014) 5:427. doi:10.3389/fimmu.2014.00427
7. Huda MN, Lewis Z, Kalanetra KM, Rashid M, Ahmad SM, Raqib R, et al. Stool microbiota and vaccine responses of infants. *Pediatrics* (2014) 134:e362–72. doi:10.1542/peds.2013-3937
8. Huang JS, Bousvaros A, Lee JW, Diaz A, Davidson EJ. Efficacy of probiotic use in acute diarrhea in children: a meta-analysis. *Dig Dis Sci* (2002) 47:2625–34. doi:10.1023/A:1020501202369
9. Engelbrektson A, Korzenik JR, Pittler A, Sanders ME, Klaenhammer TR, Leyer G, et al. Probiotics to minimize the disruption of faecal microbiota in healthy subjects undergoing antibiotic therapy. *J Med Microbiol* (2009) 58:663–70. doi:10.1099/jmm.0.47615-0
10. Pagnini C, Saeed R, Bamias G, Arseneau KO, Pizarro TT, Cominelli F. Probiotics promote gut health through stimulation of epithelial innate immunity. *Proc Natl Acad Sci U S A* (2010) 107:454–9. doi:10.1073/pnas.0910307107
11. Walker CLF, Rudan I, Liu L, Nair H, Theodoratou E, Bhutta ZA, et al. Global burden of childhood pneumonia and diarrhoea. *Lancet* (2013) 381:1405–16. doi:10.1016/S0140-6736(13)60222-6
12. Lamberti LM, Ashraf S, Walker C, Black RE. A systematic review of the effect of rotavirus vaccination on diarrhea outcomes among children younger than 5 years. *Pediatr Infect Dis J* (2016) 35(9):992–8. doi:10.1097/INF.0000000000001232
13. Round JL, Mazmanian SK. The gut microbiota shapes intestinal immune responses during health and disease. *Nat Rev Immunol* (2009) 9:313–23. doi:10.1038/nri2515
14. Majamaa H, Isolauri E, Saxelin M, Vesikari T. Lactic acid bacteria in the treatment of acute rotavirus gastroenteritis. *J Pediatr Gastroenterol Nutr* (1995) 20:333–8. doi:10.1097/00005176-199504000-00012
15. Nagata S, Asahara T, Ohta T, Yamada T, Kondo S, Bian L, et al. Effect of the continuous intake of probiotic-fermented milk containing *Lactobacillus casei* strain Shirota on fever in a mass outbreak of norovirus gastroenteritis and the faecal microflora in a health service facility for the aged. *Br J Nutr* (2011) 106:549–56. doi:10.1017/S000711451100064X
16. McFarland LV. Meta-analysis of probiotics for the prevention of antibiotic associated diarrhea and the treatment of *Clostridium* difficile disease. *Am J Gastroenterol* (2006) 101:812–22. doi:10.1111/j.1572-0241.2006.00465.x
17. Sindhu KN, Sowmyanarayanan TV, Paul A, Babji S, Ajjampur SS, Priyadarshini S, et al. Immune response and intestinal permeability in children with acute gastroenteritis treated with *Lactobacillus rhamnosus* GG: a randomized, double-blind, placebo-controlled trial. *Clin Infect Dis* (2014) 58:1107–15. doi:10.1093/cid/ciu065
18. Sanders ME, Guarner F, Guerrant R, Holt PR, Quigley EM, Sartor RB, et al. An update on the use and investigation of probiotics in health and disease. *Gut* (2013) 62:787–96. doi:10.1136/gutjnl-2012-302504
19. Vlasova AN, Kandasamy S, Chattha KS, Rajashekara G, Saif LJ. Comparison of probiotic lactobacilli and bifidobacteria effects, immune responses and rotavirus vaccines and infection in different host species. *Vet Immunol Immunopathol* (2016) 172:72–84. doi:10.1016/j.vetimm.2016.01.003
20. Szajewska H, Kotowska M, Mrukowicz JZ, Arma M, Mikolajczyk W. Efficacy of *Lactobacillus* GG in prevention of nosocomial diarrhea in infants. *J Pediatr* (2001) 138:361–5. doi:10.1067/mpd.2001.111321
21. Chattha KS, Vlasova AN, Kandasamy S, Rajashekara G, Saif LJ. Divergent immunomodulating effects of probiotics on T cell responses to oral attenuated human rotavirus vaccine and virulent human rotavirus infection in a neonatal gnotobiotic piglet disease model. *J Immunol* (2013) 191:2446–56. doi:10.4049/jimmunol.1300678
22. Rosenfeldt V, Michaelsen KF, Jakobsen M, Larsen CN, Møller PL, Pedersen P, et al. Effect of probiotic *Lactobacillus* strains in young children hospitalized with acute diarrhea. *Pediatr Infect Dis J* (2002) 21:411–6. doi:10.1097/00006454-200205000-00012
23. Kaila M, Isolauri E, Saxelin M, Arvilommi H, Vesikari T. Viable versus inactivated *Lactobacillus* strain GG in acute rotavirus diarrhoea. *Arch Dis Child* (1995) 72:51–3. doi:10.1136/adc.72.1.51
24. Guandalini S, Pensabene L, Zikri MA, Dias JA, Casali LG, Hoekstra H, et al. *Lactobacillus* GG administered in oral rehydration solution to children with acute diarrhea: a multicenter European trial. *J Pediatr Gastroenterol Nutr* (2000) 30:54–60. doi:10.1097/00005176-200001000-00018
25. Sarker SA, Sultana S, Fuchs GJ, Alam NH, Azim T, Brüssow H, et al. *Lactobacillus paracasei* strain ST11 has no effect on rotavirus but ameliorates the outcome of nonrotavirus diarrhea in children from Bangladesh. *Pediatrics* (2005) 116:e221–8. doi:10.1542/peds.2004-2334
26. Henker J, Laass M, Blokhin BM, Bolbot YK, Maydannik VG, Elze M, et al. The probiotic *Escherichia coli* strain Nissle 1917 (EcN) stops acute

diarrhoea in infants and toddlers. *Eur J Pediatr* (2007) 166:311–8. doi:10.1007/s00431-007-0419-x

27. Lodinová–Žaadniková R, Tlaskalová–Hogenová H, Sonnenborn U. Local and serum antibody response in full–term and premature infants after artificial colonization of the intestine with *E. coli* strain Nissle 1917 (Mutaflor®). *Pediatr Allergy Immunol* (1992) 3:43–8. doi:10.1111/j.1399-3038.1992.tb00026.x
28. Cukrowska B, Lodínová-Žádníková R, Enders C, Sonnenborn U, Schulze J, Tlaskalová-Hogenová H. Specific proliferative and antibody responses of premature infants to intestinal colonization with nonpathogenic probiotic *E. coli* strain Nissle 1917. *Scand J Immunol* (2002) 55:204–9. doi:10.1046/j.1365-3083.2002.01005.x
29. Lodinová-Žádníková R, Sonnenborn U. Effect of preventive administration of a nonpathogenic *Escherichia coli* strain on the colonization of the intestine with microbial pathogens in newborn infants. *Neonatology* (1997) 71:224–32. doi:10.1159/000244421
30. Splichalova A, Trebichavsky I, Rada V, Vlkova E, Sonnenborn U, Splichal I. Interference of *Bifidobacterium choerinum* or *Escherichia coli* Nissle 1917 with *Salmonella typhimurium* in gnotobiotic piglets correlates with cytokine patterns in blood and intestine. *Clin Exp Immunol* (2011) 163:242–9. doi:10.1111/j.1365-2249.2010.04283.x
31. Kandasamy S, Vlasova AN, Fischer D, Kumar A, Chattha KS, Rauf A, et al. Differential effects of *Escherichia coli* Nissle and *Lactobacillus rhamnosus* strain GG on human rotavirus binding, infection, and B cell immunity. *J Immunol* (2016) 196:1780–9. doi:10.4049/jimmunol.1501705
32. Vlasova AN, Shao L, Kandasamy S, Fischer DD, Rauf A, Langel SN, et al. *Escherichia coli* Nissle 1917 protects gnotobiotic pigs against human rotavirus by modulating pDC and NK-cell responses. *Eur J Immunol* (2016) 46(10):2426–37. doi:10.1002/eji.201646498
33. Kreuzer S, Machnowska P, Aßmus J, Sieber M, Pieper R, Schmidt MF, et al. Feeding of the probiotic bacterium *Enterococcus faecium* NCIMB 10415 differentially affects shedding of enteric viruses in pigs. *Vet Res* (2012) 43:1. doi:10.1186/1297-9716-43-58
34. Schroeder B, Duncker S, Barth S, Bauerfeind R, Gruber A, Deppenmeier S, et al. Preventive effects of the probiotic *Escherichia coli* strain Nissle 1917 on acute secretory diarrhea in a pig model of intestinal infection. *Dig Dis Sci* (2006) 51:724–31. doi:10.1007/s10620-006-3198-8
35. Von Buenau R, Jaekel L, Schubotz E, Schwarz S, Stroff T, Krueger M. *Escherichia coli* strain Nissle 1917: significant reduction of neonatal calf diarrhea. *J Dairy Sci* (2005) 88:317–23. doi:10.3168/jds.S0022-0302(05)72690-4
36. Dogi C, Galdeano CM, Perdigón G. Gut immune stimulation by non pathogenic Gram (+) and Gram (−) bacteria. Comparison with a probiotic strain. *Cytokine* (2008) 41:223–31. doi:10.1016/j.cyto.2007.11.014
37. Ukena SN, Singh A, Dringenberg U, Engelhardt R, Seidler U, Hansen W, et al. Probiotic *Escherichia coli* Nissle 1917 inhibits leaky gut by enhancing mucosal integrity. *PLoS One* (2007) 2:e1308. doi:10.1371/journal.pone.0001308
38. Cross ML, Ganner A, Teilab D, Fray LM. Patterns of cytokine induction by Gram-positive and Gram-negative probiotic bacteria. *FEMS Immunol Med Microbiol* (2004) 42:173–80. doi:10.1016/j.femsim.2004.04.001
39. Hessle C, Hanson L, Wold AE. Lactobacilli from human gastrointestinal mucosa are strong stimulators of IL-12 production. *Clin Exp Immunol* (1999) 116:276–82. doi:10.1046/j.1365-2249.1999.00885.x
40. Boyle RJ, Robins-Browne RM, Tang ML. Probiotic use in clinical practice: what are the risks? *Am J Clin Nutr* (2006) 83:1256–64.
41. Özdemir Ö. Various effects of different probiotic strains in allergic disorders: an update from laboratory and clinical data. *Clin Exp Immunol* (2010) 160:295–304. doi:10.1111/j.1365-2249.2010.04109.x
42. Ménard O, Butel M-J, Gaboriau-Routhiau V, Waligora-Dupriet A-J. Gnotobiotic mouse immune response induced by *Bifidobacterium* sp. strains isolated from infants. *Appl Environ Microbiol* (2008) 74:660–6. doi:10.1128/AEM.01261-07
43. Karlsson H, Hessle C, Rudin A. Innate immune responses of human neonatal cells to bacteria from the normal gastrointestinal flora. *Infect Immun* (2002) 70:6688–96. doi:10.1128/IAI.70.12.6688-6696.2002
44. Qi H, Denning TL, Soong L. Differential induction of interleukin-10 and interleukin-12 in dendritic cells by microbial toll-like receptor activators and skewing of T-cell cytokine profiles. *Infect Immun* (2003) 71:3337–42. doi:10.1128/IAI.71.6.3337-3342.2003
45. Sonnenborn U, Schulze J. The non-pathogenic *Escherichia coli* strain Nissle 1917–features of a versatile probiotic. *Microb Ecol Health Dis* (2009) 21:122–58. doi:10.3109/08910600903444267
46. Arribas B, Rodríguez-Cabezas M, Camuesco D, Comalada M, Bailón E, Utrilla P, et al. A probiotic strain of *Escherichia coli*, Nissle 1917, given orally exerts local and systemic anti-inflammatory effects in lipopolysaccharide-induced sepsis in mice. *Br J Pharmacol* (2009) 157:1024–33. doi:10.1111/j.1476-5381.2009.00270.x
47. Macpherson AJ, Harris NL. Interactions between commensal intestinal bacteria and the immune system. *Nat Rev Immunol* (2004) 4:478–85. doi:10.1038/nri1373
48. Hessle C, Andersson B, Wold AE. Gram-positive bacteria are potent inducers of monocytic interleukin-12 (IL-12) while Gram-negative bacteria preferentially stimulate IL-10 production. *Infect Immun* (2000) 68:3581–6. doi:10.1128/IAI.68.6.3581-3586.2000
49. Surbatovic M, Popovic N, Vojvodic D, Milosevic I, Acimovic G, Stojicic M, et al. Cytokine profile in severe Gram-positive and Gram-negative abdominal sepsis. *Sci Rep* (2015) 5:11355. doi:10.1038/srep11355
50. Cerutti A, Rescigno M. The biology of intestinal immunoglobulin A responses. *Immunity* (2008) 28:740–50. doi:10.1016/j.immuni.2008.05.001
51. Güttsches A-K, Löseke S, Zähringer U, Sonnenborn U, Enders C, Gatermann S, et al. Anti-inflammatory modulation of immune response by probiotic *Escherichia coli* Nissle 1917 in human blood mononuclear cells. *Innate Immun* (2012) 18:204–16. doi:10.1177/1753425910396251
52. Christensen HR, Frøkiaer H, Pestka JJ. Lactobacilli differentially modulate expression of cytokines and maturation surface markers in murine dendritic cells. *J Immunol* (2002) 168:171–8. doi:10.4049/jimmunol.168.1.171
53. Zeuthen LH, Christensen HR, Frøkiaer H. Lactic acid bacteria inducing a weak interleukin-12 and tumor necrosis factor alpha response in human dendritic cells inhibit strongly stimulating lactic acid bacteria but act synergistically with Gram-negative bacteria. *Clin Vaccine Immunol* (2006) 13:365–75. doi:10.1128/CVI.13.3.365-375.2006
54. Macpherson AJ, Uhr T. Induction of protective IgA by intestinal dendritic cells carrying commensal bacteria. *Science* (2004) 303:1662–5. doi:10.1126/science.1091334
55. Ruane D, Chorny A, Lee H, Faith J, Pandey G, Shan M, et al. Microbiota regulate the ability of lung dendritic cells to induce IgA class-switch recombination and generate protective gastrointestinal immune responses. *J Exp Med* (2016) 213:53–73. doi:10.1084/jem.20150567
56. Pone EJ, Lou Z, Lam T, Greenberg ML, Wang R, Xu Z, et al. B cell TLR1/2, TLR4, TLR7 and TLR9 interact in induction of class switch DNA recombination: modulation by BCR and CD40, and relevance to T-independent antibody responses. *Autoimmunity* (2015) 48:1–12. doi:10.3109/08916934.2014.993027
57. Zeuthen LH, Fink LN, Frokiaer H. Epithelial cells prime the immune response to an array of gut-derived commensals towards a tolerogenic phenotype through distinct actions of thymic stromal lymphopoietin and transforming growth factor-β. *Immunology* (2008) 123:197–208. doi:10.1111/j.1365-2567.2007.02687.x
58. Iliev ID, Kitazawa H, Shimosato T, Katoh S, Morita H, He F, et al. Strong immunostimulation in murine immune cells by *Lactobacillus rhamnosus* GG DNA containing novel oligodeoxynucleotide pattern. *Cell Microbiol* (2005) 7:403–14. doi:10.1111/j.1462-5822.2004.00492.x
59. Krieg AM, Yi A-K, Matson S, Waldschmidt TJ, Bishop GA, Teasdale R, et al. CpG motifs in bacterial DNA trigger direct B-cell activation. *Nature* (1995) 374:546–9. doi:10.1038/374546a0
60. Blaas S, Stieber-Gunckel M, Falk W, Obermeier F, Rogler G. CpG-oligodeoxynucleotides stimulate immunoglobulin A secretion in intestinal mucosal B cells. *Clin Exp Immunol* (2009) 155:534–40. doi:10.1111/j.1365-2249.2008.03855.x
61. Diana J, Moura IC, Vaugier C, Gestin A, Tissandie E, Beaudoin L, et al. Secretory IgA induces tolerogenic dendritic cells through SIGNR1 dampening autoimmunity in mice. *J Immunol* (2013) 191:2335–43. doi:10.4049/jimmunol.1300864
62. Monteiro R. Immunoglobulin A as an anti-inflammatory agent. *Clin Exp Immunol* (2014) 178:108–10. doi:10.1111/cei.12531
63. Salerno-Goncalves R, Safavie F, Fasano A, Sztein MB. Free and complexed-secretory immunoglobulin A triggers distinct intestinal epithelial responses. *Clin Exp Immunol* (2016) 185(3):338–47. doi:10.1111/cei.12801

64. Vlasova AN, Chattha KS, Kandasamy S, Liu Z, Esseili M, Shao L, et al. Lactobacilli and bifidobacteria promote immune homeostasis by modulating innate immune responses to human rotavirus in neonatal gnotobiotic pigs. *PLoS One* (2013) 8:e76962. doi:10.1371/journal.pone.0076962
65. Zhang B, Chassaing B, Shi Z, Uchiyama R, Zhang Z, Denning TL, et al. Prevention and cure of rotavirus infection via TLR5/NLRC4-mediated production of IL-22 and IL-18. *Science* (2014) 346:861–5. doi:10.1126/science.1256999
66. Hernández PP, Mahlakõiv T, Yang I, Schwierzeck V, Nguyen N, Guendel F, et al. Interferon-[lambda] and interleukin 22 act synergistically for the induction of interferon-stimulated genes and control of rotavirus infection. *Nat Immunol* (2015) 16:698–707. doi:10.1038/ni.3180
67. Shao L, Fischer DD, Kandasamy S, Rauf A, Langel SN, Wentworth DE, et al. Comparative in vitro and in vivo studies of porcine rotavirus G9P [13] and human rotavirus Wa G1P [8]. *J Virol* (2016) 90:142–51. doi:10.1128/JVI.02401-15
68. Ichinohe T, Pang IK, Kumamoto Y, Peaper DR, Ho JH, Murray TS, et al. Microbiota regulates immune defense against respiratory tract influenza A virus infection. *Proc Natl Acad Sci U S A* (2011) 108:5354–9. doi:10.1073/pnas.1019378108
69. Smits HH, Van Beelen AJ, Hessle C, Westland R, De Jong E, Soeteman E, et al. Commensal Gram-negative bacteria prime human dendritic cells for enhanced IL-23 and IL-27 expression and enhanced Th1 development. *Eur J Immunol* (2004) 34:1371–80. doi:10.1002/eji.200324815
70. Adam E, Delbrassinne L, Bouillot C, Reynders V, Mailleux AC, Muraille E, et al. Probiotic *Escherichia coli* Nissle 1917 activates DC and prevents house dust mite allergy through a TLR4-dependent pathway. *Eur J Immunol* (2010) 40:1995–2005. doi:10.1002/eji.200939913
71. Ganal SC, Sanos SL, Kallfass C, Oberle K, Johner C, Kirschning C, et al. Priming of natural killer cells by nonmucosal mononuclear phagocytes requires instructive signals from commensal microbiota. *Immunity* (2012) 37:171–86. doi:10.1016/j.immuni.2012.05.020
72. Fábrega MJ, Aguilera L, Giménez R, Varela E, Cañas MA, Antolin M, et al. Activation of immune and defense responses in the intestinal mucosa by outer membrane vesicles of commensal and probiotic *Escherichia coli* strains. *Front Microbiol* (2016) 7:705. doi:10.3389/fmicb.2016.00705
73. Jones MK, Watanabe M, Zhu S, Graves CL, Keyes LR, Grau KR, et al. Enteric bacteria promote human and mouse norovirus infection of B cells. *Science* (2014) 346:755–9. doi:10.1126/science.1257147
74. Karst SM. The influence of commensal bacteria on infection with enteric viruses. *Nat Rev Microbiol* (2016) 14:197–204. doi:10.1038/nrmicro.2015.25
75. Pfeiffer JK, Virgin HW. Transkingdom control of viral infection and immunity in the mammalian intestine. *Science* (2016) 351:aad5872. doi:10.1126/science.aad5872
76. Robinson CM, Pfeiffer JK. Viruses and the microbiota. *Annu Rev Virol* (2014) 1:55. doi:10.1146/annurev-virology-031413-085550
77. Kane M, Case LK, Kopaskie K, Kozlova A, Macdearmid C, Chervonsky AV, et al. Successful transmission of a retrovirus depends on the commensal microbiota. *Science* (2011) 334:245–9. doi:10.1126/science.1210718
78. Robinson CM, Jesudhasan PR, Pfeiffer JK. Bacterial lipopolysaccharide binding enhances virion stability and promotes environmental fitness of an enteric virus. *Cell Host Microbe* (2014) 15:36–46. doi:10.1016/j.chom.2013.12.004
79. Miura T, Sano D, Suenaga A, Yoshimura T, Fuzawa M, Nakagomi T, et al. Histo-blood group antigen-like substances of human enteric bacteria as specific adsorbents for human noroviruses. *J Virol* (2013) 87:9441–51. doi:10.1128/JVI.01060-13

2

Gut Microbiota Species can Provoke both Inflammatory and Tolerogenic Immune Responses in Human Dendritic Cells Mediated by Retinoic Acid Receptor Alpha Ligation

Krisztian Bene[1], Zsofia Varga[1], Viktor O. Petrov[2], Nadiya Boyko[2†] and Eva Rajnavolgyi[1†]*

[1] *Faculty of Medicine, Department of Immunology, University of Debrecen, Debrecen, Hungary,* [2] *Faculty of Medicine, R&D Centre of Molecular Microbiology and Mucosal Immunology, Uzhhorod National University, Uzhhorod, Ukraine*

Edited by:
Haruki Kitazawa,
Tohoku University, Japan

Reviewed by:
Zoltan Simandi,
Sanford-Burnham Institute for Medical Research, USA
Hervé M. Blottiere,
INRA/Micalis Institute & INRA/MetaGenoPolis, France

***Correspondence:**
Eva Rajnavolgyi
evaraj@med.unideb.hu

[†]*These authors have contributed equally to this work.*

Dendritic cells are considered as the main coordinators of both mucosal and systemic immune responses, thus playing a determining role in shaping the outcome of effector cell responses. However, it is still uncovered how primary human monocyte-derived DC (moDC) populations drive the polarization of helper T (Th) cells in the presence of commensal bacteria harboring unique immunomodulatory properties. Furthermore, the individual members of the gut microbiota have the potential to modulate the outcome of immune responses and shape the immunogenicity of differentiating moDCs *via* the activation of retinoic acid receptor alpha (RARα). Here, we report that moDCs are able to mediate robust Th1 and Th17 responses upon stimulation by *Escherichia coli Schaedler* or *Morganella morganii*, while the probiotic *Bacillus subtilis* strain limits this effect. Moreover, physiological concentrations of all-*trans* retinoic acid (ATRA) are able to re-program the differentiation of moDCs resulting in altered gene expression profiles of the master transcription factors RARα and interferon regulatory factor 4, and concomitantly regulate the cell surface expression levels of CD1 proteins and also the mucosa-associated CD103 integrin to different directions. It was also demonstrated that the ATRA-conditioned moDCs exhibited enhanced pro-inflammatory cytokine secretion while reduced their co-stimulatory and antigen-presenting capacity thus reducing Th1 and presenting undetectable Th17 type responses against the tested microbiota strains. Importantly, these regulatory circuits could be prevented by the selective inhibition of RARα functionality. These results altogether demonstrate that selected commensal bacterial strains are able to drive strong effector immune responses by moDCs, while in the presence of ATRA, they support the development of both tolerogenic and inflammatory moDC in a RARα-dependent manner.

Keywords: monocyte-derived dendritic cell, gut microbiota, all-*trans* retinoic acid, retinoic acid receptor alpha, interferon regulatory factor 4, T cell, CD1a, CD1d

INTRODUCTION

The development and the metabolic activity of the human immune system critically depend on the amount and the diversity of the human microbiota acquired from the actual tissue microenvironment (1, 2). Upon birth, the human gastrointestinal tract becomes colonized by commensal microbes co-evolved with humans in a symbiotic or at least mutualistic manner together with the immune system

(3, 4). The local dendritic cell (DC) network involves a highly heterogeneous population of cells of myeloid and bone marrow origin (5), and in the course of this balancing regulation, moDCs also act as potent organizers of adaptive immunity leading to the maintenance of peripheral tolerance against the gut resident microbes. However, our knowledge about the interplay of molecular interactions during diet involving vitamin A supplementation, and the presence of gut microbiota species in the course of an ongoing human immune system is still limited in both health and diseases.

The uncontrolled disruption of the gut microbiota can be provoked by dysbiosis due to excessive hygiene conditions and/or the presence of antibiotics. This microbial perturbation may play role in the pathogenesis of chronic inflammatory and autoimmune diseases such as inflammatory bowel diseases (IBD), celiac disease, allergy, and metabolic and neurobehavioral diseases. For example, in Crohn's disease, the ratio of *Proteobacteria* could be increased (6), while the diversity and the fraction of *Firmicutes* in the gut microbiota are decreased (7). Colonization with commensal *Escherichia coli* 083 and *Lactobacillus rhamnosus* strains in early life is able to decrease the incidence of allergies and atopic dermatitis, respectively (8, 9). The various effects of probiotic gut bacteria also may prevent infection by pathogens such as the probiotic *E. coli Nissle* 1917 strain, which is able to inhibit the growth of enteropathogenic *E. coli*, which also may serve as a safe strain in IBD treatment (10–12).

Here, we focus to the underlying mechanisms involved in the recognition and processing of different species of gut commensal and beneficial bacteria and to their ability to polarize helper T (Th) lymphocytes. Considering that the human commensal microbiota is personalized (13) and exhibits high heterogeneity, it also contributes to the development of protective immune responses against pathogens *via* modulating the type and the composition of gut resident effector T cells (13–15). It is well established that pathogenic microbes or pathobionts, including fungal and bacterial species, are able to induce different types of immune responses (16, 17), which are modulated by external and internal signals. However, the means how non-pathogenic gut commensal species contribute to the coordination and fine tuning of immune responses by moDCs is not completely uncovered. In line with this, the primary goal of this study was to characterize a selected set of the normal gut microbiota including *Escherichia coli var. mutabilis* (*E. coli Schaedler*), *Morganella morganii* from *Proteobacteria*, and probiotic *Bacillus subtilis* 090 from *Firmicutes*, all with individual immunogenic and/or modulatory potential during moDC maturation and T-lymphocyte polarization. As it has previously been described, *E. coli Schaedler* and *M. morganii* exert unique stimulatory effects on the developing immune system and are also able to induce oral tolerance in mice (18), while *B. subtilis* is widely used in veterinary practice based on the active constituents of probiotic Monosporyn™ developed at the Uzhhorod National University. Upon interaction with the mucosal immune system, tolerogenic immune responses are raised against commensal and beneficial microbes. However, it is still poorly understood how the special but highly complex and dynamic intestinal milieu impacts the differentiation program of moDCs and the outcome of moDC-mediated immunological processes initiated by normal

The differentiation program of monocytes during moDC generation is initiated by granulocyte-macrophage colony-stimulating factor (GM-CSF) and interleukin (IL)-4 and is regulated by the peroxisome proliferator-activated receptor gamma (PPARγ) (19). PPARγ is known to collaborate with retinoid receptors and acts as a master transcriptional regulator in human moDC differentiation and function (19). In addition, a set of genes encoding proteins related to metabolism, lipid antigen processing and presentation, invariant natural killer T (iNKT) cell activation, and RA synthesis are regulated by PPARγ and overlaps with those regulated by retinoic acid receptor alpha (RARα) (20–23), showing that RARα also serves as a master regulator of moDC functions. In humans, the vitamin A derivate all-*trans* retinoic acid (ATRA) is produced endogenously from retinol by DCs, macrophages, and epithelial and stromal cells (20, 24–27) and binds to RARα and retinoic X receptor alpha (RXRα) with different affinities (28) and enables to follow up the modulatory effects of the retinoid pathways in moDC-mediated immune responses. Besides targeting the highly conserved receptor RARα (29), ATRA also serves as a potential therapeutic drug in anticancer settings (30) and in combinations with other therapeutic agents such as GM-CSF (31) able to promote myelomonocytic differentiation.

We hypothesize that human monocytes migrating from the blood to the intestinal *lamina propria* have access to these special microenvironments, which are conditioned by growth factors and metabolites, including GM-CSF, exogenous and/or endogenous ATRA, and take part in the coordination of immune responses raised against the targeted gut commensal species. Intestinal mononuclear cells express mucosa-associated cell surface molecules such as CX_3CR1 and/or CD103 (32, 33). The main sources of human intestinal CX_3CR1^+ DCs are circulating monocytes, which lose this marker within 24 h (34). In contrast to this event, the CX_3CR1 chemokine receptor remains expressed on the cell surface of intestinal mononuclear phagocytes and acts directly as an inflammatory and migratory cell population with high phagocytic capacity (34–37), while mucosal $CD103^+$ DCs have been described as a dominant migratory population involved in triggering regulatory T cell responses raised against commensal bacteria *via* producing RA (38).

Based on this concept, *in vitro* conditions were designed to analyze the canonical pathways leading to the ATRA-modulated expression of the contributing master transcription factors including retinoid receptors, PPARγ and interferon regulatory factor 4 (IRF4) playing role in moDC differentiation in line with the impact of different, individual commensal bacteria exerted on moDC-mediated inflammation and effector T-lymphocyte priming. In this context, we will follow up the phenotypic changes and the functional activities of moDC populations by monitoring their phagocytic potential, inflammatory nature, and immunogenicity. Taken the unique intestinal microenvironment and the complex interplay of various exogenous effects, we sought to demonstrate how external and internal stimuli derived from the engulfed commensal *E. coli Schaedler*, *M. morganii*, and the probiotic *B. subtilis* bacteria may impact on the development of effector T-lymphocyte activation and polarization followed up by the production of interferon gamma (IFNγ) and IL-17

MATERIALS AND METHODS

Bacterial Strains and Reagents

The experiments were performed with the commensal bacteria as follows: *E. coli var. mutabilis (Schaedler)* (O83:K24:H31, member of the original Schaedler's flora), *M. morganii*, and *B. subtilis* 090. *M. morganii* was kindly provided by Michael Potter, National Institutes of Health, strain *E. coli Schaedler* was obtained from Russel Schaedler, USA, and *B. subtilis* 090 was provided by Nadiya Boyko, National University of Uzhhorod, Ukraine. Both commensal gut microbiota strains were received by the R&D Centre for Molecular Microbiology and mucosal immunology from Pennsylvania University in the framework of a research cooperation agreement. ATRA, the selective RARα antagonist BMS-195614 (BMS614), the vehicle dimethyl-sulfoxide (DMSO), and the anti-hβ-actin mAb were from Sigma-Aldrich, Schnelldorf, Germany. The anti-hIRF4 antibody was from Cell Signaling Technology, Inc. (Trask Lane, Danvers, MA, USA).

Human moDC Cultures

Peripheral blood mononuclear cells (PBMCs) were separated by a standard density gradient centrifugation with Ficoll-Paque Plus (Amersham Biosciences, Uppsala, Sweden). Monocytes were purified from PBMCs by positive selection using immunomagnetic cell separation and anti-CD14 microbeads, according to the manufacturer's instruction (Miltenyi Biotec, Bergisch Gladbach, Germany). After separation on a VarioMACS magnet, 96–99% of the cells were shown to be $CD14^+$ monocytes, as measured by flow cytometry. Isolated monocytes were cultured for 2 days in 12-well tissue culture plates at a density of 5.0×10^5 cells/ml in Gibco's serum-free AIM-V medium (Thermo Fischer Scientific, Waltham, MA, USA) supplemented with 80 ng/ml GM-CSF (Gentaur Molecular Products, Brussels, Belgium) and 100 ng/ml IL-4 (PeproTech EC, London, UK). The cells were differentiated in the presence or absence of 1 nM ATRA followed by a 75-min incubation period with or without 1 μM BMS614 specific RARα-antagonist at 37°C atmosphere containing 5% CO_2.

Bacterial Growth for moDC Activation

Selected gut commensal bacteria were grown in 2% lysogeny broth medium (Serva Electrophoresis GmbH, Heidelberg, Germany) for overnight with shaking at 37°C. Bacterial suspensions were washed with 25 ml sterile phosphate-buffered saline (PBS) three times and OD_{600nm} was measured by spectrophotometry and converted to cell/ml following $OD_{600nm} \times 2.5 \times 10^8$ CFU/ml. Human moDC cultures were activated with the specific toll-like receptor ligand bacterial lipopolysaccharide (LPS) (250 ng/ml ultrapure LPS, InvivoGen, San Diego, CA, USA) and with live commensal bacteria at a non-toxic ratio of 1:0.4 and were co-cultured for another 24 h.

Phagocytosis Assay

Live bacterial cells were centrifuged at 1,000 × *g* for 5 min and washed three times in 25 ml PBS. Suspensions of bacterial cells were heat inactivated by heating at 65°C for 45 min and were re-suspended in 0.25 M carbonate–bicarbonate buffer (pH 9.0). The heat-killed bacterial cell suspensions (900 μl) were stained with 100 μl fluorescein-isothiocyanate (FITC) used at 5 mg/ml dissolved in DMSO and were rotated overnight at 4°C in dark. FITC-labeled bacteria were washed three times with cold PBS and were co-incubated for 3 h with moDCs at 37 or 4°C at a moDC:bacteria ratio of 1:20. moDCs positive for FITC-labeled bacteria were analyzed by flow cytometry using FACSCalibur (BD Biosciences, Franklin Lakes, NJ, USA).

Flow Cytometry

Phenotyping of resting and activated moDCs was performed by flow cytometry using anti-human CD1d-phycoerythrin (PE), CD103-FITC, HLA-DQ-FITC, PD-L1-PE (BD Biosciences, Franklin Lakes, NJ, USA), CD1a-allophycocyanin (APC), CD40-FITC (BioLegend, San Diego, CA, USA), CX_3CR1-PE, CD80-FITC, CD83-FITC, CD86-PE, DC-SIGN-FITC, CCR7-PE, CD14-PE (R&D Systems, Minneapolis, MN, USA), B7RP1 (ICOSL)-PE (EBiosciences, Santa Clara, CA, USA), and isotype-matched control antibodies. The ratio of regulatory T-lymphocytes was measured by flow cytometry using anti-human CD25-PE (BD Pharmingen), CD4-FITC (BioLegend), FoxP3-APC (R&D Systems), and anti-IL-10-AlexaFluor488 (BioLegend). The viability of moDCs was determined with 2 μg/ml 7-amino-actinomycin D (LKT Laboratories Inc., St. Paul, MN, USA) dye followed by a 24-h activation period with live bacteria or LPS. Fluorescence intensities were measured by FACSCalibur (BD Biosciences), and data were analyzed by the FlowJo software (Tree Star, Ashland, OR, USA).

RNA Isolation, cDNA Synthesis, and Real-time Quantitative PCR

Briefly, total RNA was isolated by TriReagent (Molecular Research Centre, Inc., Cincinnati, OH, USA). Total RNA (1 μg) was reverse-transcribed using High-Capacity cDNA Reverse Transcription Kit (Thermo Fischer Scientific). Gene-specific TaqMan assays (Thermo Fischer Scientific) were used to perform qPCR in a final volume of 12.5 μl in triplicates using DreamTaq DNA polymerase and ABI StepOnePlus real-time PCR instrument. Amplification of h36B4 was used as normalizing controls using specific primers and probe (Integrated DNA Technologies, Coralville, IA, USA). Cycle threshold values were determined using the StepOne Software, version 2.1 (Thermo Fischer Scientific). The sequences of the primers and probes are available upon request.

Measurement of Cytokine Concentration

Culture supernatants of moDCs were harvested 24 h after moDC activation, and the concentration of TNF-α, IL-1β, IL-6, IL-10, IL-12(p70), IL-23(p19) cytokines, and chemokine CXCL8 was measured using OptEIA kits (BD Biosciences) following the manufacturer's instructions.

Stimulation of moDCs to Measure T-Lymphocyte Polarization

To analyze the polarized effector T cells, immature and activated moDCs were washed and co-cultured with peripheral blood lymphocytes (PBLs) for 4 days in AIM-V medium at a moDC:T-cell ratio of 1:20. The T cells were analyzed for IFNγ and IL-17 secretion by the avidin-horseradish peroxidase (HRP)-based enzyme-linked ImmunoSpot system (NatuTec GmbH, Frankfurt am Main, Germany). The co-cultures containing resting moDCs and T-cells as well as T-cells alone served as negative controls. To detect IL-17 secretion, the plates were coated with 0.5 μg/ml mouse anti-hCD3 antibody (BD Biosciences). The plates were analyzed by using the ImmunoScan plate reader (Cell Technology Limited, Shaker Heights, OH, USA). To detect regulatory T-lymphocytes, activated and resting moDCs were washed and co-cultured with PBL or naïve $CD4^+$ T-lymphocytes for 6 days in serum-free AIM-V medium at a moDC:T-cell ratio of 1:10. On day 6, cells were harvested, permeabilized, and fixed with Citofix/Cytoperm intracellular staining kit (BD Biosciences). The ratio of $CD4^+CD25^+FoxP3^+$ T cells was measured by flow cytometry. To detect the presence of intracellular IL-10, T cells were treated on day 6 with Golgi-Stop™ containing monensin (BD Biosciences) for 6 h followed by the surface CD25, CD4, and intracellular FoxP3 and IL-10 staining of cells. Naïve $CD4^+$ T-lymphocytes were isolated by the Naïve $CD4^+$ T Cell Isolation Kit II, human (Miltenyi Biotec).

Stimulation of moDCs to Measure iNKT Cell Expansion

Two-day moDCs were co-incubated with live bacteria, LPS, or 100 ng/ml α-galactosylceramide (α-GalCer, KRN7000, Funakoshi, Tokyo, Japan) for 24 h in AIM-V medium. Activated and resting moDCs were washed and co-cultured with PBL for 5 days in AIM-V medium at a moDC:T cell ratio of 1:10 in 24-well plates in AIM-V medium. On day 5, cells were labeled with anti-human CD3-PECy5, T cell receptor (TCR) Vα24-FITC, TCR Vβ11-PE monoclonal antibodies (Beckman Coulter, Brea, CA, USA), and the double-positive iNKT population was monitored by flow cytometry using FACSCalibur.

Western Blotting

Cells were lysed in Laemmli buffer, and the protein extracts were tested by antibody specific for IRF4 diluted to 1:1,000; secondary antibodies were used at 1:10,000. Anti-rabbit antibody, conjugated to HRP (GE Healthcare Life Sciences, Little Chalfont Buckinghamshire, UK), was used as a secondary antibody. The SuperSignal ECL system was used for probing target proteins (Thermo Fischer Scientific). After the membranes had been probed for the target protein, they were stripped and re-probed for β-actin.

Statistical Analysis

Student's unpaired two-tailed *t*-test or ANOVA followed by Bonferroni's multiple comparison tests were used as indicated in the relevant experiments. In case of significantly different variances ($P < 0.05$) between the two sets of samples, the Welch's correction was applied in the *t*-test. The results were expressed as mean + SD. All analyses were performed by using the GraphPad Prism software, version 6.0 (GraphPad Software Inc., La Jolla, CA, USA). Differences were considered to be statistically significant at $P < 0.05$. Significance was indicated as $^*P < 0.05$; $^{**}P < 0.01$; $^{***}P < 0.005$; and $^{****}P < 0.0001$.

RESULTS

The Expression Profile of Master Transcription Factors and the Cell Surface Expression of CD1 Glycoprotein Receptors Differ in Human moDCs

We found that in the presence of 1 nM ATRA, monocytes generated in the presence of GM-CSF and IL-4 induced the differentiation of monocytes to moDCs within 2 days accompanied by the increasing expression levels of genes encoding the nuclear hormone receptor RXRα as well as its dimerization partners RARα and PPARγ in line with the aldehyde dehydrogenase-1 family member A2 (ALDH1A2)/retinaldehyde-dehydrogenase 2 (RALDH2) gene (**Figure 1A**) playing role in the regulation of retinoic acid production in moDCs. In the absence of ATRA, the CD1d gene was expressed in moDCs at low levels, but the CD1d gene transcripts and the cell surface expression of the translated protein was upregulated, while in ATRA-conditioned moDCs, the cell surface expression of CD1a decreased (**Figure 1B**). Moreover, on days 2 and 3, the differentiation of moDCs could be re-programmed to induce CD1d but inhibited CD1a expression, respectively (data not shown). Importantly, the cell surface expression of the DC-specific intercellular adhesion molecule-3-grabbing non-integrin (DC-SIGN) remained constant at these conditions (**Figure 1C**), while ATRA maintained the expression level of CD14 (**Figure 1D**) suggesting a decelerated differentiation phase of moDCs.

Dendritic cells can also be classified according to the expression levels of the transcription factors guiding both DC differentiation and re-programming (39, 40). Murine models suggested that $CD11b^+$ bone marrow-derived DCs cultured in the presence of GM-CSF and IL-4 express IRF4 and regulate the cell surface expression of the major histocompatibility gene complex II (MHC class II), while IRF4 increases the antigen-presenting capacity of moDCs resulting in potent T helper cell priming (41). In this human *in vitro* model system, we also found that moDCs express CD11b independent on the presence of ATRA (**Figure 1E**). Interestingly, ATRA was able to downmodulate the gene expression levels of IRF4 (**Figure 1F**) while upregulated the cell surface expression of CD103 (**Figures 3D,E**). Importantly, the relative mRNA level of interferon regulatory factor (IRF)8, responsible for regulating CD103 protein expression in DCs (41), remained unaffected by ATRA (**Figure 1G**). Collectively, these results demonstrate that nanomolar concentration of ATRA has the potential to modify the moDC differentiation program in a coordinated manner leading to increased mRNA levels of PPARγ, retinoid receptors, ALDH1A2, and CD1d, while the expression of CD1a and IRF4 remained inhibited. Based on this finding, we were able to identify two separate moDC subsets exhibiting distinct phenotypic characteristics based on the expression patterns of CD1 and CD103 proteins and transcription factors. The ATRA-primed $CD1a^-CD103^+CD1d^+$ cells are the $RAR\alpha^{hi}IRF4^{lo}$ subpopulation, and in contrast to this combination, the $CD1a^{+/-}$ $CD103^-CD1d^-$ cells are identified as a resting $RAR\alpha^{lo}IRF4^{hi}$ cell population.

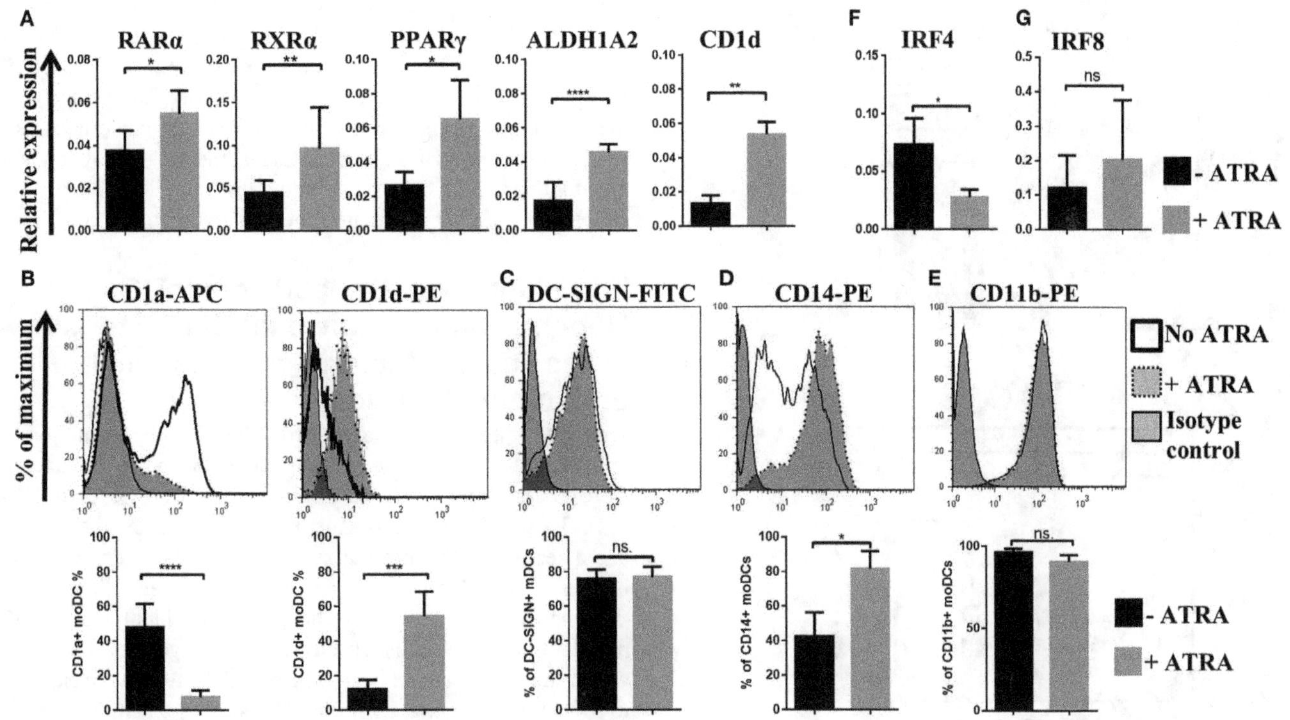

FIGURE 1 | The effects of all-*trans* retinoic acid (ATRA) on human monocyte-derived dentritic cell (moDC) differentiation. Two-day moDCs were differentiated in the absence or presence of 1 nM ATRA. The relative gene expression levels of retinoic acid receptor alpha (RARα), retinoic X receptor alpha (RXRα), peroxisome proliferator-activated receptor gamma (PPARγ), ALDH1A2, and CD1d **(A)**, interferon regulatory factor (IRF)4 **(F)**, and IRF8 **(G)** were measured by quantitative real-time PCR, and the cell surface expression level of CD1a, CD1d **(B)**, DC-SIGN **(C)**, CD14 **(D)**, and CD11b **(E)** was measured by flow cytometry. Mean values of relative mRNA levels and the ratio of moDCs positive for the measured cell surface proteins were calculated from five independent experiments +SD. Student's unpaired two-tailed *t*-test was used in the statistical analysis with significance defined as $^*P < 0.05$, $^{**}P < 0.01$, $^{***}P < 0.001$, and $^{****}P < 0.0001$.

Stimulation of $RAR\alpha^{lo}IRF4^{hi}$ moDCs by Non-Pathogenic Commensal Bacteria Polarize Effector T-Lymphocytes Differently as Compared to $RAR\alpha^{hi}IRF4^{lo}$ Cells

Besides the novel finding showing that the outcome of the inflammatory response of DCs to engulfed commensal bacteria is determined by the unique characteristics of the tested microbes (42), we were able to follow-up the immunomodulatory properties of a given microbe though monitoring the activation state and the direction of cell polarization of moDC-mediated autologous T-lymphocytes. In this experimental setting, moDCs were activated by live *E. coli Schaedler* or *M. morganii* both of them being capable to increase the number of IFNγ-producing T-lymphocytes (**Figure 2A**). By contrast, the Th17 response could be activated by all of the tested species (**Figure 2B**). In addition, ATRA-conditioned moDCs exhibited a completely different T-lymphocyte stimulatory potential as compared to moDCs manipulated in the absence of ATRA. In this case, the number of IFNγ-secreting T cells was decreased, while that of the Th17 cells remained undetectable in the moDC–T cell co-cultures. Taken the individual features of commensal bacteria, the $RAR\alpha^{lo}IRF4^{hi}$ moDCs could be activated by both *E. coli Schaedler* and *M. morganii* leading to the differentiation of $CD4^+CD25^+FoxP3^+$ regulatory T-lymphocytes, while the $RAR\alpha^{hi}IRF4^{lo}$ reduced this effect (Figures S1A,B in Supplementary Material). To confirm this unexpected observation, we validated the existence of the regulatory T-cell population by detecting the level of the IL-10 cytokine derived from $CD4^+CD25^+FoxP3^+$ T-lymphocytes co-cultured with moDCs upon the prior activation by commensal bacteria (Figure S1C in Supplementary Material). Based on these results, we were able to identify two moDC populations, which respond to gut commensal species differently, but in a strain- and ATRA-dependent manner. To get further insight how microbiota species guide immune responses of distinct characteristics, we sought to analyze the impact of selected bacterial strains driving the differentiation and functional activities of moDCs by using various experimental approaches.

The Commensal *E. coli Schaedler* and the Probiotic *B. subtilis* Modulate the Cell Surface Expression of CD1, CX_3CR1, and CD103 Proteins in an ATRA-Dependent Manner

To test how gut microbiota strains may act on human moDC differentiation at *in vitro* culture conditions mimicking the intestinal milieu, the cells were exposed to stimulatory signals such as LPS and selected live commensal bacteria. At this experimental

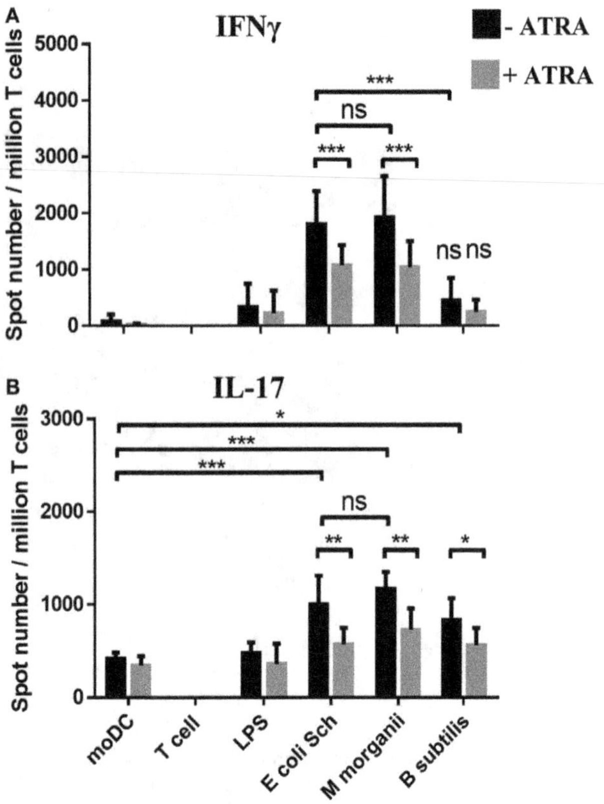

FIGURE 2 | Monitoring monocyte-derived dentritic cell (moDC)-mediated T-lymphocyte polarization induced by commensal stimuli. The T cell polarizing capacity of moDCs was monitored in moDC stimulated with *Escherichia coli Schaedler*, *Morganella Morganii*, and *Bacillus subtilis* or lipopolysaccharide (LPS) followed by co-culturing the cells with freshly isolated autologous T cells for 4 days. The number of cytokine producing T-lymphocytes induced by LPS or by moDCs exposed to commensal bacteria was measured by interferon gamma (IFNγ) **(A)** and interleukin (IL)-17 **(B)** enzyme-linked ImmunoSpot assays. T corresponds to T cells cultured without dendritic cells as negative control. The mean value of spot numbers was calculated from five independent experiments +SD. ANOVA followed by Bonferroni's multiple comparison tests was used in the statistical analysis with significance defined as $^{*}P < 0.05$, $^{**}P < 0.01$, and $^{***}P < 0.001$.

setting, exclusively *E. coli Schaedler* was capable to reduce the ratio of CD1a$^+$ moDCs indicating the potential of this commensal bacterium to reduce CD1a expression selectively, but it had no effect on CD1d expression (**Figure 3A**), even though the viability of moDCs remained intact as compared to the immature cells (Figure S2 in Supplementary Material). Interestingly, *B. subtilis* exerted an opposing effect on the cell surface expression pattern of CD1 proteins, and LPS reduced the levels of both CD1d and CD1a in moDCs, while *M. morganii* had no effect on the cell surface expression level of CD1 proteins. These results indicated that lipid antigen presentation by moDCs *via* CD1a and CD1d proteins is regulated by both ATRA and the gut microbiota in a species-specific manner.

Using the *in vitro* system, we established the live commensal bacteria were able to upregulate the cell surface expression of CX_3CR1 within 24 h (**Figures 3B,C**) but had no effect on CD103 expression in the absence of ATRA (**Figures 3D,E**). Moreover, ATRA-conditioned moDCs downregulated the cell surface expression of CD103, but stimulation by commensal bacteria upregulated the CX_3CR1 receptor. These data altogether confirmed that in the presence of live commensal bacteria, ATRA drives the differentiation of moDCs leading to either synergistic or inhibitory directions, thus modulating the cell surface expression pattern of CD1 and that of the gut-tropic proteins.

The Phagocytic Capacity of moDCs Depends on the Individual Characteristics of the Tested Bacteria and on Actual Environmental Cues

The very first steps of moDC activation and the induction of antigen-induced immune responses are assisted by the phagocytic potential and the standby physiological activities of moDCs (42). These events can be further modulated by the unique characteristics of the internalized corpuscular antigens as well as by the cell surface receptor repertoire of the given cell. To assess the phagocytic potential of the previously identified moDC populations, we established an *in vitro* phagocytosis assay in which the FITC-labeled heat-inactivated bacteria were exposed to 37°C for 3 h, or were kept at 4°C as control (**Figures 3F,G**). As expected, the engulfment of commensal bacteria could be enhanced significantly and was found to be mediated by the RARα^{hi}IRF4^{lo} moDC population. When the moDCs were co-incubated with FITC-labeled bacteria at 4°C, background fluorescence intensities varied remarkably indicating differences in the individual functional characteristics of the tested commensal bacteria upon penetrating through the moDC membrane. These results altogether confirmed that in the presence of gut-derived microbial stimuli ATRA supports the differentiation of phagocytic CD1a$^-$CD1d$^+$ moDCs, while the expression of the gut-tropic protein CD103 is partially downmodulated. It was also observed that in the absence of ATRA, the gated CD1a$^-$ and CD1a$^+$ moDC fractions engulfed the tested bacteria with similar activities as the CD1a$^+$ cells (data not shown). Consequently, the median fluorescence intensity values within the gated moDC populations of the FITC-labeled bacteria remained similar demonstrating that the efficacy of moDC-mediated phagocytosis depends on both the unique features and the species of the engulfed bacteria, and this effector mechanism can be further enhanced by ATRA.

Activation of RARα^{hi}IRF4^{lo} moDCs by Commensal Bacteria Provokes Exacerbated Inflammation as Compared to RARα^{lo}IRF4^{hi} moDCs

Next, we continued to monitor the inflammatory potential of the selected commensals. Exposure of moDCs to live commensal bacteria such as *E. coli Schaedler* and *B. subtilis* or LPS for 24 h was found to increase the cell surface expression of CD83, while ATRA could downmodulate this response significantly (**Figure 4A**). The cell surface expression of the chemokine receptor CCR7, playing an essential role in driving DC migration to reach the secondary

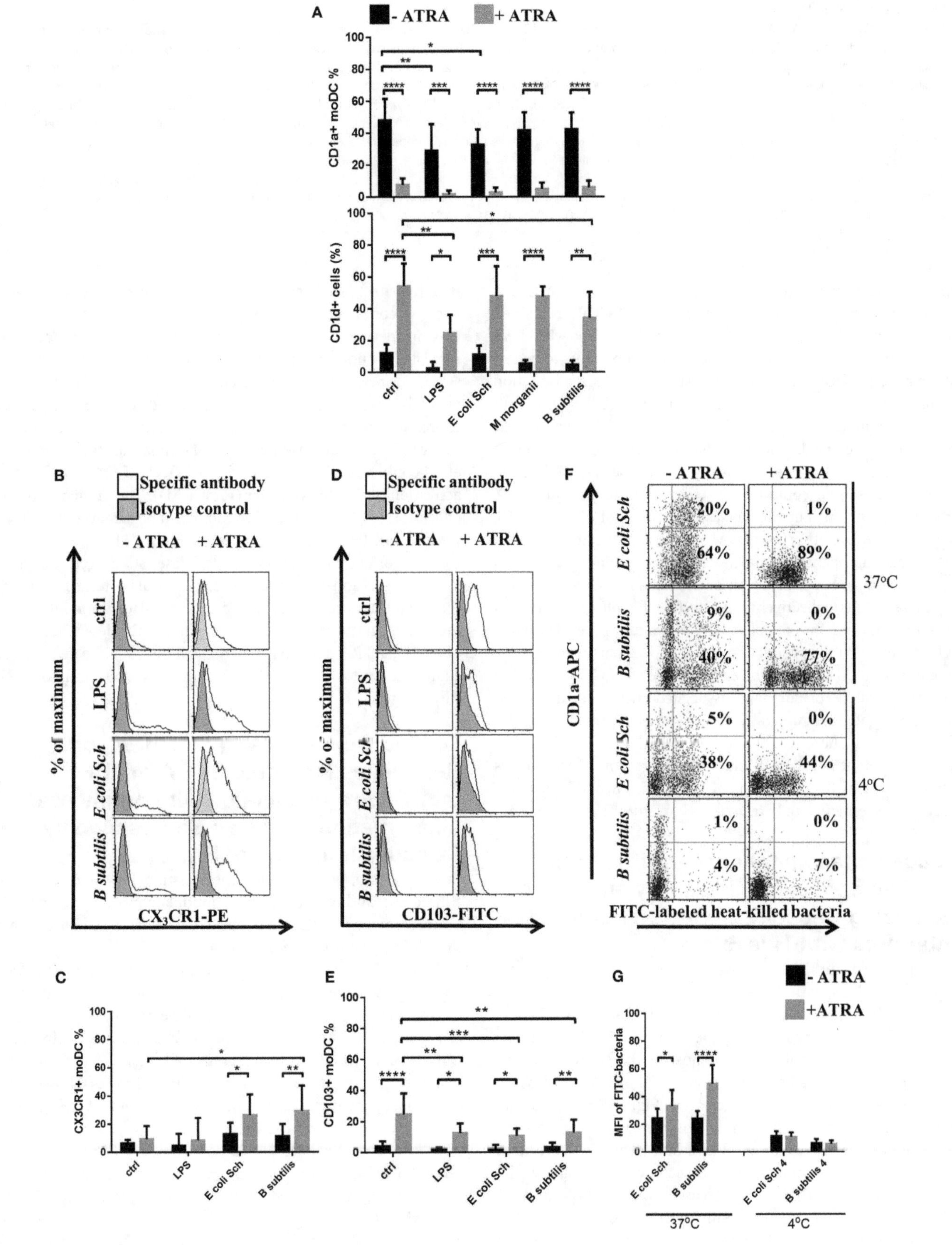

FIGURE 3 | Continued

FIGURE 3 | Continued
All-*trans* retinoic acid (ATRA) shifts the cell surface expression pattern of CD1, gut-related receptors, and the phagocytic capacity of monocyte-derived dentritic cells (moDCs) in an ATRA and commensal strain-dependent manner. Human moDCs were differentiated in the presence of granulocyte-macrophage colony-stimulating factor and interleukin-4 with or without 1 nM ATRA for 2 days. The surface expression level of CD1a and CD1d was measured on resting cells and moDCs activated with live commensal bacteria for 24 h **(A)** by flow cytometry. Histogram overlays show results derived from 1 representative donor of 10. The cell surface expression level of the mucosa-related CX_3CR1 **(B,C)** and CD103 **(D,E)** was measured by flow cytometry followed by a 24-h activation period with live commensal bacteria or lipopolysaccharide (LPS) served as a positive control. Mean values showing the ratio of moDCs positive for the measured surface protein were calculated from five independent experiments +SD. To monitor the phagocytic capacity of moDCs, on day 2, moDCs were co-cultured with heat-inactivated and fluorescein-isothiocyanate (FITC)-labeled bacteria at 37°C or at 4°C for 3 h at a moDC:bacteria ratio of 1:20. **(F,G)** Dot plots show one of four independent experiments. The ratio of moDC positive for heat-inactivated and FITC-labeled bacteria was measured by flow cytometry. The number of moDCs carrying FITC-labeled bacteria was calculated from four independent experiments +SD. ANOVA followed by Bonferroni's multiple comparison tests was used in the statistical analysis with significance defined as $^*P < 0.05$, $^{**}P < 0.01$, $^{***}P < 0.001$, and $^{****}P < 0.0001$.

lymphoid organs, could also be induced in the presence of LPS or *E. coli Schaedler*, but the expression level of CCR7 remained inhibited in ATRA-treated moDC (**Figure 4B**). In line with these results showing the potential of microbial components to generate mature moDCs, we detected the species-specific production of inflammatory cytokines including TNF-α, IL-1β, IL-6, and CXCL8 chemokine (**Figure 4C**). Furthermore, *B. subtilis* was found to induce negligible pro-inflammatory cytokine production as compared to Gram-negative *E. coli Schaedler*, but the effects of *B. subtilis* could be boosted significantly upon ATRA treatment confirmed by the increased secretion of TNF-α, IL-1β, and IL-6. We also observed that *M. morganii* induced the expression of a similar panel of moDC-derived inflammatory cytokines as compared to that of *E. coli Schaedler* (data not shown).

These results collectively indicate that *E. coli Schaedler* and *B. subtilis* harbor individual moDC-provoking potential, while ATRA can boost the production of pro-inflammatory mediators. In contrast to this finding, the expression level of CCR7 becomes downmodulated presumably associated with its decreased migratory potential guided by the $RAR\alpha^{hi}IRF4^{lo}$ moDC population. Based on these results, we conclude that *E. coli Schaedler* acts as a potent inducer of inflammatory responses in moDCs accompanied by the production of TNF-α, IL-1β, and IL-6, while *B. subtilis* is less efficient to trigger TNF-α and/or IL-1β secretion.

E. coli Schaedler and *B. subtilis* Increase the T-Lymphocyte Stimulatory and Polarizing Capacity of moDCs but ATRA Interferes with This Effect

The first signal for Th cell activation derives from the interaction of the TCR with MHC class II–peptide complexes presented by antigen-presenting proteins such as HLA-DQ and HLA-DR inducible by LPS or by the selected microbiota strains (**Figure 5A**). When moDCs were exposed to LPS or to commensal bacteria, the cell surface expression of the CD80 and CD86 co-stimulatory molecules was increased (**Figure 5B**). In such an experimental system, the secretion of the regulatory cytokine IL-10 was independent on ATRA in case of moDC activation by bacteria. More importantly, the secretion level of the Th1 polarizing cytokine IL-12 was decreased, while that of the IL-23 cytokine was enhanced significantly in the $RAR\alpha^{hi}IRF4^{lo}$ moDC population (**Figure 5C**). Interestingly, *B. subtilis* was unable to induce IL-23 secretion and the level of IL-12 also remained lower than the effect provoked by moDCs in the presence of the Gram-negative commensal bacterium *E. coli Schaedler*.

Considering that the differentiation of T-lymphocytes is regulated by both co-stimulatory and inhibitory signals, the cell surface expression of known co-stimulators of T-lymphocytes were also monitored. The results revealed that the cell surface expression of the co-stimulatory molecule CD40 could be induced by LPS and also by the two commensal strains, and this effect could be slightly enhanced in $PPAR\gamma^{hi}IRF4^{low}$ moDCs upon activation by *E. coli Schaedler* (**Figure 5D**). The induction of the effector T cell inhibitor PD-L1 could also be achieved if moDCs were stimulated by *E. coli Schaedler* (**Figure 5E**), in contrast to *B. subtilis* or LPS with no such effects. These data altogether suggest that both LPS and gut-associated commensal bacteria can induce the cell surface expression of T cell co-stimulatory and inhibitory molecules on the moDC cell surface in a strain-dependent manner, while ATRA-activated moDCs exhibit impaired cell surface expression of MHC class II, co-stimulatory, and inhibitory cell surface proteins.

Limited Commensal-Induced Effector Responses Mediated by $RAR\alpha^{hi}IRF4^{lo}$ moDCs Are Associated with Augmented Inflammation That Can Be Rescued by the Selective Inhibition of RARα

In a next step, we addressed the question how T-lymphocyte stimulation and maturation may modulate moDC responses in the presence of ATRA or commensal bacteria. Taken the fact that differentiation of moDCs can be modified in the presence of 1 nM ATRA, we also confirmed that the blockade of RARα signaling by a specific antagonist resulted in the prevention of CD1d and CD103 expression, while in the presence of ATRA, the cell surface expression of CD1a remained similar as control cells (**Figure 6A**). The chemical antagonist of RARα, i.e., BMS614 was unable to increase the cell surface expression level of CD1a on the cell surface showing that a minimal concentration of endogenous ATRA is presented by moDCs.

In a further step, we also demonstrated that the enhanced secretion of the pro-inflammatory cytokines (**Figure 6B**) and IL-23 (**Figure 6C**) induced by commensal bacteria could be ameliorated by the prior blockade of RARα. Moreover, the reduced antigen-presenting capacity of the ATRA-conditioned moDCs could be restored by the inhibition of RARα (**Figure 6D**).

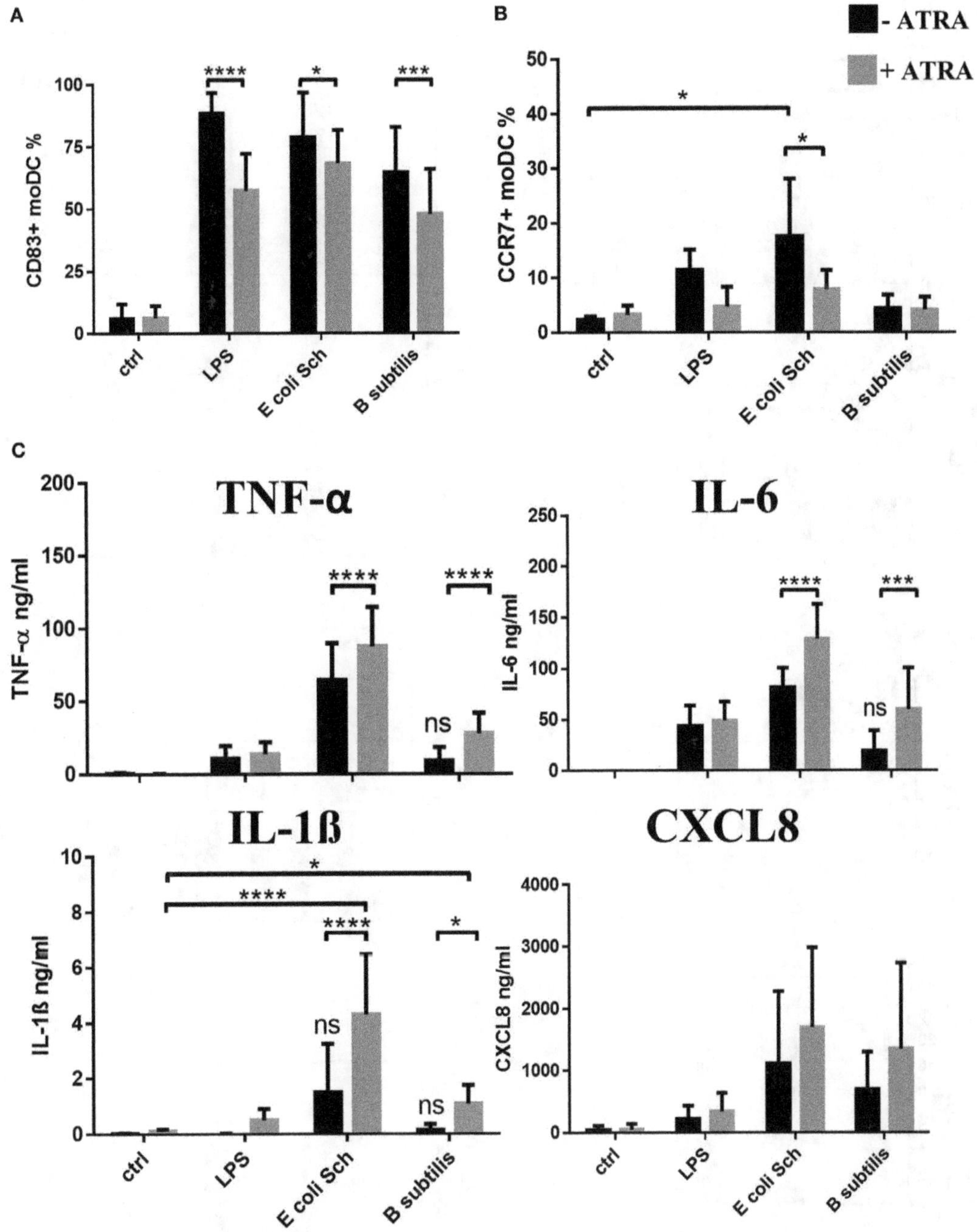

FIGURE 4 | Characteristics of the inflammatory and migratory potential of monocyte-derived dendritic cell (moDC) populations induced by commensal bacteria. Two-day moDCs were co-incubated with live commensal strains or with 250 ng/ml lipopolysaccharide (LPS) used as control for 24 h. Expression of the moDC-associated activation marker CD83 **(A)** and CCR7 **(B)** was measured by flow cytometry. Mean values were calculated from five to seven independent experiments +SD. The concentration of TNF-α, interleukin (IL)-1β, IL-6 pro-inflammatory cytokines, and the chemokine CXCL8 **(C)** was measured by ELISA followed by a 24-h activation of moDC in five independent experiments. Mean values +SD are shown. ANOVA followed by Bonferroni's multiple comparison tests was used in the statistical analysis with significance defined as $^{*}P < 0.05$, $^{***}P < 0.001$, and $^{****}P < 0.0001$.

Considering that the IRF4 transcription factor plays a pivotal role in setting the degree of DC-mediated antigen presentation (41), in a final experimental setting, we described for the first time in human moDCs that the protein level of IRF4 could be upregulated by live commensal bacteria and this effect could be decreased in a RARα-dependent manner (**Figure 6E**). As we expected, the decreased effector T-lymphocyte polarizing capacity of moDCs could be recovered by the selective blockade of RARα leading to strong Th1 (**Figure 6F**) and Th17 (**Figure 6G**) responses against the selected microbiota strains.

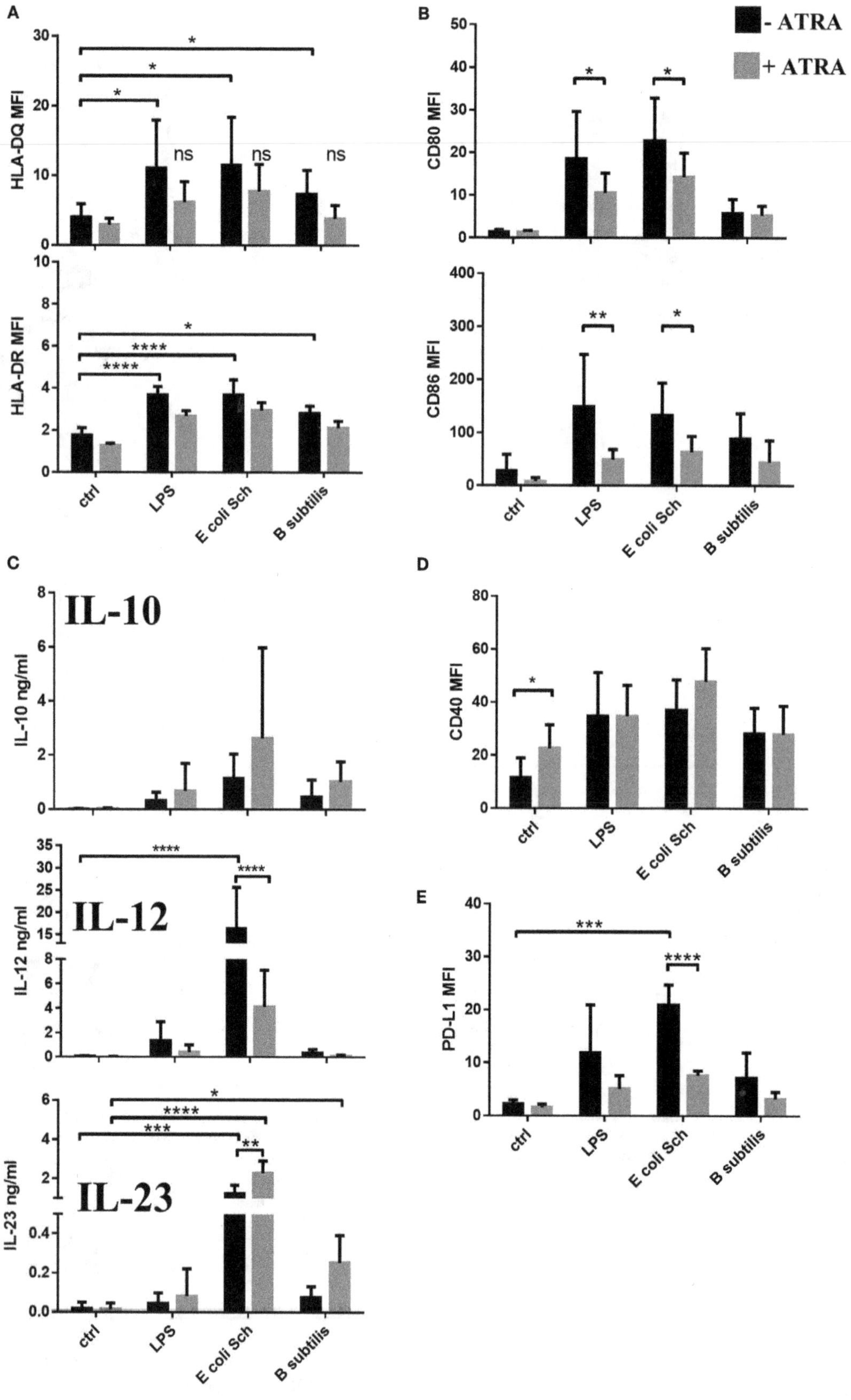

FIGURE 5 | Continued

FIGURE 5 | Continued
The T-lymphocyte activating and polarizing capacity of monocyte-derived dentritic cells (moDCs) activated by selected commensal bacteria. Two-day moDCs were co-incubated with live commensal strains or with 250 ng/ml lipopolysaccharide (LPS) used as control for 24 h. The expression levels of HLA-DQ and HLA-DR **(A)**, the co-stimulatory proteins CD80 and CD86 **(B)**, CD40 **(D)**, and the inhibitory molecule PD-L1 **(E)** was measured by flow cytometry. Mean values of median fluorescence intensities (MFIs) were calculated from five to seven independent experiments +SD. The concentration of interleukin (IL)-12, IL-23, and IL-10 cytokines was measured by ELISA followed by a 24-h activation of moDC and was tested in seven independent experiments **(C)**. Mean values +SD are shown. ANOVA followed by Bonferroni's multiple comparison tests was used in the statistical analysis with significance defined as $^{*}P < 0.05$, $^{**}P < 0.01$, $^{***}P < 0.001$, and $^{****}P < 0.0001$.

Based on these results, we propose that the differentiation program of moDC initiated by GM-CSF and IL-4 can readily be modulated by ATRA, and this effect is associated specifically to the RARα nuclear receptor. In line with the results showing that ATRA is able to downmodulate the gene expression of IRF4 in both resting and ATRA-conditioned activated moDCs in the presence of commensal bacteria, the cell surface expression of antigen-presenting HLA-DQ molecules is decreased in a RARα-dependent manner.

DISCUSSION

This study focuses to the interplay of moDCs differentiated *in vitro* and designed to accommodate to various microenvironments having the potential to guide autologous effector T-lymphocyte functional activities. In this context, the polarization and the actual expression patterns of the cell surface molecules exhibiting co-stimulatory and/or inhibitory potential were monitored in the presence and absence of selected members of the gut microbiota exemplified by *E. coli Schaedler*, *M. morganii*, and *B. subtilis*. Based on our concept, the outcome of moDC differentiation is able to accommodate to unique cellular microenvironments (21, 44) and remains remarkably plastic until the terminal differentiation of the moDCs ensues. In line with this, we also demonstrated that during the very early phase of moDC differentiation, the cells remain programmable at physiologically relevant doses of environmental cues such as in the presence of nanomolar ATRA (45). Importantly, these events can be prevented by the selective ligation of RARα acting through its natural antagonist resulting in a moDC phenotype similar to that of the "gold standard" of moDCs (43) differentiated by GM-CSF and IL-4.

In a retinoid-rich milieu, moDCs shift the cell surface expression pattern of CD1 proteins, and in resting moDCs, the expression level of CD103 remains inducible supporting the development of a mucosa-related phenotype (46, 47). This observation allowed us to distinguish the characteristics of the expressed cell surface molecules such as CD1 and CD103 on various moDC types. These proteins can be expressed by the $CD1a^{+/-}CD1d^{-}CD103^{-}$ and the $CD1a^{-}CD1d^{+}CD103^{+}$ cell populations, respectively (**Figure 7A**).

We first characterized and compared the expression levels of the contributing transcription factors, including IRF4, PPARγ, and RARα in moDCs. DCs expressing IRF4 were shown to be the less potent inducers of cytotoxic T-lymphocytes as compared to cells expressing IRF8, a DC subset localized to the gut mucosa (39, 48). The results revealed that $IRF4^{hi}$ moDCs can be characterized as immunogenic cells provoking commensal-induced Th1 and Th17 immune responses, but this pattern could be reduced in case the T cells were primed with microbiota-stimulated $RAR\alpha^{hi}PPAR\gamma^{hi}IRF4^{lo}$ moDCs supporting the notion that these cells remain highly inflammatory, lose their potential to activate autologous effector T helper cells, and also lack molecular interactions, which may play role in preventing effector T cell responses induced by commensal bacteria (**Figure 7B**). This observation is further supported by previous studies showing that the increased expression level and activity of PPARγ is associated with CD1d expression and the development of tolerogenic moDCs (20). Ligation of the CD40 cell surface molecule enhances the inflammatory potential of DCs (49) and the resting moDCs concomitantly conditioned with ATRA upregulate the cell surface expression of CD40, which can be further increased by *E. coli Schaedler* as compared to moDCs differentiated in the absence of ATRA. This observation is also confirmed by the concept that resting DCs express high levels of CD40 on the cell surface representing a semi-activated DC population with tolerogenic features (50, 51).

It has also been demonstrated that in the presence of heat-killed *E. coli Schaedler* and *B. subtilis* bacteria, the phagocytic capacity of moDCs could be facilitated by ATRA, similar to a previous work showing increased PPARγ activity in moDCs upon internalizing corpuscular antigens more efficiently than moDCs with low PPARγ activity (52). In addition to these findings, we also demonstrated that the stimulation of moDC with selected commensal bacteria resulted in moDCs expressing CX_3CR1 supported by ATRA and showing a phenotype similar to that of the $CD11b^{+}CX_3CR1^{+}CD103^{-}$ mononuclear mucosal phagocytes of myeloid origin. Moreover, in the presence of selected bacterial strains, the ATRA-primed moDCs induced the secretion of pro-inflammatory cytokines including TNF-α, IL-1β, IL-6, and IL-23 at high levels. Considering that these inflammatory cytokines play central role in the maintenance and/or disruption of mucosal integrity, exemplified by secreted IL-23 of both DC and macrophage origin. These regulatory circuits may serve as double-edged swords in the maintenance of balance in health and disease. The increased level of secreted IL-23 could directly be associated with several chronic inflammatory diseases including IBD (53). However, the presence of microbiota provide signals for both CX_3CR1^{+} inflammatory cells and $CD11b^{+}CD103^{+}$ DCs in the *lamina propria* to produce IL-23 and induce IL-22 secretion by innate lymphoid cells, thus playing a critical role in promoting mucosal healing in colitis (37, 54). Pro-inflammatory *lamina propria*-derived TNF-α can also exacerbate colitis through CX_3CR1^{+} DCs indicating that this DC subset also plays role in the maintenance of balanced inflammatory and/or standby conditions upon gut homeostasis (32).

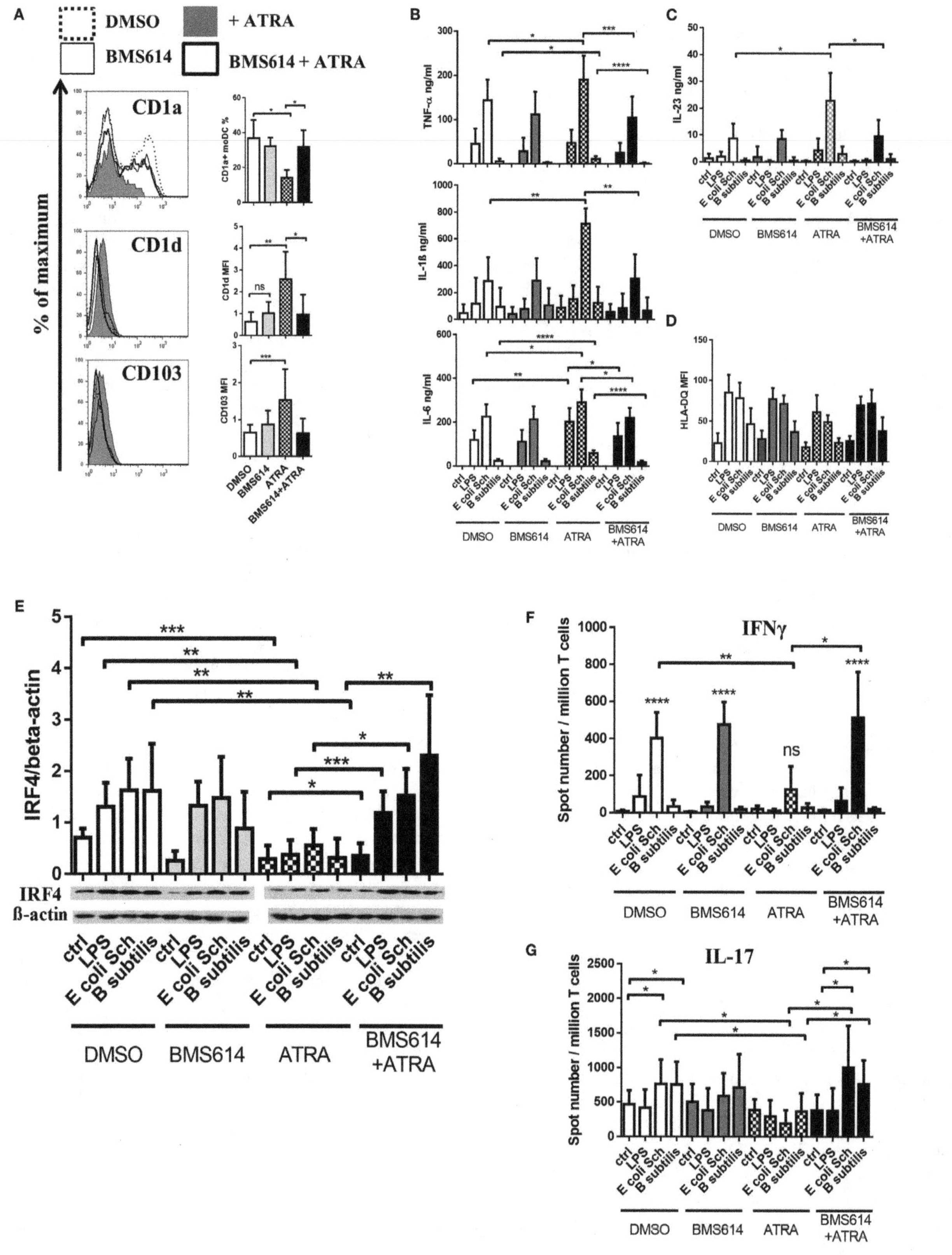

FIGURE 6 | Continued

FIGURE 6 | Continued
The selective inhibition of retinoic acid receptor alpha (RARα) prevents the all-*trans* retinoic acid (ATRA)-induced signature of microbiota-generated immune responses mediated by monocyte-derived dentritic cells (moDCs). To analyze how ATRA acts on the moDC-mediated immune response against microbiota species, the cells were treated with the RARα antagonist BMS614 prior to treating the cell culture medium with ATRA. The cell surface expression level of CD1a, CD1d, and CD103 was measured by flow cytometry in 2-day moDCs **(A)**. The concentration of TNF-α, interleukin (IL)-6, and IL-1β **(B)** and IL-23 **(C)** was measured by ELISA followed by a 24-h activation of moDC performed in seven independent experiments. Mean values +SD are shown. The cell surface expression level of HLA-DQ was measured by flow cytometry followed by a 24-h incubation period with live commensal bacteria. **(D)** Mean values of cells positive for the measured cell surface molecules were calculated from the results of seven independent donors +SD. Analysis of interferon regulatory factor 4 (IRF4) expression in moDCs. **(E)** Two-day moDCs were activated by live commensal bacteria for 24 h, and the relative expression levels of IRF4 protein was measured by Western blotting. Bar graphs show IRF4/β-actin ratios measured after 24 h of stimulation. Mean values of protein densities were calculated from five independent experiments +SD. The T cell polarizing capacity of moDCs was monitored in moDCs activated with the selected commensal strains or with lipopolysaccharide (LPS) followed by co-culturing the cells with autologous T cells. Freshly isolated peripheral blood lymphocytes were co-cultured with autologous moDCs for 4 days. The number of cytokine producing T-lymphocytes, induced by LPS or moDCs exposed to *Escherichia coli Schaedler* and *Bacillus Subtilis*, was measured by interferon gamma (IFNγ) **(F)** and IL-17 **(G)** enzyme-linked ImmunoSpot assays. The mean value of spot numbers was calculated from five independent experiments +SD. Statistical analysis was performed by the Student's unpaired two-tailed *t*-test with significance defined as $^*P < 0.05$, $^{**}P < 0.01$, $^{***}P < 0.001$, and $^{****}P < 0.0001$.

In the presence of live bacteria, ATRA boosts the secretion of Th17 polarizing cytokines; however, the polarizing capacity of these moDCs is reduced. This observation is also supported by our previous study showing that moDCs "educated" by the supernatant of ATRA-primed colonic epithelial cells were able to reduce CCR7-dependent cell migration as well as their Th17 polarizing capacity as compared to control moDCs (44). Interestingly, in a murine model, Th17 differentiation was found to be dependent on IRF4 and IL-6 secreted by CD11b$^+$CD103$^+$ DCs derived from the mesenteric lymph nodes (55). The same group also showed that the human equivalent of these DCs could be identified as the intestinal IRF4 protein expressing CD103$^+$SIRPα^{hi} DCs.

Based on the known regulatory functions of DCs, this study demonstrates that the selected commensal bacteria also secrete IL-10, an inhibitory cytokine acting independently on the bacterial species. At our experimental conditions, the cell surface expression of PD-L1 protein became upregulated in a bacterial strain dependent manner, which could be demonstrated also in the ATRA-primed moDCs, even though its expression level was significantly lower as compared to the respective ATRA free moDC counterpart. In addition to these results, the secretion of IL-12 cytokine with known inflammatory properties was downmodulated by ATRA as shown before by others (56). In contrast to these findings, we demonstrated that ATRA had no effect on IL-10 secretion in moDCs. Collectively, these data indicate that the decreased levels of IL-12, the reduced co-stimulatory and antigen-presenting capacity of RARα^{hi}IRF4^{lo} moDCs, together with the production inhibitory IL-10 create a local milieu, which is inefficient to induce potent effector T helper cell responses upon targeting the selected gut microbiota species.

Our results clearly demonstrated that in resting moDCs, ATRA is able to upregulate the relative mRNA levels of RARα, previously confirmed also by others (56). In addition, we can exclude the effects of other RAR isoforms such as RARβ, as it is not expressed and the expression of RARβ could not be induced in moDCs in the presence of ATRA. It has also been shown that the effects of ATRA on the differentiation and the microbiota-induced stimulation of moDCs could be prevented by the selective inhibition of RARα, a transcription factor playing critical role in regulating moDC differentiation and guiding mucosal immune responses. It has also been found that the gut microbiota has an impact on retinoid signaling-mediated immune homeostasis transmitted by microbial metabolites such as short-chain fatty acids (57). Furthermore, retinoid supplementation through diet also acts on the composition of the gut microbiota and on energy metabolism of the host (58). For example, vitamin A deficiency causes perturbations in the gut microbiota by reducing the ratio of *Firmicutes* and *Proteobacteria* on a Myd88- and TRIF-dependent manner (59). It has previously been demonstrated that RA is associated to inflammatory macrophages, as patients with Crohn's disease exhibit an increased capacity to generate RALDH-derived RA, which is associated with CD14$^+$ macrophages derived from the intestinal mucosa, thus maintaining an inflammatory phenotype mediated by RARα (26). This group also showed that clinical samples derived from Crohn's disease patients involve both CD103$^+$ and CD103$^-$ DCs with elevated expression levels of the ALDH1A2 gene, which is undetectable in RA-producing macrophages. Retinoids involving ATRA also improves the antitumor immunity in microbiota-induced colorectal cancer, as it increases the efficacy of tumor-specific cytotoxic T-lymphocytes by increasing RARα-mediated MHCI expression in tumor cells (60).

Human moDCs not only provoke antigen-specific immune responses but also induce the activation and expansion of innate lymphoid cells; among them, iNKT cells (20, 61) and also present lipid antigens *via* cell surface CD1 glycolipid receptors. Remarkably, the level of CD1a and CD1d expression can be modified by commensal bacteria to different extents supporting the notion that this effect is not even related to the local lipid/retinoid environment, the activity of PPARγ (21), or the presence of pathogenic microbes (62), but their activities may resemble some microbiota species such as *E. coli Schaedler* and *B. subtilis.* moDCs with increased PPARγ activity also induce the expansion of IFNγ-secreting iNKT cell at high levels as compared to moDCs with low PPARγ activity (52). Surprisingly, we were unable to detect changes in the number of iNKT cells in moDCs stimulated by commensal bacteria, when the activated moDC–T cell cultures were tested. Instead, moDCs generated processed lipid antigens derived from commensal bacteria indicating that these lipids are unable to provide ligands for CD1a or CD1d proteins (Figure S3 in Supplementary Material). However, it was previously reported that bacterial colonization of the murine colon

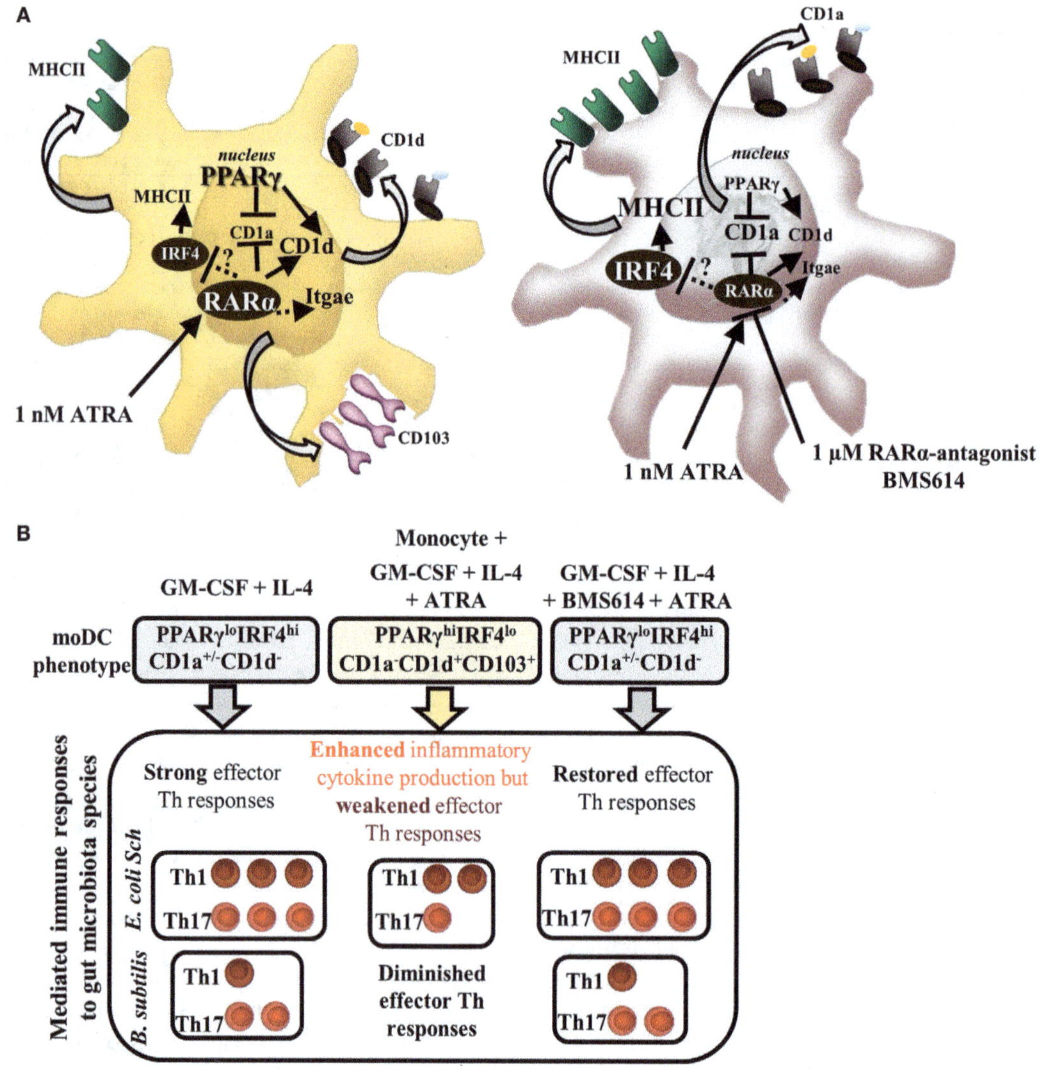

FIGURE 7 | The role of retinoic acid receptor alpha (RARα) in guiding monocyte-derived dentritic cell (moDC) development and microbiota-induced immune responses. All-*trans* retinoic acid (ATRA) modifies the differentiation of moDCs that could be prevented by the selective inhibition of RARα. **(A)** In the presence of granulocyte-macrophage colony-stimulating factor (GM-CSF) and interleukin (IL)-4, monocytes differentiate to $CD1d^-CD1a^+$ DCs (43). Peroxisome proliferator-activated receptor gamma (PPARγ) and RARα regulate the gene expression of CD1d and ALDH1A2 both directly and indirectly in human moDCs (20). Interferon regulatory factor 4 (IRF4) mediates the differentiation and antigen-presenting capacity of human moDCs, which is downregulated by the ligation of RARα resulting in decreased mRNA and protein levels of IRF4 together with CD1a. Selected microbiota species provoke different types of immune responses mediated by moDCs. **(B)** *Escherichia coli Schaedler* induces full maturation in moDCs leading to strong inflammatory and microbiota-induced effector helper T (Th) responses, while *Bacillus subtilis* induces inflammation in the absence of IL-12 and IL-23 and provokes decreased effector Th1/Th17 immune responses. ATRA downmodulates the immunogenicity of moDCs resulting in diminished Th1 and undetectable Th17 responses, which effect can be restored in moDCs by the prior inhibition of RARα in moDCs. Solid lines represent known mechanisms; dotted lines indicate unknown molecular interactions.

with *E. coli Schaedler* stimulates intestinal epithelial cells and intraepithelial innate lymphoid cells (63) independently, and this effect may play role in the pathogenesis of colitis as demonstrated in adoptive transfer models using SCID mice, which may also operate in patients with IBD.

Collectively, we offer a sensitive *in vitro* assay system appropriate for the comparative analysis of selected individual microbes in the course of collaboration with human phagocytic cells such as primary moDCs, playing essential roles in orchestrating the outcome of immune responses. We also confirmed that the vitamin A derivative ATRA has the potential to drive the differentiation program of moDCs in a RARα-dependent manner and thus confers suppressive signals during gut commensal bacteria-induced effector T-lymphocyte responses in line with enhancing their local inflammatory potential.

The interactions of diet, gut microbiota and the host build up a highly complex network of regulatory circuits to drive the development of both mucosal and systemic immune responses. Preferentially in early childhood, imbalances in food supplementation together with the acquired perturbance of the gut microbiota increase the risk of chronic immune and metabolic disorders; however, how the environmental and genetic factors determine the outcome of such immune failures requires further analysis.

ETHICS STATEMENT

Leukocyte-enriched buffy coats were obtained from healthy blood donors drawn at the Regional Blood Center of the Hungarian National Blood Transfusion Service (Debrecen, Hungary) in accordance with the written approval of the Director of the National Blood Transfusion Service of the University of Debrecen, Faculty of Medicine (Hungary) and from the Regional and Institutional Research Ethical Committee of the University of Debrecen (DEOEC RKEB/IKEB 3855-2013). Written, informed consent was obtained from the blood donors prior blood donation, their data were processed and stored according to the directives of the European Union.

AUTHOR CONTRIBUTIONS

KB designed and performed the experiments, analyzed the results, organized the data, and wrote the manuscript. ZV contributed to protein-based experiments. VP contributed to the isolation and cultivation of commensal microbes. NB provided initial experimental idea and revised the manuscript. ER designed the concept, developed the interpretation, and revised the manuscript.

ACKNOWLEDGMENTS

This research was supported by the "Host/bacterial interaction—mechanisms of the regulation of mucosal immune response by the commensal bacteria," State Found of Fundamental Research (SFFR in Ukraine with the International Participation), 20/451-2007, 0107U008933, the Ukrainian-Hungarian Intergovernmental S&T Project: "Nosocomial Infections of population in Hungarian-Ukrainian Transborders Regions: current state and effective ways for their prevention," M/220-20070107U007971 and "Immunomodulatory role of the commensal microflora: new mechanisms, potential target cells and the prosperity of their usage," M/27-2009. This research was also supported by the TORNADO FP7-KBBE-2007-2A "Molecular targets open for regulation by the gut flora: *New avenues for improved diet to optimize European health*," a project supported by the European Union and the State of Hungary, co-financed by the European Social Fund in the framework of TAMOP 4.2.4.A/2-11-1-2012-0001 and TAMOP 4.2.2.A-11/1/KONV-2012-0023. The authors thank Istvan Szatmari for revising the manuscript, Peter Gogolak for his valuable experimental advices, and Zsuzsanna Biro-Debreceni and Erzsebet Nagyne Kovacs for their excellent technical assistance.

SUPPLEMENTARY MATERIAL

The Supplementary Material for this article can be found online at http://journal.frontiersin.org/article/10.3389/fimmu.2017.00427/full#supplementary-material.

FIGURE S1 | Regulatory T-lymphocyte polarizing capacity of monocyte-derived dendritic cell (moDC) populations stimulated by *Escherichia coli* Schaedler, *Morganella morganii*, and *Bacillus subtilis*. To detect the number of regulatory T-lymphocytes, resting and stimulated moDCs were co-cultured with peripheral blood lymphocyte for 6 days. The ratio of $CD25^+FoxP3^+$ Treg cells **(A,B)** and the interleukin (IL)-10-producing Treg cells **(C)** were analyzed by flow cytometry, respectively. Dot plots show one out of five independent experiments. The mean value of Treg cell numbers was calculated from five independent experiments +SD. In the statistical analysis, ANOVA followed by Bonferroni's multiple comparison tests were used with significance defined as $^*P < 0.05$.

FIGURE S2 | Monitoring the viability of monocyte-derived dendritic cells (moDCs) exposed to live commensal bacteria in the absence or presence of all-*trans* retinoic acid (ATRA). moDCs were differentiated with or without ATRA for 2 days in serum-free culture medium. On day 2, moDCs were co-incubated with live commensal bacteria for 24 h followed by labeling the cells with 7-amino-actinomycin D (7-AAD) dye. Mean values of moDCs positive for 7-AAD staining were calculated from five independent experiments +SD.

FIGURE S3 | The invariant natural killer T (iNKT) cell inducing capacity of monocyte-derived dendritic cell (moDC) populations stimulated by *Escherichia coli* Schaedler and *Bacillus subtilis*. To detect the number of iNKT cells, moDCs were stimulated with live bacteria or with lipopolysaccharide (LPS) followed by co-incubation with autologous peripheral blood lymphocyte for 5 days, and the moDC cultures were incubated with the CD1d ligand α-GalCer served as a positive control. The ratio of $CD3^+$ cells expressing Vα24Vβ11 T cell receptors was analyzed by flow cytometry. The mean values of iNKT cell numbers were calculated from three independent experiments +SD.

REFERENCES

1. Round JL, Mazmanian SK. The gut microbiota shapes intestinal immune responses during health and disease. *Nat Rev Immunol* (2009) 9(5):313–23. doi:10.1038/nri2515
2. Blanton LV, Barratt MJ, Charbonneau MR, Ahmed T, Gordon JI. Childhood undernutrition, the gut microbiota, and microbiota-directed therapeutics. *Science* (2016) 352(6293):1533. doi:10.1126/science.aad9359
3. Rooks MG, Garrett WS. Gut microbiota, metabolites and host immunity. *Nat Rev Immunol* (2016) 16(6):341–52. doi:10.1038/nri.2016.42
4. Belkaid Y, Hand TW. Role of the microbiota in immunity and inflammation. *Cell* (2014) 157(1):121–41. doi:10.1016/j.cell.2014.03.011
5. Persson EK, Scott CL, Mowat AM, Agace WW. Dendritic cell subsets in the intestinal lamina propria: ontogeny and function. *Eur J Immunol* (2013) 43(12):3098–107. doi:10.1002/eji.201343740
6. Rhodes JM. The role of *Escherichia coli* in inflammatory bowel disease. *Gut* (2007) 56(5):610–2. doi:10.1136/gut.2006.111872
7. Sokol H, Seksik P, Furet JP, Firmesse O, Nion-Larmurier I, Beaugerie L, et al. Low counts of *Faecalibacterium prausnitzii* in colitis microbiota. *Inflamm Bowel Dis* (2009) 15(8):1183–9. doi:10.1002/ibd.20903
8. Lodinova-Zadnikova R, Cukrowska B, Tlaskalova-Hogenova H. Oral administration of probiotic *Escherichia coli* after birth reduces frequency of allergies and repeated infections later in life (after 10 and 20 years). *Int Arch Allergy Immunol* (2003) 131(3):209–11. doi:10.1159/000071488
9. Kalliomaki M, Salminen S, Arvilommi H, Kero P, Koskinen P, Isolauri E. Probiotics in primary prevention of atopic disease: a randomised placebo-controlled trial. *Lancet* (2001) 357(9262):1076–9. doi:10.1016/S0140-6736(00)04259-8
10. Boudeau J, Glasser AL, Julien S, Colombel JF, Darfeuille-Michaud A. Inhibitory effect of probiotic *Escherichia coli* strain Nissle 1917 on adhesion

to and invasion of intestinal epithelial cells by adherent-invasive *E. coli* strains isolated from patients with Crohn's disease. *Aliment Pharmacol Ther* (2003) 18(1):45–56. doi:10.1046/j.1365-2036.2003.01638.x
11. Kamada N, Maeda K, Inoue N, Hisamatsu T, Okamoto S, Hong KS, et al. Nonpathogenic *Escherichia coli* strain Nissle 1917 inhibits signal transduction in intestinal epithelial cells. *Infect Immun* (2008) 76(1):214–20. doi:10.1128/IAI.01193-07
12. Schultz M. Clinical use of *E. coli* Nissle 1917 in inflammatory bowel disease. *Inflamm Bowel Dis* (2008) 14(7):1012–8. doi:10.1002/ibd.20377
13. Ahern PP, Faith JJ, Gordon JI. Mining the human gut microbiota for effector strains that shape the immune system. *Immunity* (2014) 40(6):815–23. doi:10.1016/j.immuni.2014.05.012
14. Goto Y, Panea C, Nakato G, Cebula A, Lee C, Diez MG, et al. Segmented filamentous bacteria antigens presented by intestinal dendritic cells drive mucosal Th17 cell differentiation. *Immunity* (2014) 40(4):594–607. doi:10.1016/j.immuni.2014.03.005
15. Wang J, Li F, Wei H, Lian ZX, Sun R, Tian Z. Respiratory influenza virus infection induces intestinal immune injury via microbiota-mediated Th17 cell-dependent inflammation. *J Exp Med* (2014) 211(12):2397–410. doi:10.1084/jem.20140625
16. Buffie CG, Pamer EG. Microbiota-mediated colonization resistance against intestinal pathogens. *Nat Rev Immunol* (2013) 13(11):790–801. doi:10.1038/nri3535
17. Wang T, Pan D, Zhou Z, You Y, Jiang C, Zhao X, et al. Dectin-3 deficiency promotes colitis development due to impaired antifungal innate immune responses in the gut. *PLoS Pathog* (2016) 12(6):e1005662. doi:10.1371/journal.ppat.1005662
18. Jiang HQ, Thurnheer MC, Zuercher AW, Boiko NV, Bos NA, Cebra JJ. Interactions of commensal gut microbes with subsets of B- and T-cells in the murine host. *Vaccine* (2004) 22(7):805–11. doi:10.1016/j.vaccine.2003.11.022
19. Nagy L, Szanto A, Szatmari I, Szeles L. Nuclear hormone receptors enable macrophages and dendritic cells to sense their lipid environment and shape their immune response. *Physiol Rev* (2012) 92(2):739–89. doi:10.1152/physrev.00004.2011
20. Szatmari I, Pap A, Ruhl R, Ma JX, Illarionov PA, Besra GS, et al. PPARgamma controls CD1d expression by turning on retinoic acid synthesis in developing human dendritic cells. *J Exp Med* (2006) 203(10):2351–62. doi:10.1084/jem.20060141
21. Szatmari I, Torocsik D, Agostini M, Nagy T, Gurnell M, Barta E, et al. PPARgamma regulates the function of human dendritic cells primarily by altering lipid metabolism. *Blood* (2007) 110(9):3271–80. doi:10.1182/blood-2007-06-096222
22. Bastien J, Rochette-Egly C. Nuclear retinoid receptors and the transcription of retinoid-target genes. *Gene* (2004) 328:1–16. doi:10.1016/j.gene.2003.12.005
23. Nakken B, Varga T, Szatmari I, Szeles L, Gyongyosi A, Illarionov PA, et al. Peroxisome proliferator-activated receptor gamma-regulated cathepsin D is required for lipid antigen presentation by dendritic cells. *J Immunol* (2011) 187(1):240–7. doi:10.4049/jimmunol.1002421
24. Vicente-Suarez I, Larange A, Reardon C, Matho M, Feau S, Chodaczek G, et al. Unique lamina propria stromal cells imprint the functional phenotype of mucosal dendritic cells. *Mucosal Immunol* (2015) 8(1):141–51. doi:10.1038/mi.2014.51
25. Sun CM, Hall JA, Blank RB, Bouladoux N, Oukka M, Mora JR, et al. Small intestine lamina propria dendritic cells promote de novo generation of Foxp3 T reg cells via retinoic acid. *J Exp Med* (2007) 204(8):1775–85. doi:10.1084/jem.20070602
26. Sanders TJ, McCarthy NE, Giles EM, Davidson KL, Haltalli ML, Hazell S, et al. Increased production of retinoic acid by intestinal macrophages contributes to their inflammatory phenotype in patients with Crohn's disease. *Gastroenterology* (2014) 146(5):1278–88.e1–2. doi:10.1053/j.gastro.2014.01.057
27. Iliev ID, Spadoni I, Mileti E, Matteoli G, Sonzogni A, Sampietro GM, et al. Human intestinal epithelial cells promote the differentiation of tolerogenic dendritic cells. *Gut* (2009) 58(11):1481–9. doi:10.1136/gut.2008.175166
28. Allenby G, Bocquel MT, Saunders M, Kazmer S, Speck J, Rosenberger M, et al. Retinoic acid receptors and retinoid X receptors: interactions with endogenous retinoic acids. *Proc Natl Acad Sci U S A* (1993) 90(1):30–4. doi:10.1073/pnas.90.1.30
29. Garcia-Manero G, Yang H, Kuang SQ, O'Brien S, Thomas D, Kantarjian H. Epigenetics of acute lymphocytic leukemia. *Semin Hematol* (2009) 46(1):24–32. doi:10.1053/j.seminhematol.2008.09.008
30. Tallman MS, Andersen JW, Schiffer CA, Appelbaum FR, Feusner JH, Ogden A, et al. All-trans-retinoic acid in acute promyelocytic leukemia. *N Engl J Med* (1997) 337(15):1021–8. doi:10.1056/NEJM199710093371501
31. Matsui W, Smith BD, Vala M, Beal N, Huff CA, Diehl LF, et al. Requirement for myeloid growth factors in the differentiation of acute promyelocytic leukaemia. *Br J Haematol* (2005) 128(6):853–62. doi:10.1111/j.1365-2141.2005.05395.x
32. Varol C, Vallon-Eberhard A, Elinav E, Aychek T, Shapira Y, Luche H, et al. Intestinal lamina propria dendritic cell subsets have different origin and functions. *Immunity* (2009) 31(3):502–12. doi:10.1016/j.immuni.2009.06.025
33. Coombes JL, Powrie F. Dendritic cells in intestinal immune regulation. *Nat Rev Immunol* (2008) 8(6):435–46. doi:10.1038/nri2335
34. Panek CA, Ramos MV, Mejias MP, Abrey-Recalde MJ, Fernandez-Brando RJ, Gori MS, et al. Differential expression of the fractalkine chemokine receptor (CX3CR1) in human monocytes during differentiation. *Cell Mol Immunol* (2015) 12(6):669–80. doi:10.1038/cmi.2014.116
35. Rescigno M, Urbano M, Valzasina B, Francolini M, Rotta G, Bonasio R, et al. Dendritic cells express tight junction proteins and penetrate gut epithelial monolayers to sample bacteria. *Nat Immunol* (2001) 2(4):361–7. doi:10.1038/86373
36. Diehl GE, Longman RS, Zhang JX, Breart B, Galan C, Cuesta A, et al. Microbiota restricts trafficking of bacteria to mesenteric lymph nodes by CX(3)CR1(hi) cells. *Nature* (2013) 494(7435):116–20. doi:10.1038/nature11809
37. Longman RS, Diehl GE, Victorio DA, Huh JR, Galan C, Miraldi ER, et al. CX(3)CR1(+) mononuclear phagocytes support colitis-associated innate lymphoid cell production of IL-22. *J Exp Med* (2014) 211(8):1571–83. doi:10.1084/jem.20140678
38. Coombes JL, Siddiqui KR, Arancibia-Carcamo CV, Hall J, Sun CM, Belkaid Y, et al. A functionally specialized population of mucosal CD103+ DCs induces Foxp3+ regulatory T cells via a TGF-beta and retinoic acid-dependent mechanism. *J Exp Med* (2007) 204(8):1757–64. doi:10.1084/jem.20070590
39. Chopin M, Allan RS, Belz GT. Transcriptional regulation of dendritic cell diversity. *Front Immunol* (2012) 3:26. doi:10.3389/fimmu.2012.00026
40. Schinnerling K, Garcia-Gonzalez P, Aguillon JC. Gene expression profiling of human monocyte-derived dendritic cells – searching for molecular regulators of tolerogenicity. *Front Immunol* (2015) 6:528. doi:10.3389/fimmu.2015.00528
41. Vander Lugt B, Khan AA, Hackney JA, Agrawal S, Lesch J, Zhou M, et al. Transcriptional programming of dendritic cells for enhanced MHC class II antigen presentation. *Nat Immunol* (2014) 15(2):161–7. doi:10.1038/ni.2795
42. Underhill DM, Goodridge HS. Information processing during phagocytosis. *Nat Rev Immunol* (2012) 12(7):492–502. doi:10.1038/nri3244
43. Sallusto F, Lanzavecchia A. Efficient presentation of soluble antigen by cultured human dendritic cells is maintained by granulocyte/macrophage colony-stimulating factor plus interleukin 4 and downregulated by tumor necrosis factor alpha. *J Exp Med* (1994) 179(4):1109–18. doi:10.1084/jem.179.4.1109
44. Chatterjee A, Gogolak P, Blottiere HM, Rajnavolgyi E. The impact of ATRA on shaping human myeloid cell responses to epithelial cell-derived stimuli and on T-lymphocyte polarization. *Mediators Inflamm* (2015) 2015:579830. doi:10.1155/2015/579830
45. Wang C, Kang SG, HogenEsch H, Love PE, Kim CH. Retinoic acid determines the precise tissue tropism of inflammatory Th17 cells in the intestine. *J Immunol* (2010) 184(10):5519–26. doi:10.4049/jimmunol.0903942
46. Jaensson-Gyllenback E, Kotarsky K, Zapata F, Persson EK, Gundersen TE, Blomhoff R, et al. Bile retinoids imprint intestinal CD103+ dendritic cells with the ability to generate gut-tropic T cells. *Mucosal Immunol* (2011) 4(4):438–47. doi:10.1038/mi.2010.91
47. Sato S, Kiyono H. The mucosal immune system of the respiratory tract. *Curr Opin Virol* (2012) 2(3):225–32. doi:10.1016/j.coviro.2012.03.009
48. Edelson BT, Wumesh KC, Juang R, Kohyama M, Benoit LA, Klekotka PA, et al. Peripheral CD103+ dendritic cells form a unified subset developmentally related to CD8alpha+ conventional dendritic cells. *J Exp Med* (2010) 207(4):823–36. doi:10.1084/jem.20091627
49. Ma DY, Clark EA. The role of CD40 and CD154/CD40L in dendritic cells. *Semin Immunol* (2009) 21(5):265–72. doi:10.1016/j.smim.2009.05.010
50. Dudek AM, Martin S, Garg AD, Agostinis P. Immature, semi-mature, and fully mature dendritic cells: toward a DC-cancer cells interface that augments anticancer immunity. *Front Immunol* (2013) 4:438. doi:10.3389/fimmu.2013.00438

51. Jaen O, Rulle S, Bessis N, Zago A, Boissier MC, Falgarone G. Dendritic cells modulated by innate immunity improve collagen-induced arthritis and induce regulatory T cells in vivo. *Immunology* (2009) 126(1):35–44. doi:10.1111/j.1365-2567.2008.02875.x
52. Majai G, Gogolak P, Ambrus C, Vereb G, Hodrea J, Fesus L, et al. PPARgamma modulated inflammatory response of human dendritic cell subsets to engulfed apoptotic neutrophils. *J Leukoc Biol* (2010) 88(5):981–91. doi:10.1189/jlb.0310144
53. Yen D, Cheung J, Scheerens H, Poulet F, McClanahan T, McKenzie B, et al. IL-23 is essential for T cell-mediated colitis and promotes inflammation via IL-17 and IL-6. *J Clin Invest* (2006) 116(5):1310–6. doi:10.1172/JCI21404
54. Kinnebrew MA, Buffie CG, Diehl GE, Zenewicz LA, Leiner I, Hohl TM, et al. Interleukin 23 production by intestinal CD103(+)CD11b(+) dendritic cells in response to bacterial flagellin enhances mucosal innate immune defense. *Immunity* (2012) 36(2):276–87. doi:10.1016/j.immuni.2011.12.011
55. Persson EK, Uronen-Hansson H, Semmrich M, Rivollier A, Hagerbrand K, Marsal J, et al. IRF4 transcription-factor-dependent CD103(+)CD11b(+) dendritic cells drive mucosal T helper 17 cell differentiation. *Immunity* (2013) 38(5):958–69. doi:10.1016/j.immuni.2013.03.009
56. Tao Y, Yang Y, Wang W. Effect of all-trans-retinoic acid on the differentiation, maturation and functions of dendritic cells derived from cord blood monocytes. *FEMS Immunol Med Microbiol* (2006) 47(3):444–50. doi:10.1111/j.1574-695X.2006.00108.x
57. Honda K, Littman DR. The microbiota in adaptive immune homeostasis and disease. *Nature* (2016) 535(7610):75–84. doi:10.1038/nature18848
58. Liu HX, Hu Y, Wan YJ. Microbiota and bile acid profiles in retinoic acid-primed mice that exhibit accelerated liver regeneration. *Oncotarget* (2016) 7(2):1096–106. doi:10.18632/oncotarget.6665
59. Cha HR, Chang SY, Chang JH, Kim JO, Yang JY, Kim CH, et al. Downregulation of Th17 cells in the small intestine by disruption of gut flora in the absence of retinoic acid. *J Immunol* (2010) 184(12):6799–806. doi:10.4049/jimmunol.0902944
60. Bhattacharya N, Yuan R, Prestwood TR, Penny HL, DiMaio MA, Reticker-Flynn NE, et al. Normalizing microbiota-induced retinoic acid deficiency stimulates protective CD8(+) T cell-mediated immunity in colorectal cancer. *Immunity* (2016) 45(3):641–55. doi:10.1016/j.immuni.2016.08.008
61. Zajonc DM, Girardi E. Recognition of microbial glycolipids by natural killer T cells. *Front Immunol* (2015) 6:400. doi:10.3389/fimmu.2015.00400
62. Sieling PA, Jullien D, Dahlem M, Tedder TF, Rea TH, Modlin RL, et al. CD1 expression by dendritic cells in human leprosy lesions: correlation with effective host immunity. *J Immunol* (1999) 162(3):1851–8.
63. Keilbaugh SA, Shin ME, Banchereau RF, McVay LD, Boyko N, Artis D, et al. Activation of RegIIIbeta/gamma and interferon gamma expression in the intestinal tract of SCID mice: an innate response to bacterial colonisation of the gut. *Gut* (2005) 54(5):623–9. doi:10.1136/gut.2004.056028

3

Visualization of Probiotic-Mediated Ca^{2+} Signaling in Intestinal Epithelial Cells *In Vivo*

Takahiro Adachi[1]*, *Shigeru Kakuta*[2], *Yoshiko Aihara*[3], *Tomonori Kamiya*[4], *Yohei Watanabe*[4], *Naomi Osakabe*[5], *Naoki Hazato*[5], *Atsushi Miyawaki*[6], *Soichiro Yoshikawa*[7], *Takako Usami*[8], *Hajime Karasuyama*[7], *Hiromi Kimoto-Nira*[9], *Kazuhiro Hirayama*[10]* and *Noriko M. Tsuji*[4]*

[1] *Department of Immunology, Medical Research Institute, Tokyo Medical and Dental University, Tokyo, Japan,* [2] *Department of Biomedical Science, Graduate School of Agricultural and Life Sciences, The University of Tokyo, Tokyo, Japan,* [3] *Department of Agrobioscience, Graduate School of Agricultural Science, Kobe University, Kobe, Japan,* [4] *Biomedical Research Institute, National Institute for Advanced Industrial Science and Technology (AIST), Tsukuba, Japan,* [5] *Department of Bio-science and Engineering, Shibaura Institute of Technology, Saitama, Japan,* [6] *Laboratory for Cell Function and Dynamics, Advanced Technology Development Group, Brain Science Institute, RIKEN, Saitama, Japan,* [7] *Department of Immune Regulation, Tokyo Medical and Dental University, Tokyo, Japan,* [8] *Laboratory of Recombinant Animals, Medical Research Institute, Tokyo Medical and Dental University, Tokyo, Japan,* [9] *NARO Institute of Livestock and Grassland Science, National Agriculture and Food Research Organization, Tsukuba, Ibaraki, Japan,* [10] *Laboratory of Veterinary Public Health, Graduate School of Agricultural and Life Sciences, The University of Tokyo, Tokyo, Japan*

Edited by:
Haruki Kitazawa,
Tohoku University, Japan

Reviewed by:
Michio Tomura,
Osaka Ohtani University, Japan
Mauro Rossi,
CNR, Italy

***Correspondence:**
Takahiro Adachi
tadachi.imm@mri.tmd.ac.jp;
Kazuhiro Hirayama
akazu@mail.ecc.u-tokyo.ac.jp;
Noriko M. Tsuji
nm-tsuji@aist.go.jp

Probiotics, such as lactic acid bacteria (LAB) and *Bacillus subtilis* var. *natto*, have been shown to modulate immune responses. It is important to understand how probiotic bacteria impact intestinal epithelial cells (IECs), because IECs are the first line of defense at the mucosal surface barrier and their activities substantially affect the gut microenvironment and immunity. However, to date, their precise mechanism remains unknown due to a lack of analytical systems available for live animal models. Recently, we generated a conditional Ca^{2+} biosensor Yellow Cameleon (YC3.60) transgenic mouse line and established 5D (x, y, z, time, and Ca^{2+}) intravital imaging systems of lymphoid tissues including those in Peyer's patches and bone marrow. In the present study, we further advance our intravital imaging system for intestinal tracts to visualize IEC responses against orally administrated food compounds in real time. Using this system, heat-killed *B. subtilis natto*, a probiotic TTCC012 strain, is shown to directly induce Ca^{2+} signaling in IECs in mice housed under specific pathogen-free conditions. In contrast, this activation is not observed in the *Lactococcus lactis* strain C60; however, when we generate germ-free YC3.60 mice and observe the LAB stimulation of IECs in the absence of gut microbiota, C60 is capable of inducing Ca^{2+} signaling. This is the first study to successfully visualize the direct effect of probiotics on IECs in live animals. These data strongly suggest that probiotic strains stimulate IECs under physiological conditions and that their activity is affected by the microenvironment of the small intestine, such as commensal bacteria.

Keywords: probiotic, Ca^{2+} signaling, intestinal epithelial cell, intravital imaging, *Lactococcus*, *Bacillus subtilis*, small intestine, germ-free mouse

INTRODUCTION

Food compounds are digested and absorbed through the gastrointestinal tract for nutrition, and probiotic bacteria and polysaccharides affect immunological homeostasis in the gut (1–6). Fermentative lactic acid bacteria (LAB) are aerobic and abundant in the environment and are very often contained in the average diet, consequently composing a major part of small intestinal commensal flora (7–9). LAB, therefore, affect the maturation of host immune cells and intestinal immune homeostasis under normal steady-state conditions (10–12). Oral administration of some LAB strains has been shown to stimulate innate immunity at mucosal sites and to potentiate systemic immune responses against pathogenic bacteria or viruses (13–17). In addition to resident LAB, orally administrated LAB, although inactive, have a substantial effect on the regulation of immunity. We recently described an anti-inflammatory mechanism exclusive to LAB strains. Most LAB strains contain large amounts of double-stranded RNA and are sensed by the endosomal toll-like receptor (TLR) 3 on intestinal dendritic cells to produce interferon-β. This innate sensing procedure contributes to anti-inflammatory and protective immune responses both locally and systemically; therefore, both live and inactive LAB can be utilized as effective probiotics (12). Functional maturation of the immune system is largely dependent on mucosal biological events, and our findings suggest a co-evolutional process through a long-term mutualism between LAB and the immune system. We have demonstrated that *Lactococci* tolerates bile acids and low pH and adheres to human enterocyte-like Caco-2 cells (18). We have not, however, determined the mechanism of interaction between LAB and intestinal epithelial cells (IECs).

Intestinal epithelial cells communicate with commensal microbes and probiotics and potentiate immune responses *via* cytokines and antigen delivery (19). Probiotics trigger signaling pathways in IECs, such as NF-κB and MAP kinase, which affect the immune response and integrity of the mucosal surface barrier. However, it is difficult to monitor their biological events in real time *in vivo*. This issue became an obstacle in our initial study on the interaction between probiotics and IECs. Thus, it would be of great value to develop a reliable analytical system for intravital imaging of IECs.

Calcium ions (Ca^{2+}) are universal second messengers performing multiple functions in most cells. In the immune system, stimulation of immunological receptors, including B-cell antigen and cytokine receptors, induces intracellular Ca^{2+} mobilization concomitant with other signaling events such as phosphorylation of cellular substrates (20–24). To visualize Ca^{2+} signaling *in vivo*, we generated a conditional Föster/fluorescent resonance energy transfer (FRET)-based calcium biosensor Yellow Cameleon 3.60 (YC3.60) transgenic mice (25). YC3.60 is a double-chromophore indicator that employs FRET between a cyan fluorescent protein (CFP) and a circularly permuted variant of the yellow fluorescent protein (YFP) Venus (26). Ca^{2+} signaling can be monitored by measuring the ratio of YFP to CFP (YFP/CFP). FRET-based ratiometric indicators including YC3.60 can be corrected for unequal sensor expression and motion-derived changes in fluorescent intensity. Therefore, ratiometric sensors, such as YC3.60, are suitable for *in vivo* whole-body imaging in mice. Accordingly, we have recently established 5D (*x*, *y*, *z*, time, and Ca^{2+} signal) live imaging of immunological tissues including those in bone marrow and Peyer's patches (25).

Here, we applied our system to detect probiotic-mediated Ca^{2+} signaling in IECs *in vivo* and found differences between the two types of Gram-positive probiotic bacteria, *Lactococcus lactis* and *Bacillus subtilis* var. *natto.* Our results suggest, for the first time, that probiotic strains stimulate small IECs *via* intravital observations; in addition, these results facilitate the understanding of probiotic-mediated immunoregulatory mechanisms.

MATERIALS AND METHODS

Mice

The conditional YC3.60 expression transgenic mouse line has been previously described (25). The floxed YC3.60 reporter ($YC3.60^{flox}$) mouse line was crossed with a CD19-Cre mouse line (27), which resulted in $CD19^{+}$ cell-specific YC3.60 expression in $YC3.60^{flox}$/CD19-Cre mice due to the loss of the loxP-flanked neomycin cassette. The $YC3.60^{flox}$ mouse line was crossed with a CAG-Cre (28) mouse line, which expresses the Cre gene ubiquitously. These mice were maintained in our animal facility under specific pathogen-free (SPF) conditions in accordance with the guidelines of the Tokyo Medical and Dental University for animal care. These procedures have been approved by the Committee of the Tokyo Medical and Dental University for animal care.

Germ-free BALB/cA mice were bred at the Laboratory of Veterinary Public Health, the University of Tokyo, and were used as foster mothers. Germ-free animals were kept in flexible vinyl isolators in a room at 24°C, relative humidity of 60%, and 12 h periods of light and dark, and were fed a CMF-pelleted diet (Oriental Yeast Co., Tokyo, Japan) sterilized by γ-irradiation at a dose of 50 kGy. For the generation of germ-free mice with ubiquitous YC3.60 expression, *in vitro* fertilization and cesarean operation were performed as described below. Female mice with ubiquitous YC3.60 expression were superovulated by an intraperitoneal injection of 7.5 IU eCG followed by 7.5 IU hCG at an interval of 48 h. Eggs were collected from sacrificed female mice and fertilized with the sperm of male mice with ubiquitous YC3.60 expression in HTF medium (ARK Resource, Kumamoto, Japan). After overnight culture in the KSOM medium (ARK Resource), two-cell embryos were transferred into the oviducts of pseudopregnant female ICR mice. The estimated delivery date was controlled by a subcutaneous injection of Progehorrmon (Mochida Pharmaceutical Co., Ltd., Tokyo, Japan). The surrogate mothers were sacrificed at the fetal age of 19.5 days by cervical dislocation, and the uterus was aseptically removed with clamps at the top of each uterine horn and the base of the uterus close to the cervix. The uterus was introduced into an isolator for operation through a germicidal trap with 2% peracetic acid solution kept at 37°C. The uterus was cut with scissors, and pups were removed. Their breathing was stimulated, and they were cleaned with dry gauze. After the pups started breathing normally, they were transferred to the isolator with their foster mothers. The germ status was checked once a month. These procedures were approved by the Committee for Care of Laboratory Animals in the Graduate School of Agricultural and Life Sciences at the University of Tokyo.

Probiotic Bacteria

Lactococcus lactis subsp. *cremoris* C60 (29) was cultured in MRS broth (BD Difco) for 20 h at 30°C (late-log phase) at the National Institute of Advanced Industrial Science and Technology (AIST). The bacteria were harvested, washed two times, and resuspended in sterile saline. The suspensions were then heated for 30 min at 70°C (heat-killed) and were stored at −80°C. Heat-killed *B. subtilis* var. *natto* TTCC12 (late-log phase) were kindly provided from Takano Foods Co. Ltd. and were stored at −80°C.

Flow Cytometry

Calcium ions mobilization was analyzed using flow cytometry. Ca^{2+} mobilization in YC3.60-expressing cells was analyzed by flow cytometry using CyAn ADP™ (Beckman Coulter) as previously described (25). Antibodies with the following specificity of CD19-Alexa647 and B220-Alexa647 (BioLegend) were used.

Intravital and *In Vitro* Microscope

Intestinal epithelial cells from anesthetized mice were imaged. Small intestinal tracts were surgically opened lengthwise, placed on a cover glass, and immobilized on a microscope stage. For image acquisition, a Nikon A1 laser-scanning confocal microscope with a 20× objective and NIS-Elements AR software was used as previously described (25). We used a dichronic mirrors (DM457/514) and two bandpass emission filters (482/35 for CFP, 540/30 for YFP). YFP/CFP ratio was obtained by excitation at 458 nm. Images of purified spleen cells in PBS were also obtained as above. Acquired images were analyzed with NIS-Elements software (Nikon).

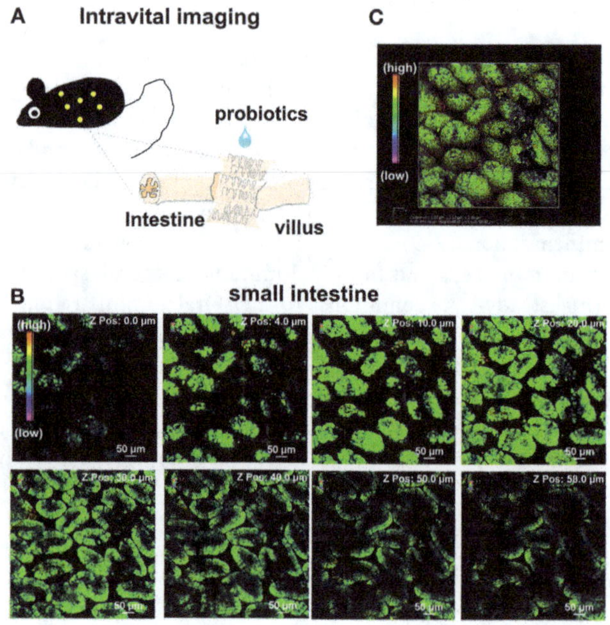

FIGURE 1 | Structure of intestinal villi in a mouse under ubiquitous YC3.60 expression. (A) Schematic method of intravital imaging of intestinal epithelial cells (IECs). **(B)** *Z*-stack analysis of epithelial cells in the intestinal tract. Intravital imaging of small intestinal villi in the jejunum was performed using confocal lazar microscopy. Ratiometric images (yellow fluorescent protein/cyan fluorescent protein at excitation of 458 nm) are shown. *Z*-stack images of 2-µm intervals up to a depth of 58 µm were obtained. Only representative images are shown. A rainbow parameter indicates relative Ca^{2+} concentration; scale bar, 50 µm. **(C)** 3D structures of small IECs with intracellular Ca^{2+} concentrations. 3D images based on *Z*-stack images **(B)** were obtained using NIS-Elements software. Shown are representative results from three mice.

RESULTS

Establishment of *In Vivo* Ca^{2+} Signaling Detection System in Intestinal Gut Epithelial Cells

We previously established an intravital imaging system of Ca^{2+} signaling in lymphoid tissues, such as in Peyer's patches, spleen, and bone marrow (25). To visualize Ca^{2+} signaling in IECs, we surgically opened the small intestinal tract of the mice with ubiquitous YC3.60 expression, fixed a cover glass on it, and placed it on the stage of the confocal microscope (**Figure 1A**). Images of the villi in the middle of the small intestine of the mice with ubiquitous YC3.60 expression are shown in **Figure 1B**. Images of over 50 µm from top of the villi to the basal were obtained. Reconstructed 3D structures showed that almost the entire length of the small intestinal villi could be visualized (**Figure 1C**). There were no salient differences in intracellular Ca^{2+} concentration among the total epithelial cells, and they included heterogeneous minor subpopulations, such as goblet cells, enteroendocrine cells, and tuft cells (30, 31).

Intravital imaging of the IECs showed sporadic but relatively minute Ca^{2+} signaling in some regions under steady-state conditions (**Figure 2A**). Less than 1% IECs exhibited spontaneous Ca^{2+} signaling (**Figure 2B**). To determine if the perceptive Ca^{2+} signaling response is observed in this system, we first tested ionomycin, as a positive control, on the stimuli. Upon the addition of ionomycin, transient Ca^{2+} elevation was observed in many IECs (**Figures 2C,D**). Thus, a system was established to detect *in vivo* real-time Ca^{2+} signaling of IECs.

Effect of Probiotics on Ca^{2+} Signaling in the IECs of the Mice with Ubiquitous YC3.60 Expression *In Vivo*

Lactococcus lactis (18, 29) regulate immune responses by inducing cytokines in dendritic cells and *B. subtilis natto* regulate gut flora and immunity (32–34). We tested whether these probiotics induce Ca^{2+} signaling in IECs. Intravital imaging of IECs exhibited Ca^{2+} signaling upon *B. subtilis natto* treatment (**Figure 3A**; Video S1 in Supplementary Material). *Bacillus subtilis natto* induced gradual and sustained elevation of intracellular Ca^{2+} concentration in most cells (**Figures 3A,B**). **Figure 3C** shows that intracellular Ca^{2+} concentration in IECs was strikingly increased after adding *B. subtilis natto*. Thus, the kinetics of *B. subtilis natto*-mediated Ca^{2+} signaling in IECs is clearly distinct from that

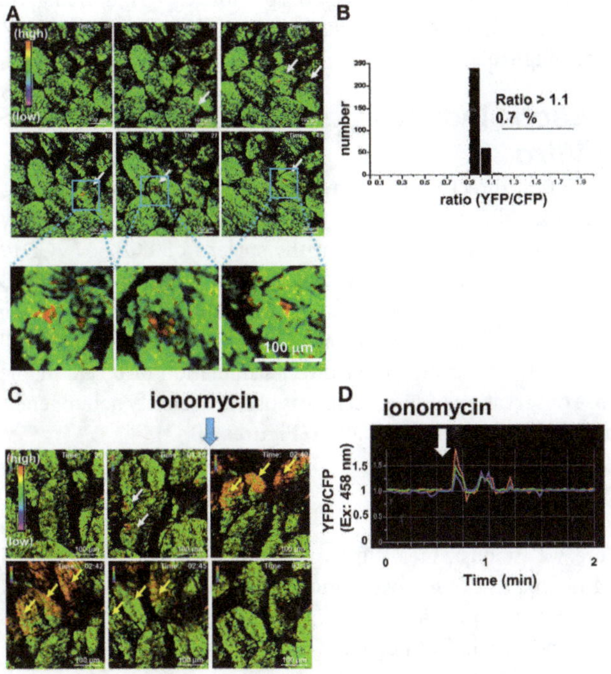

FIGURE 2 | Intravital Ca^{2+} signaling images mediated by ionomycin in the intestinal tract of a mouse under ubiquitous YC3.60 expression. **(A)** Representative Ca^{2+} signaling images in the intestinal tract of a mouse under ubiquitous YC3.60 expression without any stimulation. Ratiometric images [yellow fluorescent protein (YFP)/cyan fluorescent protein (CFP) at excitation of 458 nm] are shown. The rainbow parameter indicates relative Ca^{2+} concentration. **(B)** Distribution of time-integrated intracellular Ca^{2+} concentrations of randomly selected regions. $N = 10$; frame = 30. **(C)** Representative Ca^{2+} signaling images in the intestinal tract of a mouse under ubiquitous YC3.60 expression with ionomycin. Ratiometric images (YFP/CFP at excitation of 458 nm) are shown. Five micromolars of ionomycin in PBS were added at the indicated time point. A rainbow parameter indicates relative Ca^{2+} concentration; scale bar, 100 µm; frame = 85. **(D)** Ratiometric intensities (YFP/CFP at excitation of 458 nm) of indicated regions, represented by yellow arrows in **(C)** ($n = 3$), were measured for 2 min at 2-s intervals. Spontaneous Ca^{2+} signals are indicated by white arrows. Shown are representative results from two mice.

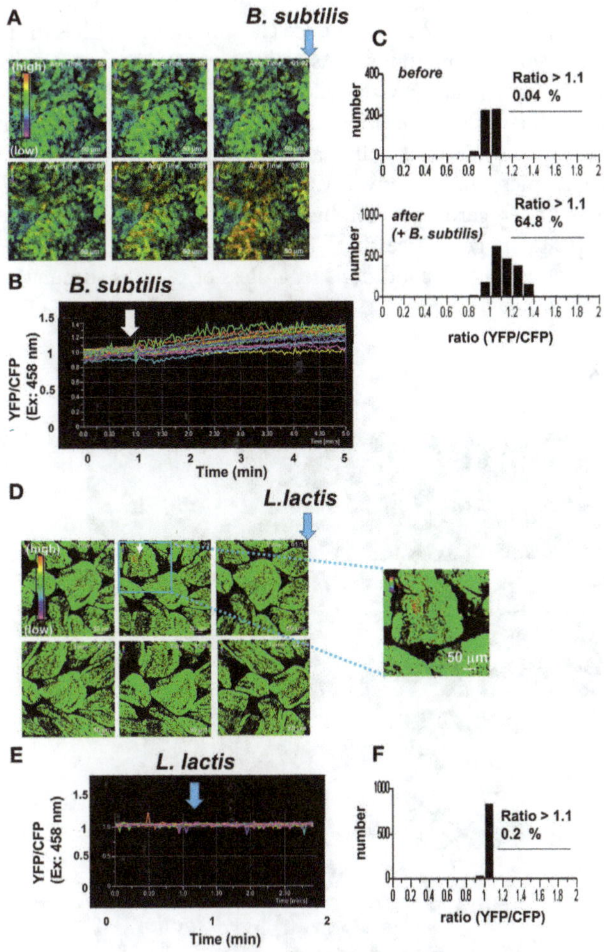

FIGURE 3 | Intravital Ca^{2+} signaling images mediated by probiotics in the intestinal tract of a mouse under ubiquitous YC3.60 expression. **(A)** Representative Ca^{2+} signaling images in the intestinal tract of a mouse under ubiquitous YC3.60 expression and specific pathogen-free (SPF) conditions. Ratiometric images [yellow fluorescent protein (YFP)/cyan fluorescent protein (CFP) at excitation of 458 nm] are shown. The 0.1 ml of *Bacillus subtilis natto* in PBS (10^9 cells/ml) was added at the indicated time point. A rainbow parameter indicates relative Ca^{2+} concentration. **(B)** Time course for fluorescence intensities of YFP/CFP on excitation at 458 nm. Randomly selected regions ($n = 10$) were measured. Scale bar, 50 µm; frame = 151. Spontaneous Ca^{2+} signals are indicated by arrows. **(C)** Distribution of time-integrated intracellular Ca^{2+} concentrations of randomly selected regions before (upper panel) and after (lower panel) stimulation; $n = 10$. **(D)** Representative Ca^{2+} signaling images in the intestinal tract of a mouse under ubiquitous YC3.60 expression and SPF conditions. Ratiometric images (YFP/CFP at excitation of 458 nm) are shown. The 0.1 ml of *Lactococcus lactis* in PBS (10^9 cells/ml) was added at the indicated time point. **(E)** Time course for fluorescence intensities of YFP/CFP on excitation at 458 nm; frame = 85. **(F)** Distribution of time-integrated intracellular Ca^{2+} concentrations of randomly selected regions; $n = 10$. Shown are representative results from three mice.

observed under steady-state conditions (**Figure 2A**). One LAB strain, *L. lactis* C60, did not induce Ca^{2+} signaling in IECs except for spontaneous signals (**Figures 3D–F**). This result is surprising as both *B. subtilis* and LAB are Gram-positive bacteria and well-known probiotics; yet the responses of IECs in SPF mice were distinct in inducing Ca^{2+} signaling. LAB compose a major part of small intestinal commensal flora, and therefore, chronic exposure to the bacteria species may have induced hyporesponsiveness of IECs against LAB.

LAB Induces Ca^{2+} Signaling in IECs under Germ-Free Conditions

As *Lactococcus* is a related genus of *Enterococcus*, a constituent of gut-resident LAB in the small intestine (7), it may constantly stimulate IECs under steady-state conditions. IECs may refrain from responding to heat-killed *L. lactis* C60 and induce Ca^{2+} signaling due to chronic microbial stimuli by *Enterococci*. We attempted to clarify whether small intestinal microenvironments, especially gut commensal flora, modulate the responsiveness of IECs against LAB.

To this end, we generated germ-free YC3.60 mice to determine whether *L. lactis* can induce Ca^{2+} signaling in IECs in the absence of gut microbiota. As shown in **Figure 4** and Video S2 in Supplementary Material, *L. lactis* C60 induced sustained intracellular Ca^{2+} elevation as *B. subtilis natto*, indicating that *L. lactis* C60 can stimulate IECs directly in the absence of gut microbiota. Many IECs were stimulated by adding *L. lactis* under germ-free conditions (**Figure 4B**). Furthermore, the IECs in germ-free mice exhibited sporadic Ca^{2+} signals under steady-state conditions regardless of *L. lactis* stimulation (**Figures 4A,C**). The frequency of sporadic Ca^{2+} signals in germ-free mice (**Figure 4B**, left panel) is higher than that in the SPF mice (**Figure 2A**).

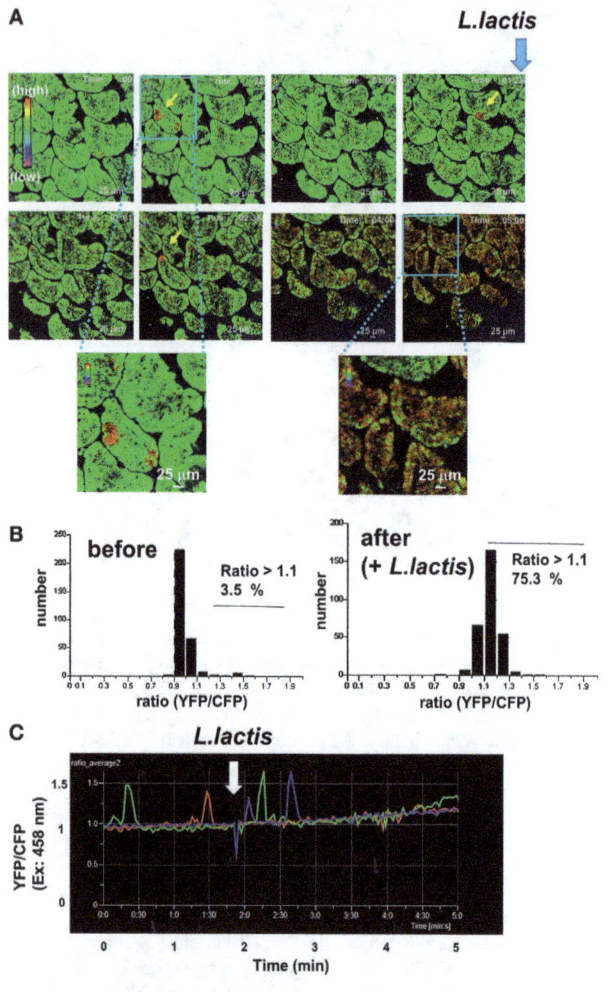

FIGURE 4 | Intravital Ca^{2+} signaling images mediated by *Lactococcus lactis* in the intestinal tract of a mouse under ubiquitous YC3.60 expression. **(A)** Representative Ca^{2+} signaling images in the intestinal tract of a mouse under ubiquitous YC3.60 expression and germ-free conditions. Ratiometric images [yellow fluorescent protein (YFP)/cyan fluorescent protein (CFP) at excitation of 458 nm] are shown. The 0.1 ml of *L. lactis* in PBS (10^9 cells/ml) was added at the indicated time point. A rainbow parameter indicates relative Ca^{2+} concentration. Scale bar, 25 μm; frame = 145. Spontaneous Ca^{2+} signals are indicated by arrows. **(B)** Distribution of time-integrated intracellular Ca^{2+} concentrations of randomly selected regions before (left) and after (right) stimulation. **(C)** Time course for fluorescence intensities of YFP/CFP on excitation at 458 nm in the indicated region is represented by the yellow arrow in **(A)**; $n = 3$. Shown are representative results from three mice.

L. Lactis Induces Ca^{2+} Signaling in B Cells *In Vitro*

Probiotics directly stimulate various immune cells such as dendritic cells, macrophages, NK cells, and T cells (11, 35). We prepared primary B cells from the spleens of YC3.60^{flox}/CD19-Cre mice and stimulated with *B. subtilis natto* (**Figures 5A,B**) or *L. lactis* (**Figures 5C,D**). Upon stimulation, both *B. subtilis natto* and *L. lactis* induced Ca^{2+} mobilization in primary B cells (**Figure 5**), confirming their direct stimulation of B cells. Time-lapse observation of single cells was useful to clarify heterogeneity in the kinetics of Ca^{2+} signaling (**Figures 5B,D**).

DISCUSSION

Here, we establish a real-time visualization system of Ca^{2+} signaling in small IECs *in vivo* to monitor food signals. By using this system, we show that *B. subtilis natto* triggers Ca^{2+} signaling in IECs and that *L. lactis* evokes Ca^{2+} signaling in gut tissue under germ-free conditions but not under SPF conditions. These results suggest that gut microbiota regulate their responses against orally administered probiotics.

In this study, we successfully visualize probiotic-mediated Ca^{2+} signaling in IECs based on the 5D (*x*, *y*, *z*, time, and Ca^{2+}) live imaging system in YC3.60 mice (25). A calcium biosensor YC3.60 is a double-chromophore indicator that employs FRET between CFP and YFP mutants (Venus) (26). Ca^{2+} signaling can be monitored by measuring YFP/CFP when CFP is excited. Motion-induced artifacts or unequal biosensor expression are corrected by an internal control in the denominator of the ratio. Thus, the ratiometric sensor YC3.60 is suitable for *in vivo* imaging of the gut, which exhibits vigorous motion with peristalsis in addition to beating and breathing. Moreover, 5D live imaging of tissues enables time-lapse monitoring of dynamic Ca^{2+} signaling in single cells, cell–cell interactions, and other segments of interests. Response of these tissues is quantified and integrated over the desired time span as shown in **Figures 2B, 3C,F** and **4B**.

Probiotic *B. subtilis natto*, but not *L. lactis*, triggers Ca^{2+} signaling in the gut epithelium in SPF mice, although both of them are capable of stimulating spleen B cells from mice with the same microbial conditions. Since *L. lactis* C60 stimulates IECs in the absence of gut microbiota in germ-free mice, the gut microbiota may shape the responsiveness of IECs against LAB.

Intestinal epithelial cells express a series of pattern recognition receptors (PRRs) including TLRs, nucleotide-binding sites, leucine-rich repeat-containing receptors, and retinoic acid-inducible gene-I-like receptors (36). Bacterial components stimulate these PRRs and regulate IRFs, NF-κB, and/or the MAP kinase signaling pathway. One study showed that IECs from germ-free mice show a reduction in TLR expression (37). Another study reported that immunobiotic strains regulate the expression and activity of TLRs in IECs (38). These findings suggest that microbial conditions shape the homeostatic regulation of functional PRRs. Since

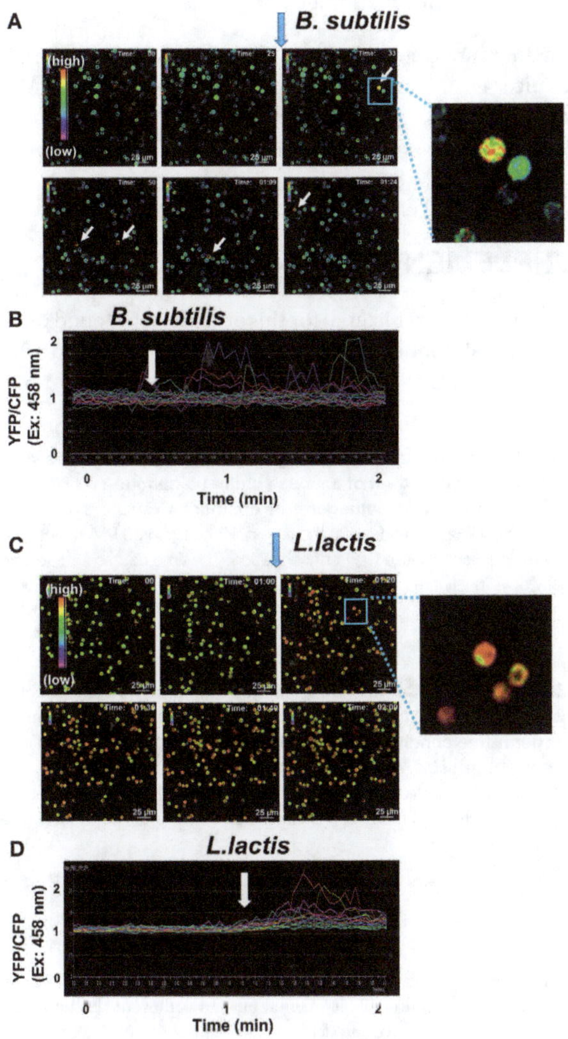

FIGURE 5 | Ca^{2+} signaling images mediated by *probiotics* in B cells *in vitro*. **(A)** Representative Ca^{2+} signaling images in spleen B cells form CD19-Cre/YC3.60 mice. Ratiometric images [YFP/cyan fluorescent protein (CFP) at excitation of 458 nm] are shown. Ten microliters of *Bacillus subtilis natto* in PBS (10^9 cells/ml) were added to the cell culture (0.2 ml) at the indicated time point. A rainbow parameter indicates relative Ca^{2+} concentration. **(B)** The time course for fluorescence intensities of YFP/CFP on excitation at 458 nm in the cells ($n = 15$). Scale bar, 25 µm; frame = 56. **(C)** Representative Ca^{2+} signaling images in spleen B cells of CD19-Cre/YC3.60 expression in mice. Ratiometric images (YFP/CFP at excitation of 458 nm) are shown. Ten microliters of *Lactococcus lactis* in PBS (10^9 cells/ml) were added to the cell culture at the indicated time point. A rainbow parameter indicates relative Ca^{2+} concentration. **(D)** The time course for fluorescence intensities of YFP/CFP on excitation at 458 nm in the cells ($n = 15$). Scale bar, 25 µm; frame = 61. Shown are representative results of three experiments.

Lactococcus is similar to *Enterococcus*, a major member of small intestinal commensal LAB, probably IECs, at least in part, is hyporesponsive to this symbiotic genus of bacteria. We hypothesize that due to this hyporesponsiveness, further stimulation with *L. lactis* does not induce visible Ca^{2+} signaling despite the expression of PRRs on the IECs. As reported, probiotic strains tolerate IECs (38, 39); such causal relationships may also explain the frequent and sporadic Ca^{2+} signaling observed in IECs of germ-free mice under steady-state conditions (**Figure 4**). The molecular mechanisms underlying these observations, however, remain unclear.

We find that IECs exhibit sporadic transient Ca^{2+} signaling, although we do not know the precise mechanism of this action. The signals appear to be more striking in the germ-free mice than in the SPF mice, suggesting that these signals are mediated by the gut microbiota or endocrine systems (40).

B cells also express PRRs and are directly stimulated by microbial components (41). Although *L. lactis* C60 fails to induce Ca^{2+} signaling in IECs under SPF conditions, it strongly induces Ca^{2+} signaling in spleen B cells from SPF mice. In contrast, *B. subtilis natto* induces Ca^{2+} signaling in both IECs *in vivo* and B cells *in vitro*. It is not known whether the different reactivity against two types of probiotics can be attributed to the difference in the methods between the intravital and *in vitro* assay, to the skewed influence of stimuli including commensal flora and diet on local and systemic immune cells, or to the outcome of strain difference of probiotics. Additional studies are required to evaluate these results further.

Understanding the function of IECs is important to evaluate immune responses, since stimulated IECs produce cytokines and/or chemokines (11, 23). Goblet cells and M cells deliver antigens to dendritic cells (42, 43). Beneficial probiotic signaling may be transferred to immune cells through these mechanisms, resulting in the regulation of immune tolerance or response. In this study, we show that an intravital imaging system using YC3.60 mice allows for the detection of real-time activation of IECs by probiotics. This system is proven here to be a powerful method for not only clarifying the effects of probiotics on epithelial cell–immune cell communication with stoichiometries but also detecting a subtle disorder before pathological onset (25) and developing preventive and therapeutic strategies with probiotics.

ETHICS STATEMENT

YC3.60 mice were maintained in our animal facility under SPF conditions in accordance with the guidelines of the Tokyo Medical and Dental University for animal care. IECs of anesthetized mice were imaged. Small intestinal tracts were surgically opened, immobilized on a microscope stage, and maintained. Then, images were obtained by a confocal laser microscopy. These procedures have been approved by the Committee of the Tokyo Medical and Dental University for animal care. Germ-free BALB/cA mice used as foster mothers were bred at the Laboratory of Veterinary Public Health, the University of Tokyo. All the germ-free animals were kept in flexible vinyl isolators in a room with 24°C, relative humidity of 60% and 12-h periods of light and dark and fed CMF-pelleted diet (Oriental Yeast Co., Tokyo, Japan) sterilized by γ-irradiation at dose of 50 kGy. For the generation of germ-free ubiquitous YC3.60 expression mice, *in vitro* fertilization and caesarean operation were performed as described below. Female ubiquitous YC3.60 expression mice were superovulated by intraperitoneal injection of 7.5 IU eCG followed by 7.5 IU hCG at an interval of 48 h. Eggs were collected from sacrificed female mice and fertilized with sperm of male ubiquitous YC3.60 expression mice in HTF medium (ARK Resource, Kumamoto, Japan). After over night culture in KSOM medium (ARK Resource), two-cell embryos were transferred into oviduct of pseudopregnant female ICR mice. Estimated delivery date was controlled by subcutaneous injection of Progehorrmon (Mochida Pharmaceutical Co., Ltd., Tokyo, Japan). The surrogate mothers were sacrificed at the fetal age of 21st day by cervical dislocation and "uterine package" was aseptically removed with clamps at the top of each uterine horn and the base of the uterus close to the cervix. The "uterine package" was introduced into isolator for operation through germicidal trap with 2% peracetic acid solution kept at 37°C. Then, "uterine package" was cut open with scissors and pups were taken out. The pups were stimulated breathing while cleaning them with dry gauze. After the pups started breathing normally, pups were transferred to the isolator with foster mothers. The germ-free status was check once a month. These procedures have been approved by the Committee for Care of Laboratory Animals in the Graduate School of Agricultural and Life Sciences at the University of Tokyo. There is no additional consideration.

AUTHOR CONTRIBUTIONS

KH, NT, YA, NO, AM, SY, HK, and TA designed the research; TA and NT wrote the manuscript; KH, SK, YA, TU, NH, TK, YW, HK-N, SY, and TA performed the experiments, analyzed the data, and prepared the figures.

ACKNOWLEDGMENTS

The authors are grateful to Dr. K. Rajewsky (MDC) for the CD19-Cre mice, Dr. M. Okabe (Osaka University) for the CAG-Cre mice, and Drs. K. Nishitani and M. Nishikawa (Takano Foods Co., Ltd.) for a *B. subtilis* strain TTCC12.

SUPPLEMENTARY MATERIAL

The Supplementary Material for this article can be found online at http://journal.frontiersin.org/article/10.3389/fimmu.2016.00601/full#supplementary-material.

VIDEO S1 | Intravital Ca^{2+} signaling images mediated by *Bacillus subtilis natto* in the intestinal tract of a mouse under ubiquitous YC3.60 expression and specific pathogen-free conditions. *B. subtilis natto* in PBS (10^9 cells/ml) in PBS was added at the time point of 1 min 30 s. A rainbow parameter indicates relative Ca^{2+} concentration. The time course for fluorescence intensity of yellow fluorescent protein/cyan fluorescent protein on excitation at 458 nm was performed. Scale bar, 50 μm; frame = 151.

VIDEO S2 | Intravital Ca^{2+} signaling images mediated by *Lactococcus lactis* in the intestinal tract of a ubiquitous YC3.60 expression mouse under germ-free conditions. *L. lactis* in PBS (10^9 cells/ml) was added at the time point of 1 min 50 s. A rainbow parameter indicates relative Ca^{2+} concentration. The time course for fluorescence intensity of yellow fluorescent protein/cyan fluorescent protein on excitation at 458 nm was performed. Scale bar, 25 μm; frame = 145.

REFERENCES

1. Mitsuoka T. Development of functional foods. *Biosci Microbiota Food Health* (2014) 33(3):117–28. doi:10.12938/bmfh.33.117
2. van Baarlen P, Wells JM, Kleerebezem M. Regulation of intestinal homeostasis and immunity with probiotic lactobacilli. *Trends Immunol* (2013) 34(5):208–15. doi:10.1016/j.it.2013.01.005
3. Tsuji NM, Kosaka A. Oral tolerance: intestinal homeostasis and antigen-specific regulatory T cells. *Trends Immunol* (2008) 29(11):532–40. doi:10.1016/j.it.2008.09.002
4. Tsuji NM, Yan H, Watanabe Y. Gut to systemic immune-homeostasis mediated by innate signals. *Nihon Rinsho Meneki Gakkai Kaishi* (2015) 38(6):448–56. doi:10.2177/jsci.38.448
5. Yan H, Kakuta S, Nishihara M, Sugi M, Adachi Y, Ohno N, et al. *Kjellmaniella crassifolia* Miyabe (Gagome) extract modulates intestinal and systemic immune responses. *Biosci Biotechnol Biochem* (2011) 75(11):2178–83. doi:10.1271/bbb.110473
6. Yan H, Ohno N, Tsuji NM. The role of C-type lectin receptors in immune homeostasis. *Int Immunopharmacol* (2013) 16(3):353–7. doi:10.1016/j.intimp.2013.04.013
7. Hao WL, Lee YK. Microflora of the gastrointestinal tract: a review. *Methods Mol Biol* (2004) 268:491–502. doi:10.1385/1-59259-766-1:491
8. Suzuki K, Meek B, Doi Y, Muramatsu M, Chiba T, Honjo T, et al. Aberrant expansion of segmented filamentous bacteria in IgA-deficient gut. *Proc Natl Acad Sci U S A* (2004) 101(7):1981–6. doi:10.1073/pnas.0307317101
9. Mitsuoka T. Establishment of intestinal bacteriology. *Biosci Microbiota Food Health* (2014) 33(3):99–116. doi:10.12938/bmfh.33.99
10. Shida K, Nanno M. Probiotics and immunology: separating the wheat from the chaff. *Trends Immunol* (2008) 29(11):565–73. doi:10.1016/j.it.2008.07.011
11. Cerf-Bensussan N, Gaboriau-Routhiau V. The immune system and the gut microbiota: friends or foes? *Nat Rev Immunol* (2010) 10(10):735–44. doi:10.1038/nri2850
12. Kawashima T, Kosaka A, Yan H, Guo Z, Uchiyama R, Fukui R, et al. Double-stranded RNA of intestinal commensal but not pathogenic bacteria triggers production of protective interferon-beta. *Immunity* (2013) 38(6):1187–97. doi:10.1016/j.immuni.2013.02.024
13. Corr SC, Gahan CG, Hill C. Impact of selected *Lactobacillus* and *Bifidobacterium* species on *Listeria monocytogenes* infection and the mucosal immune response. *FEMS Immunol Med Microbiol* (2007) 50(3):380–8. doi:10.1111/j.1574-695X.2007.00264.x
14. Kawashima T, Hayashi K, Kosaka A, Kawashima M, Igarashi T, Tsutsui H, et al. *Lactobacillus plantarum* strain YU from fermented foods activates Th1 and protective immune responses. *Int Immunopharmacol* (2011) 11(12):2017–24. doi:10.1016/j.intimp.2011.08.013
15. Chiba E, Tomosada Y, Vizoso-Pinto MG, Salva S, Takahashi T, Tsukida K, et al. Immunobiotic *Lactobacillus rhamnosus* improves resistance of infant mice against respiratory syncytial virus infection. *Int Immunopharmacol* (2013) 17(2):373–82. doi:10.1016/j.intimp.2013.06.024
16. Kosaka A, Yan H, Ohashi S, Gotoh Y, Sato A, Tsutsui H, et al. *Lactococcus lactis* subsp. cremoris FC triggers IFN-gamma production from NK and T cells via IL-12 and IL-18. *Int Immunopharmacol* (2012) 14(4):729–33. doi:10.1016/j.intimp.2012.10.007
17. Tohno M, Shimosato T, Moue M, Aso H, Watanabe K, Kawai Y, et al. Toll-like receptor 2 and 9 are expressed and functional in gut-associated lymphoid tissues of presuckling newborn swine. *Vet Res* (2006) 37(6):791–812. doi:10.1051/vetres:2006036
18. Kimoto H, Kurisaki J, Tsuji NM, Ohmomo S, Okamoto T. Lactococci as probiotic strains: adhesion to human enterocyte-like Caco-2 cells and tolerance to low pH and bile. *Lett Appl Microbiol* (1999) 29(5):313–6. doi:10.1046/j.1365-2672.1999.00627.x

19. Thomas CM, Versalovic J. Probiotics-host communication: modulation of signaling pathways in the intestine. *Gut Microbes* (2010) 1(3):148–63. doi:10.4161/gmic.1.3.11712
20. Scharenberg AM, Humphries LA, Rawlings DJ. Calcium signalling and cell-fate choice in B cells. *Nat Rev Immunol* (2007) 7(10):778–89. doi:10.1038/nri2172
21. Oh-hora M, Rao A. Calcium signaling in lymphocytes. *Curr Opin Immunol* (2008) 20(3):250–8. doi:10.1016/j.coi.2008.04.004
22. Kurosaki T, Shinohara H, Baba Y. B cell signaling and fate decision. *Annu Rev Immunol* (2010) 28:21–55. doi:10.1146/annurev.immunol.021908.132541
23. Feske S. Calcium signalling in lymphocyte activation and disease. *Nat Rev Immunol* (2007) 7(9):690–702. doi:10.1038/nri2152
24. Engelke M, Engels N, Dittmann K, Stork B, Wienands J. Ca(2+) signaling in antigen receptor-activated B lymphocytes. *Immunol Rev* (2007) 218:235–46. doi:10.1111/j.1600-065X.2007.00539.x
25. Yoshikawa S, Usami T, Kikuta J, Ishii M, Sasano T, Sugiyama K, et al. Intravital imaging of Ca(2+) signals in lymphocytes of Ca(2+) biosensor transgenic mice: indication of autoimmune diseases before the pathological onset. *Sci Rep* (2016) 6:18738. doi:10.1038/srep18738
26. Nagai T, Yamada S, Tominaga T, Ichikawa M, Miyawaki A. Expanded dynamic range of fluorescent indicators for Ca(2+) by circularly permuted yellow fluorescent proteins. *Proc Natl Acad Sci U S A* (2004) 101(29):10554–9. doi:10.1073/pnas.0400417101
27. Rickert RC, Roes J, Rajewsky K. B lymphocyte-specific, Cre-mediated mutagenesis in mice. *Nucleic Acids Res* (1997) 25(6):1317–8. doi:10.1093/nar/25.6.1317
28. Matsumura H, Hasuwa H, Inoue N, Ikawa M, Okabe M. Lineage-specific cell disruption in living mice by Cre-mediated expression of diphtheria toxin A chain. *Biochem Biophys Res Commun* (2004) 321(2):275–9. doi:10.1016/j.bbrc.2004.06.139
29. Tsuji MN, Kimoto H. Lactic acid bacteria and their cellular components inducing immunoregulatory function, and method of obtaining the same. EP 1538198 A2 (2005).
30. Gerbe F, Legraverend C, Jay P. The intestinal epithelium tuft cells: specification and function. *Cell Mol Life Sci* (2012) 69(17):2907–17. doi:10.1007/s00018-012-0984-7
31. Howitt MR, Lavoie S, Michaud M, Blum AM, Tran SV, Weinstock JV, et al. Tuft cells, taste-chemosensory cells, orchestrate parasite type 2 immunity in the gut. *Science* (2016) 351(6279):1329–33. doi:10.1126/science.aaf1648
32. Hosoi T, Ametani A, Kiuchi K, Kaminogawa S. Improved growth and viability of lactobacilli in the presence of *Bacillus subtilis* (*natto*), catalase, or subtilisin. *Can J Microbiol* (2000) 46(10):892–7. doi:10.1139/cjm-46-10-892
33. Kim S, Yang JY, Lee K, Oh KH, Gi M, Kim JM, et al. *Bacillus subtilis*-specific poly-gamma-glutamic acid regulates development pathways of naive CD4(+) T cells through antigen-presenting cell-dependent and -independent mechanisms. *Int Immunol* (2009) 21(8):977–90. doi:10.1093/intimm/dxp065
34. Ozawa N, Shimojo N, Suzuki Y, Ochiai S, Nakano T, Morita Y, et al. Maternal intake of natto, a Japan's traditional fermented soybean food, during pregnancy and the risk of eczema in Japanese babies. *Allergol Int* (2014) 63(2):261–6. doi:10.2332/allergolint.13-OA-0613
35. Rescigno M. Dendritic cell-epithelial cell crosstalk in the gut. *Immunol Rev* (2014) 260(1):118–28. doi:10.1111/imr.12181
36. Lavelle EC, Murphy C, O'Neill LA, Creagh EM. The role of TLRs, NLRs, and RLRs in mucosal innate immunity and homeostasis. *Mucosal Immunol* (2010) 3(1):17–28. doi:10.1038/mi.2009.124
37. Lundin A, Bok CM, Aronsson L, Bjorkholm B, Gustafsson JA, Pott S, et al. *Gut flora*, toll-like receptors and nuclear receptors: a tripartite communication that tunes innate immunity in large intestine. *Cell Microbiol* (2008) 10(5):1093–103. doi:10.1111/j.1462-5822.2007.01108.x
38. Hosoya S, Villena J, Chiba E, Shimazu T, Suda Y, Aso H, et al. Advanced application of porcine intestinal epithelial cells for the selection of immunobiotics modulating toll-like receptor 3-mediated inflammation. *J Microbiol Immunol Infect* (2013) 46(6):474–81. doi:10.1016/j.jmii.2012.04.005
39. Shimazu T, Villena J, Tohno M, Fujie H, Hosoya S, Shimosato T, et al. Immunobiotic *Lactobacillus jensenii* elicits anti-inflammatory activity in porcine intestinal epithelial cells by modulating negative regulators of the Toll-like receptor signaling pathway. *Infect Immun* (2012) 80(1):276–88. doi:10.1128/IAI.05729-11
40. El Aidy S, van den Bogert B, Kleerebezem M. The small intestine microbiota, nutritional modulation and relevance for health. *Curr Opin Biotechnol* (2015) 32:14–20. doi:10.1016/j.copbio.2014.09.005
41. Michallet MC, Rota G, Maslowski K, Guarda G. Innate receptors for adaptive immunity. *Curr Opin Microbiol* (2013) 16(3):296–302. doi:10.1016/j.mib.2013.04.003
42. Honda K, Littman DR. The microbiome in infectious disease and inflammation. *Annu Rev Immunol* (2012) 30:759–95. doi:10.1146/annurev-immunol-020711-074937
43. McDole JR, Wheeler LW, McDonald KG, Wang B, Konjufca V, Knoop KA, et al. Goblet cells deliver luminal antigen to CD103+ dendritic cells in the small intestine. *Nature* (2012) 483(7389):345–9. doi:10.1038/nature10863

4

Effects of Microbial Aerosol in Poultry House on Meat Ducks' Immune Function

Guanliu Yu [1], Yao Wang [1], Shouguo Wang [2], Changmin Duan [2], Liangmeng Wei [1], Jing Gao [3], Tongjie Chai [1] and Yumei Cai [1*]*

[1] College of Animal Science and Veterinary Medicine, Shandong Agricultural University, Sino-German Cooperative Research Centre for Zoonosis of Animal Origin Shandong Province, Tai'an, China, [2] Deizhou People's Hospital, Deizhou, China, [3] The Central Hospital of Tai'an, Tai'an, China

Edited by:
Haruki Kitazawa,
Tohoku University, Japan

Reviewed by:
Graciela Alicia Cremaschi,
Institute of Biomedical Research, National Research Council of Argentina, Argentina
Jessica Lynn Humann,
Florida A&M University, USA

***Correspondence:**
Tongjie Chai
chaitj117@163.com
Yumei Cai
caiyum@163.com

The aim of this study was to evaluate effects of microbial aerosols on immune function of ducks and shed light on the establishment of microbial aerosol concentration standards for poultry. A total of 1800 1-d-old cherry valley ducks were randomly divided into five groups (A, B, C, D, and E) with 360 ducks in each. To obtain objective data, each group had three replications. Concentrations of airborne bacteria, fungi, endotoxin in different groups were created by controlling ventilation and bedding cleaning frequency. Group A was the control group and hygienic conditions deteriorated progressively from group B to E. A 6-stage Andersen impactor was used to detect the aerosol concentration of aerobes, gram-negative bacteria, fungi, and AGI-30 microbial air sampler detect the endotoxin, and Composite Gas Detector detect the noxious gas. In order to assess the immune function of meat ducks, immune indicators including H5 AIV antibody titer, IgG, IL-2, T-lymphocyte transformation rate, lysozyme and immune organ indexes were evaluated. Correlation coefficients were also calculated to evaluate the relationships among airborne bacteria, fungi, endotoxin, and immune indicators. The results showed that the concentration of airborne aerobe, gram-negative bacteria, fungi, endotoxin have a strong correlation to H5 AIV antibody titer, IgG, IL-2, T-lymphocyte transformation rate, lysozyme, and immune organ indexes, respectively. In addition, when the concentration of microbial aerosol reach the level of group D, serum IgG (6–8 weeks), lysozyme (4 week) were significantly higher than in group A ($P < 0.05$); serum IL-2 (7 and 8 weeks), T-lymphocyte transformation rate, lysozyme (7 and 8 weeks), spleen index (6 and 8 weeks), and bursa index (8 week) were significantly lower than in group A ($P < 0.05$ or $P < 0.01$). The results indicated that a high level of microbial aerosol adversely affected the immune level of meat ducks. The microbial aerosol values in group D provide a basis for recommending upper limit concentrations of microbial aerosols for healthy meat ducks.

Keywords: microbial aerosol, immune indicators, stress, cherry valley ducks, poultry houses

INTRODUCTION

The air in poultry houses is usually heavily contaminated by large quantities of airborne microorganisms, endotoxins and toxic gases (NH_3, H_2S), etc. (Nimmermark et al., 2009; Cambra-López et al., 2010; Lawniczek-Walczyk et al., 2013). In airborne microorganisms, there is a high concentration of non-pathogenic microorganisms leading to animal immunosuppression (Douwes et al., 2003; Fiegel et al., 2006). The high level of airborne aerobe could reduce animal immunity and growth rate (Wolinsky, 2006). Many studies have documented that exposure to fungal aerosol may be associated with asthma, acute toxic and allergic, and it may threaten caretakers and external ambient in animal houses as well (Bush and Portnoy, 2001; Pavan and Manjunath, 2014). The percentage of airborne gram-negative bacteria in the bacterial aerosol is small, but it contains a lot of pathogenic bacteria (Zucker et al., 2000). Endotoxins are ubiquitous in the environment. They are a biologically active lipopolysaccharide that is a component of the outer membrane of gram-negative bacteria (Balasubramanian et al., 2012). According to Pirie, inhaled endotoxin contributes significantly to the induction of airway inflammation and dysfunction (Pirie et al., 2003). Many occupational studies have shown positive associations between endotoxin exposure and respiratory disorders including asthma-like syndrome, chronic airway obstruction, organic duct toxic syndrome, byssinosis, bronchitis, etc. (Madsen, 2006). Zucker et al. have used it as an important symbol of organic dust in the air of poultry house (Zucker et al., 2000). Endotoxin also affects human humoral and cellular immunity (Burrell, 1990). Furthermore, in terms of toxic gases in animal house, ammonia and hydrogen sulfide are two well-known toxic components (Yao and Li, 2010). They can cause respiratory, eye diseases and even poisoning death (Teye et al., 2008; Yao and Li, 2010; Barrasa et al., 2012).

To date, numerous correlation studies have focused on microbial aerosol composition, concentration and mechanisms of spread to the surrounding ambient (Zucker et al., 2000; Madsen, 2006; Duan et al., 2007; Masclaux et al., 2013; Matković et al., 2013). However, studies of microbial aerosol on immune function have not been found. Therefore, the aim of this study was to clarity the effect of microbial aerosol on the immune function of ducks, which was based on comparing the significance between control group and the treatment groups of ducks' specific immune indexes (e.g., IgG, H5 AIV antibody titer, IL-2, etc.) and the non-specific immune factors (e.g., lysozyme), as well as the relationship between major microbial aerosol concentration and immune indicators. Moreover, this study also could enlighten future studies on the establishment of microbial aerosol concentration standards for poultry breeding.

MATERIALS AND METHODS

Experimental Design

This study was conducted at the Animal Husbandry & Veterinary Station of Shandong Agricultural University, China during January–March, 2014. Five groups were set up, with a control group A and 4 treatment groups (B, C, D, and E, with hygienic conditions deteriorating progressively from group B to E). Each group had three replications with each in a separate poly-tunnel. The poly-tunnel is covered by a double layer of clear plastic with 2 cm insulation in between and with steel or wood arch frames and bedding on the ground. It is naturally ventilated and the duck feces are cleaned manually. All 15 poly-tunnels were identical, equipped with similar exhaust fan, radiator and incandescent light bulb (80 W). Air warmed by the heat from the sun in the day and the bulb at night was retained in the building by the roof and walls. Temperature of each group was maintained between 20 and 24°C using radiators and exhaust fan. A regime of 16 h light (between 05:00 and 21:00) and 8 h darkness was used, with a 25 min twilight phase at the end of each day, and light intensity was about 60 lx at bird-eye height. The size of poly-tunnel was 4.0 × 4.0 × 3.0 m, with a window (2.0 × 1.5 m) facing the sun. A glass door (0.8 × 1.8 m) was used to observe the behavior of ducks in each poly-tunnel. A total of 1800 1-day old cherry valley ducks were placed in the ducks houses, with 360 ducks in each poly-tunnel. The ducks were reared on the floor with thick bedding (wood-shavings), and food and water were automatically refilled. Phosphoric acid (H_3PO_4), calcium superphosphate [$Ca(H_2PO_4)_2$], ferrous sulfate ($FeSO_4{\cdot}7H_2O$), caustic lime (CaO), acticarbon and alum [$Al_2(SO_4)_3{\cdot}18H_2O$] were used to absorb noxious gases (such as NH_3; Moore et al., 1996; Do et al., 2005; Yao and Li, 2010). Before the trial began, environmental management measures under rearing conditions in poly-tunnels in North China were investigated, while health management measures in different groups were examined. Based on these findings, the health management measures of all treatment groups in this experiment are listed (**Table 1**; Yu et al., 2016). All animal experiments were performed according to the guidelines of the Committee on the Ethics of Animals of Shandong and the appropriate biosecurity guidelines, and the protocol was approved by Shandong Agricultural University Animal Care and Use Committee (No. SDAUA-2014-066).

Sample Collection and Analysis

Determination of Airborne Aerobe, Fungi, and Gram-Negative Bacteria

A 6-stage Andersen impactor (airflow 28.3 L/min), at a height of about 0.2 m (duck's breathing zone) above the ground in the central part of each poly-tunnel, was used to sample airborne aerobe, fungi and gram-negative bacteria weekly at 7:00, 14:00,

TABLE 1 | Management regimes in different groups.

Groups	Ventilation method	Ventilation time (h)	Frequency of troughs cleaning, sterilization, and bedding replacement
A (Control)	Natural and mechanical	24	Once/day
B (Treatment)	Mechanical	24	Once/2 days
C (Treatment)	Mechanical	18	Once/3 days
D (Treatment)	Mechanical	12	Once/4 days
E (Treatment)	Mechanical	10	Once/5 days

and 20:00 h, respectively. The samples were selected three times for 1–2 min a time in every poly-tunnel. Soy agar medium with 5% defibrinated sheep blood, Sabouraud's medium (HB0253-8, Hope Bio-Technology Co., Ltd, Qingdao, China) and a gram-negative bacteria selective medium (HB8643, Hope Bio-Technology Co., Ltd, Qingdao, China) were used as sampling media for aerobes, fungi, and gram-negatives, respectively. For Sabouraud's medium, after high temperature steam sterilization, add Chloramphenicol (dose is 0.2 g/L) into it. The samples were taken to the microbe laboratory and cultured in incubators (aerobic condition)–the aerobes at 37°C for 1 day, fungi at 25°C for 4 days and gram-negative bacteria at 37°C for 3 days. After incubation, the numbers of colonies on plates were determined with a Colony Star counter and concentrations were expressed as colony forming units per m^3 (CFU/m^3; Andersen, 1958).

Determination of Airborne Endotoxin

Air samples for endotoxin were collected by the AGI-30 Sampler (airflow 12.5 L/min) weekly at the height of 0.2 m (Duck's breathing zone) for 20 min, with 50 mL pyrogen-free water as media (Brachmann et al., 1964). Sampling sites were set in the central part of each poly-tunnel. Endotoxin content was determined by Limulus amebocyte lysate (LAL) assay (QLC2100 Bio Whittaker, Walkersville, MD, USA). A standard curve obtained from an *Escherichia* was used to express concentrations as endotoxin units (EU) which were presented as EU/m^3.

Determination of Noxious Gas

Noxious gas was detected by Composite Gas Detector (GC310, Chicheng Electric Co., Ltd, Henan, China) in all groups in real time. The instrument was hung 0.2 m above the ground on the wall. The concentration of noxious gas was presented as mg/Kg.

Determination of Immune Indicators

At the age of 10 days, ducks were immunized with H5 AIV vaccine (Reassortant Avian Influenza Virus H5 Subtype Vaccine, Inactivated Strain Re-6+Strain Re-4, Qingdao Yebio Biological Engineering Co., Ltd., Qingdao, China) by neck subcutaneous, 1.5 mL of each one.

Five mL of blood sample was collected in EDTA vacuum tubes through vena digitalis from each duck of 4-, 5-, 6-, 7- and 8-week old (60 ducks in each group). After centrifugation for 10 min at 800 g, serum samples were stored at −20°C until analysis. Duck IgG detection kit, duck IL-2 detection kit (both of them were purchased from Nanjing SenBenJia Biological Technology Co., Ltd. Nanjing, China), lysozyme detection kit (Nanjing Jiancheng Bioengineering Institute, Nanjing, China) and hemagglutination-inhibition (HI) test were used to detect the serum IgG, IL-2, lysozyme and H5 AIV antibody titer, respectively.

MTT (Methy Thiazolyl Tetrazolium) colorimetric assay was used to detect T lymphocytes transformation rate (Lazar et al., 2010; Hsiao and Huang, 2011; Yin et al., 2015). The procedure as follows:

One mL of blood sample was collected in EDTA vacuum tubes through vena digitalis from each duck of 4-, 5-, 6-, 7-, and 8-week old (60 ducks in each group).

One mL whole blood dilution (Shanghai Yanjin Biotechnology Co.Ltd. Shanghai, China) was added to the above blood sample (1 mL), then mixed. The mixture was added on 4 mL lymphocyte separation fluid (Beijing Dingguo Chengsheng Biotechnology Co., Ltd. Beijing, China) for 15 min centrfugation at 800 g. The white coat that under the plasma layer was sucked out and washed 2 times with 3–5 times volume RPMI 1640 culture liquid (Sigma, USA) without calf serum, each time with centrfugation for 10 min at 800 g.

Counting with Trypan Blue (Sigma, USA), the living cells was more than 95%. Single cell suspensions (final concentration was 3×10^6 /mL) were prepared by RPMI 1640 complete culture liquid containing 10% calf serum. The single cell suspension was cultured in a cell incubator at 37°C, 6.5% CO_2 for 14 h. Peripheral blood lymphocyte were obtain and then prepared for lymphocyte suspension (final concentration was 2×10^6 /mL).

Cells are grown in microtiter plates (tissue culture grade, 96 wells, flat bottom). 100 µL of the lymphocyte suspension and 100 µL of the PHA (phytohaemagglutinin; Beijing Baiaosentai Biotechnology Co., Ltd. Beijing, China; final concentration was 25 µg / mL) was added (final concentration was 2×10^6 /mL) into each test well. 100 µL of the lymphocyte suspension and 100 µL of the RPMI 1640 was added into each control well. The replications is five. After the incubation in a cell incubator at 37°C, 6.5% CO_2 for 44 h, 20 µL of MTT (5 mg/mL) was added into each well and then continued to incubate for 4 h. The supernatant of each well was discarded carefully.

After that, 150 µL of dimethyl sulfoxide was added into each well and then oscillated for 10 min on microoscillator. The value of OD 570 nm was measured by Microplate Reader (Antai AY-858, Shanghai, China).

$$\text{T-lymphocyte transformation rate} = \frac{\text{Mean value of test } OD_{570}}{\text{Mean value of control } OD_{570}} \times 100\%$$

Determination of Immune Organ Indexes

The ducks of 4-, 6-, 8-week were weighed and recorded (60 ducks in each group). After that, thymus, spleen and bursa were collected from those ducks, respectively, and then weighed and recorded. At last, the immune organ indexes were calculated according to the follow formula.

$$\text{Immune organ indexes} = \frac{\text{Immune organ (g)}}{\text{Body weight (Kg)}} \times 100\%$$

Statistical Analysis

Data collection ran from week 4 to week 8. Data for each group were expressed as the mean of three replications. The maximum, minimum and median value were used for the air ambient parameter (Duan et al., 2007). All statistical analyses were performed using SAS 9.1 Software (SAS Institute, Inc., Cary, NC, USA). One-way ANOVA analysis with multiple-range test was used to evaluate the difference among groups (Duncan, 1955). Results are expressed as mean ± standard deviation (SD). Correlation between major microbial concentrations and immune indicators were analyzed by Pearson's. $P < 0.05$ was considered statistically significant.

RESULTS

The Concentrations of Microbial Aerosol and Noxious Gas under Different Hygienic Conditions

Over time, the concentrations of airborne aerobe, airborne fungi, airborne gram-negative, airborne endotoxin, and NH_3 showed an overall trend of increase with the deteriorating of hygienic conditions, however, concentration of NH_3 in each group was lower than the poultry harmless criterion (10 ppm, GB/T 18407.3–2001), and H_2S was not found in all groups (**Table 2**; Yu et al., 2016).

The Effect of Microbial Aerosol on Specific Immunity of Meat Ducks

H5 AIV Antibody Titer

Under the condition without booster immunization, the H5 AIV antibody titer in serum of meat ducks of groups A and B reached a peak at week 5 (6.00 ± 1.00 and 6.33 ± 1.53, respectively), however, groups C, D, and E reached the peak at weeks 6, 7, and 8 (5.00 ± 1.00, 4.33 ± 1.53, and 3.00 ± 2.00, respectively; **Figure 1**). At the same week age, with the microbial aerosol concentrations increasing, the concentration of H5 AIV antibody titer in the serum of meat ducks generally showed a tendency of decline.

Serum H5 AIV antibody titers were lower in groups E than in group A ($P < 0.01$) at weeks 4 and 7; groups E were lower than group A ($P < 0.05$) at weeks 5 and 6.

TABLE 2 | Airborne aerobe, airborne fungi, airborne gram-negative bacteria, airborne endotoxin, and noxious gas concentrations under different hygienic conditions.

Parameter	Value	Groups				
		A	B	C	D	E
Aerobe (×10E5 CFU/mE3)	Minimum	0.46	0.69	0.68	0.59	0.71
	Maximum	2.00	5.10	5.76	5.06	8.96
	Mean	1.05	2.45	2.94	**2.96**	4.31
Fungi (×10E4 CFU/mE3)	Minimum	0.11	0.21	0.19	0.85	0.78
	Maximum	3.49	3.54	3.95	5.73	8.05
	Mean	1.02	1.32	1.44	**2.63**	3.07
Gram-negative bacteria (×10E4 CFU/mE3)	Minimum	0.20	0.32	0.36	0.89	0.98
	Maximum	2.04	1.95	3.62	8.87	5.03
	Mean	0.93	1.24	1.68	**3.09**	2.64
Endotoxin (×10E3 EU/mE3)	Minimum	0.20	0.40	0.28	0.13	0.56
	Maximum	25.6	72.4	102.4	144.8	144.8
	Mean	6.49	10.48	23.03	**41.78**	47.79
NH_3 (mg/Kg)	Minimum	0	0	2	4	4
	Maximum	4	12	10	15	14
	Mean	2.56	2.42	5.67	**9.48**	8.97
H_2S (mg/Kg)	Minimum	–[a]	–	–	–	–
	Maximum	–	–	–	–	–
	Mean	–	–	–	–	–

All value for total experimental period.
[a]Below the limit of detection.
The bold values could be used as a basis for recommending upper limit concentrations of microbial aerosols for healthy meat ducks.

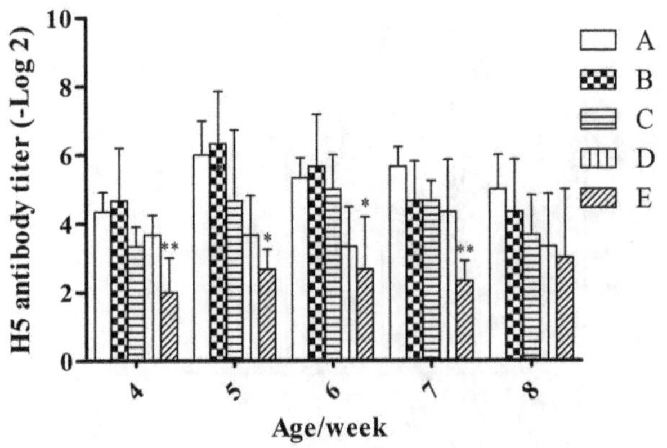

FIGURE 1 | H5 AIV antibody titer under different hygienic conditions ($n = 60$). Note: The comparison was between treatment groups (B–E) and control group (A) at the same age/week, *$P < 0.05$ and **$P < 0.01$. The same as below. *Means that the difference between treatment groups (B–E) and control group (A) was significant.

IgG

At the same week age, with the increase of the microbial aerosol concentrations, the concentration of IgG in serum of meat ducks generally showed a tendency of increase (**Figure 2**).

Concentration of serum IgG were higher in groups E than in groups A ($P < 0.05$) at week 4 and 5; groups D were higher than

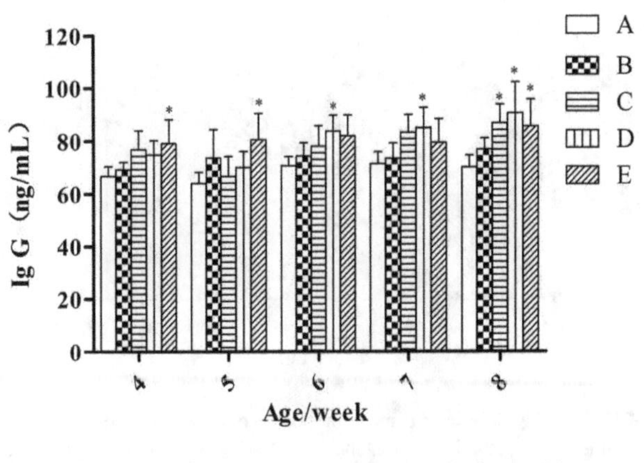

FIGURE 2 | IgG concentration under different hygienic conditions ($n = 60$). *Means that the difference between treatment groups (B–E) and control group (A) was significant.

group A ($P < 0.05$) at week 6 and 7; groups C, D, and E were higher than group A ($P < 0.05$) at week 8.

IL-2

At the same week age, with the increase of the microbial aerosol concentrations, the concentration of IL-2 in serum of meat ducks generally showed a tendency of decline (**Figure 3**).

Serum IL-2 in groups E were lower than in group A ($P < 0.05$) at week 4 and 6; groups D and E were lower than group A ($P < 0.01$) at week 7; groups D and E were lower than group A ($P < 0.05$ and $P < 0.01$, respectively) at week 8.

T-Lymphocyte Transformation Rate

At the same week age, with the increase of the microbial aerosol concentrations, T-lymphocyte transformation rate of meat ducks generally showed a tendency of decline (**Figure 4**), and the decline range was obvious.

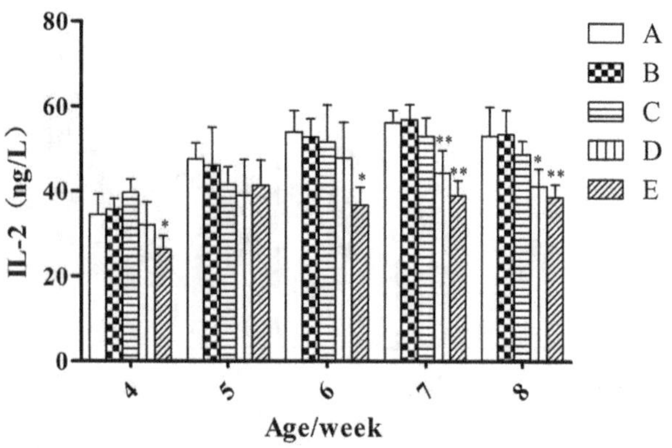

FIGURE 3 | IL-2 concentration under different hygienic conditions ($n = 60$). *Means that the difference between treatment groups (B–E) and control group (A) was significant. **Means that the difference between treatment groups (B–E) and control group (A) was extremely significant.

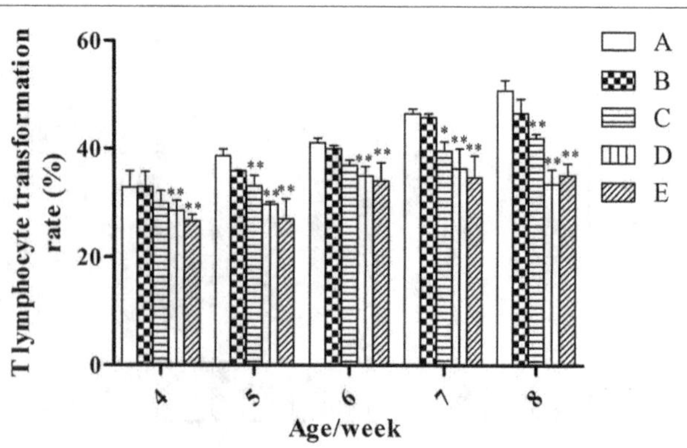

FIGURE 4 | T-lymphocyte transformation rate under different hygienic conditions ($n = 60$). *Means that the difference between treatment groups (B–E) and control group (A) was significant. **Means that the difference between treatment groups (B–E) and control group (A) was extremely significant.

T-lymphocyte transformation rates of groups D and E were lower than that of group A ($P < 0.01$) at weeks 4 and 6; groups C, D, and E were lower than that of group A ($P < 0.01$) at weeks 5 and 8; groups C, D, and E were lower than that of group A ($P < 0.05$, $P < 0.01$ and $P < 0.01$, respectively) at week 7.

The Effect of Microbial Aerosol on Non-specific Immunity of Meat Ducks

Lysozyme

At the same week age, as microbial aerosol concentrations increasing, the concentration of lysozyme in serum of meat ducks generally showed a tendency of increase at first (at weeks 4 and 5) and then showed a tendency of decline (at weeks 6, 7, and 8; **Table 3**).

Serum lysozyme in groups D and E were higher than group A ($P < 0.05$) at week 4; groups B, C, D and E were lower than group A ($P < 0.01$) at week 7; groups D and E were lower than group A ($P < 0.01$), but the group B was higher than group A ($P < 0.01$) at week 8.

Immune Organ Indexes

At the same week age, with the increase of the microbial aerosol concentrations, the index of thymus, spleen and bursa of meat ducks generally showed a tendency of decline (**Table 4**).

For thymus index, there was no significant effect ($P > 0.05$). As for spleen index, groups D and E were lower than group A ($P < 0.05$) at week 6; groups D and E were lower than group A ($P < 0.05$ and $P < 0.01$, respectively) at week 8. For bursa index, groups C, D and E were lower than group A ($P < 0.05$) at week 8.

Relationships between Microbial Aerosol Constituents and Immune Indicators

The correlation between microbial aerosol and immune indicators is shown in **Table 5**.

The concentration of aerobe showed a strong correlation to IgG, H5 AIV antibody titer, T-lymphocyte transformation rate, Thymus Index, Spleen Index and Bursa Index ($r = 0.91$ at $P < 0.05$, $r = -0.90$ at $P < 0.05$, $r = -0.89$ at $P < 0.05$, $r = -0.92$ at $P < 0.05$, $r = -0.94$ at $P < 0.05$, $r = -0.88$ at $P < 0.05$, respectively).

As for fungi, a significant negative correlation was recorded between fungi and H5 AIV antibody titer, IL-2, T-lymphocyte transformation rate, Lysozyme, Thymus Index, Spleen Index and Bursa Index ($r = 0.95$ at $P < 0.05$, $r = -0.99$ at $P < 0.01$, $r = -0.95$ at $P < 0.05$, $r = -0.97$ at $P < 0.01$, $r = -0.96$ at $P < 0.01$, $r = -0.96$ at $P < 0.01$, $r = -0.93$ at $P < 0.05$, respectively).

The concentration of endotoxin revealed the same dependency on H5 AIV antibody titer, IL-2, T-lymphocyte transformation rate, Lysozyme, Thymus Index, Spleen Index, and Bursa Index ($r = 0.98$ at $P < 0.01$, $r = -0.99$ at $P < 0.01$, $r = -0.95$ at $P < 0.05$, $r = -0.97$ at $P < 0.01$, $r = -0.98$ at $P < 0.01$, $r = -0.95$ at $P < 0.05$, $r = -0.89$ at $P < 0.05$, respectively).

However, the gram-negative bacteria correlated negatively with IgG, IL-2, T-lymphocyte Transformation Rate, Lysozyme,

TABLE 3 | Lysozyme concentration (U/mL) under different hygienic conditions (n = 60).

Weeks	Groups				
	A	B	C	D	E
4	120.14 ± 4.22	126.10 ± 4.99	124.60 ± 9.73	130.62 ± 7.99*	133.62 ± 6.14*
5	148.32 ± 5.21	150.85 ± 5.79	149.22 ± 6.68	152.30 ± 7.76	156.83 ± 9.35
6	153.72 ± 6.77	152.80 ± 11.29	158.16 ± 8.43	145.65 ± 7.03	148.98 ± 9.43
7	176.42 ± 6.43	158.47 ± 6.92**	162.38 ± 9.68**	151.90 ± 7.56**	141.37 ± 5.98**
8	166.31 ± 4.46	180.53 ± 6.65**	156.90 ± 8.21	144.82 ± 8.60**	139.43 ± 7.34**

*The comparison was between treatment groups (B–E) and control group (A) at the same age/week, * $P < 0.05$ and ** $P < 0.01$. The same as below. *Means that the difference between treatment groups (B–E) and control group (A) was significant. **Means that the difference between treatment groups (B–E) and control group (A) was extremely significant.*

TABLE 4 | Immune organ indexes under different hygienic conditions (n = 60).

Items	Weeks	Groups				
		A	B	C	D	E
Thymus index	4	2.81 ± 0.17	2.60 ± 0.11	2.49 ± 0.63	2.16 ± 0.33	2.09 ± 0.51
	6	2.44 ± 0.47	2.16 ± 0.38	1.95 ± 0.13	1.98 ± 0.48	1.80 ± 0.34
	8	2.21 ± 0.45	2.19 ± 0.28	1.96 ± 0.26	1.56 ± 0.33	1.57 ± 0.41
Spleen index	4	1.32 ± 0.12	1.24 ± 0.26	1.25 ± 0.33	1.03 ± 0.38	0.96 ± 0.08
	6	1.26 ± 0.22	1.06 ± 0.14	0.90 ± 0.14	0.79 ± 0.28*	0.69 ± 0.20*
	8	1.19 ± 0.21	0.96 ± 0.08	0.98 ± 0.18	0.80 ± 0.20*	0.72 ± 0.12**
Bursa index	4	1.84 ± 0.39	1.74 ± 0.56	1.86 ± 0.17	1.49 ± 0.47	1.54 ± 0.33
	6	1.44 ± 0.08	1.27 ± 0.16	1.31 ± 0.25	1.16 ± 0.20	1.19 ± 0.19
	8	1.46 ± 0.23	1.16 ± 0.16	1.03 ± 0.20*	0.97 ± 0.23*	0.89 ± 0.23*

**Means that the difference between treatment groups (B–E) and control group (A) was significant. **Means that the difference between treatment groups (B–E) and control group (A) was extremely significant.*

TABLE 5 | Correlation between concentrations of major microbial aerosol components and values of immune indicators.

Immune index	Aerobe	Fungi	Gram-negative bacteria	Endotoxin
IgG	**r = 0.91***	r = 0.86	**r = −0.90***	r = 0.86
H5 AIV antibody titer	**r = −0.90***	**r = −0.95***	r = −0.87	**r = −0.98****
IL-2	r = −0.84	**r = −0.99****	**r = −0.88***	**r = −0.99****
T-lymphocyte trans-formation rate	**r = −0.89***	**r = −0.95***	**r = −0.95***	**r = −0.95***
Lysozyme	r = −0.79	**r = −0.97****	**r = −0.95***	**r = −0.97****
Thymus index	**r = −0.92***	**r = −0.96****	r = −0.83	**r = −0.98****
Spleen index	**r = −0.94***	**r = −0.96****	**r = −0.92***	**r = −0.95***
Bursa index	**r = −0.88***	**r = −0.93***	**r = −0.94***	**r = −0.89***

Significant relationships ($P < 0.05$, **$P < 0.01$) expressed as Pearson correlation coefficients (**r**) in bold.*

Spleen Index, and Bursa Index ($r = -0.90$ at $P < 0.05$, $r = -0.88$ at $P < 0.05$, $r = -0.95$ at $P < 0.05$, $r = -0.95$ at $P < 0.05$, $r = -0.92$ at $P < 0.05$, $r = -0.94$ at $P < 0.05$, respectively).

The prediction models are as follows:

$Y = 75.49 - 2.78 \times 10E\text{-}6\ X_1 + 2.13 \times 10E\text{-}5\ X_2$, $R^2 = 0.3414$, $p = 0.5086 > 0.05$

Y: IgG (ng/mL); X_1: airborne aerobe (CFU/mE3); X_2: airborne gram-negative bacteria (CFU/mE3)

$Y = 4.76 + 2.41 \times 10E\text{-}6\ X_1 + 1.00 \times 10E\text{-}4\ X_2 - 1.03 \times 10E\text{-}4\ X_3$, $R^2 = 0.9760$, $p = 0.0230$

Y: H5 AIV antibody titer (−Log 2); X_1: airborne aerobe (CFU/mE3); X_2: airborne fungi (CFU/mE3); X_3: airborne endotoxin (EU/mE3)

$Y = 55.61 - 5.01 \times 10E\text{-}4\ X_1 + 6.01 \times 10E\text{-}6\ X_2 - 1.03 \times 10E\text{-}4\ X_3$, $R^2 = 0.8795$, $p = 0.0141$

Y: IL-2 (ng/mL); X_1: airborne fungi (CFU/mE3); X_2: airborne gram-negative bacteria (CFU/mE3); X_3: airborne endotoxin (EU/mE3)

$Y = 43.77 - 5.53 \times 10E\text{-}6\ X_1 + 1.01 \times 10E\text{-}4\ X_2 + 3.69 \times 10E\text{-}6\ X_3 - 3.03 \times 10E\text{-}4\ X_4$, $R^2 = 0.8417$, $p = 0.0392$

Y: T-lymphocyte transformation rate (%); X_1: airborne aerobe (CFU/mE3); X_2: airborne fungi (CFU/mE3); X_3: airborne gram-negative bacteria (CFU/mE3); X_4: airborne endotoxin (EU/mE3)

$Y = 155.45 - 8.35 \times 10E\text{-}6\ X_1 - 1.99 \times 10E\text{-}6\ X_2 - 2.00 \times 10E\text{-}4\ X_3$, $R^2 = 0.9097$, $p = 0.0517 > 0.05$

Y: Lysozyme (U/mL); X_1: airborne fungi (CFU/mE3); X_2: airborne gram-negative bacteria (CFU/mE3); X_3: airborne endotoxin (EU/mE3)

From the analysis above, it could be concluded that the concentration of airborne aerobe, fungi, gram-negative bacteria, endotoxin have a strong correction with the value of H5 AIV antibody titer, IgG, IL-2, T-lymphocyte rate, lysozyme, and immune organ indexes, respectively. Thus, it can provide a substantial evidence to confirm the effect of microbial aerosol on immune level.

DISCUSSION

Microbial aerosol originates from feed, manure, litter, as well as microorganisms, their byproducts and fragments in poultry houses (Millner, 2009; Just et al., 2011). Airborne aerobes, fungi, gram-negative bacteria and their bioproducts or biological fragments (such as endotoxins) are major components (Yu et al., 2016). The concentrations and components of it could reflect the condition of ambient sanitation in animal houses (Zucker and Muller, 2000; Kaliste et al., 2002). High concentrations of microbial aerosol and its metabolites (endotoxin, NH_3, H_2S, etc) are important factors affecting the health and productivity of animals (Prazmo et al., 2003; Banhai et al., 2008).

In this study, four treatment groups with gradually deteriorating hygienic conditions and one control group under standard hygienic sanitary management were set up by changing the frequency of trough cleaning, sterilization, bedding replacement, and ventilation (**Table 1**). The concentrations of airborne aerobes, fungi, gram-negative bacteria, and endotoxin in groups B, C, D increased both over time and as hygienic conditions deteriorated (**Table 2**). The results show that routine hygienic management measures, such as ventilation, bedding replacement and sterilization can reduce bioaerosols in duck poly-tunnels, which is important in order to maintain optimal microclimate and hygiene. Phosphoric acid, calcium superphosphate, ferrous sulfate, caustic lime, acticarbon, and alum were effective in absorbing noxious gases.

To the best of our knowledge, this study is the first to evaluate the effects of microbial aerosol on duck immunity. As we all known, immunity of animal can be divided into specific and non-specific immunity, and specific immunity can be divided into humoral and cellular immunity. In order to explore the effects of microbial aerosol on the immune function of duck. We chose IgG, H5 AIV antibody titer as reliable indicators for humoral immunity; took IL-2, T-lymphocyte transformation rate as representativeness indexes for cellular immunity; and took lysozyme, Immune organ indexes as non-specific immune factors.

Immunity to avian influenza is mainly based on humoral immunity, and detection of antibody titer of avian influenza contributes to indicating the condition of specific immune system protection (Ellis et al., 2004; Liu et al., 2006). As for serum IgG, it is the highest level of immunoglobulin in the blood of bodies. The activity of anti-bacteria, anti-virus and anti-toxin of IgG can be embodied in animal blood, and it plays essential roles in "Main Immune" (Borghesi et al., 2014). IL-2, also called T-cell growth factor, is the main cytokine in regulating cellular immune (Bayer et al., 2013). It is mainly produced by activated T-lymphocytes, and also can activate a variety of immune cells, regulate the body's immunity and enhance the body's anti-inflammatory effects, etc. (Song et al., 2005). In the process of the immune response, T-lymphocyte transformation rate is involved in the cellular immune response, therefore, it is often used to assess the functional status of lymphocytes and the status of body's immunity (Toivanen and Toivanen, 1973; Hovi et al., 1978; Kim et al., 1996).

Lysozyme is a kind of hydrolase that has special effects on the microbial cytoderm, which relaxes cytoderm and loses the protective effect on cells, and results in bacteria dissolution eventually (Sung et al., 2011). In the process of anti-bacterial infection, lysozyme often used as an important indicator that reflects strength of non-specific immunity (Fiolka et al., 2012; Zhao et al., 2014). The weight of thymus, spleen and bursa can be used to evaluate the immune status of poultry. It also reflects the strength of immune function intuitively (Rivas and Farbricant, 1985).

Over the experimental period, as microbial aerosol concentration increasing, serum IgG and lysozyme (4 and 5 weeks) increased, whereas H5 AIV antibody titer, IL-2, T-lymphocyte transformation rate, lysozyme (6 and 8 weeks), and immune organ indexes decreased. When the concentration of microbial aerosol reach the level of group D, serum IgG (6–8 weeks), serum lysozyme (4 week) were significantly higher than in group A ($P < 0.05$); serum IL-2 (7 and 8 weeks), T-lymphocyte transformation rate, serum lysozyme (7 and 8 weeks), spleen index (6 and 8 weeks), and bursa index (8 week) were significantly lower than in group A ($P < 0.05$ or $P < 0.01$).

Microbial aerosols at certain concentrations can stimulate the stress response, and stress can have serious adverse effects on welfare (Yu et al., 2016). Under stress, animals have to activate energy to combat the stressor, which can enhance catabolism and weaken the anabolism of protein and fat. Where animals are reared in environments contaminated with microorganisms, the nutrient status of organs may be compromised (Benson et al., 1993). This might be the reason for the decreasing tendency of immune organ indexes.

Moreover, if the stress in a long period of time, and it could lead to chronic stress, which could lead to cellular immune inhibition (Schedlowski, 1993; Bartolomucci et al., 2003), cutting down the production of IL-2 in serum (McEwen et al., 1997). This might be the reason for the tendency of serum IL-2 and T-lymphocyte transformation rates.

As for the tendency of serum IgG and lysozyme, after the initial increase it later decreased (6–8 weeks; **Figure 2** and **Table 3**), this may be due to the appearance of "malignant stress" in the late stages of this study, that is, under the short-term and mild stress, animals could adapt to it by compensatory reaction, but the long-term stress at any intensity will result in harmful effects, such as deterioration of physiological function in animals, etc. (He et al., 2011).

In addition, high level of microbial aerosol also affected the humoral immunity level of meat ducks, and it not only reduced the H5 AIV antibody titer of ducks, but also delayed the emergence of the antibody titer peak (**Figure 1**). This result is analogous to that of Witter (1998). Witter argued that weakened immune function reduces the immune protective effect of the vaccine.

CONCLUSIONS

In conclusion, a high level of airborne aerobe, gram-negative bacteria, fungi, and endotoxin adversely affected the immune level of meat ducks. This study indicates that good ventilation, bedding replacement and sterilization can decrease microbial aerosol concentration effectively. The present findings suggest that the microbial aerosol concentrations of group D provide a basis for recommending upper limit concentrations of microbial aerosols for healthy meat ducks.

AUTHOR CONTRIBUTIONS

GY and YC designed the experiment and completed most of the works. YW, SW, CD, and JG analyzed some test results and collected materials. TC and LW gave experiment instruction. Thank all the authors' contribution to the experiment.

ACKNOWLEDGMENTS

This research was funded by The National Science and Technology Support Project "Research of airborne microorganisms of animal houses and their impact on the Animal Health and Control Technology" [2012BAD39B0205]; Natural Science Foundation of Shandong Province [ZR2012CM041]; Natural Science Foundation of Shandong Province [ZR2011HM032]; State Environmental Protection Key Laboratory of Microorganism Application and Risk Control (MARC), Tsinghua University, China [SMARC2013D001].

REFERENCES

Andersen, A. A. (1958). New sampler for collection, sizing and enumeration of viable airborne particles. *J. Bacteriol.* 76, 471–484.

Balasubramanian, R., Nainar, P., and Rajasekar, A. (2012). Airborne bacteria, fungi, and endotoxin levers in residential microenvironments: a case study. *Aerobiologia* 28, 375–390. doi: 10.1007/s10453-011-9242-y

Banhai, T. M., Seedorf, J., Laffrique, M., and Rutley, D. L. (2008). Identification of the risk factors for high airborne particle concentrations in broiler buildings using statistical modeling. *Biosyst. Eng.* 101, 100–110. doi: 10.1016/j.biosystemseng.2008.06.007

Barrasa, M., Lamosa, S., Fernandez, M. D., and Fernandez, E. (2012). Occupational exposure to carbon dioxide, ammonia and hydrogen sulphide on livestock farms in the north-west Spain. *Ann. Agric. Environ. Med.* 19, 17–24.

Bartolomucci, A., Sacerdote, P., and Panerai, A. E. (2003). Chronic psychosocial stress induced down-regulation of immunity depends upon individual factors. *J. Neuroimmunol.* 141, 58–64. doi: 10.1016/S0165-5728(03)00220-0

Bayer, A. L., Pugliese, A., and Malek, T. R. (2013). The IL-2/IL-2R system: from basic science to therapeutic applications to enhance immune regulation. *Immunol. Res.* 57, 197–209. doi: 10.1007/s12026-013-8452-5

Benson, B. N., Calvert, C. C., Roura, E., and Klasing, K. C. (1993). Dietary energy source and density modulate the expression of immunologic stress in chicks. *J. Nutr.* 123, 1714–1723.

Borghesi, J., Lara, C. M., Rodrigues, M. N., Favaron, P. O., and Miglino, M. A. (2014). Immunoglobulin transport during gestation in domestic animals and humans-a review. *Open J. Anim. Sci.* 4, 323–336. doi: 10.4236/ojas.2014.45041

Brachmann, P. S., Ehrlich, R., Eichenwald, H. F., Heninz, F., Gabelli, V. J., Kethley, T. W., et al. (1964). Standard sampler for assay of airborne microorganisms. *Science* 144, 1295.

Burrell, R. (1990). Immunomodulation by bacterial endotoxin. *Crit. Rev. Microbiol.* 17, 189–208. doi: 10.3109/10408419009105725

Bush, R. K., and Portnoy, J. M. (2001). The role and abatement of fungal allergens in allergic diseases. *J. Allergy Clin. Immunol.* 107, 430–440. doi: 10.1067/mai.2001.113669

Cambra-López, M., Aarnink, A. J. A., Zhao, Y., Calvet, S., and Torres, A. G. (2010). Airborne particulate matter from livestock production systems: a review of an air pollution problem. *Environ. Pollut.* 158, 1–17. doi: 10.1016/j.envpol.2009.07.011

Do, J. C., Choi, I. H., and Nahm, K. H. (2005). Effects of chemically amended litter on broiler performance, atmospheric ammonia concentration, and phosphorus solubility in litter. *Poult. Sci.* 84, 679–689. doi: 10.1093/ps/84.5.679

Douwes, J., Thorne, P., Pearce, N., and Heederik, D. (2003). Bioaerosol health effects and exposure assessment: progress and prospects. *Ann. Occup. Hyg.* 47, 187–200. doi: 10.1093/annhyg/meg032

Duan, H., Chai, T., Zhang, X., and Ma, R. (2007). Microbiological aerosols in poultry house and its ambience. ISAH-2007 Tartu. *Estonia* 2007, 526–232.

Duncan, D. B. (1955). Multiple range and multiple F tests. *Biometrics* 11, 1–42. doi: 10.2307/3001478

Ellis, T. M., Leung, C. Y., Chow, M. K., Bissett, L. A., Wong, W., and Guan, Y. (2004). Vaccination of chickens against H5N1 avian influenza in the face of an outbreak interrupts virus transmission. *Avian Pathol.* 33, 405–412. doi: 10.1080/03079450410001724012

Fiegel, J., Clarke, R., and Edwarde, D. A. (2006). Airborne infectious disease and the suppression of pulmonary bioaerosols. *Drug Discov. Today* 11, 51–57. doi: 10.1016/S1359-6446(05)03687-1

Fiolka, M. J., Zagaja, M. P., Hulas-Stasiak, M., and Wielbo, J. (2012). Activity and immunodetection of lysozyme in earthworm *Dendrobaena veneta* (Annelida). *J. Invertebr. Pathol.* 109, 83–90. doi: 10.1016/j.jip.2011.10.002

He, Z. M., Li, G. P., Li, G. M., Chen, Z. W., and Wang, L. Z. (2011). "Laboratory animal welfare and animal experimental science," in *Laboratory Animal Welfare*, eds Z. M. He and G. P. Li (Beijing: Science Press), 104–106.

Hovi, T., Suni, J., Hortling, L., and Vaheri, A. (1978). Stimulation of chicken lymphocytes by T and B cell mitogens. *Cell. Immunol.* 39, 70–78. doi: 10.1016/0008-8749(78)90084-9

Hsiao, I. L., and Huang, Y. J. (2011). Improving the interferences of methyl thiazolyl tetrazolium and IL-8 assays in assessing the cytotoxicity of nanoparticles. *J. Nanosci. Nanotechnol.* 11, 5228–5233. doi: 10.1166/jnn.2011.4132

Just, N., Kirychuk, S., Gilbert, Y., Letourneau, V., Veillette, M., and Singh, B. (2011). Bacterial diversity characterization of bioaerosols from cage-housed and floor-housed poultry operations. *Environ. Res.* 11, 492–498. doi: 10.1016/j.envres.2011.01.009

Kaliste, E., Linnainmaa, M., Meklin, T., and Nevalainen, A. (2002). Airborne contaminants in conventional laboratory rabbit rooms. *Lab. Anim.* 36, 43–50. doi: 10.1258/0023677021911759

Kim, H. M., Han, S. B., Oh, G. T., Kim, Y. H., Hong, D. H., Hong, N. D., et al. (1996). Stimulation of humoral and cell mediated immunity by polysaccharide from mushroom *Phellinus linteus*. *Int. J. Immunopharmacol.* 18, 295–303. doi: 10.1016/0192-0561(96)00028-8

Lawniczek-Walczyk, A., Górny, R. L., Golofit-Szymczak, M., Niesler, A., and Wlazlo, A. (2013). Occupational exposure to airborne microorganisms, endotoxins and β-glucans in poultry houses at different stages of the production cycle. *Ann. Agric. Environ. Med.* 20, 259–268.

Lazar, V., Chifiriuc, M. C., Steward-Tull, D. E., Bleotu, C., Candlich, D., and Wardlaw, A. C. (2010). Investigation of the cytotoxic capacity of some adherent opportunistic enterobacterial strains by the MTT assay and transmission electron microscopy. *Roum. Arch. Microbiol. Immunol.* 69, 35–40.

Liu, C. N., Liu, M., Zhang, Y., Liu, C. G., and Gao, X. L. (2006). Pathogenicity of H5N1 influenza virus for ducks. *Sci. Agric. Sin.* 39, 412–417.

Madsen, A. M. (2006). Airborne endotoxin in different background environments and seasons. *Ann. Agric. Environ. Med.* 13, 81–86.

Masclaux, F. G., Sakwinska, O., Charrière, N., Semaani, E., and Oppliger, A. (2013). Concentration of airborne *Staphylococcus aureus* (MRSA and MSSA), total bacteria, and endotoxins in pig farms. *Ann. Occup. Hyg.* 57, 550–557. doi: 10.1093/annhyg/mes098

Matković, K., Vučemilo, M., Štoković, I., Šimić, R., Marušić, D., Vinković, B., et al. (2013). Concentrations of airborne bacteria and fungi in a livestock building with caged laying hens. *Vet. Arh.* 83, 413–424.

McEwen, B. S., Biron, C. A., and Brunson, K. W. (1997). The role of Adrenocorticoids as modulates of immune function in health and disease: neural, endocrine and immune interactions. *Brain Res. Rev.* 23, 79–133. doi: 10.1016/S0165-0173(96)00012-4

Millner, P. D. (2009). Bioaerosols associated with animal production operations. *Bioresour. Technol.* 100, 5379–5385. doi: 10.1016/j.biortech.2009.03.026

Moore, P. A., Daniel, T. C., Edwards, D. R., and Miller, D. M. (1996). Evaluation of chemical amendments to reduce ammonia volatilization from poultry litter. *Poult. Sci.* 75, 315–320. doi: 10.3382/ps.0750315

Nimmermark, S., Lund, V., Gustafsson, G., and Eduard, W. (2009). Ammonia, dust and bacteria in welfare-oriented systems for laying hens. *Ann. Agric. Environ. Med.* 16, 103–113.

Pavan, R., and Manjunath, K. (2014). Qualitative analysis of indoor and outdoor airborne fungi in cowshed. *J. Mycol.* 2014, 1–8. doi: 10.1155/2014/985921

Pirie, R. S., Collie, D. D., and Dixon, P. M. (2003). Inhaled endotoxin and organic dust particulates have synergistic proinflammatory effects in equine heaves (organic dust-induced asthma). *Clin. Exp. Allergy* 33, 676–683. doi: 10.1046/j.1365-2222.2003.01640.x

Prazmo, Z., Dutkiewicz, J., Skórska, C., Sitkowska, J., and Cholewa, G. (2003). Exposure to airborne Gram-negative bacteria, dust and endotoxin in paper factories. *Ann. Agric. Environ. Med.* 10, 93–100.

Rivas, A. L., and Farbricant, J. (1985). Indication of Immundepression in chicken infected with various of Marek's Disease Virus. *Avian Dis.* 32, 1–8. doi: 10.2307/1590941

Schedlowski, M. (1993). Psychophysiological neuroendocrine and cellular immune reactions under psychological stress. *Neuropsychobiology* 28, 87–90. doi: 10.1159/000119006

Song, Q. Y., Guo, X., and Yang, H. C. (2005). Porcine cytokines (In Chinese). *Chinese J. Vet. Med.* 41, 33–38.

Sung, K., Khan, S. A., Nawaz, M. S., Cerniglia, C. E., Tamplin, M. L., Phillips, R. W., et al. (2011). Lysozyme as a barrier to growth of *Bacillus anthracis* strain sterne in liquid egg white, milk and beef. *Food Microbiol.* 28, 1231–1234. doi: 10.1016/j.fm.2011.03.002

Teye, F. K., Hautala, M., Pastell, M., Praks, J., Veermae, I., Poikalainen, V., et al. (2008). Microclimate and ventilation in Estonian and Finnish dairy buildings. *Energy Build.* 40, 1194–1201. doi: 10.1016/j.enbuild.2007.10.017

Toivanen, P., and Toivanen, A. (1973). Selective activation of chicken T lymphocytes by Concanavalin A. *J. Immunol.* 111, 1602–1603.

Witter, R. L. (1998). Control strategies for Marek's Disease: a perspective for the future. *Poult. Sci.* 77, 1197–1203. doi: 10.1093/ps/77.8.1197

Wolinsky, S. M. (2006). Public health: chicken monster or chicken little? *Science* 311, 780–781. doi: 10.1126/science.1123435

Yao, Z. Q., and Li, Y. C. (2010). Effects of harmful gas in poultry house on livestock and its control measures (In Chinese). *Livestock and Poultry Industry*, 258, 22–23.

Yin, W., Ma, Q. H., Jiang, J. B., Fan, K. H., Sun, N., and Sun, Y. G. (2015). Effects of *Astragalus* Polysaccharides (APS) on T Lymphocyte proliferation regulated by red blood cells (In Chinese). *Prog. Vet. Med.* 36, 53–58.

Yu, G. L., Wei, L. M., Liu, Y. Y., Liu, J. Y., Wang, Y., Gao, J., et al. (2016). Influence of indoor microbial aerosol on the welfare of meat ducks. *Br. Poult. Sci.* 57, 12–22. doi: 10.1080/00071668.2015.1122739

Zhao, M., Song, Q. R., Dai, G. Z., and Wang, L. (2014). Influence of long-term high-temperature environment on immune system of rats. *Occup. Health* 18, 2568–2570.

Zucker, B. A., and Muller, W. (2000). Investigation on airborne microorganisms in animals stables. 3: relationship between inhalable endotoxin, inhalable dust and airborne bacteria in a hen house. *Berl. Munch. Tierarztl. Wochenschr.* 113, 279–283.

Zucker, B. A., Trojan, S., and Muller, W. (2000). Airborne gram-negative bacterial flora in animal houses. *J. Vet. Med. Ser. B* 47, 37–46. doi: 10.1046/j.1439-0450.2000.00308.x

5

Dysbiosis of the Urinary Microbiota Associated with Urine Levels of Proinflammatory Chemokine Interleukin-8 in Female Type 2 Diabetic Patients

Zongxin Ling[1†], Fengping Liu[1,2†], Li Shao[1], Yiwen Cheng[1] and Lanjuan Li[1*]*

[1] Collaborative Innovation Center for Diagnosis and Treatment of Infectious Diseases, State Key Laboratory for Diagnosis and Treatment of Infectious Diseases, The First Affiliated Hospital, College of Medicine, Zhejiang University, Hangzhou, China,
[2] Nursing School, Jiangsu Vocational College of Medicine, Yancheng, China

Edited by:
Haruki Kitazawa,
Tohoku University, Japan

Reviewed by:
Maryam Dadar,
Razi Vaccine and Serum Research Institute, Iran
Ashok Munjal,
Barkatullah University, India

***Correspondence:**
Fengping Liu
11418229@zju.edu.cn;
Lanjuan Li
ljli@zju.edu.cn

†These authors have contributed equally to this work.

Evidence has shown that dysbiosis of the urinary microbiota existed in female type 2 diabetes mellitus (T2DM) patients. Perturbations of intestinal microbiota are linked to proinflammatory chemokine interleukin-8 (IL-8); however, the correlations between urinary microbiota and IL-8 are not well studied. Here, we investigated the associations between the altered urinary microbiota and urinary IL-8 in female T2DM patients. A modified four-tube midstream urine technique was used to collect urine specimens from 70 female T2DM patients and 70 matched healthy controls (HCs). Bacterial genomic DNA from urine specimens was isolated using magnetic beads and the urinary microbiota was assessed using Illumina MiSeq platform targeting on the 16S rRNA gene V3–V4 region. Urinary IL-8 was determined by enzyme linked immunosorbent assay. Subsequently, the T2DM patients were separated into urine IL-8 detectable (WIL8) and undetectable (NIL8) groups, and the composition of urinary microbiota between the two groups was compared. Meanwhile, the levels of IL-8 between the "≥HCs" group (those specific bacterial genera were more than or equal to the HCs) and the "<HCs" group (those specific bacterial genera were less than the HCs) was also compared. Of 70 urine samples from T2DM patients without urinary tract infections, 46 patients had detectable IL-8 in their urine (64.31 ± 70.43 pg/mL), while 24 patients had undetectable IL-8. Compared to the NIL8 group, 11 bacterial genera increased in the WIL8 group, including *Corynebacterium*, *Akkermansia*, *Enterococcus*, etc., whereas 10 genera, such as *Faecalibacterium*, *Bacteroides*, and *Pseudomonas* decreased. One species of *Lactobacillus*, *Lactobacillus iners*, increased obviously in the WIL8 group. The "≥HCs" group showed 17 genera increased and 16 genera decreased. In addition, 18 genera contributed to the presence of urinary IL-8 in T2DM patients, which explained 95.60% of the total variance of urinary microbiota. Our study demonstrated that dysbiosis of the urinary microbiota with several key bacteria was associated with urinary IL-8 in female T2DM patients, which might be useful to explore the interactions between urinary microbiota and inflammatory responses and shed light on novel diagnosis and therapy for urinary microbiota associated with infections in T2DM patients.

Keywords: *Akkermansia*, interleukin-8, *Lactobacillus*, type 2 diabetes mellitus, urinary microbiota

INTRODUCTION

Diabetes mellitus (DM) is a common, serious, and costly disease, which is a major public health issue (1). In recent decades, the global prevalence of DM has increased from 4.7% in 1980 to 8.5% in 2014, while the number of people with diabetes has risen from 108 million in 1980 to 422 million in 2014 (1). In 2012, 1.5 million deaths were directly caused by DM, which has been projected as the seventh leading cause of death in 2030 (1). A previous study has reported that type 2 diabetes mellitus (T2DM) comprises the majority of the people with DM around the world, approximately 90% of DM patients are T2DM patients (2).

Patients with DM are prone to various infections, with the urinary tract as the most common infection site (3, 4). Urinary tract infection (UTI) in hospitalized DM patients was nearly two times higher than that caused by other factors (5). The probability of UTIs in T2DM patients was 60% higher than that in non-DM individuals. A survey showed that the incidence of UTIs in T2DM patients was 46.9 per 1,000 person-years, compared with 29.9 for non-T2DM subjects (6).

Cytokines are small, soluble proteins produced by various cells in response to infections and inflammation (7). Interleukin (IL)-8, a potent proinflammatory chemokine and activator of neutrophils, can be stimulated by lipopolysaccharide, IL-1, and tumor necrosis factor alpha (TNF-α). Previous studies have found that interleukin-8 (IL-8) causes migration of neutrophils to the place of inflammation, leading to pyuria in patients with UTIs (8, 9). Elevated urine levels of IL-8 were detected in febrile children with UTIs compared to children with asymptomatic bacteriuria (7). It is reported that urinary IL-8 can be identified as a potential novel biomarker for the diagnosing of UTIs with 93% sensitivity and 90% specificity (10, 11). Ko et al. found that confirmation of the presence of bioactive IL-8 in urine suggests the participation of IL-8 in UTI, providing additional evidence of the role of IL-8 in inflammation (12). Consequently, the measurement of urinary IL-8 is thought to be a potential bioindicator of the localization and severity of inflammation within the urinary tract (9). Epithelial cell lines secrete interleukin in response to stimulation with bacteria (13). Therefore, it is possible that urinary microbiota modulate the presence and levels of IL-8 in the urinary tract.

Previous studies show that the production of cytokines is related to human microbiota. For instance, Schueller et al. found that Veillonellaceae and Neisseriaceae are the most abundant indicators for high IL-8 status, whereas Erysipelotrichaceae is the most abundant bacteria in low IL-8 subjects in an oral microbiota study (14). One study that explores the cytokine secretion of vaginal epithelial cells induced by commensal bacteria shows that colonization of parallel multilayer cultures with *Staphylococcus epidermidis* resulted in a significant increase in IL-8 relative to non-colonized cultures (15). Cervicovagina those dominated by *Gardnerella* and *Prevotella* induced higher levels of IL-8, whereas *Lactobacillus iners* induced moderate IL-8 secretion and *Lactobacillus crispatus* did not elicit IL-8 secretion (16). On the other hand, IL-8 in combination with other cytokines plays crucial roles in regulating the microbiota. Previous studies have shown that IL-6 and IL-10 play essential roles for the maintenance of intestinal homeostasis and the prevention of colitis (17, 18), while proinflammatory cytokines, such as IL-17 and IL-15 promote intestinal dysbiosis associated with increased susceptibility to colitis (19, 20). In addition, levels of IL-α, IL-β, and IL-6 are able to stimulate the expression of antimicrobial peptides, which help to shape the skin microbiota and have a protective role against potential pathogen attack (21).

Seventy female T2DM patients were recruited in our previous study, since female patients are known to have higher prevalence of UTI than males (22). We explored whether dysbiosis of urinary microbiota was related to T2DM females. We found that both diversity and richness of urinary microbiota declined in T2DM patients. *Actinobacteria*, *Flavobacteriales*, and *Flavobacteria* were recognized as potential distinguishing biomarkers for T2DM patients. Fourteen bacterial genera, including *Lactobacillus*, *Prevotella*, and *Streptococcus*, were enriched in the T2DM patients, while 19 bacterial genera, such as *Pseudomonas*, *Klebsiella*, and *Akkermansia*, decreased. Meanwhile, the relative abundance of *Actinobacteria*, *Lactobacillus*, and *Akkermansia muciniphila* correlated to the levels of fasting blood and urine glucose (23). The correlations between cytokines and microbiota from intestine, oral cavity, vagina, and skin have been extensively investigated, while the relationship between IL-8 and urinary microbiota remains poorly studied. Here, we investigated whether dysbiosis of urinary microbiota was associated with the presence of urinary IL-8, which might be useful to explore the interactions between the urinary microbiota and immune system and shed light on potential novel diagnosis and therapy for UTIs in T2DM patients.

MATERIALS AND METHODS

Recruitment of Subjects

We used an individually matched case–control design in our previous study, with one control for each T2DM patient. The matching attributes were age in years (based on decade) and marital and menstrual status. In this study, 70 female T2DM patients and 70 healthy controls (HCs) were recruited from the First Affiliated Hospital, School of Medicine, Zhejiang University from June 28, 2015 to January 2, 2016. Both groups ranged from 26 to 85 years old. The body mass index (BMI) in the HCs was 23.10 ± 4.49 kg/m^2 and in the T2DM group was 23.87 ± 3.65 kg/m^2. Subjects with the following attributes were excluded: UTIs in the previous month; use of antibiotics, probiotics, prebiotics, or synbiotics in the previous 3 months; unable to complete the questionnaire; menstruation; urinary incontinence; known anatomic urinary tract abnormalities (e.g., cystoceles, hydronephrosis, renal atrophy, or neurogenic bladder); urinary catheter (23). The Ethics Committee of the First Affiliated Hospital, School of Medicine, Zhejiang University approved the study (reference number: 295). Written informed consent based on the Declaration of Helsinki was obtained from each patient before enrollment, and all patients were given informed consent.

Collection of Urinary Specimens and DNA Sequencing

A modified four-tube midstream urine collection technique was used for the first urine of the day, which guaranteed that the real midstream urine was collected. A urine sample was discarded when it was confirmed to be contaminated. Samples were given anonymous identification codes and were transferred immediately to the laboratory and stored at −80°C until DNA extraction. For urinary microbiota analysis, total DNA was extracted from the pellet of urine from tubes 2 and 3, and 40 mL of urine was aspirated from each tube, separated into three sections, and injected into three 15 mL sterile centrifuge tubes. Each tube was pelleted by centrifugation at 4,000 × *g* for 15 min at 4°C. 10 mL of the supernatant was decanted, and the pellet was obtained by centrifugation for 15 min at 4,000 × *g* at 4°C. The pellet was transferred into a 2 mL sterile centrifugation tube which contained 500 μL of lysis buffer. Magnetic bead isolation of genomic DNA from bacteria was applied according to the manufacturer's protocol with minor modifications (Supplementary Material: Protocol of DNA Isolation). The 16S rRNA gene V3–V4 regions were amplified from microbial genomic DNA (forward primer, 5'-ACTCCTACGGGAGGCAGCAG-3'; reverse primer, 5'-GGACTACHVGGGTWTCTAAT-3') (23). Urinary IL-8 was determined by enzyme-linked immunosorbent assay kits (RayBiotech, Inc., Norcross, GA, USA), following the manufacturer's instructions. All measurements were performed in duplicate wells. The lower limit of detection for each assay was 1 pg/mL. Standard curves were generated for every plate and the average 0 standard optical densities were subtracted from the rest of the standards, controls and samples to obtain a corrected concentration.

Bioinformatic Analysis

Sequencing reads were processed using QIIME (version 1.9.0), and included additional quality trimming, demultiplexing, and taxonomic assignments. KW rank sum test and pairwise Wilcoxon test were used for the identification of the different markers, and LDA was used to score each feature in the LEfSe analysis. An index of alpha diversity was calculated with QIIME based on sequence similarity at 97%. Beta diversity was measured by unweighted UniFrac distance, which was also calculated by QIIME. Diversity and richness of bacteria in the urine specimens were calculated using several estimates. These consisted of the level of operational taxonomic units (which provides a measure of bacterial richness), Chao1 (which is also an estimate of bacteria richness) and the Shannon and Simpson indices (which are measures of bacterial diversity). The output file was further analyzed using Statistical Analysis of Metagenomic Profiles software package (version 2.1.3) (24). Sequence data from this study are deposited in the GenBank Sequence Read Archive with accession number SRP 087709.

Grouping

From the concentration of urinary IL-8, the T2DM patients were separated into "with IL-8" (WIL8) group, indicating there was detectable IL-8 in their urine; and "no IL-8" (NIL8) group, indicating there was no detectable IL-8 in their urine. Our previous study showed that the relative abundance of 33 bacterial genera in urine were significantly different between the HCs and the T2DM patients (Figure S1 in Supplementary Material) (23). After obtaining the results of differences in relative abundance of bacterial genera in urine between the HCs and T2DM patients ($p < 0.05$) (23), the patients were divided into two groups: "≥HCs" group, indicating relative abundance of bacterial genera were not less than the HCs; and "<HCs" group, indicating the relative abundance of bacterial genera were less than the HCs. Thereafter, the levels of IL-8 in the "≥HCs" group and "<HCs" group were compared.

Statistical Analysis

Statistical analysis was performed using the SPSS data analysis program (version 21.0) and Statistical Analysis of Metagenomic Profiles software. For continuous variables, independent *t*-test, Welch's *t*-test, and White's non-parametric *t*-test were applied. For categorical variables between groups, either the Pearson chi-square or Fisher's exact test was used depending on assumption validity. For taxon among subgroups, ANOVA test was applied (Tukey–Kramer was used in *Post hoc* test, effect size was Eta-squared) with Benjamini–Hochberg FDP false discovery rate correction (25, 26). All tests of significance were two-sided, and $p < 0.05$, or corrected $p < 0.05$, was considered statistically significant. In addition, stepwise multiple linear regression analysis was used to determine the factors that significantly affected urine microbiota in T2DM patients. All potential variables ($p < 0.05$) were entered into the analysis.

RESULTS

Characteristics of T2DM Patients in NIL8 and WIL8 Groups

There were significant differences in age, BMI, urine pH, urine white blood cells, urine leukocyte esterase, urine protein, urine glucose, and urine nitrite between T2DM patients with detectable IL-8 in their urine (WIL8) and those without detectable urine IL-8 (NIL8) ($p < 0.05$, **Table 1**).

Sequencing Data and Concentrations of Urinary IL-8

Briefly, we obtained 3,981,519 reads for microbiota analysis, which accounted for 76.93% of the valid reads. The mean read length was 438 bp (range 423–486 bp). The Good's coverage estimator was 98% (23).

The average urinary IL-8 concentration in the 70 patients was 42.26 ± 64.66 pg/mL. Urinary IL-8 was found in 46 samples and concentration was 64.31 ± 70.43 pg/mL. No significant difference was found in Shannon and Simpson indices between the NIL8 and WIL8 group ($p > 0.05$, Table S1 in Supplementary Material). However, principal coordinate analysis (PCoA) indicated that most of the samples from NIL8 and WIL8 groups could be clustered together (**Figure 1**).

Urinary IL-8 Associated Biomarkers

To identify the specific bacterial taxa associated with urinary IL-8, the urinary microbiota in the WIL8 and NIL8 groups were compared using LEfSe. A cladogram representative of the structure of the urinary microbiota and their predominant bacteria is shown in **Figure 2**. The greatest differences in taxa between

TABLE 1 | Descriptive data of participants.

Parameter	Value for cohort (n^a)^b or statistic		p-Value^c
	NIL8 (n = 24)	WIL8 (n = 46)	
Age (years)	59.25 ± 11.06	65.78 ± 13.58	0.046
Duration of type 2 diabetes mellitus (T2DM)	7.63 ± 5.67	10.89 ± 8.11	0.083
UTIs in the last year	0.57 ± 1.20	0.70 ± 1.11	0.656
Body mass index (kg/m^2)	22.46 ± 3.26	24.61 ± 3.65	0.018
Menstrual status [no. (%)]			0.955
Premenopausal	19 (79.17)	38 (90.94)	
Postmenopausal	3 (12.50)	6 (13.04)	
Hysterectomy	2 (8.33)	3 (6.52)	
Fasting blood glucose (mmol/L)	7.81 ± 2.33	7.84 ± 2.39	0.959
Urine pH	5.58 ± 0.55	5.92 ± 0.63	0.028
Urine white blood cells	2.27 ± 2.93	11.38 ± 24.25	0.015
Urine leucocyte esterase [no. (%)]			0.000
Negative	23 (95.83)	34 (73.91)	
Positive	1 (4.17)	12 (26.09)	
Urine protein [no. (%)]			0.000
Negative	23 (95.83)	33 (71.74)	
Positive	1 (4.17)	13 (28.26)	
Urine culture [no. (%)]			0.094
Negative	24 (100.00)	41 (89.13)	
Positive	0 (0.00)	5 (10.87)	
Urine glucose [no. (%)]			0.000
Negative	21 (87.50)	35 (79.09)	
Positive	3 (12.50)	11 (23.91)	
Urine nitrite [no. (%)]			0.000
Negative	24 (100.00)	40 (86.97)	
Positive	0 (0.00)	6 (13.04)	

NIL8, no interleukin-8 (IL-8) detected in urine samples from T2DM patients; WIL8, IL-8 detected in urine samples; UTIs, urinary tract infections.

[a]*No. of subjects.*

[b]*Values are mean ± SD or no. (%).*

[c]*Pearson's chi-square and Fisher's exact tests were used with categorical variables. Independent t-test was used with continuous variables.*

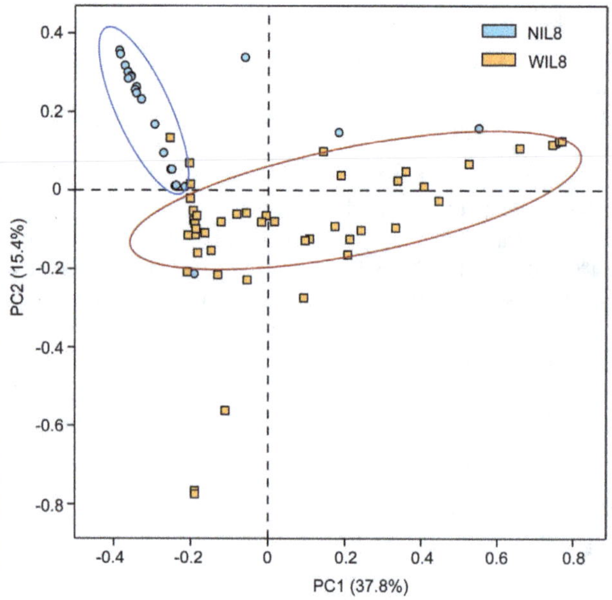

FIGURE 1 | Principal coordinate analysis (PCoA) plot. PCoA plot of the urinary microbiota based on the unweighted UniFrac metric. Blue and yellow dots represent NIL8 and WIL8 specimens, respectively.

two groups are displayed. Bifidobacteriaceae, *Shuttleworthia*, *Thermus*, Thermales, and Thermaceae could be used as potential distinguishing biomarkers between the WIL8 and NIL8 groups.

Associations between Urinary Microbiota and IL-8

At the phylum level, *Proteobacteria* was significantly higher in the WIL8 group than the NIL8 group, while Bacteroidetes was dramatically decreased in the WIL8 group ($p < 0.05$, **Figure 3**). At the genus level, 11 genera were enriched in the WIL8 group compared to the NIL8 group, including *Shuttleworthia*, *Mobiluncus*, *Peptoniphilus*, *Corynebacterium*, *Thermus*, *Gemella*, *Enterococcus*, *Acinetobacter*, *Akkermansia*, *Aquaspirillum*, and *Geobacillus*, while 10 genera were decreased, including *Faecalibacterium*, *Megamonas*, *Comamonas*, *Bacteroides*, *Coprococcus*, *Sutterella*, *Pseudomonas*, *Phascolarctobacterium*, *Prevotella*, and *Parabacteroides* ($p < 0.05$, **Figure 4**). Five bacterial species, *Streptococcus anginosus*, *Acinetobacter rhizosphaerae*, *Acinetobacter schindleri*, *L. iners*, and *A. muciniphila*, showed a significant increase in the WIL8 group than the NIL8 group, while another five species showed a significant decrease, including *Prevotella copri*, *Faecalibacterium prausnitzii*, *Prevotella stercorea*, and *Bacteroides uniformis*, and *Coprococcus eutactus* ($p < 0.05$, Figure S2 in Supplementary Material). *L. iners* dramatically increased in the WIL8 group. In addition, the *Lactobacillus* species including *Lactobacillus mucosae* and *Lactobacillus reuteri* showed a trend increase in the WIL8 group, whereas *Lactobacillus ruminis* showed a trend decrease, but these species did not reach statistical differences (Figure S3 in Supplementary Material).

Interestingly, 17 bacterial genera were enriched in the "≥HCs" group, while 16 genera were enriched in the "<HCs" group. Specifically, those patients with *Bacteroides* "≥HCs" group, *Klebsiella* "≥HCs" group, *Pseudomonas* "≥HCs" group and *Akkermansia* "≥HCs" group had higher concentrations of urinary IL-8, while those patients with *Lactobacillus* "<HCs" group, *Megamonas* "<HCs" group and *Microbacterium* "<HCs" group had higher levels of IL-8 (**Figure 5**).

Multiple regression analysis showed that the genera *Ruminococcus*, *Limnohabitans*, *Cytophaga*, *Providencia*, *Anaerotruncus*, *Giesbergeria*, *Solitalea*, *Actinomyces*, *Meiothermus*, *Luteibacter*, *Flavisolibacter*, *Dysgonomonas*, *Ureaplasma*, *Exiguobacterium*, *Zoogloea*, *Cloacibacterium*, *Lactobacillus*, and *Dokdonella* significantly affected urinary microbiota in T2DM patients and explained 95.60% of the total variance of urinary microbiota in this population (**Table 2**). In addition, the relative abundance of *Ruminococcus* was significantly positively associated with the levels of urinary IL-8 (Figure S4 in Supplementary Material).

DISCUSSION

Type 2 diabetes mellitus patients are prone to a higher occurrence of certain infections compared with the healthy population (27).

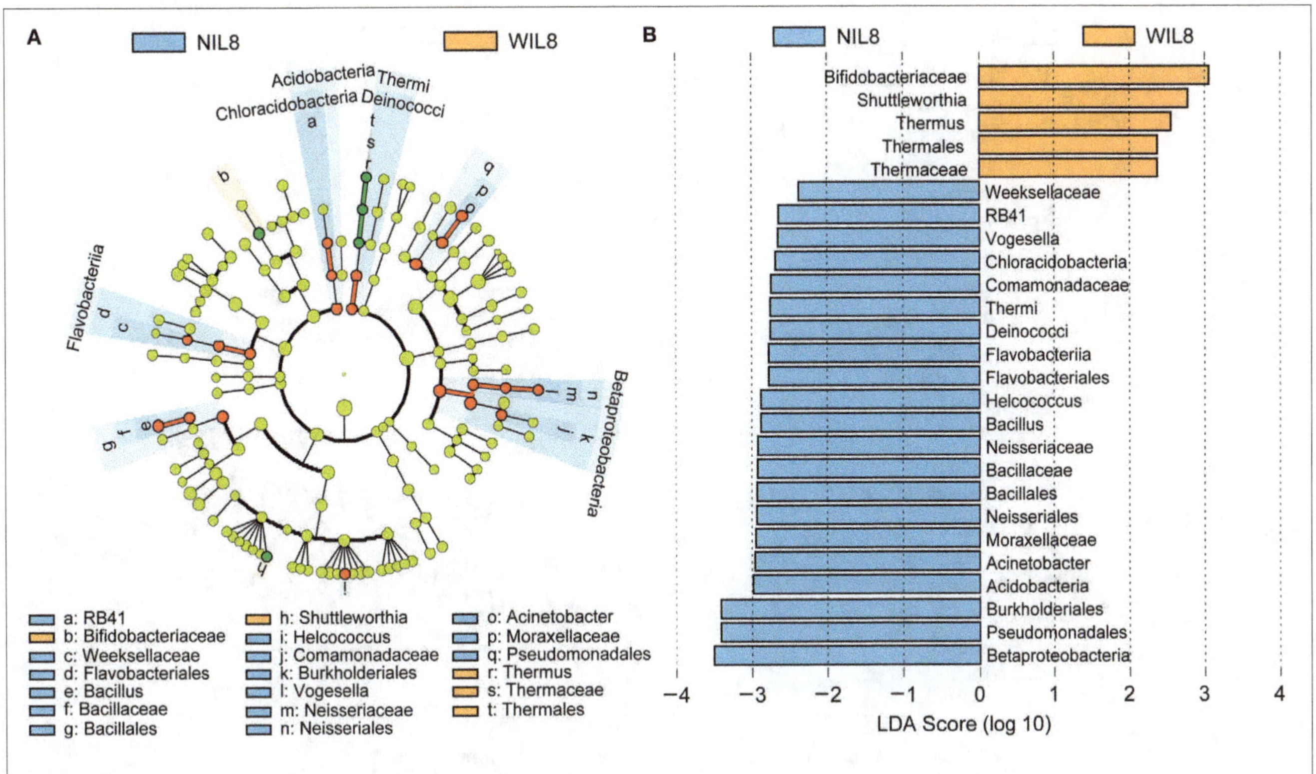

FIGURE 2 | Cladogram showing differentially abundant taxa of urinary microbiota in type 2 diabetes mellitus patients. **(A)** LEfSe cladogram showed the most differentially abundant taxa between WIL8 and NIL8 groups. Taxonomic cladogram obtained from LEfSe analysis of 16S rDNA sequences. Taxa enriched for WIL8 in yellow; NIL8 enriched taxa in blue. The size of each dot is proportional to its effect size. **(B)** Only taxa meeting an LDA threshold > 2.0 are shown.

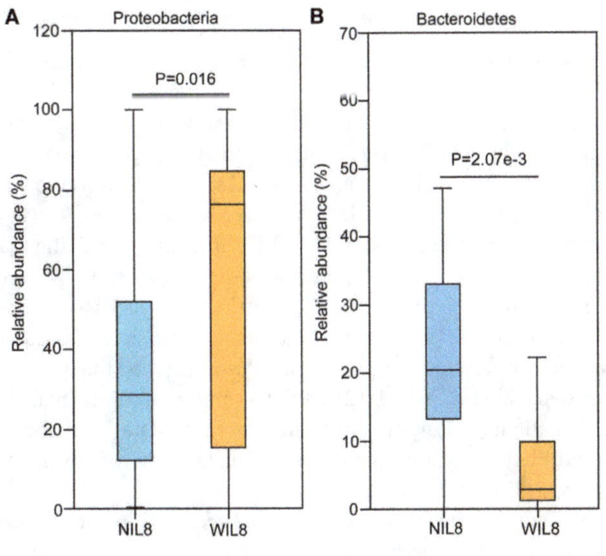

FIGURE 3 | Phylum-level operational taxonomic units different between NIL8 and WIL8 groups. STAMP software was used to calculate the bacterial phylum proportions in the two groups: Proteobacteria **(A)** and Bacteroidetes **(B)**. Welch's *t*-test was used to compare abundance at the bacterial phylum level for NIL8 urine samples and WIL8 samples. The different phyla were assigned only to those presenting a minimum variation at a significant level [p (corrected) < 0.05].

The hospitalization rate for UTIs caused by diabetes is over twice those caused by other factors (5). Defects in maintaining the integrity of mucosal barriers can result in systemic endotoxemia that contributes to chronic low-grade inflammation (28). Recent advances in understanding the pathophysiology of T2DM have established the involvement of low-grade inflammation due to an increased production of proinflammatory cytokines (29, 30). This study focused on the correlations between urinary microbiota and the proinflammatory chemokine IL-8 for the first time, with the aim of providing new insights on host–urinary microbiota interactions in T2DM patients.

Urine specimens from 46 T2DM patients had detectable levels of IL-8 (WIL8 group), while IL-8 was not detected in 24 T2DM patients (NIL8 group). The alpha diversity indices, such as Shannon and Simpson, did not show significant differences between the NIL8 and WIL8 groups, indicating that bacterial diversity was not affected by the presence of IL-8 in urine. The beta diversity index such as PCoA analysis indicated that most of the patients with urinary IL-8 formed their own cluster, which reflected a contribution from IL-8 was prominent in differentiating urinary microbiota in groups.

Interestingly, the distinguishing biomarker, Bifidobacteriaceae, which is associated with diabetic patients with higher BMIs (31), had a higher abundance in WIL8 subjects, and those patients also had higher BMIs than NIL8 participants in our study. Elfeky et al.

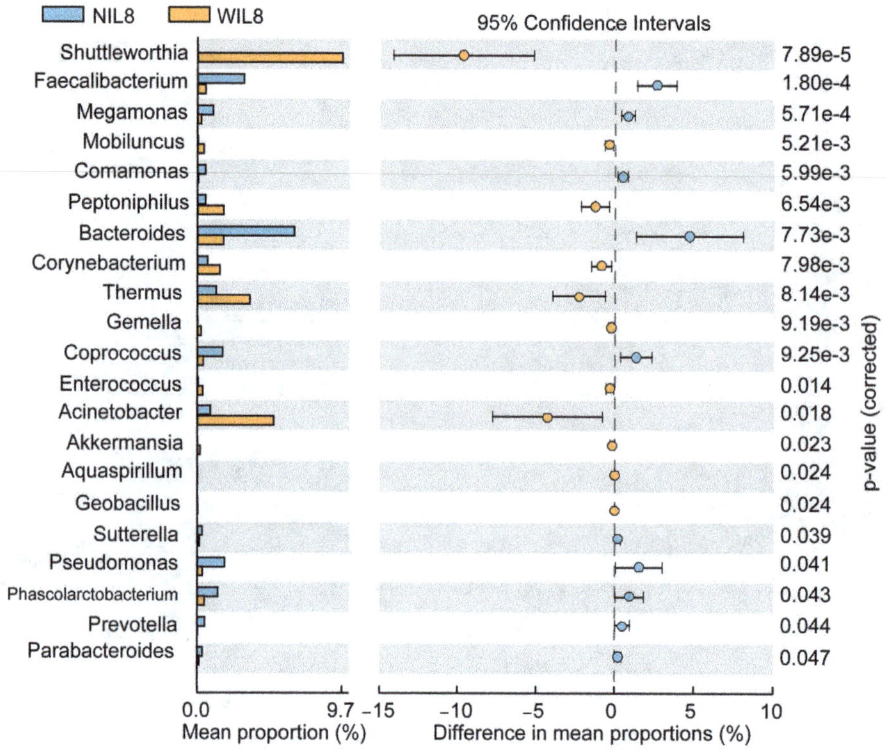

FIGURE 4 | Genus-level operational taxonomic units different between NIL8 and WIL8 groups. STAMP software was used to calculate the genus proportions in the two groups. Welch's *t*-test was used to compare abundance at the genus level for NIL8 and WIL8 specimens. The different genera were assigned only to those presenting a minimum variation at a significant level [*p* (corrected) < 0.05].

reported that exosomes increased IL-8 release from endothelial cells, and the effect was even higher when exosomes were isolated from obese women compared to lean subjects (32). Thus, BMI might play a role in regulating IL-8 levels, and subsequently IL-8 modulates the abundance of urinary Bifidobacteriaceae.

A higher abundance of *Proteobacteria* was found in the WIL8 group in this study. Fricke et al. and Rani et al. have demonstrated that *Proteobacteria* in urine decreased in patients that had renal transplantation and were exposed to high dose immunosuppressant (33, 34), during which cytokine production might be inhibited by the suppressing T cells induced by administrating the immunosuppressant. In addition, a recent study on intestinal microbiota reported that *Proteobacteria* was detected in feces of rats at the peak of experimental autoimmune encephalomyelitis (35). Demmer et al. demonstrated that inflammation explained 30–98% of the observed associations between levels of microbiota in a subgingival microbiome study, and the percentages of the overall phyla associations with inflammation were 27% for *Proteobacteria* (36). The above findings illustrated that *Proteobacteria* might be correlated to the onset or development of the inflammatory process. It is demonstrated that a rise in species belonging to the phylum *Proteobacteria* may have a larger impact on host autoimmunity which may make a protein molecule non-functional and thereby may be involved in the onset of inflammatory disorders, including diabetes (37).

The relative abundance of Bacteroidetes was lowered in the WIL8 group. A similar alteration was found in a study that showed that patients with urgency urinary incontinence had decreased abundance of Bacteroidetes compared to HCs (38). The patients suffering from renal transplantation and successive immunosuppressing therapy also had lowered levels of Bacteroidetes (34). Bacteroidetes can suppress enteric inflammation, suggesting that members of the phylum play a similar role in regulating the level of IL-8 in urinary tract system. Interestingly, there was a noticeable decrease in the phylum Bacteroidetes in newly diagnosed diabetics (39), and in our present study, we observed that patients with detectable IL-8 had T2DM for a longer duration than the NIL8 patients, suggesting that in the early state of diabetes, Bacteroidetes play a minor role in regulating the inflammatory process in diabetes.

We found that the genus of *Corynebacterium* in the urinary microbiota was enriched in WIL8 patients. A recent study reported that the prevalence of *Corynebacterium* correlated with concentrations of IL-6 and C-reaction protein in cancer patients (40). In our present study, the WIL8 group had a higher level of urine white blood cells, more leukocyte esterase and urine nitrite-positive cases, which indicated an inflammatory reaction was present in the urinary tract system, although no UTI was diagnosed currently. This might suggest that an inflammatory reaction and its correlation with urinary microbiota

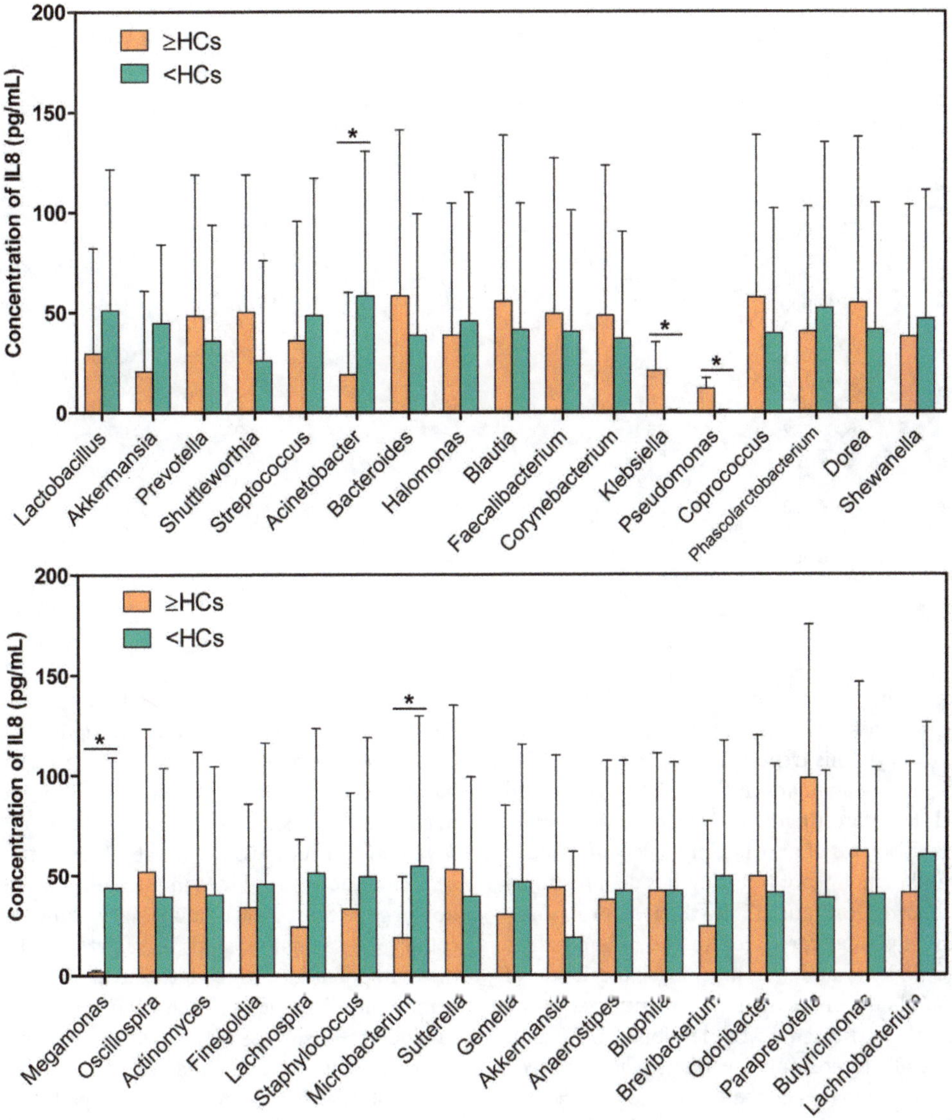

FIGURE 5 | Comparison of interleukin-8 (IL-8) levels between genus "≥HCs" group and "<HCs" group. SPSS software was used to calculate the difference in IL-8 concentrations between bacterial genus "≥HCs" group and "<HCs" group. "≥HCs" group indicates the relative abundance of a bacterial genus in this group was not less than the healthy controls (HCs), and "<HCs" group indicates relative abundance of a bacterial genus was less than the HCs. Asterisks indicate significant differences between the two groups ($p < 0.05$).

is established before a patient is diagnosed with UTI and the presence of obvious clinical manifestation, thus early detection of the interaction of the inflammatory response with urinary microbiota is valuable for clinicians to diagnose and treat UTIs in the early stages.

A higher abundance of *A. muciniphila* was correlated with a higher concentration of IL-8. Moreover, *Akkermansia* in the "≥HCs" group had a higher level of IL-8 than the "<HC" group. An *in vitro* model demonstrated that *A. muciniphila* could induce IL-8 production by enterocytes at cell concentrations 100-fold higher than those for *Escherichia coli* (41). Another study demonstrated that mice with low levels of inflammation were enriched for *Akkermansia* (42). Surprisingly, the patients from the WIL8 group had higher levels of urine leukocyte esterase and nitrite than the NIL8 patients, suggesting *Akkermansia* might play important roles in protecting patients away from UTIs, since patients in either WIL8 or NIL8 groups were not currently diagnosed with UTIs while they were recruited to the present study.

Lin et al. reported that the overgrowth of *Enterococcus* in diabetic mice was accompanied with increased IL-1β and TNF-α expression from Kupffer cells in intestine (43). Interestingly, our data indicated that *Enterococcus* was dramatically increased in the WIL8 group. Therefore, the abundance of *Enterococcus* might be regulating the level of cytokines in diabetic populations. Nienhouse et al. reported that *Pseudomonas* was enriched in positive urine culture specimens comparing to negative specimens.

TABLE 2 | Predictors of urine IL-8 by stepwise regression (*n* = 70, where *n* is number of patients).

Independent variables	Unstandardized coefficient		Standardized coefficient	*t*	*p*-Value	*F*	*p*-Value
	B	SE	β				
Constant	7.610	3.204		2.375	0.021	57.478	0.000
Ruminococcus	9.051	0.749	0.380	12.085	0.000		
Limnohabitans	4242.295	353.48	0.360	12.002	0.000		
Cytophaga	4204.23	330.817	0.481	12.709	0.000		
Providencia	13214.688	1239.622	0.319	10.66	0.000		
Anaerotruncus	800.311	71.947	0.333	11.124	0.000		
Giesbergeria	296.428	29.784	0.355	9.953	0.000		
Solitalea	849.692	74.052	0.352	11.474	0.000		
Actinomyces	24.412	4.197	0.205	5.816	0.000		
Meiothermus	20.241	2.496	0.249	8.110	0.000		
Luteibacter	2307.744	347.269	0.199	6.645	0.000		
Flavisolibacter	−105.620	24.71	−0.155	−4.274	0.000		
Dysgonomonas	5080.332	1180.355	0.144	4.304	0.000		
Ureaplasma	13.178	2.615	0.162	5.039	0.000		
Exiguobacterium	−258.281	67.919	−0.15	−3.803	0.000		
Zoogloea	−3614.663	807.044	−0.147	−4.479	0.000		
Cloacibacterium	−76.561	23.057	−0.105	−3.320	0.002		
Lactobacillus	0.304	0.092	0.107	3.292	0.002		
Dokdonella	−1478.647	617.393	−0.075	−2.395	0.020		

Also, *Pseudomonas* might cause the most severe inflammation which was accompanied by an increase in the number of inflammatory cells and IL-6 (44). This trend was similar to our study, in which patients with *Pseudomonas* in the "≥HCs" group had a higher level of IL-8. Interestingly, *Pseudomonas aeruginosa* were the predominant isolates of non-healing ulcers in diabetic foot patients (45), and diabetic foot infection has demonstrated higher concentrations of IL-6 and IL-1β than controls (46). Thus, *Pseudomonas* might be correlated to the inflammatory process in diabetic patients and might regulate the levels of cytokines. *Klebsiella*, being a recognized uropathogen (47), was enriched in female participants who developed UTIs after pelvic floor surgery (48). Interestingly, patients with *Klebsiella* in the "≥HCs" group had a higher concentration of IL-8. Huang et al. reported that diabetic patients was associated with relapse of recurrent bacteremia caused by *Klebsiella pneumonia* (49), suggesting that this bacteria is responsible for the inflammation process in diabetes. *S. anginosus* was also increased in the WIL8 group compared to the NIL8 group. A similar result was reported in the study conducted by Price et al., in which *S. anginosus* increased in subjects with UTIs compared to the non-UTI participants (50).

Members of the genus *Lactobacillus* exhibit probiotic effects in epithelial attachment, pathogen inhibition, and intestinal immunomodulation (51–53). However, their relative abundance was increased in the WIL8 group compared to the NIL8 group. Furthermore, *Lactobacillus* was one of the predictors of the presence of IL-8 in urine in our study. It was reported that *Lactobacillus* showed a rise in interstitial cystitis patients than HCs (54). However, a recent study reported that there were no associations between the presence of *Lactobacillus* and urinary cytokine levels in patients with interstitial cystitis (55). Therefore, *Lactobacillus* might play distinctive roles in regulating cytokine production in urine in different health statuses. *L. iners*, which may induce moderate IL-8 secretion and has moderate proinflammatory activity in the cervicovaginal bacterial community (16), was also increased in the WIL8 group. *L. mucosae* which has been demonstrated to possess IL-6 induction ability in macrophages (56), was found enriched in the WIL8 group. *L. reuteri* can suppress intestinal inflammation in a trinitrobenzene sulfonic acid-induced mouse colitis model *via* downregulation of gene expression of mucosal cytokine IL-6 and IL-1β in the colon (57). In another study, *L. reuteri* could produce molecules that had potential anti-TNF-α activity *in vitro* and antimicrobial compounds in diabetes (58, 59). Furthermore, intake of *L. reuteri* can increase insulin secretion, which might be due to augmented incretin release (60). Low-grade chronic inflammation is accepted as an internal metabolic adaptation pathway in T2DM, so the increased levels of members of the genus *Lactobacillus* might be believed to be players in controlling the development of inflammation in diabetes. Moreover, patients with the *Lactobacillus* "≥HCs" group had lower levels of IL-8 than the "<HCs" group, which also demonstrated that *Lactobacillus* contributed to inhibit the inflammatory process in the bladder.

In total, 18 bacterial genera contributed to the presence of IL-8 in the urine of T2DM patients. Most of these genera have not been reported by human urinary microbiota studies, except for *Actinomyces* (61) and *Lactobacillus* (47, 50, 61–65). Furthermore, very few of these genera have been reported in terms of their correlations with inflammatory cytokines. Interestingly, the abundance of *Ruminococcus* was positively correlated with the concentration of urinary IL-8, and can be considered as an important contributor to the presence of IL-8 as well. *Ruminococcus* spp. could induce dominant effector *ex vivo* mesenteric lymph node T-helper 17 responses (66), which is correlated to inducing the expression of IL-8 (67). In addition, *Ruminococcus* was more abundant in diabetic mice, and correlated negatively with delayed diabetes onset age (68). Thus, *Ruminococcus* might play a role in diabetes development by regulating the level of cytokines. *Actinomyces* spp. has been demonstrated to induce inflammatory cytokines by researchers (69), which were linked to the presence of urinary IL-8 in the present study suggesting therapy for inflammatory development in diabetes involving urinary microbiota should take a considerable to the 18 bacteria included in multiple analysis model.

There were several limitations in our study. First, the sample size in the WIL8 and NIL8 groups was not equal, which might affect the reliability of the results. Second, although all participants were not currently diagnosed with UTIs, we could not completely rule out the influence caused by previous occurrence of UTIs since it takes 6 months for diabetic patients to revert to normal glomerular filtration rate trends after an infection is cured (70); this might affect the growth environment of urinary microbiota and urine IL-8.

CONCLUSION

To our knowledge, this is the first study focused on the associations between urinary microbiota and concentrations of urine IL-8 in T2DM patients. The bacterial community showed differences in the WIL8 and the NIL8 groups, and the concentrations of IL-8 were different in the "≥HCs" group and "<HCs" group. Findings from this study indicated that urine IL-8 is interplayed with urinary microbiota among T2DM patients. Future studies should focus on how the urinary microbiota affects the inflammatory cytokine excretion in the urinary tract, which might be conducive to explore novel therapies to regulate inflammation in T2DM patients.

AUTHOR CONTRIBUTIONS

LL and FL conceived and designed the study. ZL generated the sequencing data. FL and SL collected the samples. FL and YC conducted urine cultures and the urinalysis. FL extracted the bacterial DNA. ZL and FL analyzed the data, carried out the computational analysis, interpreted the data, and drafted the manuscript.

ACKNOWLEDGMENTS

The authors gratefully acknowledge the volunteers who participated in our study.

MATERIALS AND METHODS

Protocol of DNA Isolation

The tube was placed in liquid nitrogen for 1 min, and transferred into a water bath at 65°C for 5 min, with vigorous mixing. This last process was repeated three times with a final bath for 30 min. 50 μL *Agencourt AMPure XP* (Beckman Coulter, USA) was added to 100 μL of the urine pellet, vortexed for 30 s, and incubated for 5 min at room temperature. The tube was placed into a magnetic separator for 5 min, and DNA was bound to magnetic beads which were drawn to the wall of the microcentrifuge tube. The supernatant was carefully removed without disrupting the magnetic beads. The sample was washed twice with 200 μL 80% ethanol for 30 s, being placed on a magnet separator between each washing. The purified DNA was eluted with 50 μL ddH_2O for 1 min. The beads, now released from the DNA, were collected with the magnet. The DNA-containing supernatant was transferred to a clean tube.

FIGURE S1 | Genus-level operational taxonomic units different between healthy controls (HCs) and type 2 diabetes mellitus (T2DM) patients. Welch's *t*-test was used to compare the abundance at the bacterial genus level between HCs and T2DM patients. The different genera were assigned only to those presenting a minimum variation at a significant level [p (corrected) < 0.05]. H and Pt represent HCs and T2DM patients, respectively.

FIGURE S2 | Species-level operational taxonomic units different between NIL8 and WIL8 groups. STAMP software was used to calculate the species proportions in the two groups. Welch's *t*-test was used to compare abundance at the species level for NIL8 and WIL8 specimens. The different species were assigned only to those presenting a minimum variation at a significant level [p (corrected) < 0.05].

FIGURE S3 | Differences of *Lactobacillus* spp. between NIL8 and WIL8 groups. STAMP software was used to calculate the proportions of *Lactobacillus* spp. in NIL8 and WIL8 groups. Welch's *t*-test was used to compare abundance of *Lactobacillus* spp. level for NIL8 and WIL8 specimens. The different levels were assigned only to those presenting a minimum variation at a significant level [p (corrected) < 0.05].

FIGURE S4 | Correlation between the relative abundance of *Ruminococcus* and the concentration of urinary IL-8. A correlation analysis was carried out and a significance level of $p < 0.05$ was used.

REFERENCES

1. World Health Organization. *Global Report on Diabetes*. Geneva, Switzerland: WHO Press (2016).
2. Rubino F. Is type 2 diabetes an operable intestinal disease? A provocative yet reasonable hypothesis. *Diabetes Care* (2008) 31:S290–6. doi:10.2337/dc08-s271
3. Shah BR, Hux JE. Quantifying the risk of infectious diseases for people with diabetes. *Diabetes Care* (2003) 26(2):510–3. doi:10.2337/diacare.26.2.510
4. Boyko EJ, Fihn SD, Scholes D, Abraham L, Monsey B. Risk of urinary tract infection and asymptomatic bacteriuria among diabetic and nondiabetic postmenopausal women. *Am J Epidemiol* (2005) 161(6):557–64. doi:10.1093/aje/kwi078
5. Korbel L, Spencer JD. Diabetes mellitus and infection: an evaluation of hospital utilization and management costs in the United States. *J Diabetes Complications* (2015) 29(2):192–5. doi:10.1016/j.jdiacomp.2014.11.005
6. Hirji I, Guo ZC, Andersson SW, Hammar N, Gomez-Caminero A. Incidence of urinary tract infection among patients with type 2 diabetes in the UK general practice research database (GPRD). *J Diabetes Complications* (2012) 26(6):513–6. doi:10.1016/j.jdiacomp.2012.06.008
7. Krzemien G, Szmigielska A, Turczyn A, Panczyk-Tomaszewska M. Urine interleukin-6, interleukin-8 and transforming growth factor beta1 in infants with urinary tract infection and asymptomatic bacteriuria. *Cent Eur J Immunol* (2016) 41(3):260–7. doi:10.5114/ceji.2016.63125
8. Gurgoze MK, Akarsu S, Yilmaz E, Godekmerdan A, Akca Z, Ciftci I, et al. Proinflammatory cytokines and procalcitonin in children with acute pyelonephritis. *Pediatr Nephrol* (2005) 20(10):1445–8. doi:10.1007/s00467-005-1941-6

9. Gokce I, Alpay H, Biyikli N, Unluguzel G, Dede F, Topuzoglu A. Urinary levels of interleukin-6 and interleukin-8 in patients with vesicoureteral reflux and renal parenchymal scar. *Pediatr Nephrol* (2010) 25(5):905–12. doi:10.1007/s00467-009-1396-2
10. Rao WH, Evans GS, Finn A. The significance of interleukin 8 in urine. *Arch Dis Child* (2001) 85(3):256–62. doi:10.1136/adc.85.3.256
11. Nanda N, Juthani-Mehta M. Novel biomarkers for the diagnosis of urinary tract infection-a systematic review. *Biomark Insights* (2009) 4:111–21.
12. Ko YC, Mukaida N, Ishiyama S, Tokue A, Kawai T, Matsushima K, et al. Elevated interleukin-8 levels in the urine of patients with urinary-tract infections. *Infect Immun* (1993) 61(4):1307–14.
13. Hedges S, Svensson M, Svanborg C. Interleukin-6 response of epithelial cell lines to bacterial stimulation in vitro. *Infect Immun* (1992) 60(4):1295–301.
14. Schueller K, Riva A, Pfeiffer S, Berry D, Somoza V. Members of the oral microbiota are associated with IL-8 release by gingival epithelial cells in healthy individuals. *Front Microbiol* (2017) 8:416. doi:10.3389/Fmicb.2017.00416
15. Rose WA, Mcgowin CL, Spagnuolo RA, Eaves-Pyles TD, Popov VL, Pyles RB. Commensal bacteria modulate innate immune responses of vaginal epithelial cell multilayer cultures. *PLoS One* (2012) 7(3):e32728. doi:10.1371/journal.pone.0032728
16. Anahtar MN, Byrne EH, Doherty KE, Bowman BA, Yamamoto HS, Soumillon M, et al. Cervicovaginal bacteria are a major modulator of host inflammatory responses in the female genital tract. *Immunity* (2015) 42(5):965–76. doi:10.1016/j.immuni.2015.04.019
17. Morrison PJ, Ballantyne SJ, Kullberg MC. Interleukin-23 and T helper 17-type responses in intestinal inflammation: from cytokines to T-cell plasticity. *Immunology* (2011) 133(4):397–408. doi:10.1111/j.1365-2567.2011.03454.x
18. Kole A, Maloy KJ. Control of intestinal inflammation by interleukin-10. *Curr Top Microbiol Immunol* (2014) 380:19–38. doi:10.1007/978-3-662-43492-5_2
19. Puel A, Cypowyj S, Bustamante J, Wright JF, Liu LY, Lim HK, et al. Chronic mucocutaneous candidiasis in humans with inborn errors of interleukin-17 immunity. *Science* (2011) 332(6025):65–8. doi:10.1126/science.1200439
20. Meisel M, Mayassi T, Fehlner-Peach H, Koval JC, O'brien SL, Hinterleitner R, et al. Interleukin-15 promotes intestinal dysbiosis with butyrate deficiency associated with increased susceptibility to colitis. *ISME J* (2017) 11(1):15–30. doi:10.1038/ismej.2016.114
21. Percoco G, Merle C, Jaouen T, Ramdani Y, Benard M, Hillion M, et al. Antimicrobial peptides and pro-inflammatory cytokines are differentially regulated across epidermal layers following bacterial stimuli. *Exp Dermatol* (2013) 22(12):800–6. doi:10.1111/exd.12259
22. Sewify M, Nair S, Warsame S, Murad M, Alhubail A, Behbehani K, et al. Prevalence of urinary tract infection and antimicrobial susceptibility among diabetic patients with controlled and uncontrolled glycemia in Kuwait. *J Diabetes Res* (2016) 2016:Article ID 65732157. doi:10.1155/2016/6573215
23. Liu FP, Ling ZX, Xiao YH, Lv LX, Yang Q, Wang BH, et al. Dysbiosis of urinary microbiota is positively correlated with type 2 diabetes mellitus. *Oncotarget* (2017) 8(3):3798–810. doi:10.18632/oncotarget.14028
24. Parks DH, Tyson GW, Hugenholtz P, Beiko RG. STAMP: statistical analysis of taxonomic and functional profiles. *Bioinformatics* (2014) 30(21):3123–4. doi:10.1093/bioinformatics/btu494
25. White JR, Nagarajan N, Pop M. Statistical methods for detecting differentially abundant features in clinical metagenomic samples. *PLoS Comput Biol* (2009) 5(4):e1000352. doi:10.1371/journal.pcbi.1000352
26. Parks DH, Beiko RG. Identifying biologically relevant differences between metagenomic communities. *Bioinformatics* (2010) 26(6):715–21. doi:10.1093/bioinformatics/btq041
27. Wilke T, Boettger B, Berg B, Groth A, Mueller S, Botteman M, et al. Epidemiology of urinary tract infections in type 2 diabetes mellitus patients: an analysis based on a large sample of 456,586 German T2DM patients. *J Diabetes Complications* (2015) 29(8):1015–23. doi:10.1016/j.jdiacomp.2015.08.021
28. Wang XT, Ota N, Manzanillo P, Kates L, Zavala-Solorio J, Eidenschenk C, et al. Interleukin-22 alleviates metabolic disorders and restores mucosal immunity in diabetes. *Nature* (2014) 514(7521):237–41. doi:10.1038/nature13564
29. Donath MY, Shoelson SE. Type 2 diabetes as an inflammatory disease. *Nat Rev Immunol* (2011) 11(2):98–107. doi:10.1038/nri2925
30. Nunemaker CS. Considerations for defining cytokine dose, duration, and milieu that are appropriate for modeling chronic low-grade inflammation in type 2 diabetes. *J Diabetes Res* (2016) 2016:2846570. doi:10.1155/2016/2846570
31. Long J, Cai Q, Steinwandel M, Hargreaves MK, Bordenstein SR, Blot WJ, et al. Association of oral microbiome with type 2 diabetes risk. *J Periodontal Res* (2017) 52(3):636–43. doi:10.1111/jre.12432
32. Elfeky O, Longo S, Lai A, Rice GE, Salomon C. Influence of maternal BMI on the exosomal profile during gestation and their role on maternal systemic inflammation. *Placenta* (2017) 50:60–9. doi:10.1016/j.placenta.2016.12.020
33. Fricke WF, Maddox C, Song Y, Bromberg JS. Human microbiota characterization in the course of renal transplantation. *Am J Transplant* (2014) 14(2):416–27. doi:10.1111/ajt.12588
34. Rani A, Ranjan R, Mcgee HS, Andropolis KE, Panchal DV, Hajjiri Z, et al. Urinary microbiome of kidney transplant patients reveals dysbiosis with potential for antibiotic resistance. *Transl Res* (2017) 181:59–70. doi:10.1016/j.trsl.2016.08.008
35. Stanisavljevic S, Lukic J, Sokovic S, Mihajlovic S, Mostarica Stojkovic M, Miljkovic D, et al. Correlation of gut microbiota composition with resistance to experimental autoimmune encephalomyelitis in rats. *Front Microbiol* (2016) 7:363–73. doi:10.3389/fmicb.2016.02005
36. Demmer RT, Breskin A, Rosenbaum M, Zuk A, Leduc C, Leibel R, et al. The subgingival microbiome, systemic inflammation and insulin resistance: the oral infections, glucose intolerance and insulin resistance study. *J Clin Periodontol* (2017) 44(3):255–65. doi:10.1111/jcpe.12664
37. Negi S, Singh H, Mukhopadhyay A. Gut bacterial peptides with autoimmunity potential as environmental trigger for late onset complex diseases: in-silico study. *PLoS One* (2017) 12(7):e0180518. doi:10.1371/journal.pone.0180518
38. Karstens L, Asquith M, Davin S, Stauffer P, Fair D, Gregory WT, et al. Does the urinary microbiome play a role in urgency urinary incontinence and its severity? *Front Cell Infect Microbiol* (2016) 6:78. doi:10.3389/Fcimb.2016.00078
39. Bhute SS, Suryavanshi MV, Joshi SM, Yajnik CS, Shouche YS, Ghaskadbi SS. Gut microbial diversity assessment of Indian type-2-diabetics reveals alterations in eubacteria, archaea, and eukaryotes. *Front Microbiol* (2017) 8:214. doi:10.3389/fmicb.2017.00214
40. Chua LL, Rajasuriar R, Azanan MS, Abdullah NK, Tang MS, Lee SC, et al. Reduced microbial diversity in adult survivors of childhood acute lymphoblastic leukemia and microbial associations with increased immune activation. *Microbiome* (2017) 5:35. doi:10.1186/s40168-017-0250-1
41. Reunanen J, Kainulainen V, Huuskonen L, Ottman N, Belzer C, Huhtinen H, et al. *Akkermansia muciniphila* adheres to enterocytes and strengthens the integrity of the epithelial cell layer. *Appl Environ Microbiol* (2015) 81(11):3655–62. doi:10.1128/Aem.04050-14
42. Borton MA, Sabag-Daigle A, Wu J, Solden LM, O'banion BS, Daly RA, et al. Chemical and pathogen-induced inflammation disrupt the murine intestinal microbiome. *Microbiome* (2017) 5(1):47. doi:10.1186/s40168-017-0264-8
43. Lin SH, Chung PH, Wu YY, Fung CP, Hsu CM, Chen LW. Inhibition of nitric oxide production reverses diabetes-induced Kupffer cell activation and *Klebsiella pneumonia* liver translocation. *PLoS One* (2017) 12(5):e0177269. doi:10.1371/journal.pone.0177269
44. Song C, Li H, Zhang Y, Yu J. Effects of *Pseudomonas aeruginosa* and *Streptococcus mitis* mixed infection on TLR4-mediated immune response in acute pneumonia mouse model. *BMC Microbiol* (2017) 17(1):82. doi:10.1186/s12866-017-0999-1
45. Noor S, Ahmad J, Maazozair IP, Ozair M. Culture-based screening of aerobic microbiome in diabetic foot subjects and developing non-healing ulcers. *Front Microbiol* (2016) 7:1792. doi:10.3389/Fmicb.2016.01792
46. Tiwari S, Pratyush DD, Gupta SK, Singh SK. Vitamin D deficiency is associated with inflammatory cytokine concentrations in patients with diabetic foot infection. *Br J Nutr* (2014) 112(12):1938–43. doi:10.1017/S0007114514003018
47. Wolfe AJ, Toh E, Shibata N, Rong RC, Kenton K, Fitzgerald M, et al. Evidence of uncultivated bacteria in the adult female bladder. *J Clin Microbiol* (2012) 50(4):1376–83. doi:10.1128/Jcm.05852-11
48. Ottman N, Reunanen J, Meijerink M, Pietila TE, Kainulainen V, Klievink J, et al. Pili-like proteins of *Akkermansia muciniphila* modulate host immune responses and gut barrier function. *PLoS One* (2017) 12(3):e0173004. doi:10.1371/journal.pone.0173004
49. Huang YT, Liao CH, Teng LJ, Hsu HS, Hsueh PR. Reinfection and relapse of recurrent bacteremia caused by *Klebsiella pneumoniae* in a medical center in Taiwan. *Future Microbiol* (2016) 11(9):1157–65. doi:10.2217/fmb-2016-0036

50. Price TK, Dune T, Hilt EE, Thomas-White KJ, Kliethermes S, Brincat C, et al. The clinical urine culture: enhanced techniques improve detection of clinically relevant microorganisms. *J Clin Microbiol* (2016) 54(5):1216–22. doi:10.1128/Jcm.00044-16
51. Pridmore RD, Berger B, Desiere F, Vilanova D, Barretto C, Pittet AC, et al. The genome sequence of the probiotic intestinal bacterium *Lactobacillus johnsonii* NCC 533. *Proc Natl Acad Sci U S A* (2004) 101(8):2512–7. doi:10.1073/pnas.0307327101
52. Watanabe M, Kinoshita H, Nitta M, Yukishita R, Kawai Y, Kimura K, et al. Identification of a new adhesin-like protein from *Lactobacillus mucosae* ME-340 with specific affinity to the human blood group A and B antigens. *J Appl Microbiol* (2010) 109(3):927–35. doi:10.1111/j.1365-2672.2010.04719.x
53. Lee JH, Valeriano VD, Shin YR, Chae JP, Kim GB, Ham JS, et al. Genome sequence of *Lactobacillus mucosae* LM1, isolated from piglet feces. *J Bacteriol* (2012) 194(17):4766. doi:10.1128/JB.01011-12
54. Siddiqui H, Lagesen K, Nederbragt AJ, Jeansson SL, Jakobsen KS. Alterations of microbiota in urine from women with interstitial cystitis. *BMC Microbiol* (2012) 12:205. doi:10.1186/1471-2180-12-205
55. Abernethy MG, Rosenfeld A, White JR, Mueller MG, Lewicky-Gaupp C, Kenton K. Urinary microbiome and cytokine levels in women with interstitial cystitis. *Obstet Gynecol* (2017) 129(3):500–6. doi:10.1097/AOG.0000000000001892
56. Chiang ML, Chen HC, Chen KN, Lin YC, Lin YT, Chen MJ. Optimizing production of two potential probiotic lactobacilli strains isolated from piglet feces as feed additives for weaned piglets. *Asian-Australas J Anim Sci* (2015) 28(8):1163–70. doi:10.5713/ajas.14.0780
57. Gao CX, Major A, Rendon D, Lugo M, Jackson V, Shi ZC, et al. Histamine H2 receptor-mediated suppression of intestinal inflammation by probiotic *Lactobacillus reuteri*. *MBio* (2015) 6(6):e1358–1315. doi:10.1128/mBio.01358-15
58. Schaefer L, Auchtung TA, Hermans KE, Whitehead D, Borhan B, Britton RA. The antimicrobial compound reuterin (3-hydroxypropionaldehyde) induces oxidative stress via interaction with thiol groups. *Microbiology* (2010) 156:1589–99. doi:10.1099/mic.0.035642-0
59. Thomas CM, Hong T, Van Pijkeren JP, Hemarajata P, Trinh DV, Hu W, et al. Histamine derived from probiotic *Lactobacillus reuteri* suppresses TNF via modulation of PKA and ERK signaling. *PLoS One* (2012) 7(2):e31951. doi:10.1371/journal.pone.0031951
60. Simon MC, Strassburger K, Nowotny B, Kolb H, Nowotny P, Burkart V, et al. Intake of *Lactobacillus reuteri* improves incretin and insulin secretion in glucose-tolerant humans: a proof of concept. *Diabetes Care* (2015) 38(10):1827–34. doi:10.2337/dc14-2690
61. Pearce MM, Hilt EE, Rosenfeld AB, Zilliox MJ, Thomas-White K, Fok C, et al. The female urinary microbiome: a comparison of women with and without urgency urinary incontinence. *MBio* (2014) 5(4):e1283–1214. doi:10.1128/mBio.01283-14
62. Lewis DA, Brown R, Williams J, White P, Jacobson SK, Marchesi JR, et al. The human urinary microbiome; bacterial DNA in voided urine of asymptomatic adults. *Front Cell Infect Microbiol* (2013) 3:41. doi:10.3389/fcimb.2013.00041
63. Nienhouse V, Gao X, Dong QF, Nelson DE, Toh E, Mckinley K, et al. Interplay between bladder microbiota and urinary antimicrobial peptides: mechanisms for human urinary tract infection risk and symptom severity. *PLoS One* (2014) 9(12):e114185. doi:10.1371/journal.pone.0114185
64. Siddiqui H, Lagesen K, Nederbragt AJ, Eri LM, Jeansson SL, Jakobsen KS. Pathogens in urine from a female patient with overactive bladder syndrome detected by culture-independent high throughput sequencing: a case report. *Open Microbiol J* (2014) 8:148–53. doi:10.2174/1874285801408010148
65. Pearce MM, Zilliox MJ, Rosenfeld AB, Thomas-White KJ, Richter HE, Nager CW, et al. The female urinary microbiome in urgency urinary incontinence. *Am J Obstet Gynecol* (2015) 213(3):347.e1–11. doi:10.1016/j.ajog.2015.07.009
66. Eun CS, Mishima Y, Wohlgemuth S, Liu B, Bower M, Carroll IM, et al. Induction of bacterial antigen-specific colitis by a simplified human microbiota consortium in gnotobiotic interleukin-10(-/-) mice. *Infect Immun* (2014) 82(6):2239–46. doi:10.1128/Iai.01513-13
67. Harris TJ, Grosso JF, Yen HR, Xin H, Kortylewski M, Albesiano E, et al. Cutting edge: an in vivo requirement for STAT3 signaling in TH17 development and TH17-dependent autoimmunity. *J Immunol* (2007) 179(7):4313–7. doi:10.4049/jimmunol.179.7.4313
68. Krych L, Nielsen DS, Hansen AK, Hansen CH. Gut microbial markers are associated with diabetes onset, regulatory imbalance, and IFN-gamma level in NOD mice. *Gut Microbes* (2015) 6(2):101–9. doi:10.1080/19490976.2015.1011876
69. Sato T, Watanabe K, Kumada H, Toyama T, Tani-Ishii N, Hamada N. Peptidoglycan of *Actinomyces naeslundii* induces inflammatory cytokine production and stimulates osteoclastogenesis in alveolar bone resorption. *Arch Oral Biol* (2012) 57(11):1522–8. doi:10.1016/j.archoralbio.2012.07.012
70. Chiu PF, Huang CH, Liou HH, Wu CL, Wang SC, Chang CC. Long-term renal outcomes of episodic urinary tract infection in diabetic patients. *J Diabetes Complications* (2013) 27(1):11–3. doi:10.1016/j.jdiacomp.2012.08.005

6

Dexamethasone Inhibits *S. aureus*-Induced Neutrophil Extracellular Pathogen-Killing Mechanism, Possibly through Toll-Like Receptor Regulation

Ting Wan[†]*, Yingying Zhao*[†]*, Fangli Fan, Renjian Hu and Xiuming Jin**

Eye Center, Second Affiliated Hospital, School of Medicine, Zhejiang University, Hangzhou, China

Edited by:
Julio Villena,
Reference Centre for Lactobacilli (CERELA-CONICET), Argentina

Reviewed by:
Susana Salva,
Reference Centre for Lactobacilli (CERELA-CONICET), Argentina
Tomonori Nochi,
Tohoku University, Japan

***Correspondence:**
Xiuming Jin
lzyjxm@zju.edu.cn

[†]*These authors have contributed equally to this article.*

Neutrophils release neutrophil extracellular traps (NETs) in a pathogen-killing process called NETosis. Excessive NETs formation, however, is implicated in disease pathogenesis. Therefore, to understand how NETosis is regulated, we examined the effect of dexamethasone (DXM), an anti-inflammatory drug, on this process and the role of toll-like receptors (TLRs). We stimulated human neutrophils with phorbol 12-myristate 13-acetate (PMA) or *Staphylococcus aureus* (*S. aureus*) and quantified NETs formation. We also examined the effect of DXM on the bactericidal effect of NETs and the role of reactive oxygen species (ROS) and nuclear factor (NF)-κB in DXM-regulated NETosis. DXM significantly inhibited *S. aureus*-induced NETosis and extracellular bacterial killing. ROS production and NF-κB activation were not involved in DXM-regulated NETosis. TLR2 and TLR4, but not TLR5 or TLR6, modified *S. aureus*-induced NETs formation. Neither DXM nor TLRs were involved in PMA-induced NETosis. Furthermore, TLR2 and TLR4 agonists rescued DXM-inhibited NETosis, and neither TLR2 nor TLR4 antagonists could further inhibit NETosis reduction induced by DXM, indicating that DXM may inhibit NETosis by regulating TLR2 and TLR4. In conclusion, the mechanisms of *S. aureus*- and PMA-induced NETosis are different. DXM decreases NETs formation independently of oxidant production and NF-κB phosphorylation and possibly *via* a TLR-dependent mechanism.

Keywords: neutrophil extracellular traps, dexamethasone, TLRs, *S. aureus*, PMA

INTRODUCTION

Neutrophils are the most abundant leukocytes in human blood and play an essential role in innate immunity since they are the first cells recruited to sites of infection and inflammation (1). They engulf microorganisms or opsonized particles and degrade them intracellularly as well as releasing microbicidal proteins and reactive oxygen species (ROS) (2). Recently, these cells have been shown to release structures called neutrophil extracellular traps (NETs), which consist of chromatin along with histones and many granular antimicrobial proteins—including elastase, myeloperoxidase, and calprotectin; this is a novel extracellular pathogen-killing mechanism described as NETosis (3–5).

Although NETosis contributes to pathogen control, it is essential for the balance between the formation and removal of NETs to be regulated to ensure tissue homeostasis, because large amounts of NETs may contribute to collateral damage within inflamed tissues. Excessive amounts of NETs are associated with the pathogenesis of inflammatory and autoimmune diseases, including preeclampsia (6), cystic fibrosis (7), and lupus (8). Moreover, NETs have been observed to act as a scaffold for thrombus formation (9, 10), which is increasingly being recognized as a critical phenomenon linking inflammation with venous thrombosis. Therefore, NETosis is a double-edged sword: while it is an effective first-line antimicrobial mechanism, it might also lead to organ failure and death if it is unregulated. Hence, it is important to understand the mechanism of NETs regulation, but little information is available about this topic thus far.

Since an inflammatory microenvironment is essential for NETs formation, we believed that using glucocorticoids, which are potent anti-inflammatory drugs, can help elucidate how NETs formation is regulated. They are commonly used to resolve inflammation and are closely related to neutrophil function. They have been shown to inhibit neutrophil apoptosis and cytokine release during inflammation (11) and are also associated with many neutrophil functions, including chemotaxis, migration, and phagocytosis (12). Therefore, we examined the effect of a commonly used glucocorticoid drug, dexamethasone (DXM), on NETs formation. On the other hand, toll-like receptors (TLRs), which are essential pattern-recognizing receptors (PRRs) that mediate the recognition of microbial structures, have been reported to activate neutrophil extracellular traps to ensnare bacteria in septic blood (13). Moreover, most of the TLRs were reported to be expressed in neutrophils and were involved in neutrophils activation (14). So, we also investigated the role of different TLRs in NETs formation.

We found that DXM significantly inhibited NETs formation induced by *Staphylococcus aureus* (*S. aureus*) but not that induced by phorbol 12-myristate 13-acetate (PMA), which suggested that DXM can serve as a potential drug to regulate NETosis. In addition, the modulation of TLR-2 and TLR4 had an effect on NETs production, thus indicating the involvement of TLRs in this process.

MATERIALS AND METHODS

Reagents

Phorbol 12-myristate 13-acetate, DXM, DNase I, cytochalasin D, and dichlorofluorescein diacetate (DCF-DA) were purchased from Sigma-Aldrich (St. Louis, MO, USA); Percoll, from GE Healthcare (Little Chalfont, UK); and TLR agonists and TLR antagonists, from InvivoGen (San Diego, CA, USA). Anti-histone H2B and neutrophil elastase antibodies, anti-glyceraldehyde-3-phosphate dehydrogenase (GAPDH) antibody, anti-phosphorylated nuclear factor κB (anti-p-NF-κB, p65) antibody, secondary antibodies coupled to AF488 or AF555, and horseradish peroxidase (HRP) secondary antibody were purchased from Santa Cruz Biotechnology (CA, USA). SYTOX Green, Luria broth, Quant-iT PicoGreen double-stranded deoxyribonucleic acid (dsDNA) assay kit and micro-plates were purchased from ThermoFisher Scientific (Basingstoke, UK).

Isolation of Human Neutrophils

Neutrophils were isolated from the peripheral blood of fasting healthy donors by Percoll gradient centrifugation, as previously described (7). For those donors, comprehensive history and physical examination were performed, basic laboratory tests were used to exclude occult disease. This study was conducted according to the principles expressed in the Declaration of Helsinki. Ethical approval was obtained from the Ethics Committee of Affiliated Second Hospital, School of Medicine, Zhejiang University, China. All participants provided written informed consent for the collection of samples and subsequent analyses. For each donor, 10–30 ml blood was drawn according to the need of different assays. Bloods from at least three donors were used to repeat the same assay. Cell suspensions contained >96% neutrophils, as determined by Wright–Giemsa staining, with 98% cell viability as determined by Trypan blue staining. The cells (4×10^5/ml) were re-suspended in RPMI 1640 medium supplemented with bovine serum albumin (2%).

Neutrophils Stimulation

Neutrophils (2×10^5 cells/well in 500 μl) were stimulated with PMA (50 nM) or *S. aureus* (multiplicity of infection = 10) and placed in a humidified incubator at 37°C with CO_2 (5%) for 120 min. In some experiments, neutrophils were first incubated for 120 min with DXM (10 μM), TLR2 agonist (HKLM, 10^8 CFU/ml), TLR4 agonist (LPS, 1 μg/ml), TLR5 agonist (FSL-ST, 1 μg/ml), TLR6 agonist (FSL-1, 1 μg/ml), TLR neutralizing antibodies as antagonists (TLR2, 4, 5, 6 antibody, 1 μg/ml), or vehicle (controls). Stock solutions of DXM, TLR agonists, and TLR antagonists were prepared in DMSO and were further diluted in RPMI 1640 medium. The final DMSO concentration (0.1% v/v) did not have a toxic effect. All drugs were freshly prepared for each experiment.

NETs Formation Assay

After stimulation, cells were fixed with 4% PFA, blocked with 3% normal donkey serum and 0.05% Tween 20 in phosphate-buffered saline (PBS), and incubated with the primary antibodies anti-H2B and anti-neutrophil elastase, which were detected with secondary antibodies coupled to AF488 or AF555. Isotype-matched controls were used. For DNA detection, 4′, 6′-diamidino-2-phenylindole (DAPI) was used. Specimens were mounted and analyzed under a confocal microscope (Olympus IX-50).

Neutrophil extracellular traps were also examined using the membrane-impermeable DNA-binding dye SYTOX green (Molecular Probes, Invitrogen Life Technologies). SYTOX green (5 μM) was added to the cultures after specific periods of incubation, and the cultures observed 5 min later. In one case, DNase I (100 U/ml) was added for 10 min to degrade the NETs structure as control. To visualize NETs, live-cell cultures were imaged with an inverted fluorescence microscope (Olympus IX-50).

Bacterial Culture

Staphylococcus aureus (ATCC 25923) was cultured overnight in Luria–Bertani (LB) broth (37°C, 200 rpm), harvested by centrifugation, washed, and suspended in PBS. Bacterial growth was quantified at A600 and the cell number determined using a standard curve based on colony counts. Stationary-phase bacteria were used for all experiments.

Quantification of Extracellular DNA

The levels of extracellular DNA in supernatants were quantified using Quant-iT PicoGreen dsDNA assay kit according to the manufacturer's instructions. PicoGreen is a cell-impermeable dye that binds to extracellular dsDNA without staining live cells. Fluorescence intensity was measured on a SpectraMax M3 (Molecular Devices) fluorescent plate reader at an excitation wavelength of 480 nm and an emission wavelength of 520 nm, with a 515-nm emission cutoff filter. The calibration curve was constructed using a standard dsDNA of a known concentration.

Bacterial Survival Assay of NETs

A bacterial survival assay was performed as described in earlier studies (15). Neutrophils (1×10^6 cells/well in 200 µl) were pre-incubated with or without DXM for 2 h and then treated with 50 nM PMA or left untreated for another 2 h at 37°C and 5% CO_2. NETs killing was examined by inhibiting phagocytic killing by the addition of 100 µg/ml cytochalasin D for 15 min before the addition of bacteria. After 1 h at 37°C, neutrophils and clumped NETs were disrupted by the addition of 0.01% Triton X-100 and three passes through a 25-gauge needle. Following serial dilution, bacteria were plated on LB plates for colony counting. After overnight incubation at 37°C, the number of colony-forming units (CFU) was determined. Zero killing was defined by control samples consisting of RPMI 1640. Killing efficacy was determined by subtracting the CFU of indicated treatment from control group.

ROS Production

Neutrophils were incubated in PBS (Ca^{2+}- and Mg^{2+}-free) with 10 µM DCF-DA (Sigma) at 37°C for 20 min. Subsequently, they were pelleted, washed in PBS three times, and transferred to a 96-well plate (1×10^6 cells/well in 100 µl). They were then stimulated with *S. aureus* for 1 h (some cells were pretreated with DXM for 120 min), and fluorescence was measured using SpectraMax M3 fluorescent plate reader at an excitation wavelength of 480 nm and an emission wavelength of 520 nm.

Immunoblotting

The neutrophils (3×10^6 cells/well in 500 µl) were pre-incubated with or without DXM for 2 h and then stimulated for another 2 h with *S. aureus*. Cell lysates were prepared using 1× loading buffer and boiled. Samples were then frozen at −80°C until use. Equal amounts of proteins were run on 12% sodium dodecyl sulphate-polyacrylamide gel and then electrotransferred onto polyvinylidenefluoride membranes. After blocking with 5% bovine serum albumin, membranes were incubated with phospho-NF-κBp65 and anti-GAPDH antibody overnight at 4°C, and then with HRP-conjugated secondary antibody for 2 h at room temperature. Protein bands were visualized by enhanced chemiluminescence. The gray degree of protein bands was detected by image J, and the value of p-NF-κB p65/GAPDH was calculated.

Statistical Analysis

Statistical analyses were performed using GraphPad Prism 6.1. Data are expressed as mean ± SE of individual samples. For two-group comparison, Student's *t*-test was applied for normally distributed data. The comparisons between multiple groups were performed using one-way ANOVA, followed by a Bonferroni's post-test. The significance threshold was set at 0.05.

RESULTS

NETs Formation in Response to PMA and Bacterial Stimulation

Microscopic observation clearly showed NETs structure, including neutrophil-derived proteins. Neutrophils were labeled with DAPI to identify DNA (blue) and with antibodies to identify neutrophil histone (green) and elastase (red) (**Figure 1A**). This confirmed PMA- or *S. aureus*-triggered NETs formation. SYTOX green staining further showed that bacteria were trapped in the web like structure and could be released when this NETs formation was degraded by Dnase I (**Figure 1B**).

DXM Inhibits NETs Formation Induced by *S. aureus* But Not That Induced by PMA

Fluorescence microscopy showed that DXM did not have any effect on the NETs formation induced by PMA but markedly inhibited that induced by *S. aureus* (**Figure 2A**). To further corroborate these, NETs formation was measured by quantifying the extracellular DNA in the supernatants. This experiment confirmed that *S. aureus*-induced formation of extracellular traps was significantly decreased by DXM ($p < 0.05$). In contrast, the amount of NETs formed after PMA induction was similar in controls and in DXM-treated neutrophils ($p > 0.05$) (**Figure 2B**). In addition, DMSO (0.1% v/v) in the solution of stimulates had no effect on NETs formation.

DXM Decreases the Bactericidal Efficacy of NETs

Dexamethasone significantly decreased the bactericidal efficacy of NETs, following abrogating phagocytic killing by the addition of cytochalasin D ($p < 0.05$; **Figure 3**). However, if neutrophils were activated to form NETs by PMA, DXM treatment had no effect on the killing efficacy of NETs ($p > 0.05$).

ROS and NF-κB Activation Are Not Involved in DXM-Regulated NETosis

Reactive oxygen species generation was first evaluated in resting neutrophils by performing a DCF-DA fluorescence assay. DCF-DA is a non-fluorescent molecule that becomes fluorescent in the presence of a wide variety of ROS, including superoxide anion and hydroxyl radicals (16). NETs formation has previously been reported to be dependent on or independent of ROS (17). In order to examine if DXM-regulated NETs formation is

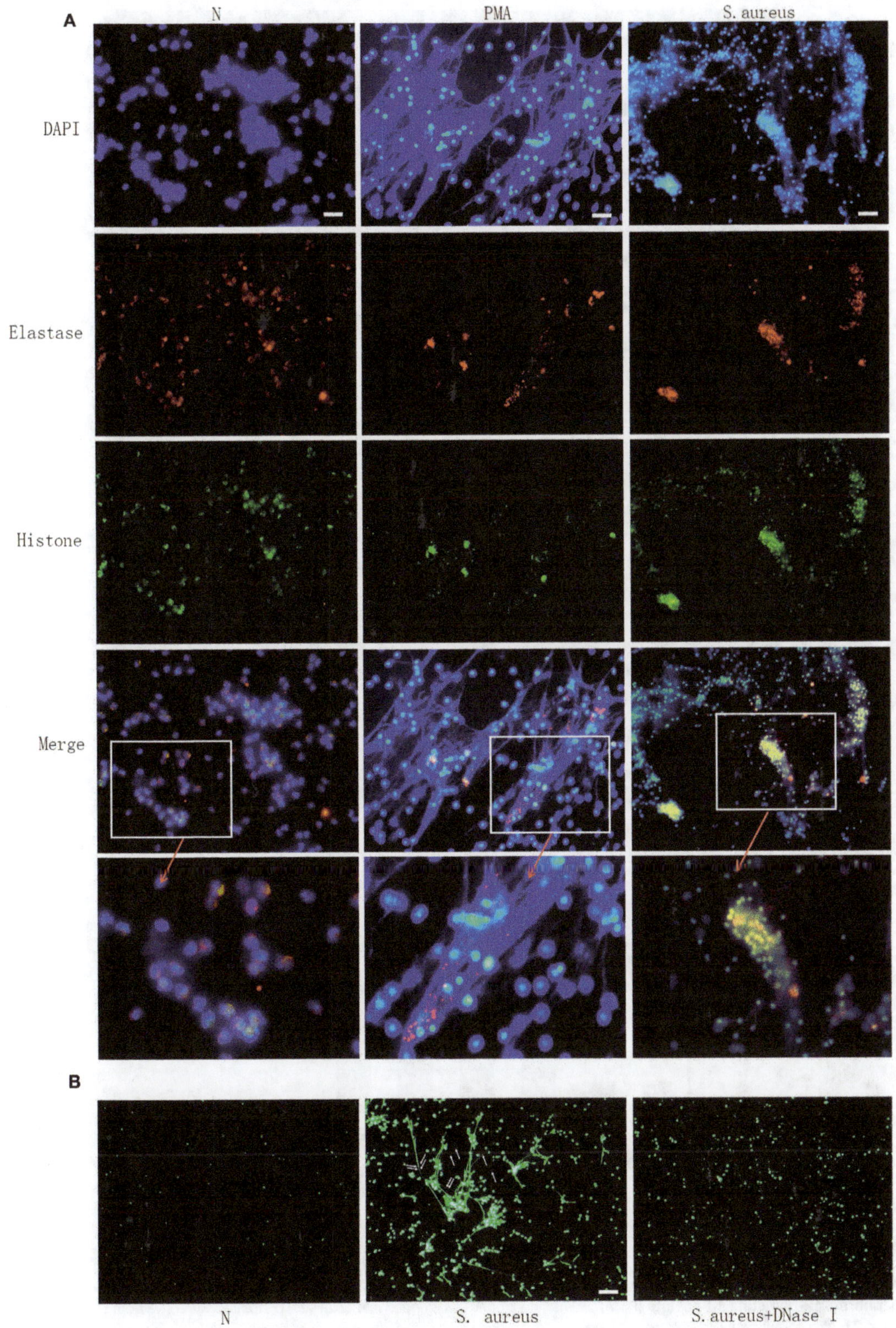

FIGURE 1 | Phorbol 12-myristate 13-acetate (PMA) and *Staphylococcus aureus* (*S. aureus*) stimulate neutrophil extracellular traps (NETs) formation in human neutrophil. Human neutrophil suspended in media were treated with PMA (50 nM) or *S. aureus* at MOI of 10. Human neutrophil without treatment (N) was used as control. NETs formation was measured at 2 h. **(A)** Neutrophils were labelled with 4′, 6′-diamidino-2-phenylindole (DAPI) to identify DNA (blue) and with antibodies to identify neutrophil histone (green) and elastase (red). PMA and *S. aureus*-induced NETs formation. **(B)** *S. aureus* (indicated with arrow) were trapped in NETs and released when NETs structure was degraded by DNase I, as observed by SYTOX green staining Bar: 50 μm.

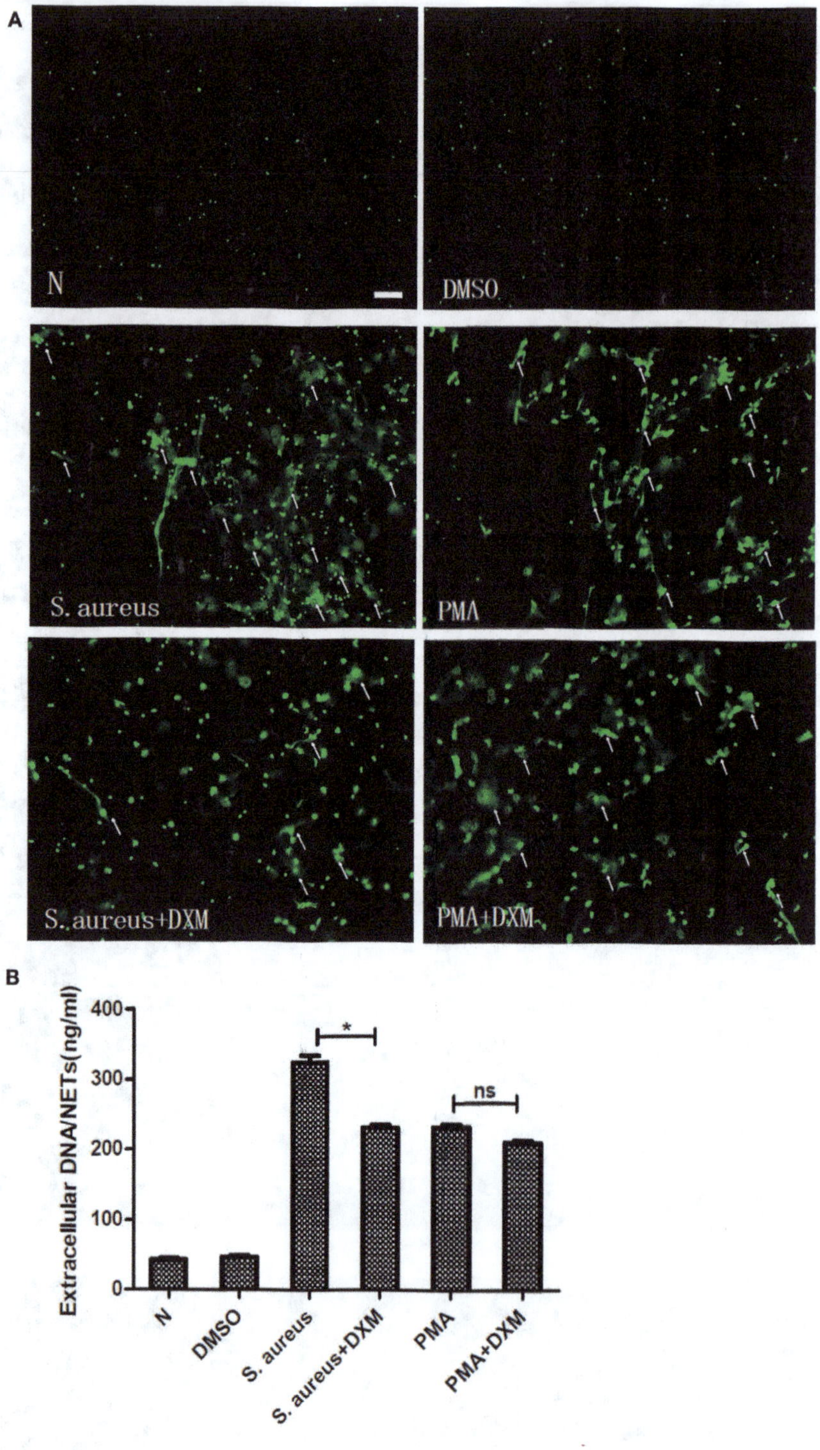

FIGURE 2 | Dexamethasone (DXM) inhibited neutrophil extracellular traps (NETs) formation induced by *Staphylococcus aureus* (*S. aureus*) but not that induced by phorbol 12-myristate 13-acetate (PMA). Human neutrophils suspended in media were pretreated with or without DXM (10 μM) for 2 h, and then NETs formation 2 h after stimulation with PMA or *S. aureus* was examined using the membrane-impermeable DNA-binding dye SYTOX green and quantified by Quant iTPicoGreen double stranded deoxyribonucleic acid assay kit. Neutrophils without any stimulation or treated with DMSO (0.1% v/v) were used as control. **(A)** DMSO (0.1% v/v) did not affect NETs formation. While dexamethasone did not modify NETs formation induced by PMA, it markedly inhibited that induced by *S. aureus*. Several typical NETs were indicated with arrows. Bar: 50 μm. **(B)** Quantification of extracellular DNA confirmed that it inhibited NETs formation induced by *S. aureus* but not that induced by PMA. Neutrophils (1×10^5cells/well in 100 μl) were stimulated to form NETs, and the mean value of NETs amount in five replicated wells was adopted. The assay was repeated for three times with bloods from three different donors; error bars represent SEM. *$p < 0.05$ by ANOVA with Bonferroni's post-test.

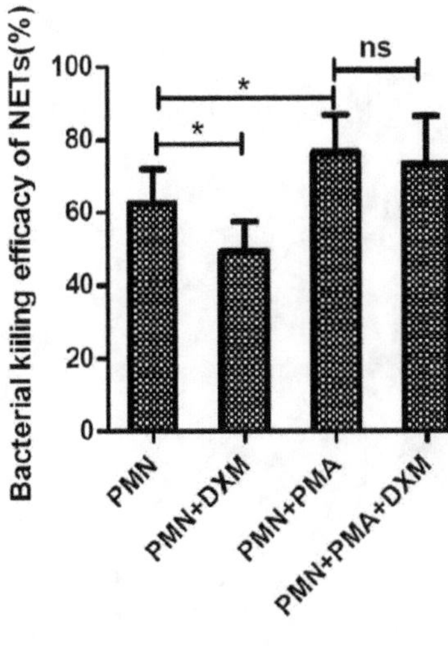

FIGURE 3 | Dexamethasone (DXM) inhibited the bactericidal efficacy of neutrophil extracellular traps (NETs). Neutrophils were pre-incubated with or without DXM for 2 h and then treated with 50 nM phorbol 12-myristate 13-acetate (PMA) or left untreated for another 2 h. One hour after addition of bacteria, colony-forming units (CFU) were determined by overnight incubation at 37°C following serial dilution. Zero killing was defined by control samples consisting of only media. Killing efficacy was determined by subtracting the CFU of indicated treatment from control groups. By using cytochalasin D to abrogate phagocytic killing, dexamethasone was found to significantly inhibit the bactericidal efficacy of NETs. However, dexamethasone could not inhibit PMA-activated bactericidal efficacy of NETs. The assay was repeated for nine times, each case in three wells; error bars represent SEM. *$p < 0.05$ by ANOVA with Bonferroni's post-test.

ROS-dependent, ROS production by activated neutrophils with or without DXM stimulation was measured. *S. aureus* infection elicited significant neutrophil oxidative burst, but DXM treatment neither increased nor decreased this response noticeably (**Figure 4A**).

The transcription factor NF-κB is a key regulator of inflammation and therefore plays a pivotal role in a wide range of inflammatory diseases (18). The phosphorylation of NF-κB has been believed to be involved in NETs generation (19). Therefore, we explored the role of DXM in the activation of NF-κB induced by *S. aureus*. The expression of p-NF-κB (p65) was significantly higher when the cells were stimulated with *S. aureus*, but this effect was not modified by DXM (**Figures 4B,C**).

TLRs Are Involved in NETs Formation Induced by *S. aureus* But Not That Induced by PMA

Toll-like receptors are key PRRs, which are important in innate immune responses. Thus, we explored the role of TLRs in the formation of NETs. None of TLR2 agonist, TLR4 agonist, TLR5 agonist, and TLR6 agonist could induce NETs formation. However, TLR2 and TLR4 agonists significantly enhanced NETs formation induced by *S. aureus* but not that induced by PMA, as shown by the quantification of extracellular DNA. Moreover, blocking TLR2 and TLR4 with neutralizing antibodies significantly reduced the NETs formation induced by *S. aureus* but not that induced by PMA, as shown by quantification of extracellular DNA (**Figure 5**). Furthermore, neither the TLR5/TLR6 agonist nor the antagonist could modulate the formation of NETs.

DXM May Modulate *S. aureus*-Induced NETs Formation through TLR2 and TLR4

To explore the mechanism of DXM-modulated NETs formation, we first pre-incubated the cells with TLR agonists to examine the effect of TLRs on DXM-inhibited NETs formation. As expected, both HKLM (TLR2 agonist) and LPS (TLR4 agonist) rescued DXM-reduced NETs formation (**Figure 6A**). Moreover, neither TLR2 nor TLR4 antagonist could further decrease DXM-induced NETosis reduction (**Figure 6B**). While these findings suggested that DXM may modulate *S. aureus*-induced NETs formation through TLR2 and TLR4, further research is required to understand the precise mechanism.

DISCUSSION

NETosis, a recently identified mechanism of pathogen killing, helps in isolating and preventing the spread of invading bacteria, but the persistent formation or insufficient degradation of NETs can also cause injury to the host (8, 20). Since regulation of NETs formation is essential for tissue homeostasis, we aimed to determine the mechanisms and molecules underlying the regulation of this process.

A variety of stimuli promote NETs formation. In our study, NETs formation could be induced in neutrophils by both pharmacologic (PMA) and pathogenic (bacterial) stimuli, a finding that is in agreement with those of previous studies (21, 22). Although several signaling mechanisms responsible for NETs formation have been reported, critical regulatory elements remain unidentified. Since the findings from different studies often vary, it is possible that more than one mechanism exists. In this study, we observed that DXM-inhibited NETs formation induced by bacteria but not that induced by PMA. In addition, it markedly decreased the bactericidal ability of NETs. Thus far, DXM has not been reported to affect NETs formation induced by *S. aureus*. Lapponi reported that treatment of neutrophils with DXM had no effect on NETs formation induced by PMA or TNF-α (19). This is consistent with our observation that DXM was not required for the regulation of PMA-induced NETs formation. Other studies have suggested that NETs formation induced by different stimuli have distinct mechanisms. For example, Riyapa et al. (23) reported that when compared to the neutrophils of diabetic patients, those of normal individuals produced less PMA-induced NETs but the same amount of *S. aureus*-induced NETs. Parker et al. (24) hypothesized that whether NADPH oxidase and myeloperoxidase are required in NETs formation depends on the stimulus. These results prompted us to investigate whether different stimuli indeed have different underlying mechanisms. Our findings strongly suggested that bacteria and PMA regulate NETs formation through different pathways and that DXM may

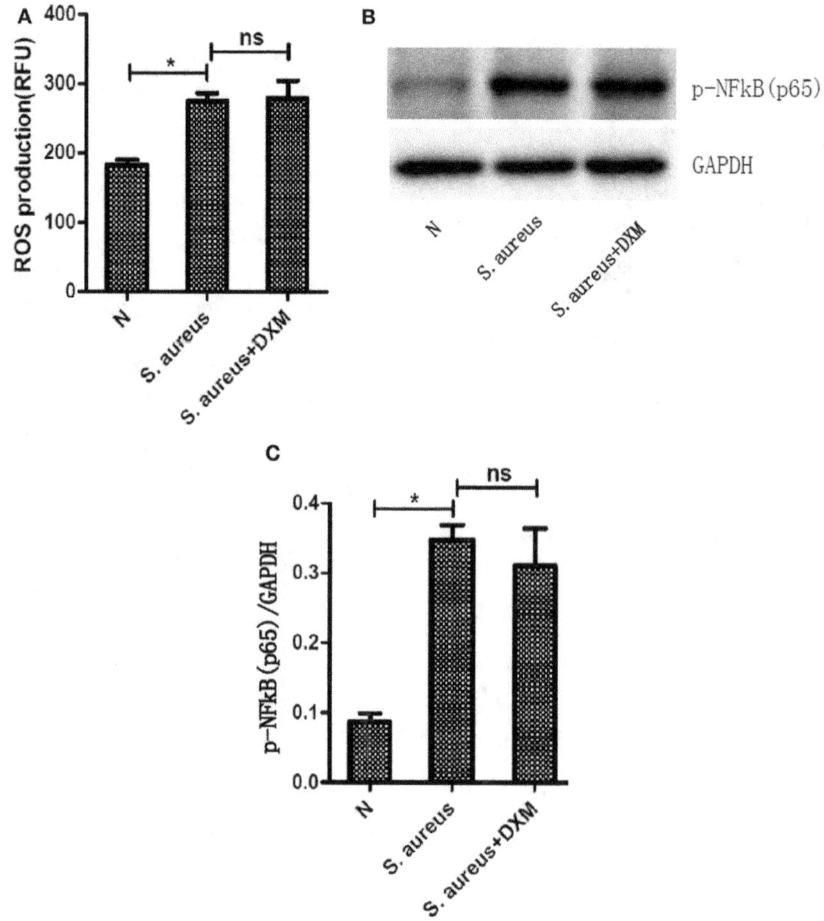

FIGURE 4 | Activation of reactive oxygen species (ROS) or nuclear factor (NF)-κB was not involved in dexamethasone-regulated NETosis. Neutrophils were pretreated with or without dexamethasone (DXM) for 2 h and then stimulated with *Staphylococcus aureus* (*S. aureus*) for 1 h. ROS production were determined by dichlorofluorescein diacetate fluorescence and NF-κB activation were determined by Western blot. **(A)** *S. aureus* infection elicited significant neutrophil oxidative burst, but DXM treatment neither increased nor decreased this response. Data represent mean ± SEM of triplicate experiments. **(B)** NF-κB was activated when stimulated with *S. aureus* but not modified by dexamethasone. **(C)** Quantification showed that p-NF-κB (p65) expression was significantly higher when the cells were stimulated with *S. aureus*, but this effect was not modified by dexamethasone. Data represent mean ± SEM of triplicate experiments, $^{*}p < 0.05$ by Student's *t*-test.

have an effect on NETs formation induced by bacteria but not on that induced by PMA.

Neutrophil extracellular traps formation has been shown to require NADPH oxidase activity as well as NF-κB activation. Our results verified the involvement of NADPH oxidase activity and NF-κB activation in the process of NETs formation. However, in contrast to our expectation, no change in ROS or pNF-κB levels was observed in DXM-treated neutrophils stimulated by *S. aureus*, which indicated that ROS and NF-κB signaling pathways were not involved in DXM-regulated NETs formation. NETosis was previously reported to be of two types: ROS dependent and ROS independent. Our study shows that DXM may modulate ROS-independent NETosis. Interestingly, DXM has been reported to inhibit calcium mobilization, which was shown to increase in LPS-treated cells (25). Therefore, DXM may regulate NETosis by modulating calcium mobilization, which is ROS independent. Moreover, our study showed that the phosphorylation of NF-κB, which has been shown to participate in NETs formation (19), is not involved in DXM-modulated NETosis. It may be because different stimuli were used, with bacteria in ours and PMA in others. Nevertheless, as we only detected the phosphorylation of NF-κB in whole cell, it could not be excluded that there were NF-κB shifting from plasma to nucleus.

The specific detection of microorganisms by innate cells is mediated by PRRs—germline-encoded receptors that recognize microbial structures referred to as pathogen-associated molecular patterns (26). TLRs are essential PRRs that mediate the recognition of microbial structures, such as those of bacteria, as well as the subsequent inflammatory and adaptive responses (27–30). Because neutrophils and TLRs are, respectively, the prototypical cells and receptors involved in innate immune responses, the effect of TLRs on NETosis was investigated. Our findings suggested that TLRs involved in inflammatory response could be key regulatory factors in NETs formation. Our results

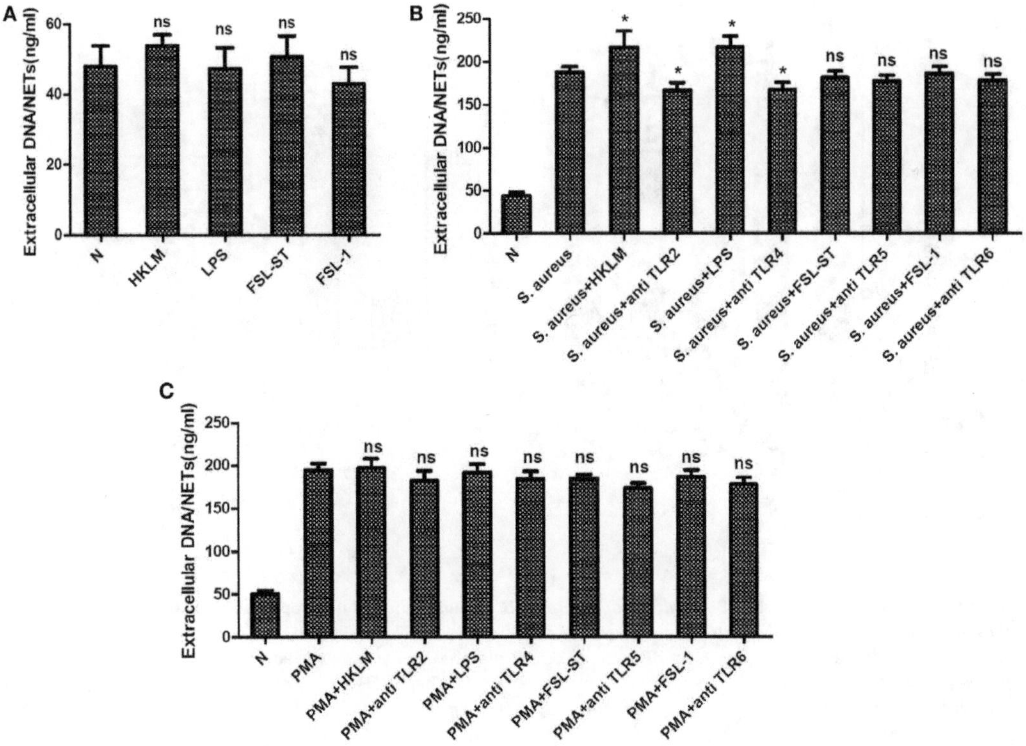

FIGURE 5 | Toll-like receptors (TLRs) were involved in *Staphylococcus aureus* (*S. aureus*)-induced but not phorbol 12-myristate 13-acetate (PMA)-induced neutrophil extracellular traps (NETs) formation. Neutrophils were pretreated with TLRs agonist or antagonist, followed by PMA or *S. aureus* stimulation. NETs formation was quantified by Quant-iT PicoGreen double-stranded deoxyribonucleic acid assay kit. **(A)** None of TLR2 agonist (HKLM), TLR4 agonist (LPS), TLR5 agonist (FSL-ST), and TLR6 (FSL-1) agonist could induce NETs formation. **(B)** Treatment with TLR2 agonist (HKLM) and TLR4 agonists (LPS) significantly enhanced NETosis, and blocking TLR2 and TLR4 with neutralizing antibodies significantly reduced *S. aureus*-induced NETs formation. None of TLR5 agonist (FSL-ST), TLR6 agonist (FSL-1), and TLR5 and TLR6 neutralizing antibodies was involved in *S. aureus*-induced NETs formation. **(C)** TLRs were not involved in PMA-induced NETs formation. The assay was repeated for three times, each case in five wells, error bars represent SEM. Compared to *S. aureus* or PMA stimulation, $^{*}p < 0.05$, ns = $p > 0.05$ by Student's *t*-test.

showed that *S. aureus*-induced NETosis was markedly inhibited by TLR2 and TLR4 antagonists and enhanced by TLR2 and TLR4 agonists. This strongly supports the role of TLR2 and TLR4 in the biogenesis of NETs, but these effects were not observed in PMA-induced NETosis. Furthermore, neither TLR5 nor TLR6 agonists/antagonists had any effect on bacteria-induced NETosis. As TLR2 is the main receptor for Gram positive, and TLR4 is for Gram-negative bacteria, respectively, it is reasonable that both of them may directly or indirectly participate in the process of NETosis triggered by *S. aureus* through the whole inflammatory network. It is further confirmed by the following results. The addition of TLR2 and TLR4 agonists (HKLM and LPS) rescued DXM-inhibited NETs formation induced by *S. aureus*, but to a lower extent than in the control group stimulated by *S. aureus*. Therefore, we believe that both TLR2 and TLR4 were involved in DXM-modulated NETosis, which is consistent with the observation in other studies that multiple receptors may together regulate NETs formation (31). Besides, we were unable to conclude whether other TLRs that mediated the interaction of neutrophils and other pathogens like viruses could also be involved.

In addition, we aimed to determine the relationship between DXM and TLRs. Both HKLM and LPS rescued DXM-reduced NETs formation. Moreover, neither TLR2 nor TLR4 antagonist could further decrease DXM induced NETosis reduction. This indicated the involvement of TLRs in DXM-reduced NETosis. A previous study showed that DXM down-regulates TLR4 mRNA expression in neutrophils (32), which implies that it may regulate NETosis by modulating TLR expression (33).

Our study has a limitation: we examined neutrophil function only *in vitro*; further *in vivo* studies are needed to characterize the fate of neutrophils. It is also not clear how DXM and TLRs cooperatively modulate NETs formation. Further research is needed to clarify these points.

In conclusion, we have demonstrated that NETs formation can be induced in neutrophils by different stimuli but not by a common mechanism. The mechanism of how DXM modulates bacteria-induced NETs formation was found to be unrelated to oxidant production and phosphorylation of NF-κB. TLR2 and TLR4 are involved in the formation of NETs. Although the specific mechanisms of how DXM regulates

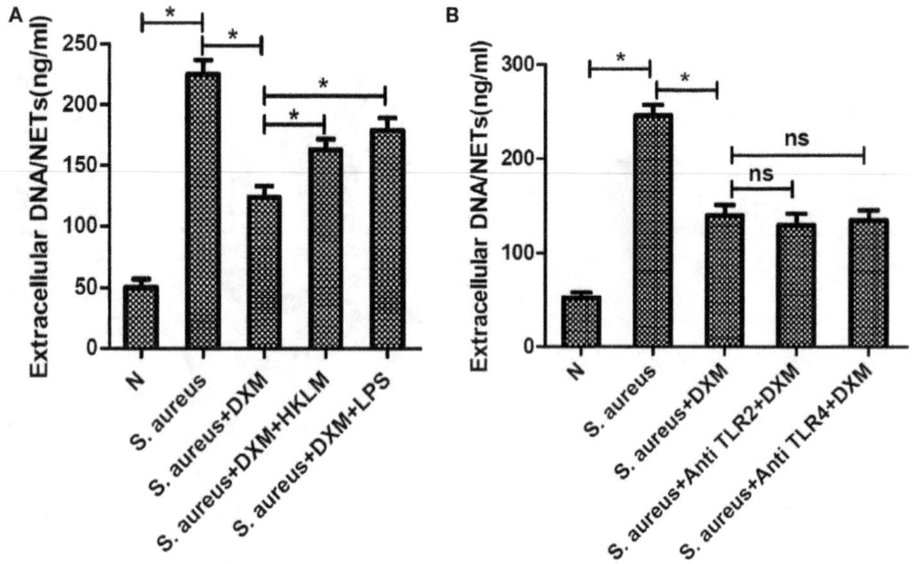

FIGURE 6 | Dexamethasone (DXM) may modulate *Staphylococcus aureus* (*S. aureus*)-induced neutrophil extracellular traps (NETs) formation through toll-like receptor (TLR)2 and TLR4. (A) Neutrophils were pretreated with HKLM (TLR2 agonist) and LPS (TLR4 agonist), followed by DXM treatment and *S. aureus* stimulation. NETs formation was quantified by Quant-iTPicoGreen double-stranded deoxyribonucleic acid (dsDNA) assay kit. Both HKLM and LPS rescued dexamethasone-reduced NETs formation. **(B)** Neutrophils were pretreated with TLR2 and TLR4 antagonist, followed by DXM treatment and *S. aureus* stimulation. NETs formation was quantified by Quant-iTPicoGreen dsDNA assay kit. Neither TLR2 nor TLR4 antagonist could further decrease DXM induced NETosis reduction. The assay was repeated for three times, each case in five wells, error bars represent SEM. $^{*}p < 0.05$ by Student's *t*-test.

NETs formation are unclear, it is possible that DXM regulates NET formation induced by *S. aureus via* a TLR-dependent mechanism.

AUTHOR CONTRIBUTIONS

TW and YZ wrote the main manuscript text. YZ, TW, FF, and RH performed the experiments. YZ and TW prepared **Figures 1–6**. XJ designed the study and provided advice on the discussion.

ACKNOWLEDGMENTS

This study was funded by National Natural Science Foundation of China (No.81270974; 81500694); Zhejiang Provincial Natural Science Foundation of China (LQ13H120003).

REFERENCES

1. Nathan C. Neutrophils and immunity: challenges and opportunities. *Nat Rev Immunol* (2006) 6(3):173–82. doi:10.1038/nri1785
2. Segal AW. How neutrophils kill microbes. *Immunology* (2005) 23(23):197–223. doi:10.1146/annurev.immunol.23.021704.115653
3. Brinkmann V, Reichard U, Goosmann C, Fauler B, Uhlemann Y, Weiss DS, et al. Neutrophil extracellular traps kill bacteria. *Science* (2004) 303(5663):1532–5. doi:10.1126/science.1092385
4. Urban CF, Reichard U, Brinkmann V, Zychlinsky A. Neutrophil extracellular traps capture and kill *Candida albicans* yeast and hyphal forms. *Cell Microbiol* (2006) 8(4):668–76. doi:10.1111/j.1462-5822.2005.00659.x
5. Urban CF, Ermert D, Schmid M, Abuabed U, Goosmann C, Nacken W, et al. Neutrophil extracellular traps contain calprotectin, a cytosolic protein complex involved in host defense against *Candida albicans*. *PLoS Pathog* (2009) 5(10):e1000639. doi:10.1371/journal.ppat.1000639
6. Gupta AK, Hasler P, Holzgreve W, Gebhardt S, Hahn S. Induction of neutrophil extracellular DNA lattices by placental microparticles and IL-8 and their presence in preeclampsia. *Hum Immunol* (2005) 66(66):1146–54. doi:10.1016/j.humimm.2005.11.003
7. Manzenreiter R, Kienberger F, Marcos V, Schilcher K, Krautgartner WD, Obermayer A, et al. Ultrastructural characterization of cystic fibrosis sputum using atomic force and scanning electron microscopy. *J Cyst Fibros* (2011) 11(2):84–92. doi:10.1016/j.jcf.2011.09.008
8. Hakkim A, Fürnrohr BG, Amann K, Laube B, Abed UA, Brinkmann V, et al. Impairment of neutrophil extracellular trap degradation is associated with lupus nephritis. *Proc Natl Acad Sci U S A* (2010) 107(21):9813–8. doi:10.1073/pnas.0909927107
9. Fuchs TA, Brill A, Duerschmied D, Schatzberg D, Monestier M, Myers DD, et al. Extracellular DNA traps promote thrombosis. *Proc Natl Acad Sci U S A* (2010) 107(36):15880–5. doi:10.1073/pnas.1005743107
10. Brühl MLV, Stark K, Steinhart A, Chandraratne S, Konrad I, Lorenz M, et al. Monocytes, neutrophils, and platelets cooperate to initiate and propagate venous thrombosis in mice in vivo. *J Exp Med* (2012) 209(4):819–35. doi:10.1084/jem.20112322
11. Saffar AS, Heather A, Gounni AS. The molecular mechanisms of glucocorticoids-mediated neutrophil survival. *Curr Drug Targets* (2011) 12(4):556–62. doi:10.2174/138945011794751555
12. Caramori G, Adcock I. Anti-inflammatory mechanisms of glucocorticoids targeting granulocytes. *Curr Drug Targets Inflamm Allergy* (2005) 4(4):455–63. doi:10.2174/1568010054526331
13. Clark SR, Ma AC, Tavener SA, McDonald B, Goodarzi Z, Kelly MM, et al. Platelet TLR4 activates neutrophil extracellular traps to ensnare bacteria in septic blood. *Nat Med* (2007) 13(4):463–9. doi:10.1038/nm1565
14. Prince LR, Whyte MK, Sabroe I, Parker LC. The role of TLRs in neutrophil activation. *Curr Opin Pharmacol* (2011) 11(4):397–403. doi:10.1016/j.coph.2011.06.007

15. Caramori G, Lasagna L, Casalini AG, Adcock IM, Casolari P, Contoli M, et al. Immune response to *Mycobacterium tuberculosis* infection in the parietal pleura of patients with tuberculous pleurisy. *PLoS One* (2011) 6(7):e22637. doi:10.1371/journal.pone.0022637
16. Walrand S, Valeix S, Rodriguez C, Ligot P, Chassagne J, Vasson MP. Flow cytometry study of polymorphonuclear neutrophil oxidative burst: a comparison of three fluorescent probes. *Clin Chim Acta* (2003) 331(331):103–10. doi:10.1016/S0009-8981(03)00086-X
17. Stoiber W, Obermayer A, Steinbacher P, Krautgartner WD. The role of reactive oxygen species (ROS) in the formation of extracellular traps (ETs) in humans. *Biomolecules* (2014) 5(2):702–23. doi:10.3390/biom5020702
18. Young RL, Malcolm KC, Kret JE, Caceres SM, Poch KR, Nichols DP, et al. Neutrophil extracellular trap (NET)-mediated killing of, *Pseudomonas aeruginosa*: evidence of acquired resistance within the CF airway, independent of CFTR. *PLoS One* (2011) 6(9):e23637. doi:10.1371/journal.pone.0023637
19. Lapponi MJ, Carestia A, Landoni VI, Rivadeneyra L, Etulain J, Negrotto S, et al. Regulation of neutrophil extracellular trap formation by anti-inflammatory drugs. *J Pharmacol Exp Ther* (2013) 345(3):430–7. doi:10.1124/jpet.112.202879
20. Caudrillier A, Kessenbrock K, Gilliss BM, Nguyen JX, Marques MB, Monestier M, et al. Platelets induce neutrophil extracellular traps in transfusion-related acute lung injury. *J Clin Invest* (2012) 122(7):2661–71. doi:10.1172/JCI61303
21. Fuchs TA, Abed U, Goosmann C, Hurwitz R, Schulze I, Wahn V, et al. Novel cell death program leads to neutrophil extracellular traps. *J Cell Biol* (2007) 176(2):231–41. doi:10.1083/jcb.200606027
22. Pilsczek FH, Salina D, Poon KK, Fahey C, Yipp BG, Sibley CD, et al. A novel mechanism of rapid nuclear neutrophil extracellular trap formation in response to *Staphylococcus aureus*. *J Immunol* (2010) 185(12):7413–25. doi:10.4049/jimmunol.1000675
23. Riyapa D, Buddhisa S, Korbsrisate S, Cuccui J, Wren BW, Stevens MP, et al. Neutrophil extracellular traps exhibit antibacterial activity against *Burkholderia pseudomallei* and are influenced by bacterial and host factors. *Infect Immun* (2012) 80(11):3921–9. doi:10.1128/IAI.00806-12
24. Parker H, Dragunow M, Hampton MB, Kettle AJ, Winterbourn CC. Requirements for NADPH oxidase and myeloperoxidase in neutrophil extracellular trap formation differ depending on the stimulus. *J Leukoc Biol* (2012) 92(4):841–9. doi:10.1189/jlb.1211601
25. Ren H, Teng Y, Tan B, Zhang X, Jiang W, Liu M, et al. Toll-like receptor-triggered calcium mobilization protects mice against bacterial infection through extracellular ATP release. *Infect Immun* (2014) 82(12):5076–85. doi:10.1128/IAI.02546-14
26. Medzhitov R. Recognition of microorganisms and activation of the immune response. *Nature* (2007) 449(7164):819–26. doi:10.1038/nature06246
27. Roeder A, Kirschning CJ, Rupec RA, Schaller M, Weindl G, Korting HC. Toll-like receptors as key mediators in innate antifungal immunity. *Med Mycol* (2004) 42(6):485–98. doi:10.1080/13693780400011112
28. Takeda K, Akira S. TLR signaling pathways. *Semin Immunol* (2004) 16:3–9. doi:10.1016/j.smim.2003.10.003
29. Beutler BA. TLRs and innate immunity. *Blood* (2008) 113(7):1399–407. doi:10.1182/blood-2008-07-019307
30. van de Veerdonk FL, Kullberg BJ, van der Meer JW, Gow NA, Netea MG. Host-microbe interactions: innate pattern recognition of fungal pathogens. *Curr Opin Microbiol* (2008) 11(4):305–12. doi:10.1016/j.mib.2008.06.002
31. Brinkmann V, Zychlinsky A. Beneficial suicide: why neutrophils die to make nets. *Nat Rev Microbiol* (2007) 5(8):577–82. doi:10.1038/nrmicro1710
32. Lecoq L, Vincent P, Lavoie-Lamoureux A, Lavoie JP. Genomic and non-genomic effects of dexamethasone on equine peripheral blood neutrophils. *Vet Immunol Immunopathol* (2009) 128(1–3):126–31. doi:10.1016/j.vetimm.2008.10.303
33. Mogensen TH, Berg RS, Paludan SR, Østergaard L. Mechanisms of dexamethasone-mediated inhibition of toll-like receptor signaling induced by *Neisseria meningitidis* and *Streptococcus pneumoniae*. *Infect Immun* (2008) 76(1):189–97. doi:10.1128/IAI.00856-07

7

Intestinal Innate Antiviral Immunity and Immunobiotics: Beneficial Effects against Rotavirus Infection

Julio Villena[1,2,3], Maria Guadalupe Vizoso-Pinto[1,4] and Haruki Kitazawa[2,3,5]**

[1] Immunobiotics Research Group, Tucuman, Argentina, [2] Laboratory of Immunobiotechnology, Reference Centre for Lactobacilli (CERELA-CONICET), Tucuman, Argentina, [3] Food and Feed Immunology Group, Laboratory of Animal Products Chemistry, Graduate School of Agricultural Science, Tohoku University, Sendai, Japan, [4] Faculty of Medicine, INSIBIO (UNT-CONICET), National University of Tucuman, Tucuman, Argentina, [5] Livestock Immunology Unit, International Education and Research Center for Food and Agricultural Immunology (CFAI), Graduate School of Agricultural Science, Tohoku University, Sendai, Japan

Edited by:
Amy Rasley,
Lawrence Livermore National Laboratory, USA

Reviewed by:
Benoit Chassaing,
Georgia State University, USA
Karl William Boehme,
University of Arkansas for Medical Sciences, USA

***Correspondence:**
Julio Villena
jcvillena@cerela.org.ar;
Haruki Kitazawa
haruki.kitazawa.c7@tohoku.ac.jp

The mucosal tissues of the gastrointestinal tract are the main portal entry of pathogens such as rotavirus (RV), which is a leading cause of death due to diarrhea among young children across the globe and a major cause of severe acute intestinal infection in livestock animals. The interactions between intestinal epithelial cells (IECs) and immune cells with RVs have been studied for several years, and now, it is known that the innate immune responses triggered by this virus can have both beneficial and detrimental effects for the host. It was demonstrated that natural RV infection in infants and experimental challenges in mice result in the intestinal activation of pattern recognition receptors (PRRs) such as toll-like receptor 3 (TLR3) and striking secretion of proinflammatory mediators that can lead to increased local tissue damage and immunopathology. Therefore, modulating desregulated intestinal immune responses triggered by PRRs activation are a significant promise for reducing the burden of RV diseases. The ability of immunoregulatory probiotic microorganisms (immunobiotics) to protect against intestinal infections, such as those caused by RVs, is among the oldest effects studied for these important group of beneficial microbes. In this review, we provide an update of the current status on the modulation of intestinal antiviral innate immunity by immunobiotics and their beneficial impact on RV infection. In addition, we describe the research of our group that demonstrated the capacity of immunobiotic strains to beneficially modulated TLR3-triggered immune response in IECs, reduce the disruption of intestinal homeostasis caused by intraepithelial lymphocytes, and improve the resistance to RV infections.

Keywords: immunobiotics, rotavirus, inflammation, TLR3, intestinal epithelial cells, intraepithelial lymphocytes

INTRODUCTION

One of the leading causes of children mortality is preventable infectious diseases (1, 2). Rotavirus (RVs), calicivirus, astrovirus, and adenovirus account to the viral etiologic agents of gastroenteritis in humans (3, 4). RV, a naked double-strand RNA (dsRNA) virus, is the most common cause of severe dehydrating diarrhea in children (5, 6). The main symptoms of RVs gastroenteritis are nausea, low-grade fever, vomit, and acute watery diarrhea. Even though two oral vaccines containing attenuated live viruses are being used globally, Rotarix (GlaxoSmithKline) and RotaTeq (Merck), the epidemic in the developing world is far from being controlled (6, 7). Vaccine effectiveness is reduced in developing areas, and some possible reasons are children infected at an early age, high viral challenge loads, and the lack of transferred maternal antibodies (8, 9).

Some lactic acid bacteria (LAB) strains are able to impact on human and animal health by modulating the mucosal and systemic immune systems. Those immunoregulatory probiotic LAB, known as immunobiotics, provide protection against viral infections by modulating innate and adaptive antiviral immunity. Thus, several reports have shown that immunobiotic LAB shorten the duration of diarrhea, reduce the number of episodes, diminish RVs shedding, normalize gut permeability, and increase the production of RVs-specific antibodies (10–12).

The purpose of this review is to provide an update of the current status on the modulation of intestinal antiviral innate immunity by immunobiotics, and their beneficial impact on RVs infection. We also highlight some results of our group, which demonstrate the capacity of immunobiotic strains to beneficially modulate toll-like receptor (TLR)-3-triggered immune response in intestinal epithelial cells (IECs), reduce the disruption of intestinal homeostasis caused by intraepithelial lymphocytes (IELs), and improve the resistance to RVs infection.

INTESTINAL ANTIVIRAL INNATE IMMUNE RESPONSE AND ROTAVIRUS

Upon RVs internalization, the capsid uncoats loosing VP4 and VP7, the outer surface proteins, and yielding a transcriptionally active double-layered particle. The eleven segments of dsRNA viral genome are transcribed directing the synthesis of structural and non-structural proteins and serving as templates for the complementary strand of genomic RNA (13). The IEC senses viral dsRNA through pattern recognition receptors (PRRs), such as TLR3, retinoic acid-inducible gene-I (RIG-I), and melanoma differentiation-associated gene-5 (MDA-5), and cellular signaling cascades are activated to react to viral infection (14–16) (**Figure 1**). One of the major innate responses against dsRNA viruses relies

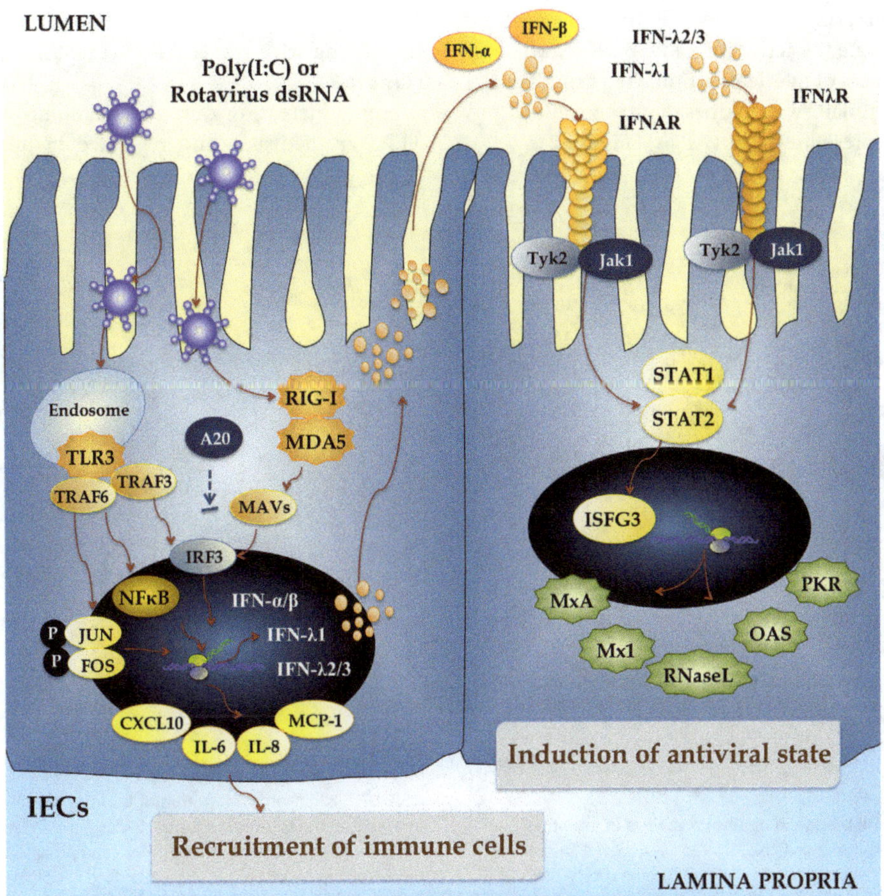

FIGURE 1 | Innate immune response against rotavirus in intestinal epithelial cells (IECs). Rotavirus double-strand genomic RNA activates toll-like receptor 3 (TLR3), retinoic acid-inducible gene-I (RIG-I), and melanoma differentiation-associated gene-5 (MDA-5), which are pattern recognition receptors (PRRs) expressed in IECs. Cellular signaling cascades are activated and converge at the level of interferon (IFN) regulatory factor-3 (IRF3) that upregulate the expression of type I (IFN-α, IFN-β) and type III (IFNλ1, IFNλ2/3) IFN, which in turn induces the synthesis of IFN-stimulated genes with antiviral activities (MxA, Mx1, RNase L, OAS, PKR). Antiviral PRRs also activate nuclear factor κB (NF-κB) pathway and induce the secretion of proinflammatory cytokines and chemokines (IL-6, IL-8, MCP-1, CXCL10). Those effects could be imitated *in vitro* and *in vivo* by administration of the dsRNA synthetic analog poly(I:C).

on the activation of those PRRs, which leads to the production of cytokines and chemokines by IECs and immune cells. Thus, RVs dsRNA triggers the production of IL-8, IP-10, IL-6, TNF-α, and IL-15 in IECs *via* the TLR3-, RIG-I-, and MDA5-activated pathways inducing recruitment and activation of macrophages and NK cells and stimulating adaptive B- and T-cell immune responses. As a result of PRRs activation, interferons (IFNs) and IFN-regulated gene products are also produced and they play a key role in establishing an antiviral state for virus clearance and restriction of spread (**Figure 1**). Type I and III IFNs limit RV infection *in vitro*, and their levels are augmented in RVs-infected children and animals (17–19). Both families of IFN are immediately produced upon RV infection, elicit responses on different types of receptors, and temporally and spatially regulated in the gastrointestinal tract (20). Another evidence suggesting that IFNs are crucial to limit RV infection relies on the fact that this virus has evolved mechanisms to manipulate IFNs signaling such as the type I IFNs damping NSP1 protein (21). While TLR3 mainly recognizes viral components such as viral nucleic acid in endosomal compartments, RIG-I and MDA-5 recognize cytoplasmatic dsRNA. These pathways converge at the level of IFN regulatory factor-3 (IRF3) (18, 22, 23). Upon IRF3 phosphorylation, antiviral responses initiate the activation of type I IFN, which in turn induces the synthesis of interferon-stimulated genes (ISGs), secretion of proinflammatory cytokines, and activation and maturation of antigen-presenting cells (APCs) (**Figure 2**).

Poly(I:C), a synthetic analog of dsRNA, when administered intraperitoneally to mice mimics the local intestinal immune response elicited by an enteric viral infection (24, 25). Both purified RVs dsRNA and poly(I:C) are able to induce severe mucosal damage in the gut *via* TLR3 activation including villous atrophy, mucosal erosion, and gut wall attenuation (24). IELs, which are mostly T cells distributed as single cells within the epithelial cell layer, play a critical role in disrupting epithelial homeostasis caused by abnormal TLR3 signaling (**Figure 3**) (24). Due to their key location at the interface between the inner intestinal tissue and the lumen, these specialized immune cells are important as a first line of defense against microbes and in maintaining the epithelial barrier homeostasis. The majority of IELs are CD8$^+$ being simply classified as CD8αα$^+$ or CD8αβ$^+$. The CD8αβ$^+$ IELs bear the hallmarks of adaptive immune cells, whereas the CD8αα$^+$ IELs are considered innate immune cells (26). When TLR3 is abnormally activated by poly(I:C) and RVs, genomic dsRNA, IL-15, and CD3$^+$NK1.1$^+$CD8αα$^+$ IELs are involved in the disruption of epithelial homeostasis. In addition, it was demonstrated that TLR3 activation in IECs induces the expression of retinoic acid early inducible-1 (RAE1), which mediates epithelial destruction and mucosal injury by interacting with the NKG2D receptor expressed on IELs (27) (**Figure 3**).

Thus, increasing our understanding of how PRRs such as TLR3 are activated and regulated in immune cells and IECs

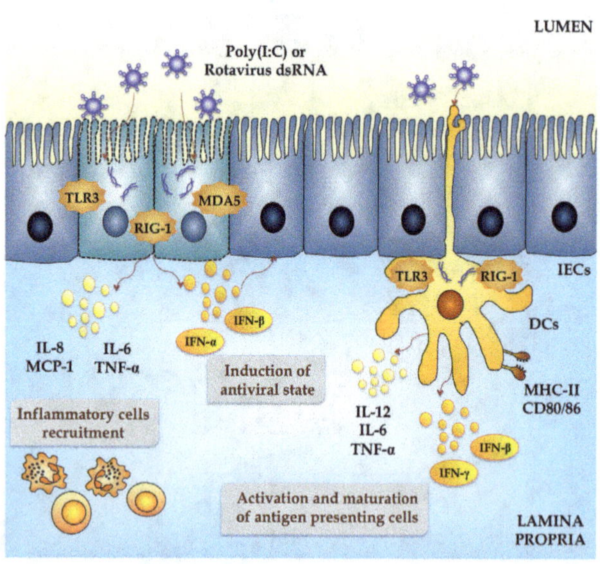

FIGURE 2 | Innate immune response against rotavirus in intestinal mucosa. Rotavirus double-strand genomic RNA activate toll-like receptor 3 (TLR3), retinoic acid-inducible gene-I (RIG-I), and melanoma differentiation-associated gene-5 (MDA-5), which are pattern recognition receptors (PRRs) expressed in intestinal epithelial cells (IECs) and dendritic cells (DCs). Activation of antiviral PRRs in the intestinal mucosa increases the production of type I IFN (IFN-α, IFN-β), IFN-γ, and proinflammatory cytokines and chemokines (TNF-α, IL-6, IL-8, IL-12, MCP-1), which improves the antiviral state in IECs, induces the recruitment and activation of immune cells and the maturation of DCs. Those effects could be imitated *in vitro* and *in vivo* by administration of the dsRNA synthetic analog poly(I:C).

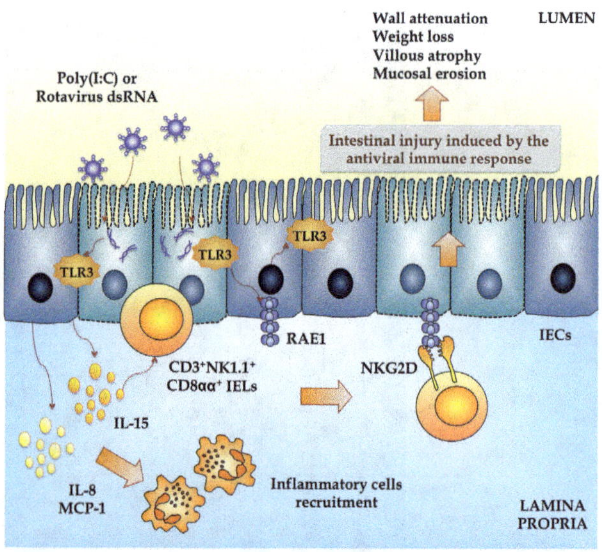

FIGURE 3 | Inflammatory damage of the intestinal mucosa induced by rotavirus in a toll-like receptor 3-deppendent manner. Both purified rotavirus double-strand genomic RNA and poly(I:C) induce severe mucosal intestinal damage *via* TLR3 activation and intestinal epithelial cells (IECs) and intraepithelial lymphocytes (IELs) interaction. Activation of TLR3 in IECs increases the expression of proinflammatory cytokines and chemokines (MCP-1, IL-8, IL-15) and retinoic acid early inducible-1 (RAE1). IL-15 produced by IECs induce the recruitment of CD3$^+$NK1.1$^+$CD8αα$^+$ IELs, which mediates epithelial destruction and mucosal injury by the NKG2D receptor expressed on these cells that is able to recognize RAE1. This intestinal TLR3-IECs-IELs interaction induces villous atrophy, mucosal erosion, and gut wall attenuation.

may help designing effective therapies for the prevention and/or treatment of viral diseases.

BENEFICIAL EFFECTS OF IMMUNOBIOTICS IN ROTAVIRUS INFECTION

Several studies have demonstrated that immunobiotics are able to improve the outcome of RV infection in human and livestock animals.

Effects of Immunobiotics in Humans

Lactobacillus rhamnosus GG is probably the most studied probiotic bacteria in the context of intestinal viral infections. Isolauri et al. (28) first described for more than 20 years, a protective effect of *L. rhamnosus* GG strain in RVs gastroenteritis in infants and children. In this study, the patients who received either a *L. rhamnosus* GG-fermented milk product or a *L. rhamnosus* GG freeze-dried powder after oral rehydration presented a significantly shorter duration of diarrhea when compared to the placebo group. Later, Majamaa et al. (29) conducted a study, in which 6- to 35-month-old children with RVs gastroenteritis received either *L. rhamnosus* GG, *Lactobacillus acidophilus* or a combination of *Streptococcus thermophilus* with *L. delbrückii* subsp. *bulgaricus* twice daily for 5 days. Only children who received *L. rhamnosus* GG had shorter diarrhea duration. The protective effect was related to augmented intestinal and serum IgA concentration, and a higher number of specific antibody-secreting cells to RVs. Additional studies showed that the consumption of *L. rhamnosus* GG is able to shorten the diarrheal phase in children suffering from RVs infection, an effect that was associated with increased concentrations of IgA antibodies as well (28–33). Furthermore, meta-analysis showed that the administration of *L. rhamnosus* GG to hospitalized children reduced the overall incidence of health care-associated diarrhea, including symptomatic RVs gastroenteritis (34). In spite of this evidence, it is important to notice that the shortening of diarrhea already at day 3 after probiotic treatment strongly suggests that the main therapeutic effect involves innate immune responses rather than the modulation of adaptive immunity (35).

Another example of probiotic treatment for alleviating RVs gastroenteritis was the use of *Lactobacillus reuteri*, which has been daily administered to hospitalized children with acute diarrhea for the length of hospitalization (up to 5 days). *L. reuteri* shortened both the duration of RVs diarrhea and the disease severity, when compared to the placebo group (36). *L. sporogenes* daily administered to newborns during 1 year, prevented the incidence and also diminished the duration of acute RVs diarrhea (37). Fang et al. (38) demonstrated that a minimal effective dose of *L. rhamnosus* significantly reduced fecal shedding RVs concentration in pediatric patients. Although the administration of lyophilized *Lactobacillus paracasei* strain ST11 daily for 5 days had a clinically significant benefit in the management of non-RVs-induced diarrhea, ST11 treatment against severe RVs diarrhea was ineffective (39). Children with RV infection who received milk-based formula supplemented with either *B. animalis* Bb12 alone or combined with *S. thermophilus* had fewer RVs infections (40).

In Argentina, mucosal infections such as bronchitis and diarrhea are the most common infectious diseases in children (41–43). In a randomized controlled trial conducted by Villena et al. (44), *L. rhamnosus* CRL1505 (administered in a yogurt formulation) improved mucosal immunity and reduced the incidence and severity of intestinal and respiratory infection in children. Hence, the incidence of infectious events was reduced from 66% in the placebo group to 34% in the group that received the probiotic yogurt. Furthermore, there was also a significant reduction in the occurrence of indicators of disease severity such as fever and the need for antibiotic treatment in children receiving the probiotic yogurt (44). Therefore, the results of this trial suggested that consumption of yogurt containing *L. rhamnosus* CRL1505 was helpful to reduce the burden of common childhood morbidities, especially those associated to viral infections including RVs (44).

Effects of Immunobiotics in Livestock Animals

Apart from the beneficial effects of immunobiotics on humans, some studies have evaluated their antiviral and anti-inflammatory activities in animals. Zhang et al. (45) reported that probiotic administration to gnotobiotic pigs challenged with RVs did not yielded differences in virus titers with respect to the placebo group. Nonetheless, LAB administration downregulated the recruitment of viral-activated monocytes/macrophages into the intestinal tract thereby limiting the inflammation induced by the virus (45).

In another study, it was shown that systemic monocyte/macrophage and APCs responses were modulated by immunobiotics in the context of a RV infection (45). Probiotic LAB induced strong TLR2-expressing APCs responses in blood and spleen, RVs induced a TLR3 response in spleen, and TLR9 responses were induced by RVs (as measured in immune cells isolated from spleen) and LAB (as determined in blood circulating immune cells). Immunobiotics and RVs had an additive effect on TLR2- and TLR9-expressing APCs responses, consistent with the adjuvant effect of LAB. Immunobiotics augmented IFN-γ and IL-4 levels in serum, but suppressed TLR3- and TLR9-expressing APCs responses in spleen and the serum IFN-α response induced by virulent RVs (46).

During RVs infections in weaned pigs, there is evidence of disruption of the barrier function as evidenced by the decreased villus height and crypt depth, lower levels of IgA, IL-4, and mucin 1 as well a reduced transcription of ZO-1, occludin, and Bcl-2 in jejunal mucosa (47). Some of these effects have been partially associated with alterations of transforming growth factor (TGF)-β production (48). Azevedo et al. (48) demonstrated that immunobiotic LAB further enhanced the Th1 and Th2 cytokine responses to RV infection as indicated by significantly higher concentrations of IL-12, IFN-γ, IL-4, and IL-10 in RVs-infected gnotobiotic pigs. LAB also helped to maintain immunological homeostasis during RV infection by regulating TGF-β production. It was also shown that treatment of pigs with *L. rhamnosus* GG modulated TGF-β and promoted the enhancement of intestinal epithelial tight junctions, which may contribute to the preservation and restoration of the gut homeostasis after RV infection (11). Further evidence was reported by Maragkoudakis et al. (12) demonstrating that *Lactobacillus casei* Shirota and *L. rhamnosus* GG protected porcine and goat epithelial cells from RVs and other transmissible gastroenteritis viruses.

CELLULAR AND MOLECULAR MECHANISMS OF IMMUNOBIOTICS ACTIONS

The interactions of IECs with luminal antigens and with immune cells play a central role in determining the type of immune response triggered by intestinal microorganisms (5, 6). A critical and virtually universal early innate response of host cells to viral infection is the secretion of factors belonging to the IFN family. The secretion of IFN results in the expression of several ISGs products with antiviral activities.

We showed in different studies that the originally established porcine intestinal epithelial cell line (PIE cells) is a useful tool for studying IFN response triggered by TLR3, RIG-I, and/or MDA-5 activation. These cells are permissive to porcine RVs and also respond to dsRNA and its synthetic analog poly(I:C) (49, 50). Furthermore, co-cultures of PIE cells with immune cells isolated from porcine Peyer's patches (PPs) provide an *in vitro* system to study the transduction of the signal from its detection by IECs to the effect on the under laying immune cells.

The response of PIE cells to poly(I:C) challenge was evaluated, and it was found that MCP-1, IL-8, TNF-α, IL-6, and both IFN-α and IFN-β were upregulated in PIE cells after stimulation (49). We also showed that after stimulation of co-cultures with poly(I:C), there was an upregulation of IFN-α, IFN-β, IFN-γ, IL-2, and IL-12p40 in immune cells (49). TLR3 was the receptor involved in the recognition of the luminal stimulus and the responsible to trigger the expression and release of cytokines, which in turn activated the underlying APCs and effector lymphocytes.

Rotavirus infection stimulates IFN-β and early antiviral gene expression by a signaling pathway that requires MAVS, an adaptor protein that is recruited to signaling complexes following activation of RIG-I or MDA-5 (51, 52). In addition, both RIG-I and MDA-5 are involved in recognizing RVs infection, as proven by the reduction of IFN-β induction when these factors are lost (51, 52). Taking into account those facts, we evaluated the suitability of PIE cells and co-cultures as models for studying this signaling pathway after RVs infection. Our results showed that PIE cells have functional TLR3, RIG-I, and MDA-5 receptors, which signal *via* IRF3 and NF-κB, inducing IFN-β and the upregulation of the ISGs MxA and RNase L (50), which are important antiviral effectors of IFN pathway.

We used PIE cells for the screening of immunobiotic LAB strains taking into consideration their ability to enhance IFN-β production upon poly(I:C) stimulation (49, 53). Thus, *L. casei* MEP221106 was selected because of its potential to impact on viral intestinal infections. *L. casei* MEP221106 had the highest capacity to improve IFN-β production in poly(I:C)-challenged PIE cells. Moreover, *in vitro* co-culture experiments showed that *L. casei* MEP221106 was able to improve not only the production of IFN-β but also the levels of other cytokines including IFN-α, TNF-α, MPC-1, and IL-6. In co-cultures of PIE cells with immune cells, we demonstrated that *L. casei* MEP221106 improved the production of inflammatory and antiviral cytokines by PPs cells when compared with control cells (49).

The PIE system was also used to screen bifidobacteria strains with anti-RVs effect (50). *Bifidobacterium infantis* MCC12 and *Bifidobacterium breve* MCC1274 were selected in the screen because they significantly upregulated IFN-β in response to poly(I:C) challenge. In addition, both MCC12 and MCC1274 strains significantly increased PIE cells resistance to RV infection (**Figure 4**), while other strains with moderate or no effect in IFN-β production did not have any influence on RVs replication (50). As a result of the enhanced IFN-β levels, there was a concomitant upregulation of the ISGs MxA and RNase L. These effectors of antiviral immunity have different mechanisms of action: RNase L degrades dsRNA and the resulting RNA fragments activate RLRs to amplify IFN production and induce apoptosis on virus infected cells (54), while MxA hijacks newly synthesized viral proteins into perinuclear complexes. Then, the upregulation of MxA, RNase L, and probably other ISGs induced by MCC12 and MCC1274 strains through IFN-β would be related to the lower RVs replication found in bifidobacteria-treated PIE cells. This is supported by the fact that IFN-β is a key factor for improving defenses against RVs since viral replication is restricted in permissive cells when they are pretreated with IFN-β (55). Accordingly, IFN-β treatment of newborn calves and piglets prior to RV infection reduces virus replication and disease severity (56).

Several cytokines are induced *via* NF-κB signaling as a result of RVs infection, including IL-8, RANTES, GM-CSF, GRO-α, MIP-1β, and IP-10 (57), as observed in both cell lines and histological intestinal samples. Secreted cytokines initiate an important primary line of host defense, but if this response lasts too long or is dysregulated, it may lead to tissue damage and epithelial barrier dysfunction. In this regard, we have reported that efficient regulation of inflammatory response induced by immunobiotic bacteria is essential to achieve full protection against pathogens (58, 59). In line with this, we also showed that bifidobacteria strains MCC12 and MCC1274 differentially modulated the production of proinflammatory mediators in RVs-infected PIE cells (**Figure 4**) (50).

Toll-like receptor negative regulators play key roles in maintaining intestinal hemostasis by regulating TLR signaling. The zinc-finger protein A20, due to its deubiquitinase and ubiquitinase E3 ligase activities, is capable to terminate TLR signaling that results in inhibition of NF-κB activation and reduction of inflammatory induced cytotoxicity (60). Saitoh et al. (61) reported that IRF3 activation is suppressed by A20. The A20 protein is able to induce the suppression of the IFN-mediated immune response and IFN-promoter-dependent transcription by physically interacting with IKK-i/IKKϵ and inhibiting dimerization of IRF3 following engagement of TLR3 by dsRNA. Moreover, A20 knock down results in enhanced IRF3-dependent transcription triggered by the stimulation of TLR3 or virus infection. Human monocyte-derived dendritic cells (DCs) stimulated

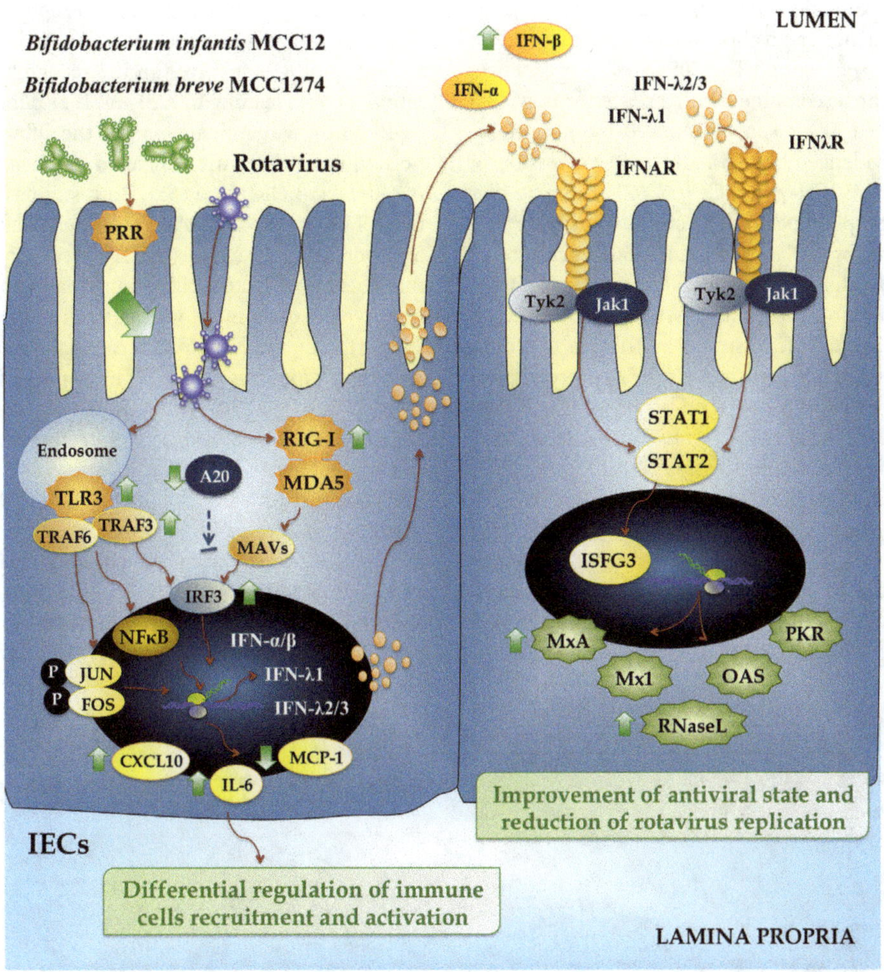

FIGURE 4 | Beneficial effects of immunobiotic bifidobacteria on the innate immune response against rotavirus in intestinal epithelial cells (IECs). Rotavirus double-strand genomic RNA activates toll-like receptor 3 (TLR3), retinoic acid-inducible gene-I (RIG-I), and melanoma differentiation-associated gene-5 (MDA-5), which are pattern recognition receptors (PRRs) expressed in IECs. Cellular signaling cascades mediated by interferon (IFN) regulatory factor-3 (IRF3) upregulate the expression of type I (IFN-α, IFN-β), and type III (IFNλ1, IFNλ2/3) IFN, which in turn induces the synthesis of IFN-stimulated genes with antiviral activities (MxA, Mx1, RNase L, OAS, PKR). Antiviral PRRs also activate nuclear factor κB (NF-κB) pathway and induce the secretion of proinflammatory cytokines and chemokines (IL-6, MCP-1, CXCL10). Preventive treatment of IECs with *Bifidobacterium infantis* MCC12 or *Bifidobacterium breve* MCC1274 reduce the expression of A20, increase the activation of IRF3, improve the production of the antiviral factors IFN-α, IFN-β, MxA, and RNase L, and differentially regulate the expression of IL-6, MCP-1, and CXCL10.

with poly(I:C) upregulate A20. When A20 is downregulated in DCs, they showed higher activation of NF-κB and AP-1, which resulted in increased and sustained production of IL-6, IL-10, and IL-12p70. Furthermore, DCs enhanced their T cell stimulatory capacity (62). Negative regulators involved in TLR signaling can be modulated by immunobiotic strains in human intestinal cell lines (63). In this regard, we also reported that both *B. infantis* MCC12 and *B. breve* MCC1274 significantly reduced the expression of A20 in RVs-infected PIE cells (**Figure 4**) (50), which is in line with the capacity of both strains to improve IRF3 activation and IFN-β production. In line with our findings, MacPherson et al. (64) also studied the effect of probiotics in the modulation of poly(I:C) induced inflammatory response in HT-29 cells. Stimulating HT29 cells with poly(I:C) alone increased the expression of A20, but the co-stimulation with poly(I:C) and probiotics significantly reduced A20 expression levels.

We also used these porcine *in vitro* systems to attain deeper knowledge into the mechanisms involved in the immunomodulatory effect of *L. rhamnosus* CRL1505 and concentrated our attention in the crosstalk between the immunobiotic strain and porcine IECs and APCs, in order to explain its capacity to reduce viral diarrhea episodes in children (44). Moreover, we performed comparative studies with another immunobiotic strain, *Lactobacillus plantarum* CRL1506, that is able stimulate intestinal immunity in animal models (65). Studies comparing the immunobiotic strains *L. rhamnosus* CRL1505 and *L. plantarum* CRL1506 in co-cultures of PIE cells and APCs, stimulated with poly(I:C), showed that both strains improved the production of type I IFNs in response to poly(I:C) challenge (66). In addition, CRL1505 and CRL1506 strains modulated the expression of proinflammatory and regulatory cytokines and influenced activation and maturation of APCs (**Figure 5**). However, *L. rhamnosus* CRL1505 had a stronger effect both when applied alone or combined with a posterior poly(I:C) challenge. The improved Th1 response induced by immunobiotic lactobacilli was evidenced by the augmented expression of MHC-II, IL-1β, IL-6, and IFN-γ in DCs (66, 67). Those studies gave scientific basis for explaining the protection against intestinal viral infections achieved by *L. rhamnosus* CRL1505 in children.

The receptors, which are activated by the immunobiotics strains with antiviral capabilities MEP221106, MCC12, MCC1274, CRL1505, and CRL1506 strains in PIE cells to reduce A20, improve IRF-3 activation and increase IFN-β production remains to be uncovered. Bifidobacteria strains with a high capacity to stimulate TLR2 such as *B. longum* BB536 and *B. breve* M-16V were able to increase the expression of A20 in PIE cells and reduce TLR4-mediated inflammatory response (68, 69). On the contrary, strains with low capacity of stimulating TLR2 did not modify the expression of the ubiquitin-editing enzyme A20 in PIE cells challenged with TLR4 agonists. In our experiments, we were unable to block the increase of IFN-β induced by the lactobacilli and bifidobacteria by using anti-TLR2 or anti-TLR9 antibodies, suggesting that other receptor(s) are involved in the immunobiotic activity (66). Further studies are needed in order to find the PRRs involved in the recognition of lactobacilli and bifidobacteria leading to A20 and IFN-β modulation in PIE cells.

Recently, we confirmed *in vivo* the differential antiviral immunomodulatory activities triggered by *L. rhamnosus* CRL1505 and *L. plantarum* CRL1506 (65). Both strains increased the production of IFNs, the CRL1505 treatment being the most effective for increasing the levels of IFN-γ. Then, our results suggest that these two lactobacilli strains have potential to be used to improve the outcome of viral gastrointestinal disease. This is also supported by the human clinical trial demonstrating the capacity of *L. rhamnosus* CRL1505 to improve the infectious disease rates in children (70). Recently, Zhang et al. (71) proposed the activation of innate immunity with flagellin as a preventive and therapeutic strategy against RVs infection. They demonstrated that intraperitoneal flagellin injection reduced severity and shedding of RVs RNA in acute and chronic infected mice *via* TLR5/NLRC4 activation, which resulted in secretion of IL-22 and IL-18 by different effector cells. Although the mechanism of action of flagellin administration is substantially different to the

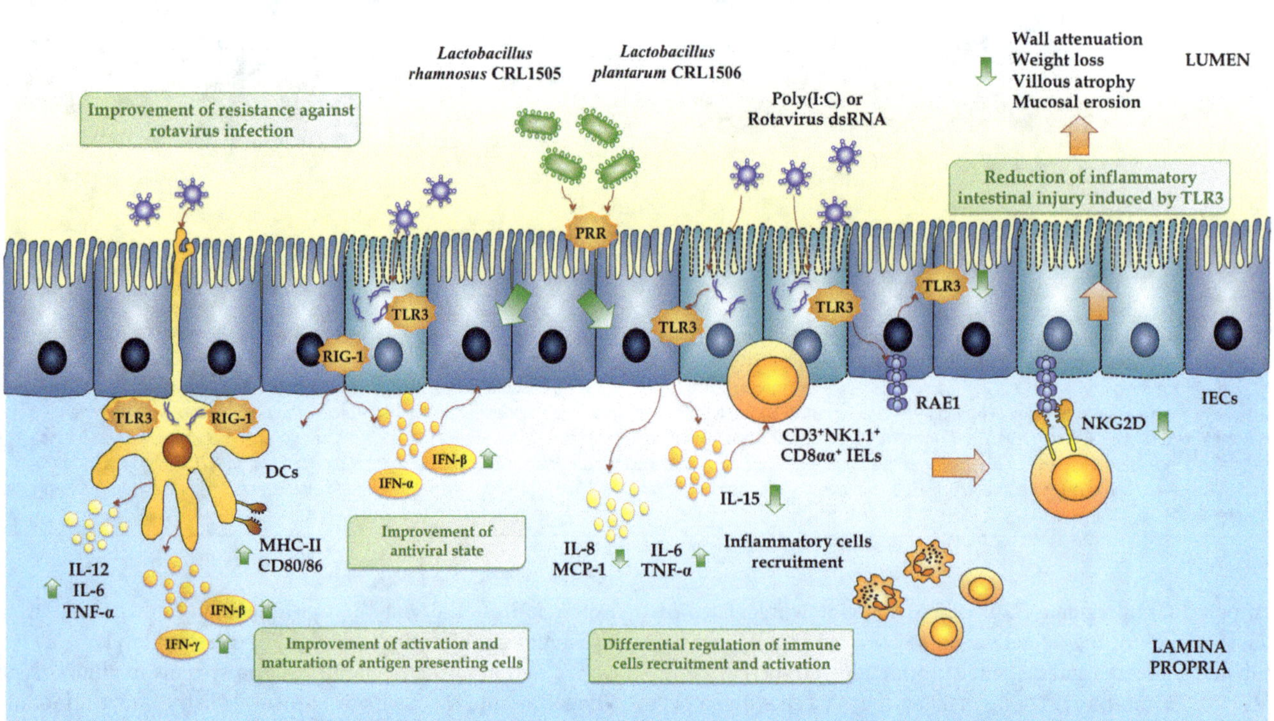

FIGURE 5 | Beneficial effects of immunobiotic lactobacilli on the innate immune response against rotavirus in intestinal mucosa. Rotavirus double-strand genomic RNA or poly(I:C) activate toll-like receptor 3 (TLR3), retinoic acid-inducible gene-I (RIG-I), and melanoma differentiation-associated gene-5 (MDA-5), which are pattern recognition receptors (PRRs) expressed in intestinal epithelial cells (IECs) and dendritic cells (DCs). Activation of antiviral PRRs increases the production of IFN-α, IFN-β, IFN-γ, and proinflammatory cytokines and chemokines (TNF-α, IL-6, IL-8, IL-12, MCP-1), which improves the antiviral state in IECs, induces the recruitment and activation of immune cells and the maturation of DCs. In addition, both purified rotavirus genomic dsRNA and poly(I:C) activate TLR3 in IECs increasing the expression of IL-15 and retinoic acid early inducible-1 (RAE1). IL-15 produced by IECs induces the recruitment of $CD3^+NK1.1^+CD8\alpha\alpha^+$ intraepithelial lymphocytes (IELs), which mediates epithelial destruction and mucosal injury by the NKG2D receptor expressed on these cells that is able to recognize RAE1. Preventive treatments with *Lactobacillus rhamnosus* CRL1505 or *Lactobacillus plantarum* CRL1506 improve the production of type I IFN and IFN-γ in the intestinal mucosa enhancing the antiviral state and differentially regulate the expression of inflammatory cytokines and chemokines reducing the intestinal damage, especially associated with the TLR3–IECs–IELs interaction.

mechanisms elicited by immunobiotics, both approaches rely on the principle of combating viral infection by enhancing innate immune defenses.

Lactobacillus rhamnosus CRL1505 and *L. plantarum* CRL1506 also reduced TLR3-induced small intestinal injury by regulation of proinflammatory cytokines production and IECs–IELs interaction (65) (**Figure 5**). IECs and IELs are the first line of defense against pathogens including viruses, and their interaction is essential for maintaining an appropriate immunological homeostasis. IECs produce a variety of cytokines and chemokines, including IL-6, IL-7, IL-8, IL-15, TNF-α, TGF-β, and GM-CSF. IL-15 functions as a mediator of TLR3-induced small intestinal injury (24). Abnormal TLR3 signaling results in elevated levels of IL-15, which regulates IECs apoptosis by activating perforin-mediated killing by $CD3^+NK1.1^+$ IELs (70). Moreover, IL-15 is able to enhance the cytotoxic activity of human IELs (72). Blocking the α receptor of IL-15 partially protected mice from poly(I:C)-induced small intestinal injury, including less villous atrophy, and mucosal erosion (24). Autologous ligands released by cells stress and infection are recognized by the NKG2D receptor in NK cells. NKG2D ligands expression is downregulated by gut microbiota, as demonstrated in germ-free mice, which had increased surface expression of these ligands (73). RAE1, a high affinity NKG2D ligand, which is minimally detected in normal cells, is upregulated upon TLR3 activation. In fact, blockade of NKG2D–RAE1 interaction avoids the cytotoxic effect of IELs on IECs and prevents acute small intestinal injury in mice challenged with dsRNA (27). Therefore, TLR3 signaling stimulates IECs to express IL-15 and RAE1 and induces $CD3^+NK1.1^+CD8\alpha\alpha^+$ IELs to express NKG2D through IEC-derived IL-15. In our hands, poly(I:C) treatment of mice increased intestinal injury in a IL-15- and $CD8\alpha\alpha^+NKG2D^+$-dependent manner (65). Poly(I:C) induced inflammatory-mediated intestinal tissue damage through the increase of $CD3^+NK1.1^+$ and $CD8\alpha\alpha^+NKG2D^+$ cells as well as proinflammatory mediators (TNF-α, IL-1β, IFN-γ, IL-15, RAE1, IL-8). Mice pretreated with immunobiotic lactobacilli before TLR3 activation responded with reduced levels of TNF-α, IL-15, RAE1, $CD3^+NK1.1^+$, $CD3^+CD8\alpha\alpha^+$, and $CD8\alpha\alpha^+NKG2D^+$ cells (**Figure 5**). The beneficial effect of these lactobacilli improved mice health as reflected by a significant reduction of body weight loss and intestinal tissue damage after poly(I:C) challenge (65).

It is well known that commensal bacteria in the gut are able to modulate IELs function. Furthermore, IELs are significantly reduced in germ-free mice (74, 75) underlying gut microbiota importance in the maintenance of IELs. These specialized lymphocytes are very important players in mucosal protection; they seem to occupy a unique temporal niche from which they are able to detect and limit bacterial penetration already in the first hours after pathogen attack (76). Ismail et al. (76) showed that IEL antibacterial response depends on bacterial stimulation in a MyD88-dependent signaling. Later, Jiang et al. (77) investigated the role of NOD2 signaling in the maintenance of IELs and found that NOD2 maintained IELs *via* recognition of gut microbiota. They demonstrated that stimulation of IEL requires activation of PRRs signaling in neighboring IECs (76, 77).

Therefore, it was shown that commensal bacteria establish a regulatory milieu in a healthy gut, with increased expression of immuno-inhibitory cytokines such as TGF-β and IL-10, which in turn downregulate NKG2D ligand surface expression (78, 79). This is in line with our findings for the immunomodulatory strains *L. rhamnosus* CRL1505 and *L. plantarum* CRL1506, which reduced expression of RAE-1 and increased levels of intestinal IL-10. Whether the immunomodulatory effects of *L. rhamnosus* CRL1505 and *L. plantarum* CRL1506 are induced by direct action on the IECs (indirectly on IELs) and/or a direct effect on IELs is an open question, which we propose to address in the near future.

CONCLUSION

The detailed characterization of the cellular and molecular mechanisms underlying the intestinal innate defense against RV infection achieved in the past years has opened new ways for developing strategies to preventing and treating this viral induced diarrhea. In this sense, the use of immunobiotic bacteria to beneficially modulate IFN and inflammatory signaling pathways in IECs and immune cells is an attractive target for preventive or therapeutic intervention against RVs infection. Furthermore, the advances in the knowledge of the molecular crosstalk between immunobiotics and the gut innate immune system have provided light into the microorganism-sensing signals that allow these beneficial microorganisms to improve intestinal immune responses. This new molecular information might be helpful to improve the development of functional foods and/or pharmabiotics using immunobiotics aimed to reduce mortality and severity of RVs disease.

AUTHOR CONTRIBUTIONS

JV, MV-P, and HK designed, wrote, and revised the review article.

REFERENCES

1. Bryce J, Black RE, Walker N, Bhutta ZA, Lawn JE, Steketee RW. Can the world afford to save the lives of 6 million children each year? *Lancet* (2005) 365(9478):2193–200. doi:10.1016/S0140-6736(05)66777-3
2. Bryce J, Victora CG. Child survival: countdown to 2015. *Lancet* (2005) 365(9478):2153–4. doi:10.1016/S0140-6736(05)66752-9
3. Ciarlet M, Estes MK. Rotavirus and calicivirus infections of the gastrointestinal tract. *Curr Opin Gastroenterol* (2001) 17(1):10–6. doi:10.1097/00001574-200101000-00003
4. Tran A, Talmud D, Lejeune B, Jovenin N, Renois F, Payan C, et al. Prevalence of rotavirus, adenovirus, norovirus, and astrovirus infections and coinfections among hospitalized children in northern France. *J Clin Microbiol* (2010) 48(5):1943–6. doi:10.1128/JCM.02181-09
5. Parashar UD, Gibson CJ, Bresee JS, Glass RI. Rotavirus and severe childhood diarrhea. *Emerg Infect Dis* (2006) 12(2):304–6. doi:10.3201/eid1202.050006
6. Greenberg HB, Estes MK. Rotaviruses: from pathogenesis to vaccination. *Gastroenterology* (2009) 136(6):1939–51. doi:10.1053/j.gastro.2009.02.076
7. Tate JE, Patel MM, Cortese MM, Lopman BA, Gentsch JR, Fleming J, et al. Remaining issues and challenges for rotavirus vaccine in preventing global childhood diarrheal morbidity and mortality. *Expert Rev Vaccines* (2012) 11(2):211–20. doi:10.1586/erv.11.184
8. Angel J, Franco MA, Greenberg HB. Rotavirus immune responses and correlates of protection. *Curr Opin Virol* (2012) 2(4):419–25. doi:10.1016/j.coviro.2012.05.003

9. Wang CM, Chen SC, Chen KT. Current status of rotavirus vaccines. *World J Pediatr* (2015) 11(4):300–8. doi:10.1007/s12519-015-0038-y
10. Basu S, Paul DK, Ganguly S, Chatterjee M, Chandra PK. Efficacy of high-dose *Lactobacillus rhamnosus* GG in controlling acute watery diarrhea in Indian children: a randomized controlled trial. *J Clin Gastroenterol* (2009) 43(3):208–13. doi:10.1097/MCG.0b013e31815a5780
11. Liu F, Li G, Wen K, Bui T, Cao D, Zhang Y, et al. Porcine small intestinal epithelial cell line (IPEC-J2) of rotavirus infection as a new model for the study of innate immune responses to rotaviruses and probiotics. *Viral Immunol* (2010) 23(2):135–49. doi:10.1089/vim.2009.0088
12. Maragkoudakis PA, Chingwaru W, Gradisnik L, Tsakalidou E, Cencic A. Lactic acid bacteria efficiently protect human and animal intestinal epithelial and immune cells from enteric virus infection. *Int J Food Microbiol* (2010) 141(Suppl 1):S91–7. doi:10.1016/j.ijfoodmicro.2009.12.024
13. Lopez S, Oceguera A, Sandoval-Jaime C. Stress response and translation control in rotavirus infection. *Viruses* (2016) 8(6):E162. doi:10.3390/v8060162
14. Frias AH, Jones RM, Fifadara NH, Vijay-Kumar M, Gewirtz AT. Rotavirus-induced IFN-beta promotes anti-viral signaling and apoptosis that modulate viral replication in intestinal epithelial cells. *Innate Immun* (2012) 18(2):294–306. doi:10.1177/1753425911401930
15. Frias AH, Vijay-Kumar M, Gentsch JR, Crawford SE, Carvalho FA, Estes MK, et al. Intestinal epithelia activate anti-viral signaling via intracellular sensing of rotavirus structural components. *Mucosal Immunol* (2010) 3(6):622–32. doi:10.1038/mi.2010.39
16. Akira S. Innate immunity and adjuvants. *Philos Trans R Soc Lond B Biol Sci* (2011) 366(1579):2748–55. doi:10.1098/rstb.2011.0106
17. Sen A, Rothenberg ME, Mukherjee G, Feng N, Kalisky T, Nair N, et al. Innate immune response to homologous rotavirus infection in the small intestinal villous epithelium at single-cell resolution. *Proc Natl Acad Sci U S A* (2012) 109(50):20667–72. doi:10.1073/pnas.1212188109
18. Meylan E, Tschopp J. Toll-like receptors and RNA helicases: two parallel ways to trigger antiviral responses. *Mol Cell* (2006) 22(5):561–9. doi:10.1016/j.molcel.2006.05.012
19. Kawai T, Akira S. Innate immune recognition of viral infection. *Nat Immunol* (2006) 7(2):131–7. doi:10.1038/ni1303
20. Lin JD, Feng N, Sen A, Balan M, Tseng HC, McElrath C, et al. Distinct roles of type I and type III interferons in intestinal immunity to homologous and heterologous rotavirus infections. *PLoS Pathog* (2016) 12(4):e1005600. doi:10.1371/journal.ppat.1005600
21. Barro M, Patton JT. Rotavirus NSP1 inhibits expression of type I interferon by antagonizing the function of interferon regulatory factors IRF3, IRF5, and IRF7. *J Virol* (2007) 81(9):4473–81. doi:10.1128/JVI.02498-06
22. Loo YM, Fornek J, Crochet N, Bajwa G, Perwitasari O, Martinez-Sobrido L, et al. Distinct RIG-I and MDA5 signaling by RNA viruses in innate immunity. *J Virol* (2008) 82(1):335–45. doi:10.1128/JVI.01080-07
23. Takeuchi O, Akira S. MDA5/RIG-I and virus recognition. *Curr Opin Immunol* (2008) 20(1):17–22. doi:10.1016/j.coi.2008.01.002
24. Zhou R, Wei H, Sun R, Tian Z. Recognition of double-stranded RNA by TLR3 induces severe small intestinal injury in mice. *J Immunol* (2007) 178(7):4548–56. doi:10.4049/jimmunol.178.7.4548
25. Araya RE, Jury J, Bondar C, Verdu EF, Chirdo FG. Intraluminal administration of poly I:C causes an enteropathy that is exacerbated by administration of oral dietary antigen. *PLoS One* (2014) 9(6):e99236. doi:10.1371/journal.pone.0099236
26. Shires J, Theodoridis E, Hayday AC. Biological insights into TCRgammadelta+ and TCRalphabeta+ intraepithelial lymphocytes provided by serial analysis of gene expression (SAGE). *Immunity* (2001) 15(3):419–34. doi:10.1016/S1074-7613(01)00192-3
27. Zhou R, Wei H, Sun R, Zhang J, Tian Z. NKG2D recognition mediates toll-like receptor 3 signaling-induced breakdown of epithelial homeostasis in the small intestines of mice. *Proc Natl Acad Sci U S A* (2007) 104(18):7512–5. doi:10.1073/pnas.0700822104
28. Isolauri E, Juntunen M, Rautanen T, Sillanaukee P, Koivula T. A human *Lactobacillus* strain (*Lactobacillus casei* sp strain GG) promotes recovery from acute diarrhea in children. *Pediatrics* (1991) 88(1):90–7.
29. Majamaa H, Isolauri E, Saxelin M, Vesikari T. Lactic acid bacteria in the treatment of acute rotavirus gastroenteritis. *J Pediatr Gastroenterol Nutr* (1995) 20(3):333–8. doi:10.1097/00005176-199504000-00012
30. Isolauri E, Kaila M, Mykkanen H, Ling WH, Salminen S. Oral bacteriotherapy for viral gastroenteritis. *Dig Dis Sci* (1994) 39(12):2595–600. doi:10.1007/BF02087695
31. Kaila M, Isolauri E, Soppi E, Virtanen E, Laine S, Arvilommi H. Enhancement of the circulating antibody secreting cell response in human diarrhea by a human *Lactobacillus* strain. *Pediatr Res* (1992) 32(2):141–4. doi:10.1203/00006450-199208000-00002
32. Shornikova AV, Casas IA, Mykkanen H, Salo E, Vesikari T. Bacteriotherapy with *Lactobacillus reuteri* in rotavirus gastroenteritis. *Pediatr Infect Dis J* (1997) 16(12):1103–7. doi:10.1097/00006454-199712000-00002
33. Guarino A, Canani RB, Spagnuolo MI, Albano F, Di Benedetto L. Oral bacterial therapy reduces the duration of symptoms and of viral excretion in children with mild diarrhea. *J Pediatr Gastroenterol Nutr* (1997) 25(5):516–9. doi:10.1097/00005176-199711000-00005
34. Szajewska H, Wanke M, Patro B. Meta-analysis: the effects of *Lactobacillus rhamnosus* GG supplementation for the prevention of healthcare-associated diarrhoea in children. *Aliment Pharmacol Ther* (2011) 34(9):1079–87. doi:10.1111/j.1365-2036.2011.04837.x
35. Vlasova AN, Kandasamy S, Chattha KS, Rajashekara G, Saif LJ. Comparison of probiotic lactobacilli and bifidobacteria effects, immune responses and rotavirus vaccines and infection in different host species. *Vet Immunol Immunopathol* (2016) 172:72–84. doi:10.1016/j.vetimm.2016.01.003
36. Shornikova AV, Casas IA, Isolauri E, Mykkanen H, Vesikari T. *Lactobacillus reuteri* as a therapeutic agent in acute diarrhea in young children. *J Pediatr Gastroenterol Nutr* (1997) 24(4):399–404. doi:10.1097/00005176-199704000-00008
37. Chandra RK. Effect of *Lactobacillus* on the incidence and severity of acute rotavirus diarrhoea in infants. A prospective placebo-controlled double-blind study. *Nutr Res* (2002) 22:65–9. doi:10.1016/S0271-5317(01)00367-0
38. Fang SB, Lee HC, Hu JJ, Hou SY, Liu HL, Fang HW. Dose-dependent effect of *Lactobacillus rhamnosus* on quantitative reduction of faecal rotavirus shedding in children. *J Trop Pediatr* (2009) 55(5):297–301. doi:10.1093/tropej/fmp001
39. Sarker SA, Sultana S, Fuchs GJ, Alam NH, Azim T, Brussow H, et al. *Lactobacillus paracasei* strain ST11 has no effect on rotavirus but ameliorates the outcome of nonrotavirus diarrhea in children from Bangladesh. *Pediatrics* (2005) 116(2):e221–8. doi:10.1542/peds.2004-2334
40. Phuapradit P, Varavithya W, Vathanophas K, Sangchai R, Podhipak A, Suthutvoravut U, et al. Reduction of rotavirus infection in children receiving bifidobacteria-supplemented formula. *J Med Assoc Thai* (1999) 82(Suppl 1):S43–8.
41. Bardach A, Ciapponi A, Garcia-Marti S, Glujovsky D, Mazzoni A, Fayad A, et al. Epidemiology of acute otitis media in children of Latin America and the Caribbean: a systematic review and meta-analysis. *Int J Pediatr Otorhinolaryngol* (2011) 75(9):1062–70. doi:10.1016/j.ijporl.2011.05.014
42. Edmond K, Scott S, Korczak V, Ward C, Sanderson C, Theodoratou E, et al. Long term sequelae from childhood pneumonia; systematic review and meta-analysis. *PLoS One* (2012) 7(2):e31239. doi:10.1371/journal.pone.0031239
43. Gentile A, Bardach A, Ciapponi A, Garcia-Marti S, Aruj P, Glujovsky D, et al. Epidemiology of community-acquired pneumonia in children of Latin America and the Caribbean: a systematic review and meta-analysis. *Int J Infect Dis* (2012) 16(1):e5–15. doi:10.1016/j.ijid.2011.09.013
44. Villena J, Salva S, Núñez M, Corzo J, Tolaba R, Faedda J, et al. Probiotics for everyone! The novel immunobiotic *Lactobacillus rhamnosus* CRL1505 and the beginning of Social Probiotic Programs in Argentina. *Int J Biotechnol Wellness Ind* (2012) 1:189–98. doi:10.6000/1927-3037/2012.01.03.05
45. Zhang W, Wen K, Azevedo MS, Gonzalez A, Saif LJ, Li G, et al. Lactic acid bacterial colonization and human rotavirus infection influence distribution and frequencies of monocytes/macrophages and dendritic cells in neonatal gnotobiotic pigs. *Vet Immunol Immunopathol* (2008) 121(3–4):222–31. doi:10.1016/j.vetimm.2007.10.001
46. Wen K, Li G, Bui T, Liu F, Li Y, Kocher J, et al. High dose and low dose *Lactobacillus acidophilus* exerted differential immune modulating effects on T cell immune responses induced by an oral human rotavirus vaccine in gnotobiotic pigs. *Vaccine* (2012) 30(6):1198–207. doi:10.1016/j.vaccine.2011.11.107
47. Mao X, Gu C, Hu H, Tang J, Chen D, Yu B, et al. Dietary *Lactobacillus rhamnosus* GG supplementation improves the mucosal barrier function in the intestine of weaned piglets challenged by porcine rotavirus. *PLoS One* (2016) 11(1):e0146312. doi:10.1371/journal.pone.0146312
48. Azevedo MS, Zhang W, Wen K, Gonzalez AM, Saif LJ, Yousef AE, et al. *Lactobacillus acidophilus* and *Lactobacillus reuteri* modulate cytokine responses in gnotobiotic pigs infected with human rotavirus. *Benef Microbes* (2012) 3(1):33–42. doi:10.3920/BM2011.0041

49. Hosoya S, Villena J, Shimazu T, Tohno M, Fujie H, Chiba E, et al. Immunobiotic lactic acid bacteria beneficially regulate immune response triggered by poly(I:C) in porcine intestinal epithelial cells. *Vet Res* (2011) 42(1):111. doi:10.1186/1297-9716-42-111
50. Ishizuka T, Kanmani P, Kobayashi H, Miyazaki A, Soma J, Suda Y, et al. Immunobiotic bifidobacteria strains modulate rotavirus immune response in porcine intestinal epitheliocytes via pattern recognition receptor signaling. *PLoS One* (2016) 11(3):e0152416. doi:10.1371/journal.pone.0152416
51. Sen A, Pruijssers AJ, Dermody TS, Garcia-Sastre A, Greenberg HB. The early interferon response to rotavirus is regulated by PKR and depends on MAVS/IPS-1, RIG-I, MDA-5, and IRF3. *J Virol* (2011) 85(8):3717–32. doi:10.1128/JVI.02634-10
52. Broquet AH, Hirata Y, McAllister CS, Kagnoff MF. RIG-I/MDA5/MAVS are required to signal a protective IFN response in rotavirus-infected intestinal epithelium. *J Immunol* (2011) 186(3):1618–26. doi:10.4049/jimmunol.1002862
53. Hosoya S, Villena J, Chiba E, Shimazu T, Suda Y, Aso H, et al. Advanced application of porcine intestinal epithelial cells for the selection of immunobiotics modulating toll-like receptor 3-mediated inflammation. *J Microbiol Immunol Infect* (2013). 46:474–81. doi:10.1016/j.jmii.2012.04.005
54. Morelli M, Ogden KM, Patton JT. Silencing the alarms: innate immune antagonism by rotavirus NSP1 and VP3. *Virology* (2015) 47(9–480):75–84. doi:10.1016/j.virol.2015.01.006
55. Papp H, Laszlo B, Jakab F, Ganesh B, De Grazia S, Matthijnssens J, et al. Review of group A rotavirus strains reported in swine and cattle. *Vet Microbiol* (2013) 165(3–4):190–9. doi:10.1016/j.vetmic.2013.03.020
56. Arnold MM, Sen A, Greenberg HB, Patton JT. The battle between rotavirus and its host for control of the interferon signaling pathway. *PLoS Pathog* (2013) 9(1):e1003064. doi:10.1371/journal.ppat.1003064
57. Casola A, Estes MK, Crawford SE, Ogra PL, Ernst PB, Garofalo RP, et al. Rotavirus infection of cultured intestinal epithelial cells induces secretion of CXC and CC chemokines. *Gastroenterology* (1998) 114(5):947–55. doi:10.1016/S0016-5085(98)70314-2
58. Chiba E, Villena J, Hosoya S, Takanashi N, Shimazu T, Aso H, et al. A newly established bovine intestinal epithelial cell line is effective for in vitro screening of potential antiviral immunobiotic microorganisms for cattle. *Res Vet Sci* (2012) 93(2):688–94. doi:10.1016/j.rvsc.2011.10.002
59. Zelaya H, Tsukida K, Chiba E, Marranzino G, Alvarez S, Kitazawa H, et al. Immunobiotic lactobacilli reduce viral-associated pulmonary damage through the modulation of inflammation-coagulation interactions. *Int Immunopharmacol* (2014) 19(1):161–73. doi:10.1016/j.intimp.2013.12.020
60. Ning S, Pagano JS. The A20 deubiquitinase activity negatively regulates LMP1 activation of IRF7. *J Virol* (2010) 84(12):6130–8. doi:10.1128/JVI.00364-10
61. Saitoh T, Yamamoto M, Miyagishi M, Taira K, Nakanishi M, Fujita T, et al. A20 is a negative regulator of IFN regulatory factor 3 signaling. *J Immunol* (2005) 174(3):1507–12. doi:10.4049/jimmunol.174.3.1507
62. Breckpot K, Aerts-Toegaert C, Heirman C, Peeters U, Beyaert R, Aerts JL, et al. Attenuated expression of A20 markedly increases the efficacy of double-stranded RNA-activated dendritic cells as an anti-cancer vaccine. *J Immunol* (2009) 182(2):860–70. doi:10.4049/jimmunol.182.2.860
63. Seifert S, Rodriguez Gomez M, Watzl B, Holzapfel WH, Franz CM, Vizoso Pinto MG. Differential effect of *Lactobacillus johnsonii* BFE 6128 on expression of genes related to TLR pathways and innate immunity in intestinal epithelial cells. *Probiotics Antimicrob Proteins* (2010) 2:211–7. doi:10.1007/s12602-010-9055-2
64. Macpherson C, Audy J, Mathieu O, Tompkins TA. Multistrain probiotic modulation of intestinal epithelial cells' immune response to a double-stranded RNA ligand, poly(i.c). *Appl Environ Microbiol* (2014) 80(5):1692–700. doi:10.1128/AEM.03411-13
65. Tada A, Zelaya H, Clua P, Salva S, Alvarez S, Kitazawa H, et al. Immunobiotic *Lactobacillus* strains reduce small intestinal injury induced by intraepithelial lymphocytes after toll-like receptor 3 activation. *Inflamm Res* (2016) 65(10):771–83. doi:10.1007/s00011-016-0957-7
66. Villena J, Chiba E, Vizoso-Pinto MG, Tomosada Y, Takahashi T, Ishizuka T, et al. Immunobiotic *Lactobacillus rhamnosus* strains differentially modulate antiviral immune response in porcine intestinal epithelial and antigen presenting cells. *BMC Microbiol* (2014) 14(1):126. doi:10.1186/1471-2180-14-126
67. Iwasaki A, Kelsall BL. Unique functions of CD11b+, CD8 alpha+, and double-negative Peyer's patch dendritic cells. *J Immunol* (2001) 166(8):4884–90. doi:10.4049/jimmunol.166.8.4884
68. Kandasamy S, Vlasova AN, Fischer D, Kumar A, Chattha KS, Rauf A, et al. Differential effects of *Escherichia coli* Nissle and *Lactobacillus rhamnosus* strain GG on human rotavirus binding, infection, and B cell immunity. *J Immunol* (2016) 196(4):1780–9. doi:10.4049/jimmunol.1501705
69. Tomosada Y, Villena J, Murata K, Chiba E, Shimazu T, Aso H, et al. Immunoregulatory effect of bifidobacteria strains in porcine intestinal epithelial cells through modulation of ubiquitin-editing enzyme A20 expression. *PLoS One* (2013) 8(3):e59259. doi:10.1371/journal.pone.0059259
70. Kinoshita N, Hiroi T, Ohta N, Fukuyama S, Park EJ, Kiyono H. Autocrine IL-15 mediates intestinal epithelial cell death via the activation of neighboring intraepithelial NK cells. *J Immunol* (2002) 169(11):6187–92. doi:10.4049/jimmunol.169.11.6187
71. Zhang B, Chassaing B, Shi Z, Uchiyama R, Zhang Z, Denning TL, et al. Viral infection. Prevention and cure of rotavirus infection via TLR5/NLRC4-mediated production of IL-22 and IL-18. *Science* (2014) 346(6211):861–5. doi:10.1126/science.1256999
72. Ebert EC. Interleukin 15 is a potent stimulant of intraepithelial lymphocytes. *Gastroenterology* (1998) 115(6):1439–45. doi:10.1016/S0016-5085(98)70022-8
73. Hansen CH, Holm TL, Krych L, Andresen L, Nielsen DS, Rune I, et al. Gut microbiota regulates NKG2D ligand expression on intestinal epithelial cells. *Eur J Immunol* (2013) 43(2):447–57. doi:10.1002/eji.201242462
74. Kawaguchi M, Nanno M, Umesaki Y, Matsumoto S, Okada Y, Cai Z, et al. Cytolytic activity of intestinal intraepithelial lymphocytes in germ-free mice is strain dependent and determined by T cells expressing gamma delta T-cell antigen receptors. *Proc Natl Acad Sci U S A* (1993) 90(18):8591–4. doi:10.1073/pnas.90.18.8591
75. Suzuki H, Jeong KI, Itoh K, Doi K. Regional variations in the distributions of small intestinal intraepithelial lymphocytes in germ free and specific pathogen-free mice. *Exp Mol Pathol* (2002) 72(3):230–5. doi:10.1006/exmp.2002.2433
76. Ismail AS, Severson KM, Vaishnava S, Behrendt CL, Yu X, Benjamin JL, et al. Gammadelta intraepithelial lymphocytes are essential mediators of host-microbial homeostasis at the intestinal mucosal surface. *Proc Natl Acad Sci U S A* (2011) 108(21):8743–8. doi:10.1073/pnas.1019574108
77. Jiang W, Wang X, Zeng B, Liu L, Tardivel A, Wei H, et al. Recognition of gut microbiota by NOD2 is essential for the homeostasis of intestinal intraepithelial lymphocytes. *J Exp Med* (2013) 210(11):2465–76. doi:10.1084/jem.20122490
78. Serrano AE, Menares-Castillo E, Garrido-Tapia M, Ribeiro CH, Hernandez CJ, Mendoza-Naranjo A, et al. Interleukin 10 decreases MICA expression on melanoma cell surface. *Immunol Cell Biol* (2011) 89(3):447–57. doi:10.1038/icb.2010.100
79. Kuhn R, Lohler J, Rennick D, Rajewsky K, Muller W. Interleukin-10-deficient mice develop chronic enterocolitis. *Cell* (1993) 75(2):263–74. doi:10.1016/0092-8674(93)80068-P

8

Applications of Genetically Modified Immunobiotics with High Immunoregulatory Capacity for Treatment of Inflammatory Bowel Diseases

Suguru Shigemori[1,2] *and Takeshi Shimosato*[3,4*]

[1] *Department of Bioscience and Food Production Science, Interdisciplinary Graduate School of Science and Technology, Shinshu University, Nagano, Japan,* [2] *Japan Society for the Promotion of Science, Tokyo, Japan,* [3] *Department of Interdisciplinary Genome Sciences and Cell Metabolism, Institute for Biomedical Sciences, Shinshu University, Nagano, Japan,* [4] *Supramolecular Complexes Unit, Research Center for Fungal and Microbial Dynamism, Shinshu University, Nagano, Japan*

Edited by:
Julio Villena,
Reference Centre for Lactobacilli (CERELA-CONICET), Argentina

Reviewed by:
Graciela Liliana Garrote,
CIDCA (CONICET-UNLP), Argentina
Susana Alvarez,
National Scientific and Technical Research Council, Argentina

****Correspondence:***
Takeshi Shimosato
shimot@shinshu-u.ac.jp

Inflammatory bowel diseases (IBDs), including ulcerative colitis and Crohn's disease, are chronic inflammatory diseases characterized by dysregulated immune responses of the gastrointestinal tract. In recent years, the incidence of IBDs has increased in developed nations, but their prophylaxis/treatment is not yet established. Site-directed delivery of molecules showing anti-inflammatory properties using genetically modified (gm)-probiotics shows promise as a new strategy for the prevention and treatment of IBD. Advantages of gm-probiotics include (1) the ability to use bacteria as a delivery vehicle, enabling safe and long-term use by humans, (2) decreased risks of side effects, and (3) reduced costs. The intestinal delivery of anti-inflammatory proteins such as cytokines and enzymes using *Lactococcus lactis* has been shown to regulate host intestinal homeostasis depending on the delivered protein-specific machinery. Additionally, clinical experience using interleukin 10-secreting *Lc. lactis* has been shown to be safe and to facilitate biological containment in IBD therapy. On the other hand, some preclinical studies have demonstrated that gm-strains of immunobiotics (probiotic strains able to beneficially regulate the mucosal immunity) provide beneficial effects on intestinal inflammation as a result of the synergy between the immunoregulatory effects of the bacterium itself and the anti-inflammatory effects of the delivered recombinant proteins. In this review, we discuss the rapid progression in the development of strategies for the prophylaxis and treatment of IBD using gm-probiotics that exhibit immune regulation effects (gm-immunobiotics). In particular, we discuss the type of strains used as delivery agents.

Keywords: probiotics, immunobiotics, IBD, gmLAB, gm-immunobiotics

INTRODUCTION

Inflammatory bowel disease (IBD) is a chronic inflammatory disease that occurs in the gastrointestinal tract (GIT); IBDs are largely classified as ulcerative colitis (UC) and Crohn's disease (CD). There has been an increase in the number of cases of IBD in recent years, mainly in Western countries (1). IBD causes inflammatory obstruction of the GIT, resulting in symptoms such as stomach cramps, pain, diarrhea, constipation, and vomiting over an extended period of time. These symptoms cause considerable reduction in quality of life. While IBD is not a direct cause of mortality, the disease can increase the risk of colorectal cancer (2). The precise etiology of IBD has yet to be clarified, but causal factors are thought to include the environment, genetics, and microorganisms (3). The chronic inflammation seen in IBD is characterized by dysregulated immune response of the host as a result of marked changes in the intestinal environment (3). Consequently, favorable regulation of the compromised immune homeostasis is effective in the prognosis and treatment of IBD. Corticosteroids, thiopurines, and anti-tumor necrosis factor (TNF) antibody (Ab), which exhibit immune-regulatory effects, can control IBD to a certain extent, and these treatments are widely used in clinical settings as therapeutic drugs (4). However, there are individual-specific differences in the effectiveness of these drugs, and there are also issues such as the possibility of serious side effects and high costs (4, 5).

There is currently a great deal of interest in the use of probiotics that have been genetically modified (gm) to produce proteins with IBD therapeutic potential as novel drug substitutes. Probiotics, defined as "live microorganisms that, when administrated in adequate amounts, confer a health benefit on the host" (6), have been reported to attenuate inflammation in the host GIT through immune system regulation, strengthening of barrier function, and improvement of the changed intestinal microbiota (7). Probiotics comprise primarily lactic acid bacteria (LAB) and bifidobacteria, and also include non-pathogenic *Escherichia coli*. Probiotics have been used in food for a long time, and many of the bacteria included in probiotics fall under the Generally Recognized As Safe assessment designated by the United States Food and Drug Administration and meet the Qualified Presumption of Safety designation of the European Food Safety Authority. Genetic modification technology has undergone considerable advances in recent years, and *Lactococcus* (*Lc.*) *lactis* in particular has been established as an efficient expression system for recombinant proteins (RPs) (8) (**Figure 1A**). Thus, probiotics, which have excellent safety and health advantages, are likely to be very useful as producers of IBD therapeutic proteins and as agents for delivering such proteins to the GIT (**Figure 1B**). gm-Probiotics that produce or secrete various different anti-inflammatory proteins have been constructed in recent years, and their anti-inflammatory effectiveness when administered orally has been verified using

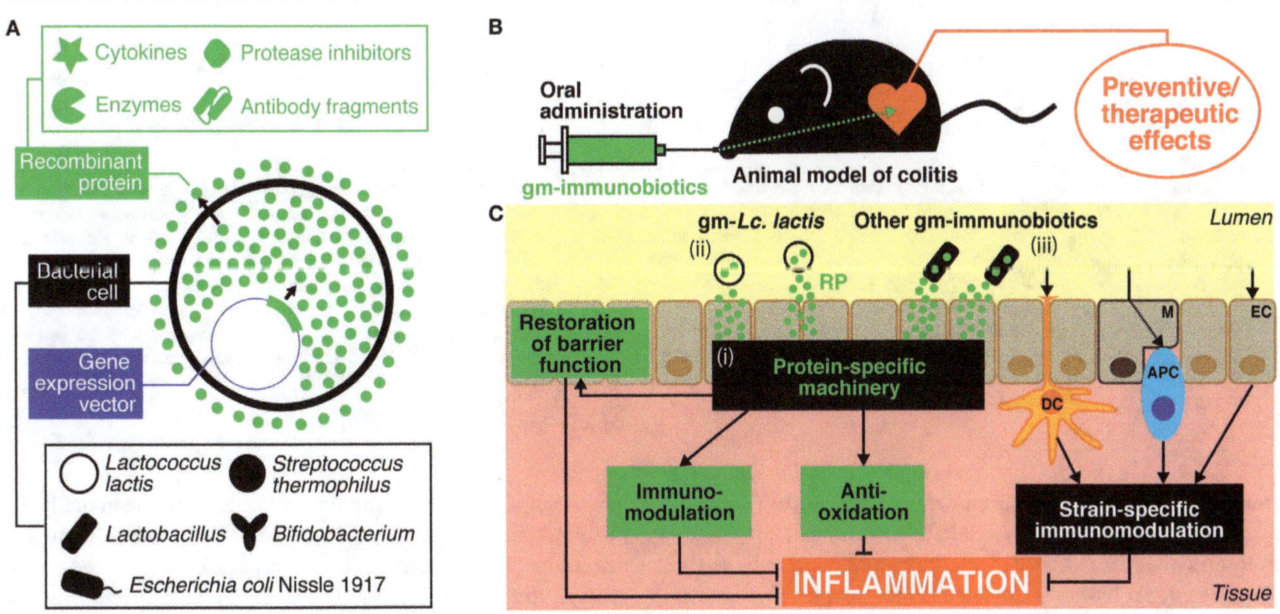

FIGURE 1 | A strategy for prevention and treatment of IBD using genetically modified (gm)-immunobiotics. (A) Different bioactive proteins such as cytokines, enzymes, protease inhibitors, and antibody fragments can be produced/secreted by gm-strains. **(B)** After oral administration, viable cells of gm-immunobiotics transit through the gastric environment and reach the intestine. Then, gm-immunobiotics provide preventive/therapeutic effects against experimental colitis in animal as a result of the exertion of anti-inflammatory effects *in situ*. **(C)** General mechanisms of action of gm-immunobiotics on anti-inflammatory effects in the intestine. Physiologically meaningful amounts of recombinant proteins are yielded by gm-immunobiotics *via* secretion or cell lysis, and exert host anti-inflammatory effects through a protein-specific machinery including immunomodulation, anti-oxidation, and restoration of epithelial barrier functions (i). *Lactococcus* (*Lc.*) *lactis* has been most widely used as a safe and effective vector in this strategy (ii). *Lc. lactis* has little or no effect on either the improvement or aggravation of the intestinal inflammation and does not colonize the intestine. Other gm-immunobiotics (including some strains of *Lactobacillus*, *Bifidobacterium*, and *Streptococcus salivarius* subsp. *thermophilus*, and *Escherichia coli* Nissle 1917) provide beneficial effects on intestinal inflammation as a result of the synergy between the immunoregulatory effects of the bacterium itself and the anti-inflammatory effects of the delivered recombinant proteins (iii). Immunobiotics interact with pattern recognition receptors of host epithelial cells and antigen-presenting cells such as dendritic cells and macrophages to exert strain-specific immunomodulatory effects. Some strains of immunobiotics may colonize the intestine. IBD, inflammatory bowel disease; RP, recombinant protein; EC, epithelial cell; M, microfold cell; DC, dendritic cell; APC, antigen-presenting cell.

TABLE 1 | Selected preclinical evidence showing beneficial effects of gm-immunobiotics in treatment of gastrointestinal tract inflammation.

Strains	Recombinant protein	Disease model	Outcome	Efficacy	Potential mechanisms	Reference
Lc. lactis MG1363/ NZ9000	IL-10	mDAC, mTAC, m*IL-10*$^{-/-}$	Reduction in MS, HS, and IM (MPO, Cox-2, SAA) Modulation of P/AICy	CC = WT/VC < Objects	Immunomodulation	(33–37)
Lc. lactis MG1363	IL-27	mTTC, mDAC	Reduction in Mo, MS, and HS Modulation of P/AICy and PTc	CC = Systemic IL-27 = VC < Object MG1363-IL-10 < Object	Immunomodulation	(38)
Lc. lactis NZ9000	Elafin/SLPI	mDAC, mDCC, mTTC, hIEC	Reduction in MS, HS, CT, IIP, and IM (PL, MPO, PICy, PIL)	CC ≤ WT < NZ9000-IL-10/ TGF-β < Objects	Reduction in elastolytic activity	(33, 39)
Lc. lactis NZ9000	HO-1	mDAC	Reduction in MS, HS, and CS Modulation of P/AICy	CC = VC < Object	Immunomodulation	(40)
Lb. casei BL23	Cat/SOD	mDAC, mTAC	Reduction in MS, HS, and LMT Modulation of P/AICy	CC ≤ WT/VC < Objects	Reduction in oxidative stress Immunomodulation	(15, 17, 18)
Lb. casei BLS	α-MSH	mDAC	Reduction in Mo, MS, HS, CS, and IM (MPO, NF-κB) Modulation of P/AICy	CC ≤ WT < Object	Immunomodulation	(23)
S. thermophilus CRL807	Cat/SOD	mTAC	Reduction in Mo, MS, HS, and LMT Modulation of CPIc	CC < WT < Objects	Reduction in oxidative stress Immunomodulation	(13)
B. longum NCC2705	IL-10	mDAC	Reduction in Mo, MS, HS, CS, and IM (MPO, NF-κB) Modulation of PTc and P/AICy	CC < WT/VC < Object	Immunomodulation	(21, 22)
EcN	AvCys	mDAC, pPWD, hIEC	Reduction in MS, HS, CS, IIP, and IM (PIM, PICh, PICy) Increase in Treg, TER	CC ≤ WT < Object	Immunomodulation Improvement of intestinal barrier function	(24)

Lc., Lactococcus; Lb., Lactobacillus; S. thermophilus, Streptococcus salivarius subsp. thermophilus; B., Bifidobacterium; EcN, Escherichia coli Nissle 1917; IL-10, interleukin 10; IL-27, interleukin 27; SLPI, secretory leukocyte protease inhibitor; HO-1, heme oxygenase-1; SOD, superoxide dismutase; Cat, catalase; α-MSH, α-melanocyte-stimulating hormone; AvCys, cystatin from Acanthocheilonema viteae; mDAC, murine dextran sulfate sodium-induced acute colitis; mTAC, murine 2,4,6-trinitrobenzene sulfonic acid-induced acute colitis; mIL-10$^{-/-}$*, spontaneous colitis in IL-10-deficient mice; mTTC, murine T-cell transfer-induced enterocolitis; mDCC, murine dextran sulfate sodium-induced chronic colitis; hIEC, human intestinal epithelial cells; pPWD, porcine post-weaning diarrhea; MS, macroscopic symptoms; HS, histological symptoms; IM, mediators of inflammation; MPO, myeloperoxidase activity; Cox-2, cyclooxygenase-2 activity; SAA, serum amyloid A; P/AICy, pro-/anti-inflammatory cytokines; Mo, mortality; PTc, phenotypes of T-cell; CT, colon thickening; IIP, intestinal epithelial permeability; PL, proteolytic activity; PICy, pro-inflammatory cytokines; PIL, pro-inflammatory leukocytes; CS, colon shortening; LMT, liver microbial translocation; NF-κB, nuclear factor-κB; CPIc, cytokine phenotypes of immune cells; PIM, pro-inflammatory macrophages; PICh, pro-inflammatory chemokines; Treg, regulatory T-cell; TER, transendothelial electrical resistance; CC, colitis control; WT, wild-type strain; VC, vector control; MG1363-IL-10, IL-10-secreting Lactococcus lactis MG1363; NZ9000-IL-10/TGF-β, IL-10- or TGF-β-secreting Lactococcus lactis NZ9000.*

in vivo experiments in animal models of IBD (9, 10) (**Table 1**; Table S1 in Supplementary Material). In this context, it is important to note that the delivery of IBD therapeutic proteins to the GIT using gm-probiotics is expected (1) to allow the therapeutic protein to act locally, with greater effectiveness and decreased risk of medical error or side effects compared to conventional systemic administration of the molecule by injection, and (2) to be considerably cheaper than refined drugs (10, 11). It is of particular interest that many of the molecules selected as anti-inflammatory proteins target the host immune system. Many studies to date have used *Lc. lactis* as a model strain, but methods using lactobacilli, bifidobacteria, streptococci, and *E. coli* Nissle 1917 (EcN), bacteria that have more beneficial health effects than *Lc. lactis*, as delivery agents have been attempted in recent years (**Figure 1A**). Many of these studies (12–26) employ bacteria that have been termed "immunobiotics," which have been defined as probiotic strains that are able to beneficially regulate mucosal immunity (27, 28). Immunobiotics are recognized by the pattern recognition receptors of epithelial and antigen-presenting cells such as dendritic cells and macrophages, and these immunobiotics are known to beneficially regulate innate and adoptive immune responses (**Figure 1C**); there have been tremendous advances in the clarification of strain-specific immune regulation functions at the cellular and molecular levels (28–32).

In this review, we describe recent developments in preventive and therapeutic strategies for the treatment of IBD using gm-probiotics. In particular, our discussion focuses on gm-probiotics that exhibit immune regulation effects (gm-immunobiotics) and bacterial species that are used as protein delivery agents.

Lactococcus lactis

Lactococcus lactis is a species of LAB used universally in cheese and other fermented dairy products. To date, *Lc. lactis* MG1363 (MG1363) and its derivatives have been widely used to produce RPs and as carriers for delivery to mucous membranes (**Figure 1**). *Lc. lactis* was the first LAB species to have its whole genome sequenced, and there exists a wealth of genetic data on this species (8, 41, 42). In addition, *Lc. lactis* genetic modification is straightforward, and there are a great number of useful gene expression systems for this organism (8). Furthermore, *Lc. lactis* is able to pass through the GIT alive but does not establish itself in the GIT and is easy to control pharmacokinetically (43, 44). It is important to note that *Lc. lactis* itself has little or no effect on either the improvement or aggravation of GIT inflammation in animals and humans and is therefore highly safe for use against IBD (14, 33–35, 38–40, 45–52) (http://ClinicalTrials.gov Identifier: NCT00729872). The research to date into gm-*Lc. lactis* has been compiled into a number of review articles (9–11, 53). In the present review, we will deal with a series of landmark studies that showed the usefulness and practicality of the present strategy, and we will examine the latest findings.

The strategy of reducing intestinal inflammation by using gm-probiotics for delivery of RPs to the GIT was first proposed in 2000 by Steidler et al. (35), who created a MG1363 strain that secreted interleukin (IL)-10 (LL-mIL10). IL-10 is a cytokine that plays a central role in the suppression of inflammation (54), and mutation of the endogenous gene has been shown to be involved in the onset of murine enterocolitis (55, 56) and infantile-onset IBD (57, 58). Steidler et al. showed that daily oral administration of LL-mIL10 resulted in a dramatic reduction of colitis onset and progression in a murine IBD model (35). Notably, the effective amount of IL-10 was 1/10,000th of the amount used in conventional systemic administration. This enhancement may be regarded as the greatest advantage of the present strategy. The reduction in the amount administered has also been demonstrated in the delivery systems of other RPs (38, 49, 50). Next, Steidler et al. constructed LL-Thy12, in which the thymidylate synthase gene (*thyA*) of the *Lc. lactis* genome was replaced by the human IL-10-encoding gene (59). The results of a phase 1 clinical study in CD patients confirmed the safety, biological containment, and significant therapeutic effect of LL-Thy12 (52). However, no statistically significant therapeutic effect was found in the subsequent phase 2a clinical study (http://ClinicalTrials.gov Identifier: NCT00729872). The authors suggested that the lack of therapeutic effect was due to low concentration of IL-10 in the intestine. Nonetheless, bearing in mind that this first clinical study using gm-LAB suggested the safety and usefulness of this delivery system, the results were remarkable.

IL-27 is an anti-inflammatory cytokine belonging to the IL-12 family, a group of molecules that has been shown to attenuate murine experimental colitis by suppressing the development of T helper 17 (Th17) cells (60). In addition, the involvement of low-expressing variants of the IL-27-encoding gene in early-onset IBD has been demonstrated (61). In 2014, Hanson et al. showed that daily oral administration of MG1363 that secretes IL-27 (LL-IL-27) almost completely cured murine T-cell transfer-induced enterocolitis and reduced the associated mortality rate (38). LL-IL-27 treatment caused a reduction in the level of inflammatory cytokines that had increased in the GIT as a result of enterocolitis and a reduction in the number of colitis pathogenic IL-17-producing T-cells. In addition, the results indicated that increased local production of IL-10 by LL-IL-27 in the GIT was effective in providing a therapeutic effect. It is important to note that oral administration of LL-IL-27 demonstrated a notably greater therapeutic effect than systemic administration of IL-27 or oral administration of IL-10-secreting MG1363.

In 2015, a study comparing *Lc. lactis* NZ9000 (NZ9000) that secreted serine protease inhibitors (elafin or secretory leukocyte protease inhibitor) to NZ9000 that secreted the anti-inflammatory cytokines IL-10 or transforming growth factor-β showed that the former significantly attenuated the symptoms of dextran sodium sulfate (DSS)-induced colitis (33). Prior to that study, Motta et al. showed that the expression of elafin was lower in IBD patients than in healthy people, and that this decreased expression correlated with the increased elastolytic activity of the colonic mucosa in IBD patients (39). Also, delivery of elafin to the GIT using a gm-NZ9000 resulted in marked improvement of acute and chronic colitis in murine models (39). Elafin-secreting NZ9000 restored the colonic elastolytic homeostasis that had broken down as a result of colitis, reduced the number of immune cells infiltrating the colon, and repaired the barrier function of the intestinal epithelium (39).

In 2015, we successfully constructed a gm-NZ9000 strain (designated NZ-HO) that secretes biologically active heme oxygenase-1 (HO-1). HO-1 is an enzyme that catalyzes heme catabolism *in vivo*. HO-1 is induced endogenously by stimuli such as inflammation or oxidative stress, and the enzyme exhibits anti-inflammatory and cytoprotective effects mediated by the generation of heme breakdown products (62, 63). We showed that daily oral administration of NZ-HO markedly attenuated the symptoms of DSS colitis (40). Interestingly, NZ-HO increased the production of IL-10, decreased inflammatory cell infiltration, and decreased expression of IL-6 and IL-1α in the colonic tissue of murine colitis models (40). In 2014, Zhang et al. showed that intraperitoneal injection of an HO-1 inducer-induced IL-10-producing regulatory T cells (Treg) (rather than IBD pathogenic Th17) by inhibiting IL-6/IL-6 receptor signaling, thus ameliorating DSS colitis (64). This result suggested that NZ-HO regulates the immune responses of the inflamed colon in a beneficial fashion to ameliorate DSS colitis.

In 2015, Aubry et al. found that preventive oral administration of MG1363 that secreted thymic stromal lymphopoietin caused a transient increase in the number of $CD4^+$ $CD25^+$ $FoxP3^+$ Treg cells in the mesenteric lymph node and attenuated DSS colitis in mice (45). Quevrain et al. found that MG1363 that secreted an anti-inflammatory protein (MAM) isolated from a strain of *Faecalibacterium prausnitzii*, a species that is deficient in CD patients and alleviated dinitrobenzene sulfonic acid-induced colitis in mice (47). MAM-secreting MG1363 markedly reduced the production of pro-inflammatory cytokines (IL-17A and interferon-γ) in the colonic tissue of colitis mice (47).

IL-6 is an important pathogenic factor in various different inflammatory diseases, including IBD. By regulating the function and proliferation of T cells, IL-6 exacerbates GIT inflammation in IBD (65). In addition, studies using murine models of colitis and CD patients showed that inhibition of IL-6 signaling using antibodies improved the symptoms (66, 67). However, the cost of Ab drugs is very high. We therefore created a NZ9000 derivative that secretes a single-chain variable fragment Ab against IL-6 (IL6scFv) (68). Importantly, we showed that the recombinant IL6scFv produced by gm-NZ9000 is immunoreactive, as demonstrated by binding to IL-6 (68). Thus, IL6scFv-secreting NZ9000 is an attractive gm-LAB for research and development of a low-cost IBD therapeutic drug that can yield site-directed delivery of anti-IL-6 antibodies.

Lactobacillus

Bacteria of the genus *Lactobacillus*, which are classified as LAB, are the best-known type of probiotics. Several strains belonging to this genus are commensal bacteria that reside within the human GIT. To date, many preclinical studies have indicated that strains belonging to genus *Lactobacillus* regulate GIT inflammation in a favorable fashion through strain-specific, health-beneficial mechanisms (9). In addition, clinical research to date has shown that a probiotic mixture containing four species of *Lactobacillus* (VSL#3) and *Lactobacillus reuteri* ATCC 55730 exhibits benefits in the treatment of active UC (69–72). Bacteria belonging to genus *Lactobacillus* are used predominantly in probiotic formulations that are useful for the prevention and drug therapy of GIT-related diseases selected by the World Gastroenterology Organization (73).

In 2007, Rochat et al. showed that daily oral administration of *Lactobacillus casei* BL23 (BL23) attenuated murine DSS colitis (17). The same year, Foligne et al. demonstrated that BL23 induced an immune reaction with dominance of anti-inflammatory IL-10 over pro-inflammatory IL-12 in human peripheral blood mononuclear cells and reduced the symptoms of murine 2,4,6-trinitrobenzenesulfonic acid (TNBS) colitis (74). In 2010, Watterlot et al. orally administered superoxide dismutase (SOD)-producing and SOD-non-producing BL23 to mice and found that the former resulted in marked amelioration of DSS-induced histological damage to the colon, while the latter gave only slight amelioration (18). An excess of reactive oxygen species causes considerable tissue damage, which suggests a link to IBD development, and the use of antioxidative enzymes to eliminate reactive oxidative species is expected to have potential as an IBD treatment strategy (75). Oral delivery of SOD using gm-LAB has actually been shown to reduce colitis in rodents (12, 14). In 2011, LeBlanc et al. orally administered BL23 that produced an antioxidative enzyme (SOD or catalase) to mice, and their results showed that the mortality rate, weight loss, histological colon damage, and liver microbial translocation induced by TNBS administration were markedly reduced (15). However, in the studies performed by Watterlot et al. (18) and LeBlanc et al. (15), wild-type (WT) BL23 had only mild anti-inflammatory properties and did not induce marked IL-10 production in colon tissue, indicating that the amelioration effects on murine colon inflammation are limited. In 2014, Hou et al. showed that oral administration of SOD-producing *Lactobacillus fermentum* I5007 (I5007) improved lipid peroxidation and immune parameters in the colon, thus ameliorating murine TNBS colitis (26). A partial, but significant, improvement effect was also observed with WT-I5007. I5007 was isolated from healthy porcine intestinal mucosa and has been used as a growth stimulator for livestock. The above series of studies proposed a novel IBD preventive strategy combining the two different intestinal inflammation amelioration mechanisms: the immunobiotic effects of lactobacilli and the antioxidative effects of delivered proteins (**Figure 1C**).

In 2008, α-melanocyte-stimulating hormone (α-MSH)-secreting *Lb. casei* BLS (BLS) was created (23). α-MSH is a neuropeptide with immunosuppressant effects that has been reported to exhibit anti-inflammatory effects in animal models of various diseases, including IBD (76). Orally administered gm-BLS shows curative effects for the symptoms of murine DSS colitis (23). This improvement involves decreased secretion of inflammatory cytokines (TNF-α, IL-1β, and IL-6) and increased secretion of immune-regulatory cytokines (IL-4 and IL-10) in *ex vivo* cultures of colonic tissue (23). It is interesting to note that gm-BLS brought about considerable improvement in a number of parameters when compared to the WT strain (23).

Streptococcus salivarius subsp. *thermophilus* (*S. thermophilus*)

Streptococcus thermophilus is a LAB that has traditionally been used as a yogurt starter. Preclinical studies to date have clarified the roles of specific *S. thermophilus* strains as immunobiotics (77–82). For example, Ogita et al. showed that *S. thermophilus* ST28 (ST28) derived from milk regulated IL-17 production in murine splenocytes in Th17-skewed conditions by induction of counteracting interferon-γ (82). Moreover, oral administration of ST28 to mice markedly decreased DSS-induced intestinal lesions, and this treatment markedly decreased IL-17 secretion and the frequency of accumulation of Th17, the numbers of which had increased in the lamina propria as a result of DSS (81). *S. thermophilus* is a component of a probiotic mixture agent (VSL#3) that has been found to be effective for induction and maintenance of remission in UC and prevention and maintenance of remission in pouchitis (73). It is interesting to note that several *S. thermophilus* strains are known to be autolytic, a useful trait for strains used as gm-immunobiotics (83).

In 2014, an immunobiotic strain, *S. thermophilus* CRL807 (CRL807), which exhibits immunosuppressant action *in vitro* and *in vivo*, was selected from a mixed yogurt starter; CRL807's usefulness as a delivery agent for SOD and catalase then was investigated (13). CRL807 significantly increased the ratios of IL-10:inflammatory cytokine (IL-12, IL-17, or interferon-γ) in human peripheral blood mononuclear cells and the digestive tract of healthy mice. Oral administration of antioxidative enzyme-producing gm-CRL807 and WT-CRL807 to mice markedly potentiated the ratio of IL-10-positive:IL-17-positive cells, a ratio that had been reduced by TNBS administration, and provided amelioration of colitis. Notably, administration of either or both SOD-producing and catalase-producing CRL807 improved antioxidative enzyme activity in the colon, demonstrating greater anti-inflammatory action than WT-CRL807 administration. Experimental long-term (30-day) oral administration of gm-CRL807 and WT-CRL807 in healthy mice showed the safety of CRL807 (84).

Bifidobacterium

The genus *Bifidobacterium* comprises indigenous bacteria that make up the intestinal flora and in particular are present in significant numbers in healthy infants. In IBD patients, on the other hand, it is known that there is a decreased number of *Bifidobacterium* and an increase in pro-inflammatory *E. coli* and *Bacteroides* in the intestinal mucosa (85–89). Preclinical studies to date have shown that various strains of genus *Bifidobacterium* bring about beneficial effects in the prevention and treatment of colitis, mediated by different effects [immunoregulation effects (90, 91), improvement of the barrier function of intestinal epithelium (92, 93), and improvement of the intestinal flora (94, 95)]. It is interesting that *Bifidobacterium longum* subsp. *infantis* 35624 has been shown to selectively drive specialization of FoxP3$^+$ Treg cells and/or induce IL-10 production in animal disease models and in humans (96–99). In addition, clinical studies of patients with UC and other inflammatory diseases showed that, compared to placebo, oral administration of this immunobiotic strain resulted in a marked decrease in the level of plasma C-type protein, an inflammatory biomarker that increases with the disease (100). It has also been shown that the symptoms of UC patients are ameliorated by a single Bifidobacteria strain (101), probiotic mixtures that include Bifidobacteria (69, 71, 72, 102, 103), and symbiotics (probiotic/prebiotic mixtures) in which Bifidobacteria is the main constituent (104–106).

In 2011, an immunobiotic strain, *B. longum* NCC2705 (NCC2705), was engineered to secrete biologically active IL-10, and the strain's curative effects in DSS colitis were investigated (21). Improvement of the symptoms of DSS colitis (aggravation of gross symptoms, colon shortening, histopathological changes accompanying tissue damage, and myeloperoxidase activation) was observed with oral administration of WT-NCC2705 alone. Considerable improvement was found with IL-10-secreting gmNCC2705 when compared to WT-NCC2705 treatment (21). In addition, this study found that WT-NCC2705 and gm-NCC2705 reduced the expression of nuclear factor-κB and pro-inflammatory cytokines in the colon and the peripheral blood, and restored the proportion of CD4$^+$ CD25$^+$ FoxP3$^+$ Treg cells (21). These effects were markedly stronger with gm-NCC2705. In 2015, Zhang et al. showed that the Treg/Th17 balance that had broken down as a result of DSS colitis was fully restored by gm-NCC2705 through the inhibition of two intracellular signaling pathways for Th17 induction (22). In 2016, the intestinal inflammation amelioration action of different strains of *B. longum* that produced human α-MSH was reported (19, 20). In the first of these reports, preventive daily oral administration of α-MSH-secreting *B. longum* HB15 (HB15) markedly reduced histopathological damage, increased myeloperoxidase activity, corrected an inflammatory/anti-inflammatory cytokine imbalance, and induced production of the pro-inflammatory factor nitrogen monoxide, overcoming effects caused by DSS colitis in rats. Administration of WT-HB15 improved all the parameters with the exception of nitrogen monoxide production, but to a considerably lower degree than that seen with the recombinant strain (19). In the second report, α-MSH-secreting *B. longum* HB25 (HB25) was created. Therapeutic daily oral administration of this recombinant strain markedly improved murine DSS colitis. Interestingly, no curative effects were observed from oral administration of the vector control strain (20). The two serial studies above indicated that immunobiotic Bifidobacteria that secrete proteins exhibiting immunomodulatory effects beneficial to IBD amelioration (IL-10 or α-MSH) are capable of stronger prevention/cure of UC-like colitis in mice than are WT strains, with effects presumably mediated through synergistic effects on various functions (**Figure 1C**).

Escherichia coli Nissle 1917

Escherichia coli Nissle 1917 has no pathogenic factors (adhesion molecules, invasiveness, enterotoxin, cytotoxins, etc.). This strain's genetics, physiology, and biological activities as a probiotics were largely characterized some time ago; as an alternative medicine (Mutaflor) for IBD and other GIT-related diseases, EcN currently serves as one of the most useful bacterial strains (104). In randomized controlled trials of UC remission maintenance, oral administration of EcN was as effective as treatment with mesalazine in preventing relapse of the disease (105–107). In studies using IBD model animals, EcN was proven to ameliorate colitis symptoms by regulation of the immune system and intestinal barrier function (108–111). In addition, the utility of this immunobiotic strain as a production platform for vaccines and pharmaceutics and as an intestinal delivery system continues to grow (112). Studies of gm-EcN that produces pathogenic bacteria/virus antigens (113–115) and immunomodulatory molecules such as cytokines and proteins derived from parasites (24, 25) have been reported, and disease preventive/curative effects have been verified in animals.

In 2012, Gardlik et al. developed IL-10-secreting EcN and verified this strain's anti-inflammatory effects using DSS colitis (25). Oral administration of IL10-secreting EcN was shown to improve inflammation parameters (reduced stool consistency, colon shortening, decreased oxidative and carbonyl stress), but these effects were of the same degree as obtained with WT-EcN or IL-10-secreting MG1363. In 2014, EcN that secretes a protease inhibitor protein derived from nematodes (AvCys) was created (24). AvCys' immune-regulatory action is mediated mainly by targeting macrophages, and this inhibitory protein exhibits anti-inflammatory action in murine models of IBD and allergies (116–119). Oral administration of AvCys-secreting EcN (EcN-AvCys) on alternate days attenuated DSS colitis by beneficial regulation of the immune system in the inflamed colon (regulation of the proportion and function of pro-inflammatory macrophages, increase in the proportion of FoxP3$^+$ Treg cells, and decrease in inflammatory cytokines and chemokines). In addition, in experiments using pigs (whose GITs closely resemble those of humans), oral administration of EcN-AvCys on alternate days to post-weaning piglets reduced spontaneous colon inflammation. Interestingly, the results of that study suggested that EcN-AvCys ameliorates inflammation in this piglet model by improving intestinal barrier function rather than by regulating the intestinal immune system. WT-EcN shows some benefits in ameliorating murine intestinal inflammation, inducing Treg cells, and increasing transepithelial resistance in a culture of a human colonic epithelial cell strain, but the efficacies were significantly milder than those obtained with EcN-AvCys.

CONCLUSION AND FUTURE PERSPECTIVES

Site-directed delivery of proteins that exhibit anti-inflammatory effects using gm-immunobiotics is extremely attractive as an effective preventive/curative strategy for IBD (**Figure 1**). A series of studies using IL-10-secreting *Lc. lactis*, ranging from basic to clinical, established a milestone by indicating the effectiveness and the feasibility of clinical application of this concept. Subsequently, gm-*Lc. lactis* strains that efficiently produce cytokines, enzymes, and protease inhibitors with a range of anti-inflammatory properties have been developed, and anti-inflammatory properties of these strains have been verified using rodent models of IBD (**Table 1**; Table S1 in Supplementary Material). Recent research into intestinal delivery of serine protease inhibitors and IL-27 has shown that these strains provide markedly more beneficial amelioration of murine intestinal inflammation than do strains that deliver IL-10. In addition, the research strongly implies that MG1363 and its derivatives do not have any negative impact on GIT inflammation or health maintenance, regardless of whether the strains are WT or recombinant. It may therefore be concluded that *Lc. lactis* is the bacterium that holds the most promise as a delivery agent for proteins with IBD therapeutic potential. In addition, work has also advanced to verify the potential for application of immunobiotics in this strategy. Interestingly, these studies show marked amelioration of GIT inflammation in animals as a result of the synergy between the immunoregulatory effects of the immunobiotic bacterium itself and the anti-inflammatory effects of the delivered RPs (**Figure 1C**; **Table 1**; Table S1 in Supplementary Material). This observation implies that the strategy of using immunobiotics is an effective means toward the development of IBD therapeutics with greater efficacy. For future work, it would be desirable to carry out comparative investigations of the therapeutic effects on GIT inflammation of different gm-strains that produce the same RP.

Clinical trials that include verification of safety and efficacy will be essential for developing gm-immunobiotics as therapeutic drugs for IBD. To date, there have been no findings that demonstrate any danger in the use of gm-probiotics including gm-immunobiotics. At the same time, there is little evidence to prove the safety of these agents in clinical use, and it remains possible that gm-probiotic organisms may be spread into the environment. Thus, there is some skepticism regarding the use of these agents. However, two clinical studies using IL-10-secreting *Lc. lactis* have demonstrated tremendous breakthroughs (59, 120, 121). In addition, in a recent phase 1b trial, oral administration of AG013 (an oral rinse containing trefoil factor 1-secreting MG1363 as the main component) was shown to be safe and well tolerated in cancer patients while also exhibiting efficacy against oral mucositis (122). Guidelines toward clinical use of gm-*Lc. lactis* have been proposed (123), and the feasibility of the clinical application of gm-*Lc. lactis* is strongly implied. With other probiotics, aspects such as the time for passage through the GIT, establishment in the GIT, health benefits, or the danger of side effects will differ from those of *Lc. lactis*, so safety evaluations will be needed and biological containment strategies will have to be developed. The establishment of effective gm-immunobiotics for prevention and treatment of IBD is near at hand, and it is to be hoped that this strategy will be facilitated by advances in the scientific understanding of gene recombination techniques in the future.

AUTHOR CONTRIBUTIONS

SS and TS conceived, designed, and wrote the manuscript.

REFERENCES

1. Molodecky NA, Soon IS, Rabi DM, Ghali WA, Ferris M, Chernoff G, et al. Increasing incidence and prevalence of the inflammatory bowel diseases with time, based on systematic review. *Gastroenterology* (2012) 142(1):46.e42–54. e42. doi:10.1053/j.gastro.2011.10.001
2. Triantafillidis JK, Nasioulas G, Kosmidis PA. Colorectal cancer and inflammatory bowel disease: epidemiology, risk factors, mechanisms of carcinogenesis and prevention strategies. *Anticancer Res* (2009) 29(7):2727–37.
3. de Souza HS, Fiocchi C. Immunopathogenesis of IBD: current state of the art. *Nat Rev Gastroenterol Hepatol* (2016) 13(1):13–27. doi:10.1038/nrgastro.2015.186
4. Zenlea T, Peppercorn MA. Immunosuppressive therapies for inflammatory bowel disease. *World J Gastroenterol* (2014) 20(12):3146–52. doi:10.3748/wjg.v20.i12.3146
5. Rutgeerts P, Van Assche G, Vermeire S. Review article: infliximab therapy for inflammatory bowel disease – seven years on. *Aliment Pharmacol Ther* (2006) 23(4):451–63. doi:10.1111/j.1365-2036.2006.02786.x
6. Hill C, Guarner F, Reid G, Gibson GR, Merenstein DJ, Pot B, et al. Expert consensus document. The International Scientific Association for probiotics and prebiotics consensus statement on the scope and appropriate use of the term probiotic. *Nat Rev Gastroenterol Hepatol* (2014) 11(8):506–14. doi:10.1038/nrgastro.2014.66
7. Gareau MG, Sherman PM, Walker WA. Probiotics and the gut microbiota in intestinal health and disease. *Nat Rev Gastroenterol Hepatol* (2010) 7(9):503–14. doi:10.1038/nrgastro.2010.117
8. Wyszynska A, Kobierecka P, Bardowski J, Jagusztyn-Krynicka EK. Lactic acid bacteria – 20 years exploring their potential as live vectors for mucosal vaccination. *Appl Microbiol Biotechnol* (2015) 99(7):2967–77. doi:10.1007/s00253-015-6498-0

9. de Moreno de LeBlanc A, Del Carmen S, Chatel JM, Miyoshi A, Azevedo V, Langella P, et al. Current review of genetically modified lactic acid bacteria for the prevention and treatment of colitis using murine models. *Gastroenterol Res Pract* (2015) 2015:146972. doi:10.1155/2015/146972
10. Wells J. Mucosal vaccination and therapy with genetically modified lactic acid bacteria. *Annu Rev Food Sci Technol* (2011) 2:423–45. doi:10.1146/annurev-food-022510-133640
11. Cano-Garrido O, Seras-Franzoso J, Garcia-Fruitos E. Lactic acid bacteria: reviewing the potential of a promising delivery live vector for biomedical purposes. *Microb Cell Fact* (2015) 14:137. doi:10.1186/s12934-015-0313-6
12. Carroll IM, Andrus JM, Bruno-Barcena JM, Klaenhammer TR, Hassan HM, Threadgill DS. Anti-inflammatory properties of *Lactobacillus gasseri* expressing manganese superoxide dismutase using the interleukin 10-deficient mouse model of colitis. *Am J Physiol Gastrointest Liver Physiol* (2007) 293(4):G729–38. doi:10.1152/ajpgi.00132.2007
13. Del Carmen S, de Moreno de LeBlanc A, Martin R, Chain F, Langella P, Bermudez-Humaran LG, et al. Genetically engineered immunomodulatory *Streptococcus thermophilus* strains producing antioxidant enzymes exhibit enhanced anti-inflammatory activities. *Appl Environ Microbiol* (2014) 80(3):869–77. doi:10.1128/aem.03296-13
14. Han W, Mercenier A, Ait-Belgnaoui A, Pavan S, Lamine F, van S II, et al. Improvement of an experimental colitis in rats by lactic acid bacteria producing superoxide dismutase. *Inflamm Bowel Dis* (2006) 12(11):1044–52. doi:10.1097/01.mib.0000235101.09231.9e
15. LeBlanc JG, del Carmen S, Miyoshi A, Azevedo V, Sesma F, Langella P, et al. Use of superoxide dismutase and catalase producing lactic acid bacteria in TNBS induced Crohn's disease in mice. *J Biotechnol* (2011) 151(3):287–93. doi:10.1016/j.jbiotec.2010.11.008
16. Qiu ZB, Chen J, Chen JJ, Rong L, Ding WQ, Yang HJ, et al. Effect of recombinant *Lactobacillus casei* expressing interleukin-10 in dextran sulfate sodium-induced colitis mice. *J Dig Dis* (2013) 14(2):76–83. doi:10.1111/1751-2980.12006
17. Rochat T, Bermudez-Humaran L, Gratadoux JJ, Fourage C, Hoebler C, Corthier G, et al. Anti-inflammatory effects of *Lactobacillus casei* BL23 producing or not a manganese-dependant catalase on DSS-induced colitis in mice. *Microb Cell Fact* (2007) 6:22. doi:10.1186/1475-2859-6-22
18. Watterlot L, Rochat T, Sokol H, Cherbuy C, Bouloufa I, Lefevre F, et al. Intragastric administration of a superoxide dismutase-producing recombinant *Lactobacillus casei* BL23 strain attenuates DSS colitis in mice. *Int J Food Microbiol* (2010) 144(1):35–41. doi:10.1016/j.ijfoodmicro.2010.03.037
19. Wei P, Yang Y, Ding Q, Li X, Sun H, Liu Z, et al. Oral delivery of *Bifidobacterium longum* expressing α-melanocyte-stimulating hormone to combat ulcerative colitis. *J Med Microbiol* (2016) 65(2):160–8. doi:10.1099/jmm.0.000197
20. Wei P, Yang Y, Liu Z, Huang J, Gong Y, Sun H. Oral *Bifidobacterium longum* expressing α-melanocyte-stimulating hormone to fight experimental colitis. *Drug Deliv* (2016) 23(6):2058–64. doi:10.3109/10717544.2015.1122672
21. Yao J, Wang JY, Lai MG, Li YX, Zhu HM, Shi RY, et al. Treatment of mice with dextran sulfate sodium-induced colitis with human interleukin 10 secreted by transformed *Bifidobacterium longum*. *Mol Pharm* (2011) 8(2):488–97. doi:10.1021/mp100331r
22. Zhang D, Wei C, Yao J, Cai X, Wang L. Interleukin-10 gene-carrying bifidobacteria ameliorate murine ulcerative colitis by regulating regulatory T cell/T helper 17 cell pathway. *Exp Biol Med (Maywood)* (2015) 240(12):1622–9. doi:10.1177/1535370215584901
23. Yoon SW, Lee CH, Kim JY, Kim JY, Sung MH, Poo H. *Lactobacillus casei* secreting α-MSH induces the therapeutic effect on DSS-induced acute colitis in Balb/c Mice. *J Microbiol Biotechnol* (2008) 18(12):1975–83. doi:10.4014/jmb.0800.445
24. Whelan RA, Rausch S, Ebner F, Gunzel D, Richter JF, Hering NA, et al. A transgenic probiotic secreting a parasite immunomodulator for site-directed treatment of gut inflammation. *Mol Ther* (2014) 22(10):1730–40. doi:10.1038/mt.2014.125
25. Gardlik R, Palffy R, Celec P. Recombinant probiotic therapy in experimental colitis in mice. *Folia Biol (Praha)* (2012) 58(6):238–45.
26. Hou CL, Zhang J, Liu XT, Liu H, Zeng XF, Qiao SY. Superoxide dismutase recombinant *Lactobacillus fermentum* ameliorates intestinal oxidative stress through inhibiting NF-κB activation in a trinitrobenzene sulphonic acid-induced colitis mouse model. *J Appl Microbiol* (2014) 116(6):1621–31. doi:10.1111/jam.12461
27. Clancy R. Immunobiotics and the probiotic evolution. *FEMS Immunol Med Microbiol* (2003) 38(1):9–12. doi:10.1016/S0928-8244(03)00147-0
28. Kitazawa H, Villena J, Alvarez S. *Probiotics: Immunobiotics and Immunogenics*. Boca Raton, FL: CRC Press (2014).
29. Kitazawa H, Villena J. Modulation of respiratory TLR3-anti-viral response by probiotic microorganisms: lessons learned from *Lactobacillus rhamnosus* CRL1505. *Front Immunol* (2014) 5:201. doi:10.3389/fimmu.2014.00201
30. Villena J, Kitazawa H. Modulation of intestinal TLR4-inflammatory signaling pathways by probiotic microorganisms: lessons learned from *Lactobacillus jensenii* TL2937. *Front Immunol* (2014) 4:512. doi:10.3389/fimmu.2013.00512
31. Villena J, Aso H, Kitazawa H. Regulation of toll-like receptors-mediated inflammation by immunobiotics in bovine intestinal epitheliocytes: role of signaling pathways and negative regulators. *Front Immunol* (2014) 5:421. doi:10.3389/fimmu.2014.00421
32. Laino J, Villena J, Kanmani P, Kitazawa H. Immunoregulatory effects triggered by lactic acid bacteria exopolysaccharides: new insights into molecular interactions with host cells. *Microorganisms* (2016) 4(3):27. doi:10.3390/microorganisms4030027
33. Bermudez-Humaran LG, Motta JP, Aubry C, Kharrat P, Rous-Martin L, Sallenave JM, et al. Serine protease inhibitors protect better than IL-10 and TGF-beta anti-inflammatory cytokines against mouse colitis when delivered by recombinant lactococci. *Microb Cell Fact* (2015) 14:26. doi:10.1186/s12934-015-0198-4
34. Foligne B, Dessein R, Marceau M, Poiret S, Chamaillard M, Pot B, et al. Prevention and treatment of colitis with *Lactococcus lactis* secreting the immunomodulatory *Yersinia* LcrV protein. *Gastroenterology* (2007) 133(3):862–74. doi:10.1053/j.gastro.2007.06.018
35. Steidler L, Hans W, Schotte L, Neirynck S, Obermeier F, Falk W, et al. Treatment of murine colitis by *Lactococcus lactis* secreting interleukin-10. *Science* (2000) 289(5483):1352–5. doi:10.1126/science.289.5483.1352
36. del Carmen S, Martin Rosique R, Saraiva T, Zurita-Turk M, Miyoshi A, Azevedo V, et al. Protective effects of lactococci strains delivering either IL-10 protein or cDNA in a TNBS-induced chronic colitis model. *J Clin Gastroenterol* (2014) 48(Suppl 1):S12–7. doi:10.1097/mcg.0000000000000235
37. Waeytens A, Ferdinande L, Neirynck S, Rottiers P, De Vos M, Steidler L, et al. Paracellular entry of interleukin-10 producing *Lactococcus lactis* in inflamed intestinal mucosa in mice. *Inflamm Bowel Dis* (2008) 14(4):471–9. doi:10.1002/ibd.20346
38. Hanson ML, Hixon JA, Li W, Felber BK, Anver MR, Stewart CA, et al. Oral delivery of IL-27 recombinant bacteria attenuates immune colitis in mice. *Gastroenterology* (2014) 146(1):210.e13–21.e13. doi:10.1053/j.gastro.2013.09.060
39. Motta JP, Bermudez-Humaran LG, Deraison C, Martin L, Rolland C, Rousset P, et al. Food-grade bacteria expressing elafin protect against inflammation and restore colon homeostasis. *Sci Transl Med* (2012) 4(158):158ra44. doi:10.1126/scitranslmed.3004212
40. Shigemori S, Watanabe T, Kudoh K, Ihara M, Nigar S, Yamamoto Y, et al. Oral delivery of *Lactococcus lactis* that secretes bioactive heme oxygenase-1 alleviates development of acute colitis in mice. *Microb Cell Fact* (2015) 14:189. doi:10.1186/s12934-015-0378-2
41. Bolotin A, Wincker P, Mauger S, Jaillon O, Malarme K, Weissenbach J, et al. The complete genome sequence of the lactic acid bacterium *Lactococcus lactis* ssp. *lactis* IL1403. *Genome Res* (2001) 11(5):731–53. doi:10.1101/gr.169701
42. Wegmann U, O'Connell-Motherway M, Zomer A, Buist G, Shearman C, Canchaya C, et al. Complete genome sequence of the prototype lactic acid bacterium *Lactococcus lactis* subsp. *cremoris* MG1363. *J Bacteriol* (2007) 189(8):3256–70. doi:10.1128/jb.01768-06
43. Drouault S, Corthier G, Ehrlich SD, Renault P. Survival, physiology, and lysis of *Lactococcus lactis* in the digestive tract. *Appl Environ Microbiol* (1999) 65(11):4881–6.
44. Kimoto H, Nomura M, Kobayashi M, Mizumachi K, Okamoto T. Survival of lactococci during passage through mouse digestive tract. *Can J Microbiol* (2003) 49(11):707–11. doi:10.1139/w03-092
45. Aubry C, Michon C, Chain F, Chvatchenko Y, Goffin L, Zimmerli SC, et al. Protective effect of TSLP delivered at the gut mucosa level by recombinant

lactic acid bacteria in DSS-induced colitis mouse model. *Microb Cell Fact* (2015) 14:176. doi:10.1186/s12934-015-0367-5

46. Liu S, Li Y, Deng B, Xu Z. Recombinant *Lactococcus lactis* expressing porcine insulin-like growth factor I ameliorates DSS-induced colitis in mice. *BMC Biotechnol* (2016) 16:25. doi:10.1186/s12896-016-0255-z
47. Quevrain E, Maubert MA, Michon C, Chain F, Marquant R, Tailhades J, et al. Identification of an anti-inflammatory protein from *Faecalibacterium prausnitzii*, a commensal bacterium deficient in Crohn's disease. *Gut* (2016) 65(3):415–25. doi:10.1136/gutjnl-2014-307649
48. Saraiva TD, Morais K, Pereira VB, de Azevedo M, Rocha CS, Prosperi CC, et al. Milk fermented with a 15-lipoxygenase-1-producing *Lactococcus lactis* alleviates symptoms of colitis in a murine model. *Curr Pharm Biotechnol* (2015) 16(5):424–9. doi:10.2174/1389201015666141113123502
49. Vandenbroucke K, de Haard H, Beirnaert E, Dreier T, Lauwereys M, Huyck L, et al. Orally administered *L. lactis* secreting an anti-TNF nanobody demonstrate efficacy in chronic colitis. *Mucosal Immunol* (2010) 3(1):49–56. doi:10.1038/mi.2009.116
50. Vandenbroucke K, Hans W, Van Huysse J, Neirynck S, Demetter P, Remaut E, et al. Active delivery of trefoil factors by genetically modified *Lactococcus lactis* prevents and heals acute colitis in mice. *Gastroenterology* (2004) 127(2):502–13. doi:10.1053/j.gastro.2004.05.020
51. Wong CC, Zhang L, Li ZJ, Wu WK, Ren SX, Chen YC, et al. Protective effects of cathelicidin-encoding *Lactococcus lactis* in murine ulcerative colitis. *J Gastroenterol Hepatol* (2012) 27(7):1205–12. doi:10.1111/j.1440-1746.2012.07158.x
52. Braat H, Rottiers P, Hommes DW, Huyghebaert N, Remaut E, Remon JP, et al. A phase I trial with transgenic bacteria expressing interleukin-10 in Crohn's disease. *Clin Gastroenterol Hepatol* (2006) 4(6):754–9. doi:10.1016/j.cgh.2006.03.028
53. Wells JM, Mercenier A. Mucosal delivery of therapeutic and prophylactic molecules using lactic acid bacteria. *Nat Rev Microbiol* (2008) 6(5):349–62. doi:10.1038/nrmicro1840
54. Moore KW, de Waal Malefyt R, Coffman RL, O'Garra A. Interleukin-10 and the interleukin-10 receptor. *Annu Rev Immunol* (2001) 19:683–765. doi:10.1146/annurev.immunol.19.1.683
55. Kuhn R, Lohler J, Rennick D, Rajewsky K, Muller W. Interleukin-10-deficient mice develop chronic enterocolitis. *Cell* (1993) 75(2):263–74. doi:10.1016/0092-8674(93)80068-P
56. Spencer SD, Di Marco F, Hooley J, Pitts-Meek S, Bauer M, Ryan AM, et al. The orphan receptor CRF2-4 is an essential subunit of the interleukin 10 receptor. *J Exp Med* (1998) 187(4):571–8. doi:10.1084/jem.187.4.571
57. Glocker EO, Frede N, Perro M, Sebire N, Elawad M, Shah N, et al. Infant colitis – it's in the genes. *Lancet* (2010) 376(9748):1272. doi:10.1016/s0140-6736(10)61008-2
58. Glocker EO, Kotlarz D, Boztug K, Gertz EM, Schaffer AA, Noyan F, et al. Inflammatory bowel disease and mutations affecting the interleukin-10 receptor. *N Engl J Med* (2009) 361(21):2033–45. doi:10.1056/NEJMoa0907206
59. Steidler L, Neirynck S, Huyghebaert N, Snoeck V, Vermeire A, Goddeeris B, et al. Biological containment of genetically modified *Lactococcus lactis* for intestinal delivery of human interleukin 10. *Nat Biotechnol* (2003) 21(7):785–9. doi:10.1038/nbt840
60. Sasaoka T, Ito M, Yamashita J, Nakajima K, Tanaka I, Narita M, et al. Treatment with IL-27 attenuates experimental colitis through the suppression of the development of IL-17-producing T helper cells. *Am J Physiol Gastrointest Liver Physiol* (2011) 300(4):G568–76. doi:10.1152/ajpgi.00329.2010
61. Imielinski M, Baldassano RN, Griffiths A, Russell RK, Annese V, Dubinsky M, et al. Common variants at five new loci associated with early-onset inflammatory bowel disease. *Nat Genet* (2009) 41(12):1335–40. doi:10.1038/ng.489
62. Abraham NG, Kappas A. Pharmacological and clinical aspects of heme oxygenase. *Pharmacol Rev* (2008) 60(1):79–127. doi:10.1124/pr.107.07104
63. Kikuchi G, Yoshida T, Noguchi M. Heme oxygenase and heme degradation. *Biochem Biophys Res Commun* (2005) 338(1):558–67. doi:10.1016/j.bbrc.2005.08.020
64. Zhang L, Zhang Y, Zhong W, Di C, Lin X, Xia Z. Heme oxygenase-1 ameliorates dextran sulfate sodium-induced acute murine colitis by regulating Th17/Treg cell balance. *J Biol Chem* (2014) 289(39):26847–58. doi:10.1074/jbc.M114.590554
65. Hunter CA, Jones SA. IL-6 as a keystone cytokine in health and disease. *Nat Immunol* (2015) 16(5):448–57. doi:10.1038/ni.3153
66. Atreya R, Mudter J, Finotto S, Mullberg J, Jostock T, Wirtz S, et al. Blockade of interleukin 6 trans signaling suppresses T-cell resistance against apoptosis in chronic intestinal inflammation: evidence in Crohn disease and experimental colitis in vivo. *Nat Med* (2000) 6(5):583–8. doi:10.1038/75068
67. Ito H, Takazoe M, Fukuda Y, Hibi T, Kusugami K, Andoh A, et al. A pilot randomized trial of a human anti-interleukin-6 receptor monoclonal antibody in active Crohn's disease. *Gastroenterology* (2004) 126(4):989–96. doi:10.1053/j.gastro.2004.01.012
68. Shigemori S, Ihara M, Sato T, Yamamoto Y, Nigar S, Ogita T, et al. Secretion of an immunoreactive single-chain variable fragment antibody against mouse interleukin 6 by *Lactococcus lactis*. *Appl Microbiol Biotechnol* (2017) 101(1):341–9. doi:10.1007/s00253-016-7907-8
69. Miele E, Pascarella F, Giannetti E, Quaglietta L, Baldassano RN, Staiano A. Effect of a probiotic preparation (VSL#3) on induction and maintenance of remission in children with ulcerative colitis. *Am J Gastroenterol* (2009) 104(2):437–43. doi:10.1038/ajg.2008.118
70. Oliva S, Di Nardo G, Ferrari F, Mallardo S, Rossi P, Patrizi G, et al. Randomised clinical trial: the effectiveness of *Lactobacillus reuteri* ATCC 55730 rectal enema in children with active distal ulcerative colitis. *Aliment Pharmacol Ther* (2012) 35(3):327–34. doi:10.1111/j.1365-2036.2011.04939.x
71. Sood A, Midha V, Makharia GK, Ahuja V, Singal D, Goswami P, et al. The probiotic preparation, VSL#3 induces remission in patients with mild-to-moderately active ulcerative colitis. *Clin Gastroenterol Hepatol* (2009) 7(11):1202–9, 1209.e1. doi:10.1016/j.cgh.2009.07.016
72. Tursi A, Brandimarte G, Papa A, Giglio A, Elisei W, Giorgetti GM, et al. Treatment of relapsing mild-to-moderate ulcerative colitis with the probiotic VSL#3 as adjunctive to a standard pharmaceutical treatment: a double-blind, randomized, placebo-controlled study. *Am J Gastroenterol* (2010) 105(10):2218–27. doi:10.1038/ajg.2010.218
73. Guarner F, Khan AG, Garisch J, Eliakim R, Gangl A, Thomson A, et al. World gastroenterology organisation global guidelines: probiotics and prebiotics October 2011. *J Clin Gastroenterol* (2012) 46(6):468–81. doi:10.1097/MCG.0b013e3182549092
74. Foligne B, Nutten S, Grangette C, Dennin V, Goudercourt D, Poiret S, et al. Correlation between in vitro and in vivo immunomodulatory properties of lactic acid bacteria. *World J Gastroenterol* (2007) 13(2):236–43. doi:10.3748/wjg.v13.i2.236
75. Piechota-Polanczyk A, Fichna J. Review article: the role of oxidative stress in pathogenesis and treatment of inflammatory bowel diseases. *Naunyn Schmiedebergs Arch Pharmacol* (2014) 387(7):605–20. doi:10.1007/s00210-014-0985-1
76. Singh M, Mukhopadhyay K. α-Melanocyte stimulating hormone: an emerging anti-inflammatory antimicrobial peptide. *Biomed Res Int* (2014) 2014:874610. doi:10.1155/2014/874610
77. Donkor ON, Ravikumar M, Proudfoot O, Day SL, Apostolopoulos V, Paukovics G, et al. Cytokine profile and induction of T helper type 17 and regulatory T cells by human peripheral mononuclear cells after microbial exposure. *Clin Exp Immunol* (2012) 167(2):282–95. doi:10.1111/j.1365-2249.2011.04496.x
78. Latvala S, Miettinen M, Kekkonen RA, Korpela R, Julkunen I. *Lactobacillus rhamnosus* GG and *Streptococcus thermophilus* induce suppressor of cytokine signalling 3 (SOCS3) gene expression directly and indirectly via interleukin-10 in human primary macrophages. *Clin Exp Immunol* (2011) 165(1):94–103. doi:10.1111/j.1365-2249.2011.04408.x
79. Shimosato T, Fujimoto M, Tohno M, Sato T, Tateo M, Otani H, et al. CpG oligodeoxynucleotides induce strong up-regulation of interleukin 33 via toll-like receptor 9. *Biochem Biophys Res Commun* (2010) 394(1):81–6. doi:10.1016/j.bbrc.2010.02.110
80. Shimosato T, Tohno M, Sato T, Nishimura J, Kawai Y, Saito T, et al. Identification of a potent immunostimulatory oligodeoxynucleotide from *Streptococcus thermophilus lacZ*. *Anim Sci J* (2009) 80(5):597–604. doi:10.1111/j.1740-0929.2009.00680.x
81. Ogita T, Nakashima M, Morita H, Saito Y, Suzuki T, Tanabe S. *Streptococcus thermophilus* ST28 ameliorates colitis in mice partially by suppression

of inflammatory Th17 cells. *J Biomed Biotechnol* (2011) 2011:378417. doi:10.1155/2011/378417

82. Ogita T, Tanii Y, Morita H, Suzuki T, Tanabe S. Suppression of Th17 response by *Streptococcus thermophilus* ST28 through induction of IFN-γ. *Int J Mol Med* (2011) 28(5):817–22. doi:10.3892/ijmm.2011.755
83. Petrarca C, Clemente E, Toto V, Iezzi M, Rossi C, Zanotta S, et al. rBet v 1 immunotherapy of sensitized mice with *Streptococcus thermophilus* as vehicle and adjuvant. *Hum Vaccin Immunother* (2014) 10(5):1228–37. doi:10.4161/hv.28155
84. de Moreno de LeBlanc A, Del Carmen S, Chatel JM, Azevedo V, Bermudez-Humaran L, Langella P, et al. Evaluation of the biosafety of recombinant lactic acid bacteria designed to prevent and to treat colitis. *J Med Microbiol* (2016) 65(9):1038–46. doi:10.1099/jmm.0.000323
85. Burke DA, Axon AT. Adhesive *Escherichia coli* in inflammatory bowel disease and infective diarrhoea. *BMJ* (1988) 297(6641):102–4. doi:10.1136/bmj.297.6641.102
86. Cummings JH, Macfarlane GT, Macfarlane S. Intestinal bacteria and ulcerative colitis. *Curr Issues Intest Microbiol* (2003) 4(1):9–20.
87. Gevers D, Kugathasan S, Denson LA, Vazquez-Baeza Y, Van Treuren W, Ren B, et al. The treatment-naive microbiome in new-onset Crohn's disease. *Cell Host Microbe* (2014) 15(3):382–92. doi:10.1016/j.chom.2014.02.005
88. Macfarlane S, Furrie E, Cummings JH, Macfarlane GT. Chemotaxonomic analysis of bacterial populations colonizing the rectal mucosa in patients with ulcerative colitis. *Clin Infect Dis* (2004) 38(12):1690–9. doi:10.1086/420823
89. Mylonaki M, Rayment NB, Rampton DS, Hudspith BN, Brostoff J. Molecular characterization of rectal mucosa-associated bacterial flora in inflammatory bowel disease. *Inflamm Bowel Dis* (2005) 11(5):481–7. doi:10.1097/01.MIB.0000159663.62651.4f
90. Jeon SG, Kayama H, Ueda Y, Takahashi T, Asahara T, Tsuji H, et al. Probiotic *Bifidobacterium breve* induces IL-10-producing Tr1 cells in the colon. *PLoS Pathog* (2012) 8(5):e1002714. doi:10.1371/journal.ppat.1002714
91. McCarthy J, O'Mahony L, O'Callaghan L, Sheil B, Vaughan EE, Fitzsimons N, et al. Double blind, placebo controlled trial of two probiotic strains in interleukin 10 knockout mice and mechanistic link with cytokine balance. *Gut* (2003) 52(7):975–80. doi:10.1136/gut.52.7.975
92. Srutkova D, Schwarzer M, Hudcovic T, Zakostelska Z, Drab V, Spanova A, et al. *Bifidobacterium longum* CCM 7952 promotes epithelial barrier function and prevents acute DSS-induced colitis in strictly strain-specific manner. *PLoS One* (2015) 10(7):e0134050. doi:10.1371/journal.pone.0134050
93. Takeda Y, Nakase H, Namba K, Inoue S, Ueno S, Uza N, et al. Upregulation of T-bet and tight junction molecules by *Bifidobacterium longum* improves colonic inflammation of ulcerative colitis. *Inflamm Bowel Dis* (2009) 15(11):1617–8. doi:10.1002/ibd.20861
94. Setoyama H, Imaoka A, Ishikawa H, Umesaki Y. Prevention of gut inflammation by *Bifidobacterium* in dextran sulfate-treated gnotobiotic mice associated with *Bacteroides* strains isolated from ulcerative colitis patients. *Microbes Infect* (2003) 5(2):115–22. doi:10.1016/S1286-4579(02)00080-1
95. Veiga P, Gallini CA, Beal C, Michaud M, Delaney ML, DuBois A, et al. *Bifidobacterium animalis* subsp. *lactis* fermented milk product reduces inflammation by altering a niche for colitogenic microbes. *Proc Natl Acad Sci U S A* (2010) 107(42):18132–7. doi:10.1073/pnas.1011737107
96. Konieczna P, Akdis CA, Quigley EM, Shanahan F, O'Mahony L. Portrait of an immunoregulatory *Bifidobacterium*. *Gut Microbes* (2012) 3(3):261–6. doi:10.4161/gmic.20358
97. Konieczna P, Groeger D, Ziegler M, Frei R, Ferstl R, Shanahan F, et al. *Bifidobacterium infantis* 35624 administration induces Foxp3 T regulatory cells in human peripheral blood: potential role for myeloid and plasmacytoid dendritic cells. *Gut* (2012) 61(3):354–66. doi:10.1136/gutjnl-2011-300936
98. O'Mahony C, Scully P, O'Mahony D, Murphy S, O'Brien F, Lyons A, et al. Commensal-induced regulatory T cells mediate protection against pathogen-stimulated NF-κB activation. *PLoS Pathog* (2008) 4(8):e1000112. doi:10.1371/journal.ppat.1000112
99. O'Mahony L, McCarthy J, Kelly P, Hurley G, Luo F, Chen K, et al. *Lactobacillus* and *Bifidobacterium* in irritable bowel syndrome: symptom responses and relationship to cytokine profiles. *Gastroenterology* (2005) 128(3):541–51. doi:10.1053/j.gastro.2004.11.050
100. Groeger D, O'Mahony L, Murphy EF, Bourke JF, Dinan TG, Kiely B, et al. *Bifidobacterium infantis* 35624 modulates host inflammatory processes beyond the gut. *Gut Microbes* (2013) 4(4):325–39. doi:10.4161/gmic.25487
101. Tamaki H, Nakase H, Inoue S, Kawanami C, Itani T, Ohana M, et al. Efficacy of probiotic treatment with *Bifidobacterium longum* 536 for induction of remission in active ulcerative colitis: a randomized, double-blinded, placebo-controlled multicenter trial. *Dig Endosc* (2016) 28(1):67–74. doi:10.1111/den.12553
102. Bibiloni R, Fedorak RN, Tannock GW, Madsen KL, Gionchetti P, Campieri M, et al. VSL#3 probiotic-mixture induces remission in patients with active ulcerative colitis. *Am J Gastroenterol* (2005) 100(7):1539–46. doi:10.1111/j.1572-0241.2005.41794.x
103. Kato K, Mizuno S, Umesaki Y, Ishii Y, Sugitani M, Imaoka A, et al. Randomized placebo-controlled trial assessing the effect of bifidobacteria-fermented milk on active ulcerative colitis. *Aliment Pharmacol Ther* (2004) 20(10):1133–41. doi:10.1111/j.1365-2036.2004.02268.x
104. Sonnenborn U, Schulze J. The non-pathogenic *Escherichia coli* strain Nissle 1917 – features of a versatile probiotic. *Microb Ecol Health Dis* (2009) 21:122–58. doi:10.3109/08910600903444267
105. Kruis W, Fric P, Pokrotnieks J, Lukas M, Fixa B, Kascak M, et al. Maintaining remission of ulcerative colitis with the probiotic *Escherichia coli* Nissle 1917 is as effective as with standard mesalazine. *Gut* (2004) 53(11):1617–23. doi:10.1136/gut.2003.037747
106. Kruis W, Schutz E, Fric P, Fixa B, Judmaier G, Stolte M. Double-blind comparison of an oral *Escherichia coli* preparation and mesalazine in maintaining remission of ulcerative colitis. *Aliment Pharmacol Ther* (1997) 11(5):853–8. doi:10.1046/j.1365-2036.1997.00225.x
107. Rembacken BJ, Snelling AM, Hawkey PM, Chalmers DM, Axon AT. Non-pathogenic *Escherichia coli* versus mesalazine for the treatment of ulcerative colitis: a randomised trial. *Lancet* (1999) 354(9179):635–9. doi:10.1016/S0140-6736(98)06343-0
108. Ukena SN, Singh A, Dringenberg U, Engelhardt R, Seidler U, Hansen W, et al. Probiotic *Escherichia coli* Nissle 1917 inhibits leaky gut by enhancing mucosal integrity. *PLoS One* (2007) 2(12):e1308. doi:10.1371/journal.pone.0001308
109. Souza EL, Elian SD, Paula LM, Garcia CC, Vieira AT, Teixeira MM, et al. *Escherichia coli* strain Nissle 1917 ameliorates experimental colitis by modulating intestinal permeability, the inflammatory response and clinical signs in a faecal transplantation model. *J Med Microbiol* (2016) 65(3):201–10. doi:10.1099/jmm.0.000222
110. Schultz M, Strauch UG, Linde HJ, Watzl S, Obermeier F, Gottl C, et al. Preventive effects of *Escherichia coli* strain Nissle 1917 on acute and chronic intestinal inflammation in two different murine models of colitis. *Clin Diagn Lab Immunol* (2004) 11(2):372–8. doi:10.1128/cdli.11.2.372-378.2004
111. Kamada N, Inoue N, Hisamatsu T, Okamoto S, Matsuoka K, Sato T, et al. Nonpathogenic *Escherichia coli* strain Nissle 1917 prevents murine acute and chronic colitis. *Inflamm Bowel Dis* (2005) 11(5):455–63. doi:10.1097/01.MIB.0000158158.55955.de
112. Ou B, Yang Y, Tham WL, Chen L, Guo J, Zhu G. Genetic engineering of probiotic *Escherichia coli* Nissle 1917 for clinical application. *Appl Microbiol Biotechnol* (2016) 100(20):8693–9. doi:10.1007/s00253-016-7829-5
113. Buddenborg C, Daudel D, Liebrecht S, Greune L, Humberg V, Schmidt MA. Development of a tripartite vector system for live oral immunization using a Gram-negative probiotic carrier. *Int J Med Microbiol* (2008) 298(1–2):105–14. doi:10.1016/j.ijmm.2007.08.008
114. Rao S, Hu S, McHugh L, Lueders K, Henry K, Zhao Q, et al. Toward a live microbial microbicide for HIV: commensal bacteria secreting an HIV fusion inhibitor peptide. *Proc Natl Acad Sci U S A* (2005) 102(34):11993–8. doi:10.1073/pnas.0504881102
115. Remer KA, Bartrow M, Roeger B, Moll H, Sonnenborn U, Oelschlaeger TA. Split immune response after oral vaccination of mice with recombinant *Escherichia coli* Nissle 1917 expressing fimbrial adhesin K88. *Int J Med Microbiol* (2009) 299(7):467–78. doi:10.1016/j.ijmm.2009.03.003

116. Danilowicz-Luebert E, Steinfelder S, Kuhl AA, Drozdenko G, Lucius R, Worm M, et al. A nematode immunomodulator suppresses grass pollen-specific allergic responses by controlling excessive Th2 inflammation. *Int J Parasitol* (2013) 43(3–4):201–10. doi:10.1016/j.ijpara.2012.10.014

117. Klotz C, Ziegler T, Figueiredo AS, Rausch S, Hepworth MR, Obsivac N, et al. A helminth immunomodulator exploits host signaling events to regulate cytokine production in macrophages. *PLoS Pathog* (2011) 7(1):e1001248. doi:10.1371/journal.ppat.1001248

118. Schierack P, Lucius R, Sonnenburg B, Schilling K, Hartmann S. Parasite-specific immunomodulatory functions of filarial cystatin. *Infect Immun* (2003) 71(5):2422–9. doi:10.1128/IAI.71.5.2422-2429.2003

119. Schnoeller C, Rausch S, Pillai S, Avagyan A, Wittig BM, Loddenkemper C, et al. A helminth immunomodulator reduces allergic and inflammatory responses by induction of IL-10-producing macrophages. *J Immunol* (2008) 180(6):4265–72. doi:10.4049/jimmunol.180.6.4265

120. Huyghebaert N, Vermeire A, Neirynck S, Steidler L, Remaut E, Remon JP. Evaluation of extrusion/spheronisation, layering and compaction for the preparation of an oral, multi-particulate formulation of viable, hIL-10 producing *Lactococcus lactis*. *Eur J Pharm Biopharm* (2005) 59(1):9–15. doi:10.1016/j.ejpb.2004.09.003

121. Huyghebaert N, Vermeire A, Neirynck S, Steidler L, Remaut E, Remon JP. Development of an enteric-coated formulation containing freeze-dried, viable recombinant *Lactococcus lactis* for the ileal mucosal delivery of human interleukin-10. *Eur J Pharm Biopharm* (2005) 60(3):349–59. doi:10.1016/j.ejpb.2005.02.012

122. Limaye SA, Haddad RI, Cilli F, Sonis ST, Colevas AD, Brennan MT, et al. Phase 1b, multicenter, single blinded, placebo-controlled, sequential dose escalation study to assess the safety and tolerability of topically applied AG013 in subjects with locally advanced head and neck cancer receiving induction chemotherapy. *Cancer* (2013) 119(24):4268–76. doi:10.1002/cncr.28365

123. Robert S, Steidler L. Recombinant *Lactococcus lactis* can make the difference in antigen-specific immune tolerance induction, the type 1 diabetes case. *Microb Cell Fact* (2014) 13(Suppl 1):S11. doi:10.1186/1475-2859-13-s1-s11

9

The Soil Bacterium *Methylococcus capsulatus* Bath Interacts with Human Dendritic Cells to Modulate Immune Function

Stine Indrelid[1,2]*, *Charlotte Kleiveland*[2]†, *René Holst*[1], *Morten Jacobsen*[1,2] *and Tor Lea*[2]

[1] *Research and Innovation, Østfold Hospital Trust, Kalnes, Norway,* [2] *Department of Chemistry, Biotechnology and Food Science, Norwegian University of Life Sciences, Aas, Norway*

Edited by:
Haruki Kitazawa,
Tohoku University, Japan

Reviewed by:
Gabriela Del Valle Perdigon,
CERELA-CONICET, Argentina
Jieliang Li,
Temple University, USA

***Correspondence:**
Stine Indrelid
stine.indrelid@nmbu.no

The prevalence of inflammatory bowel disease (IBD) has increased in Western countries during the course of the twentieth century, and is evolving to be a global disease. Recently we showed that a bacterial meal of a non-commensal, non-pathogenic methanotrophic soil bacterium, *Methylococcus capsulatus* Bath prevents experimentally induced colitis in a murine model of IBD. The mechanism behind the effect has this far not been identified. Here, for the first time we show that *M. capsulatus*, a soil bacterium adheres specifically to human dendritic cells, influencing DC maturation, cytokine production, and subsequent T cell activation, proliferation and differentiation. We characterize the immune modulatory properties of *M. capsulatus* and compare its immunological properties to those of another Gram-negative gammaproteobacterium, the commensal *Escherichia coli* K12, and the immune modulatory Gram-positive probiotic bacterium, *Lactobacillus rhamnosus* GG *in vitro*. *M. capsulatus* induces intermediate phenotypic and functional DC maturation. In a mixed lymphocyte reaction *M. capsulatus*-primed monocyte-derived dendritic cells (MoDCs) enhance T cell expression of CD25, the γ-chain of the high affinity IL-2 receptor, supports cell proliferation, and induce a T cell cytokine profile different from both *E. coli* K12 and *Lactobacillus rhamnosus* GG. *M. capsulatus* Bath thus interacts specifically with MoDC, affecting MoDC maturation, cytokine profile, and subsequent MoDC directed T cell polarization.

Keywords: dendritic cells (DC), old friends hypothesis, immune modulation, environmental bacteria, DC activation, T cell polarization, immunobiotics, soil bacteria

IMPORTANCE

There has been a growing interest in probiotics for treating both IBD, allergies, and autoimmune diseases, and considerable effort has been invested in identifying novel probiotics aimed for treating immune pathologies. Typically, candidate probiotic bacteria has been of human or animal origin, and a host-associated lifestyle is assumed to be a prerequisite for developing immune-regulatory functions. Here we describe immune modulatory functions of a non-commensal soil bacterium previously shown to exhibit anti-inflammatory effects in a murine colitis model pointing to environmental bacteria as a new and untapped source of bacteria for modulating immune responsiveness.

INTRODUCTION

Although microbes are associated with all epithelial surfaces of animal hosts, the highest number, and most diverse microbial populations are found in the intestines. Some 10–100 trillion microbes colonizes the human gastrointestinal tract, with the highest numbers present in the colon (Turnbaugh et al., 2007). The physiology of these microbes and their hosts is closely connected and mutually regulated (Brown et al., 2013). The host shapes the composition of the intestinal microbiota at species and community levels by supplying nutrients and by producing antimicrobial peptides. The human microbiota in return, adds to the metabolic, and biochemical activities of the host and play essential roles in the development and differentiation of the host intestinal epithelium, the immune system, and in the maintenance of mucosal homeostasis (Nicholson et al., 2012; Sommer and Backhed, 2013).

Only a single layer of epithelial cells separates the luminal contents and microbial community from underlying tissues, and the epithelial barrier therefore provides a possible entry point for opportunistic pathogens into the body. The host must maintain a mutualistic relationship with the commensal microbiome, while retaining protective responsiveness against pathogenic bacteria. To achieve this it must preserve epithelial integrity and regulate pro- and anti-inflammatory signaling, in an appropriate manner. Homeostasis is maintained through continuous and dynamic interactions and communication between the intestinal microbiota, the epithelium, and immune cells in the intestinal mucosa.

The regulatory interactions that exist between multicellular organisms and the microbial world are not necessarily limited to those between commensals and their hosts. The increasing prevalence of inflammatory bowel disease and autoimmune diseases in the western world has been associated with reduced exposure to helminths and environmental microorganisms from soil, water, and fermenting vegetables (Rook, 2007). The "hygiene hypothesis" was forwarded as a result of studies coherent with the idea that postnatal infections may be protective against allergy later in life, and that such protection may be lost in the presence of modern hygiene (Strachan, 1989, 2000). The related "old-friend hypothesis" explains the striking increase in chronic inflammatory disorders as largely being due to reduced contact with microorganisms that we have coevolved with, and therefore depend on, for proper immune development and regulation (Rook, 2010). In this context both pathogenic bacteria, the commensal microbiota, pseudo-commensals, and even the environmental microbiota may be essential regulatory components of the mammalian immune system. An increased mechanistic understanding of how such microbes and microbial products affect immune homeostasis may form a basis for developing novel tools for modulating immune responses in chronic inflammatory disorders.

Recently we demonstrated that a bacterial meal of the Gram-negative soil bacterium, *Methylococcus capsulatus* Bath, ameliorates dextran sulfate sodium (DSS) induced colitis in mice (Kleiveland et al., 2013). The study points to a potential for non-commensal environmental bacteria in protecting against experimental colitis in mammals, but the mechanisms behind these effects have not been identified. Both live and heat-killed probiotic bacteria have previously been shown to protect against experimental colitis (Mileti et al., 2009; Sang et al., 2014; Toumi et al., 2014; Souza et al., 2016). Proposed modes of action include competitive pathogen exclusion, production of antimicrobial substances, gut flora modulation, modulatory effects on epithelial barrier integrity, regulatory effects on innate, and adaptive immunity and effects on epithelial development and survival (Bermudez-Brito et al., 2012). However, direct effects on dendritic cells (DCs) with subsequent effects on cytokine production and T cell development is expected to be a common mode of action for those probiotic strains able to modulate adaptive immunity (Bienenstock et al., 2013).

DCs are professional antigen presenting cells that play a key role in both innate and adaptive immune responses (Steinman, 2012). Intestinal DCs expresses pattern recognizing receptors (PRRs) to recognize various microbial structures and can distinguish between microbe-associated molecular patterns (MAMPs) of even closely related organisms to initiate specific and appropriate response. The capacity of DCs to activate naïve T cells inducing T cell expansion and polarization, position DCs as critical mediators of host immune tolerance, and inflammatory responses (Mann et al., 2013).

The dietary inclusion of *M capsulatus* Bath in DSS-colitis model affected the intestinal epithelium through increased cell proliferation and mucin production, suggesting beneficial effects on gut barrier function. However, direct effects on cells of the immune system was not evaluated in that study. Here, for the first time, we show that *M. capsulatus* Bath, a non-commensal environmental bacterium, specifically and strongly adheres to murine and human DCs, an immune cell type central in regulating both innate and adaptive immunity. We compare the immune modulatory effects of *M. capsulatus* Bath to those of the Gram-negative commensal *Escherichia coli* K12, a non-pathogenic *E. coli* strain originally isolated from stool of a diphtheria patient (Agency USEP, 1997), and the well characterized Gram-positive probiotic bacterium *Lactobacillus rhamnosus* GG. The interaction between DC and *M. capsulatus* leads to functional activation of the DCs, affects DC cytokine profile, improves T cell activation, and proliferation and drive T effector cell polarization *in vitro*.

MATERIALS AND METHODS

Bacterial Strains and Culture Conditions

M. capsulatus strain (Bath) (NCIMB 11132, Aberdeen, UK) were grown in nitrate mineral salts medium (Whittenbury et al., 1970) with a head-space of 75% air, 23.75% CH_4, and 1.25% CO_2 at 45°C and 200 rpm. *E. coli* strain K12 was kindly provided by Department of Bacteriology, the Norwegian Veterinary Institute, Norway. *E. coli* K12 (Blattner et al., 1997) was grown in LB medium (Oxoid Ltd., Basingstoke, United Kingdom) at 37°C and 200 rpm. *L. rhamnosus* GG was grown in MRS medium (Oxoid Ltd.) anaerobically at 37°C without shaking.

Cells and Culture Conditions

Human erythrocyte- and plasma depleted blood were obtained from healthy volunteers from Ostfold Hospital Trust, Fredrikstad, Norway in accordance with institutional ethical guidelines and with approval from the Regional Committee of Medical and Health Research Ethics with written informed consent from all subjects. All subjects gave written informed consent in accordance with the Declaration of Helsinki. Peripheral blood mononuclear cells (PBMCs) were isolated by density gradient centrifugation on a Lymphoprep gradient (Fresenius Kabi). Human T cells were isolated from PBMCs by negative selection using Dynabeads Untouched Human T Cells Kit (Thermo Fisher). $CD14^+$ cells were isolated by positive selection using human CD14 MicroBeads (Miltenyi Biotech). To develop immature monocyte-derived dendritic cells (MoDCs) $CD14^+$ cells were cultivated for 6 days in RPMI 1640 medium supplemented with 10% heat inactivated fetal calf serum and 25 μg/ml gentamicin sulfate (Lonza), 1 mM sodium pyruvate and 100 μM non-essential amino acids (both from PAA Laboratories), 25 ng/ml interleukin 4 and 50 ng/ml granulocyte macrophage colony stimulating factor (both from ImmunoTools).

Bacterial Stimulation, Cytokine Analysis, and Immune Phenotyping of MoDCs

For immune phenotyping and DC cytokine analysis MoDCs were primed for 24 h by bacteria in a ratio of 1:10 (MoDC: bacteria) or by a maturation cocktail of 15 ng/ml TNF-α (ImmunoTools), 100 ng/ml LPS and 5 μg/ml PGE2 (Sigma-Aldrich). Culture supernatants were harvested and stored at −20°C then analyzed for cytokines by ProcartaPlex Multiplex immunoassay (eBioscience). TGF-β and IL-6 was measured by ELISA kits (eBiosciences and PeproTech respectively). MoDCs were also harvested and stained using PE-conjugated mouse anti-human CD80 antibodies, PE-Cy5 conjugated mouse anti-human CD83, and PE-Cy5 conjugated mouse anti-human CD40 (all from BD Biosciences). For viability testing cells were stained by 1μg/ml PI and analyzed by flow cytometry.

DC-T Cell Co-cultures for Cytokine Analysis and Immunophenotyping

To induce antigen specific T cell responses a modified mixed leukocyte culture system (MLC) were used with MoDC as stimulator cells and purified peripheral blood T cells as responder cells. MoDCs, either unprimed or primed by UV-inactivated bacteria in a ratio of 1:100 (MoDC:bacteria) for 24 h, were co-incubated with allogeneic T cells from two different donors (1:10 ratio between MoDCs and T cells). For cytokine analysis cells were grown in 48 well plates. After 5 days culture supernatants were harvested and T cells phenotyped by flow cytometry using FITC-conjugated anti-human CD4 and APC-conjugated anti-CD25 (both from Miltenyi Biotech). Fluorescence was detected by a MACSQuant flowcytometer and analyzed using the MACSQuantify software (both from Miltenyi Biotech). Cytokine concentrations in culture supernatant were measured by ProcartaPlex Multiplex immunoassay (eBioscience).

T Cell Proliferation Assay

MoDCs were primed for 24 h with UV-inactivated *M. capsulatus* 1:100 (DC:bacteria) in Nunc™ UpCell™ plates (Thermo Fisher). After 24 of stimulation the MoDCs were harvested, washed and co-incubated with allogenic human T cells in 96-well plates in a ratio of 1:10 (DC:T cells). Next day recombinant human IL-2 was added to each well to a final concentration of 10 U/ml. After 96 h of co-culture cells were pulsed by $[^3H]$-thymidine (1 μCi, Perkin Elmer) for 18.5 h. Cells were harvested onto glass-fiber filters and incorporated thymidine determined by liquid scintillation counting using a TopCount NXT™ Luminometer (Packard BioScience Company).

Scanning Electron Microscopy (SEM)

Immature MoDCs were co-cultivated with *M. capsulatus* Bath in 1:100 ratio (cells:bacteria) in medium free of antibiotics for 2–4 h in a humified atmosphere with 5% CO_2. Cells were washed twice by phosphate buffered saline (PAA Laboratories), fixed with 4% PFA and 2.5% glutaraldehyde (1:1) for 20 min at room temperature. Cells were washed again, dehydrated in a graded ethanol series and dried using a critical point dehydrator (CPD030 BalTec). Samples were coated with ∼500 Å Pt in a sputter coater (Polaron SC7640, Quorum technologies) and analyzed using an EVO-50 Zeiss microscope (Carl Zeiss AG).

Confocal Imaging

Immature MoDCs were generated from $CD14^+$ monocytes as described above. 1×10^8/ml *M. capsulatus* Bath were stained by 10 μM CFSE in PBS. CFSE-stained bacteria were co-incubated with immature MoDCs in a ratio of 1: 100 cells-bacteria. Cells were washed, fixated in PBS with 1% formalin then washed twice before coverslip was mounted on object slide with ProLong Diamond Antifade Mountant with DAPI (Thermo Fisher Scientific). Samples were scanned under a Zeiss LSM510 META confocal microscope (Carl Zeiss). Confocal stacks were acquired with z-spacing of 0.2 μm.

Statistical Analysis

Data were sampled in hierarchical structure, with multiple measurements per individual. This violates the assumption of independent measurements underlying ANOVA and conventional linear regression. This issue was remedied by analyzing the data using a mixed effects linear model, in which each individual acted as a random effect. Box-Cox analyses were used for finding suitable normalizing transformations. Data were analyzed on the log-scale and subsequently back-transformed for interpretation. All analyses were controlled by residual plots and Shapiro-Wilks test for normality.

RESULTS

M. capsulatus Bath Adheres Specifically to MoDC

A bacterial protein preparation of *M. capsulatus* Bath was previously found to have anti-inflammatory effects in a murine model of colitis (Kleiveland et al., 2013). When studying possible immune modulatory effects on immune cells, we observed that bacteria clustered around a small subset of cells in peripheral blood mononuclear cell preparations (**Figure 1A**). The appearance and low frequency of the target cells were consistent with the size and expected frequency of DCs among PBMCs. To determine whether the target cells were in fact DCs we incubated *M. capsulatus* Bath with $CD14^+$ monocytes or MoDCs generated from $CD14^+$ monocytes in the presence of IL-4 and GM-CSF. *M. capsulatus* did not bind to $CD14^+$ monocytes (**Figure 1B**), but quickly associated with dendritic cells (**Figure 1C**). The interaction between *M. capsulatus* Bath and MoDCs was further visualized by scanning electron microscopy (SEM) showing *M. capsulatus* Bath in large clusters on MoDCs after 3 h of co-incubation, even after several washes with PBS (**Figure 1D**).

To study binding kinetics we co-incubated CFSE-stained bacteria with MoDCs. Cells were counterstained with DAPI and confocal microscopy was used to visualize interactions over time (**Figure 2**). *M. capsulatus* Bath were found in scattered association with cells after just 30 min of co-incubation, and after 2 h a large number of bacteria associated with most cells. Strikingly, after around 3 h of co-incubation *M. capsulatus* were typically found to cluster around the nucleus of the MoDCs. A large number of bacteria could be seen associated with cells up to 20 h after co-incubation. At 48 h bacteria were cleared from most cells although a few intact bacteria was found associated with cells up to 72 h after co-incubation (**Figure 2**).

M. capsulatus Bath Induces Phenotypic and Functional Maturation of MoDCs

Upon microbial stimulation, DCs undergo a program of maturation that endows them with capacity to activate naïve T cells, induce T cell expansion, and to polarize T cells toward effector subpopulations appropriate to the stimulus encountered. Mature DCs are characterized by expression of co-stimulatory molecules required for efficient T cell activation. We compared the ability of *M. capsulatus* Bath, Gram-positive, and Gram-negative control bacteria to induce MoDC activation as assessed by expression of costimulatory molecules like CD40, CD80, and CD83. MoDCs, either left unprimed or co-incubated with bacteria (*M. capsulatus* Bath, *L. rhamnosus* GG, or *E. coli* K12) were stained for co-stimulatory molecules and maturation markers and analyzed by flow cytometry (**Figure 3**). Cells activated by a maturation cocktail containing TNF-α, LPS, and PGE_2 were used as a positive control. The maturation cocktail, *E. coli* K12, and *M. capsulatus* Bath induced upregulation of CD40, CD83, and CD80 in immature MoDCs. *E. coli* K12 was found to represent the most potent bacterial stimulus for inducing a mature DC phenotype compared to unprimed control cells, and induced expression of all activation markers. *M. capsulatus* Bath showed intermediate ability to induce MoDC maturation and elicited CD40 and CD80 expressions comparable to positive control, but a lower expression of CD83 compared to *E. coli* and the maturation cocktail (**Figure 3**). *L. rhamnosus* GG was a weak inducer of MoDC maturation, and produced a phenotype similar to unprimed cells. Cell viability, determined by PI staining, was similar between treatments suggesting that none of the strains asserted toxic effects on MoDCs (Data not shown).

MoDCs Respond to Bacterial Stimulation by Eliciting Distinct Cytokine Profiles

Depending on the nature of the stimuli, functionally mature DCs release cytokines promoting differentiation of naïve T cells into specific effector cell subsets. Since *M. capsulatus* and *E. coli* induced phenotypic maturation of MoDCs we wanted to see whether the bacteria also resulted in functional maturation characterized by cytokine release. Multiplex immunoassay and enzyme-linked immunosorbent assay (ELISA) was used to measure select cytokines in culture supernatants of MoDCs co-cultivated with bacteria for 24 h (**Figure 4**). In general, and in accordance with the observed phenotypic activation of MoDC, *E. coli* K12 was the most potent inducer of cytokine production, and resulted in increased release of IL-1β, IL-12p70, IL-10, TNF-α, IL-2, IL-23, IFN-γ, and IL-6 compared to unprimed control. *L. rhamnosus* GG in comparison was the least potent inducer of cytokine production in MoDCs of the three tested bacteria (**Figure 4**). Incubation with *M. capsulatus* Bath resulted in intermediate levels of cytokines. Similar to *E. coli*-primed MoDCs, incubation with *M. capsulatus* enhanced the production of IL-12p70, IL-10, TNF-α, IL-2, and IL-23 compared to unprimed MoDCs. However, *M. capsulatus* treatment in general resulted in lower cytokine levels than *E. coli* K12. *M. capsulatus*-primed cells produced substantially less IL-1β, IL-6, IL-10, IL-12p70, IL-23, and TNF-α than *E. coli*-primed cells, but the two bacteria induced similar levels of IL-2 from the MoDCs. TGF-β could not be detected in any of the co-cultures (data not shown). Thus, the interaction between *M. capsulatus* Bath and MoDCs resulted in both quantitative and qualitative differences in cytokine production compared to *E. coli* K12.

M. capsulatus Bath Increases DC-Induced T Cell Activation and Proliferation

Antigen recognition and a co-stimulatory signal through CD28 on T cells is required to induce functional T cell activation and clonal expansion. As the bacteria differently induced expression of DC co-stimulatory molecules, we examined the ability of bacteria-primed MoDCs to activate and induce proliferation in peripheral blood T cells. We co-incubated bacteria-primed MoDCs with allogenic T cells and measured expression of CD25 by flow cytometry. T cells co-cultivated with *M. capsulatus*-primed MoDCs expressed increased levels of CD25 compared to T cells cultivated with unprimed MoDCs or MoDCs primed by any of the control bacteria (**Figure 5A**). To test the ability of bacteria-treated MoDCs to induce proliferation in allogeneic T cells we measured DNA synthesis by [^{3}H] thymidine incorporation. MoDCs activated by *M. capsulatus* were stronger supporters of T cell proliferation than MoDCs primed by any of the control bacteria (**Figure 5B**).

MoDCs Primed by Different Bacteria Have Different Ability to Drive T Cell Differentiation

Cytokines produced by mature DCs contribute to drive T cell differentiation into specific effector cell subsets. In order to evaluate functional effects of bacteria-treated MoDCs on T cell polarization, activated MoDCs were co-incubated with

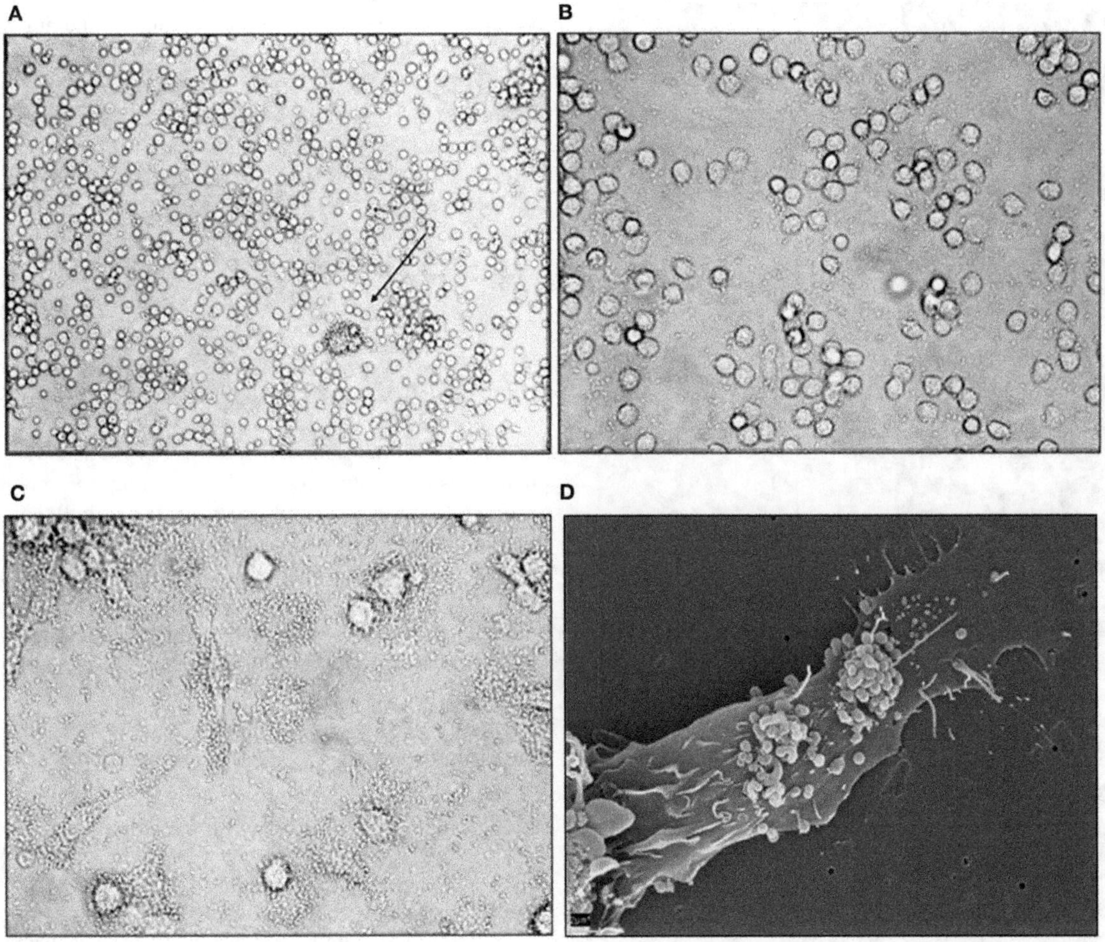

FIGURE 1 | *M. capsulatus* Bath interacts specifically with human MoDCs. (A–C) Light microscopy image of *M. capsulatus* Bath co-incubated (1:100 cells:bacteria) with human PBMC, CD14$^+$ monocytes, or monocyte-derived dendritic cells without washing. *M. capsulatus* Bath clusters around low frequency-cells in PBMC **(C)** (arrow), but not CD14$^+$ monocytes **(B)**. In co-culture with MoDCs bacteria cluster around a majority of cells **(C)**. **(D)** SEM electrograph showing *M. capsulatus* Bath adhering to human MoDCs after 3 h co-incubation.

allogeneic T cells. Culture medium was collected and analyzed for cytokines associated with different effector T cell subsets (**Figure 6**). MoDCs primed by any of the bacteria resulted in markedly reduced levels of typical Th2 cytokines like IL-5 and IL-13. All bacteria further resulted in increased release of the Th1 cytokine IFN-gamma and IL-10, an anti-inflammatory cytokine produced by several effector T cell lineages, compared to the basal level produced by T cells co-incubated with unprimed MoDCs.

Although all bacteria shifted T cells toward a Th1 rather that a Th2 phenotype, a major difference was found between Gram-negative *M. capsulatus* Bath and *E. coli* K12 on the one hand and Gram-positive *L. rhamnosus* GG on the other. Compared to T cells co-cultivated with unprimed MoDCs only *L. rhamnosus*-treated MoDCs resulted in significantly reduced release of IL-18, a proinflammatory cytokine that enhances innate immunity as well as Th1- and Th2-driven immune responses depending on cytokine milieu.

Conversely, only the Gram-negative bacteria *M. capsulatus* Bath and *E. coli* K12 gave significantly higher levels of the proinflammatory cytokines IL-6, TNF-α, IL-1β, and IL-1α. Both bacteria also increased IL-23, a cytokine linked to the generation and maintenance of Th17 cells, Th17 cytokines (IL-17A, IL-21, IL-22), Th22 cytokines (IL-22, TNF-α), and Th9 cytokines (IL-9 and IL-21).

Not all differences could be attributed to dissimilarities between Gram-positive vs. Gram-negative bacteria, however. No significant difference was found between *E. coli* and *M. capsulatus* in their ability to induce Th1, Th22, or Th9 cells, as evaluated by IFN-γ, TNF-α, IL-9, and IL-21, but compared to *E. coli*, *M. capsulatus* resulted in significantly less IL-23, Th17- associated cytokines IL-17A, and IL-22 as well as pro-inflammatory cytokines IL1-α, IL-1β, and IL-6 and the anti-inflammatory cytokine IL-10. Furthermore, reduction in Th2 cytokines IL-5 and IL-13 was lowest for *M. capsulatus* Bath primed co-cultures and *E. coli* and *L. rhamnosus*, but not *M.*

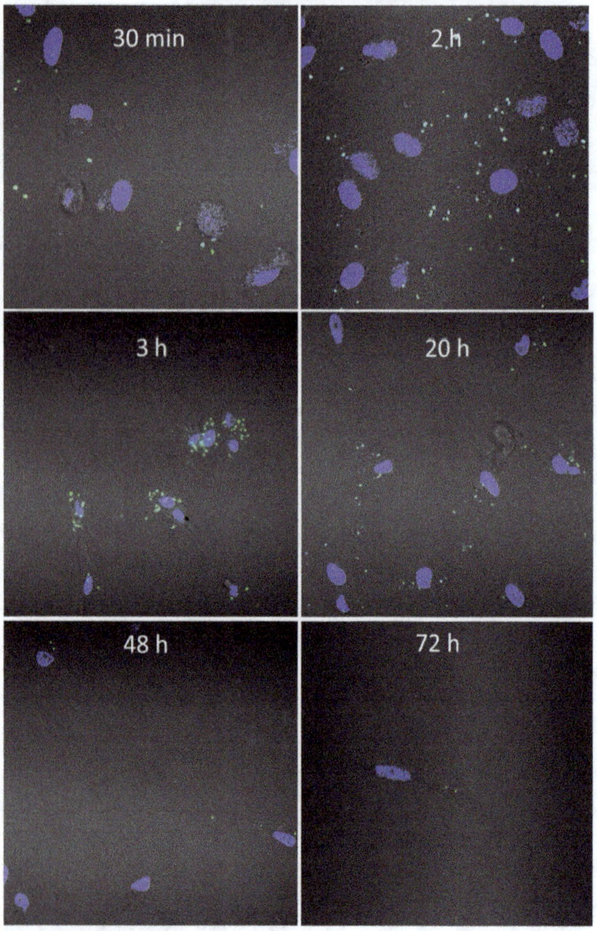

FIGURE 2 | *Methylococcus capsulatus*—DC interaction kinetics. Figure shows CFSE labeled *M. capsulatus* Bath (green) co-incubated with human MoDCs for 30 min to 72 h. MoDC nuclei were counterstained with DAPI (blue) to aid visualization and interactions were visualized by confocal microscopy.

capsulatus Bath, reduced IL-1RA and lymphotoxin-α levels in the cultures. *M. capsulatus* thus induces a T cells response functionally distinct from both *E. coli* K12 and *L. rhamnosus* GG.

DISCUSSION

Previous studies have described protective properties of probiotic bacteria, commensals, and their metabolites against experimental colitis in animal models (Pils et al., 2011; Qiu et al., 2013; Toumi et al., 2014; Souza et al., 2016). Although a connection between chronic intestinal inflammation and a reduced exposure to bacteria from soils and water has been made (Rook, 2007), few studies have focused on immune modulatory effects of non-commensal environmental bacteria. Here we show that a soil bacterium previously shown to reduce symptoms of chemically induced colitis in mice (Kleiveland et al., 2013) specifically targets human dendritic cells *in vitro,* affecting DC maturation, T cell activation, proliferation, and differentiation. *M. capsulatus* Bath was found to adhere specifically to human DCs. To our knowledge, this is the first report of an environmental bacterium to target mammalian DCs to modulate immune function.

The realization that a soil bacterium interacts specifically with human DCs raises some important questions. The significance of the commensal microbiome in health and disease is increasingly recognized, and there is a growing interest in probiotics within the scientific and public community. However, the role of environmental bacteria in immune regulation has been underappreciated for understandable reasons. It is not difficult to imagine that commensals living in close connection with humans are also closely connected to human physiology (Sommer and Backhed, 2013). Similarly, there is a long history of probiotics in fermented food associated with longevity and health. In a modern world of reduced microbial diversity it may be less intuitive to connect environmental bacteria to regulation of human health. However, as emphasized by the "old friends" hypothesis, mammals are evolutionary linked not only to commensals and probiotics, but also to ambient microbes in both soil and water (Rook, 2010).

Not only have mammals evolved from environmental bacteria, but the mammalian immune system has developed in the presence of such microbes. Throughout evolution some of these microbes may have taken on functions for us, some may relay signals necessary for immune development, while others, because of our long evolutionary association, are recognized by the immune system as harmless and have taken on regulatory roles (Rook et al., 2004). For example, chronic exposure to environmental LPS and other bacterial components present in farm dust may protect against asthmatic disease (Schuijs et al., 2015) possibly by reducing the overall reactivity of the immune system.

M. capsulatus Bath is an environmental bacterium that has been isolated from soil, water, sewage, mud, and lake sediments. It does not require a host to survive and may therefore face no obvious selection pressure to express immune modulatory molecules. Nevertheless, as discussed by Casadevall and Pirofski (2007), soil is an extreme environment with rapidly changing conditions, and bacteria living in soils will encounter an enormous number of predators of different types: unicellular amoebas, slime molds, protists, nematodes, snails as well as larger animals. As they are likely to meet ever-changing conditions as well as predatory hosts with different types of receptors and antimicrobial defenses, soil dwellers have to carry a diverse array of characteristics including host cell adhesins and immune modulatory molecules as defense mechanisms against predators. It was beyond the scope of our study to identify the bacterial factors involved in adhesion. However, a computational and experimental analysis of the *M. capsulatus* secretome has previously identified *M. capsulatus* Bath protein homologs of adhesion proteins that are involved in microbe adhesion to host cells in other bacterial species (Indrelid et al., 2014), showing that candidate host interaction proteins are present in *M. capsulatus* Bath and may facilitate adhesion to DC.

The maturation state and cytokine profile of DCs is functionally important. Although DCs represent a heterogeneous group of antigen-presenting cells, they have traditionally been divided into immature and mature differentiation stages

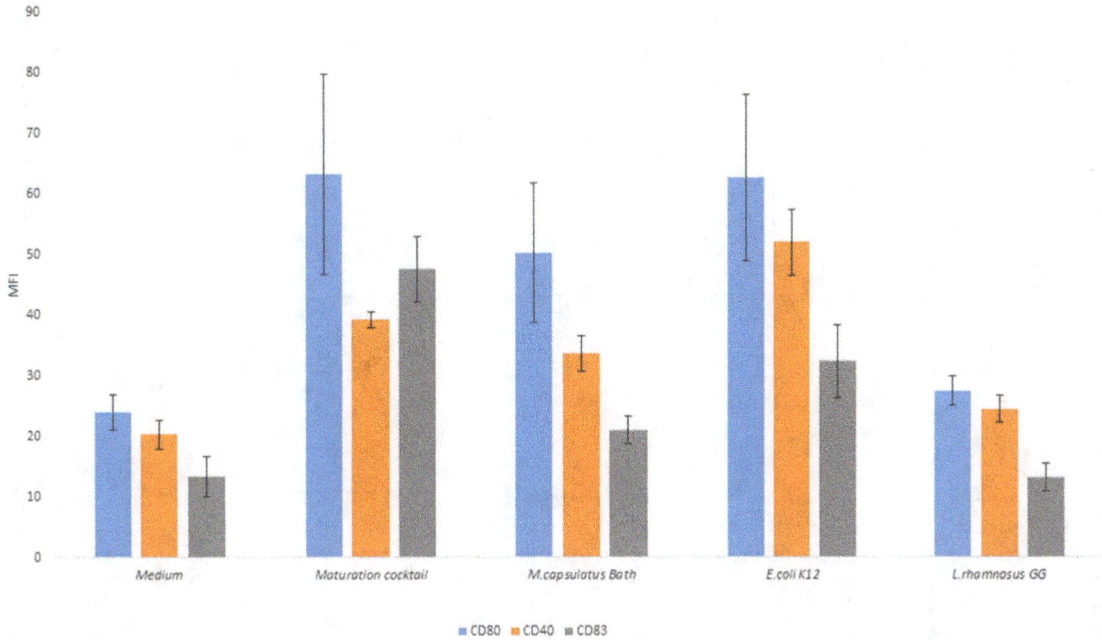

FIGURE 3 | *M. capsulatus* Bath and *E. coli* K12 induce maturation of MoDCs. Human MoDCs were either activated by a maturation cocktail of TNF-α, PGE2, and LPS or co-incubated with bacteria (*M. capsulatus* Bath, *E. coli* K12, or *L. rhamnosus* GG) for 24 h. Cells were stained for CD80, CD83, and CD40 and analyzed by flow cytometry in this figure. Median fluorescence intensity (MFI) is reported. Error bars indicate standard error on median fluorescence intensity values from 6 different donors.

(Reis e Sousa, 2006). Immature DCs are characterized by low surface expression of major histocompatibility complex (MHC) class II molecules and co-stimulatory molecules (e.g., CD80, CD86, and CD40). However, when DCs encounter microbes, pattern-recognition receptors (PRRs) are triggered by microbe-associated molecular patterns resulting in major changes in gene expression and acquisition of a number of functional properties: antigen processing and presentation, migration, and T-cell co-stimulation (Dalod et al., 2014).

It has been proposed that pathogen, probiotic, and commensal bacteria can be divided into three distinct classes based on the extent of host response by DCs and other PRR expressing cells. MAMPs of pathogenic microorganisms tend to induce a strong host response, probiotics induce an intermediate response whereas commensal bacteria exhibit homeostatic control of the response (Lebeer et al., 2010). In the present study the non-commensal, non-pathogenic *M. capsulatus* Bath induced a DC response intermediate between the Gram-positive probiotic *Lactobacillus rhamnosus* GG and the commensal Gram-negative *E. coli* K12. Substantial differences were found between *M. capsulatus* Bath, *L. rhamnosus* GG and the *E. coli* K12 in their ability to induce phenotypical and functional maturation of monocyte-derived DCs. Toll like receptor 4 is expressed on MoDCs and recognize lipopolysaccharide (LPS), the major component of the outer membrane of Gram-negative bacteria (Schreibelt et al., 2010). LPS represents a strong stimulatory signal for inducing expression of co-stimulatory molecules and cytokine production in DCs (Verhasselt et al., 1997). Concordantly, *E. coli* K12 and *M. capsulatus* Bath were found to be stronger inducers of DC maturation and cytokine release compared to the Gram-positive *L. rhamnosus*. It has been suggested that probiotic bacteria modulate immune response by controlling the maturation of DCs and thereby the release of proinflammatory cytokines (Foligne et al., 2007). Both the Gram-negative bacteria tested in our study induced phenotypical and functional maturation. However, *M. capsulatus* Bath produced a less mature phenotype and substantially lower cytokine levels than *E. coli* K12. The fact that the Gram-negative *M. capsulatus* Bath results in a less mature phenotype and low levels of proinflammatory cytokines, suggests that similarly to probiotic bacteria *M. capsulatus* may modulate immunity through directing the maturation of DCs.

Interestingly, although priming with *M. capsulatus* resulted in a less mature MoDC phenotype than *E. coli* K12, it was found more efficient than both *E. coli* K12 and *L. rhamnosus* GG bacteria in inducing T cell activation and proliferation in the presence of interleukin 2, a growth factor necessary for cell cycle progression and clonal expansion (Smith, 1988). *M. capsulatus*-primed MoDCs enhanced T cell expression of CD25, the α-chain of the trimeric high affinity IL-2 receptor explaining the increased proliferative T cell response compared to the other bacteria.

Whereas, co-stimulatory molecules on DCs and T cells are necessary for T cell activation and proliferation, DC cytokines are central in polarizing effector T cell development. In addition to antigen presentation and signaling through co-stimulatory molecules, cytokines provide a third signal for activation and differentiation of naïve T cells to effector cells. The nature of signal 3 depends on the triggering of particular PRRs by MAMPs

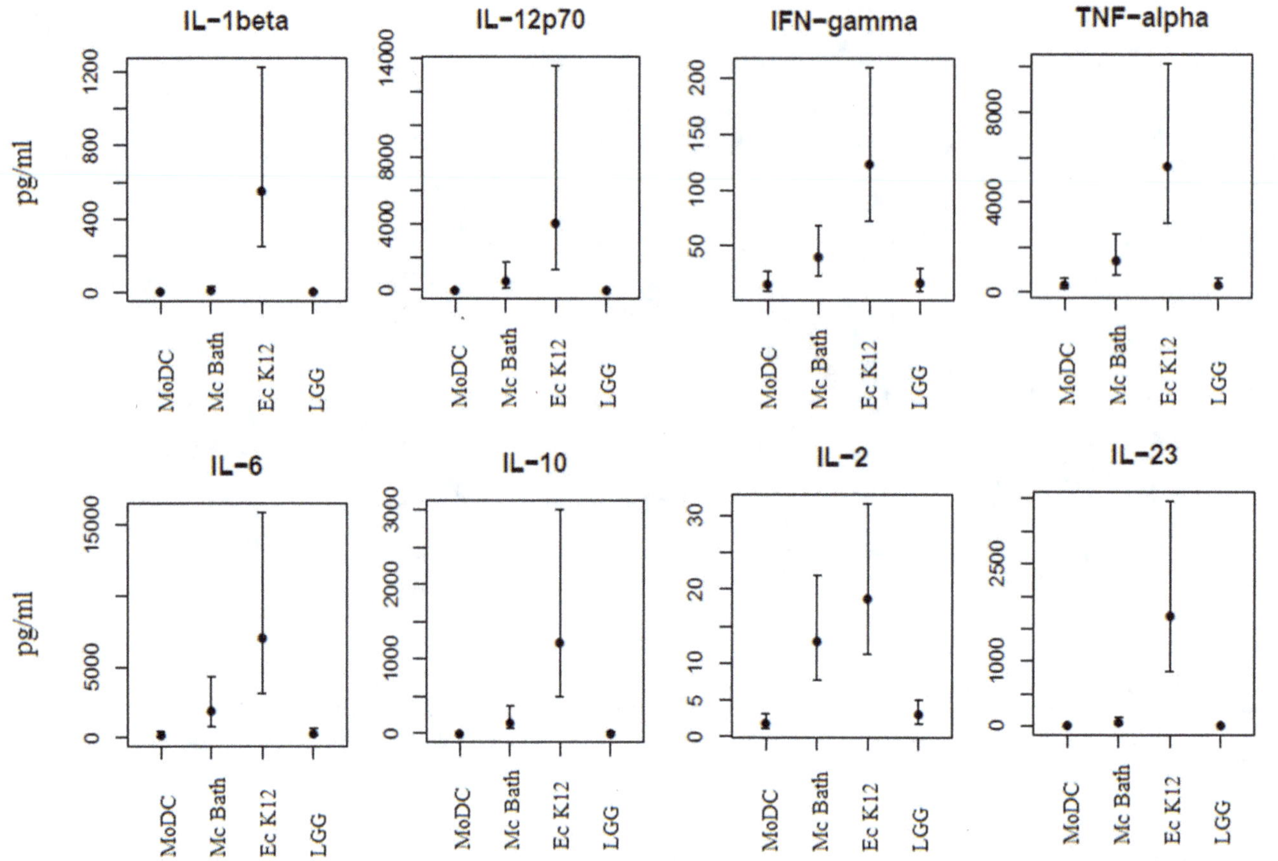

FIGURE 4 | MoDCs produce distinct cytokine profiles in response to different bacteria. MoDCs were incubated with bacteria *(M. capsulatus* Bath, *E. coli* K12, *L. rhamnosus* GG) for 24 h in a ration of 1:10 (DC: bacteria). Culture supernatants were collected and analyzed for cytokines by multiplex immunoassay or ELISA. Cytokine concentrations are given in picogram/milliliter. Bars represents 95% confidence intervals on cytokine concentrations from 4 different donors.

specific to the microbe encountered (Kapsenberg, 2003). Several DC-derived cytokines are important for T cell polarization into specific T cell subsets, e.g., IFNγ and IL-12p70 are known to be important for Th1 polarization, IL-4 is essential for the Th2 differentiation process, and TGF-β to TH17 and Tregs. Although *M. capsulatus* behaved more similar to *E. coli* than *L. rhamnosus* in its ability to induce cytokine production from MoDCs, both the magnitude and cytokine profiles of the two strains were different. Both strains for example induced similar levels of IL-2, but *E. coli* induced considerably higher levels of IL-23, a cytokine linked to the generation and maintenance of Th17 functions. *M. capsulatus* induced negligible IL-1β, and compared to *E. coli* substantially less of Th1 polarizing factors IL12p70 and IFN-γ as well as reduced IL-6 levels. IL-6 is a cytokine that plays a role in proliferation and survival of both Th1 and Th2 cells, is important for the commitment of $CD4^+$ cells to the Th17 and Th22 lineages and has an inhibitory role in Treg development (Hunter and Jones, 2015).

Bacteria-induced differences in MoDC cytokine production were also functionally reflected in different T cell polarizing ability in MoDC-T cell co-cultures. In response to bacteria-primed MoDCs, T cells produced increased levels of the anti-inflammatory cytokine IL-10. IL-10 plays important roles both in preventing inflammatory responses to intestinal microbiota under steady state conditions, and in limiting T cell-driven inflammation in pathogen clearance (Maynard and Weaver, 2008). Notably, MoDC-priming with all three bacteria significantly increased concentration of the Th1 signature cytokine IFN-γ and reduced the levels of typical Th2 cytokines IL-13 and IL-5. Th2 development has previously been suggested to be a "default pathway" in the absence of IL-12 (Moser and Murphy, 2000). In agreement with that, in our experiments unprimed MoDCs tended to induce Th2 cell responses compared to MoDCs primed by bacteria. The observation that even the Gram-positive *L. rhamnosus* drives Th1 development suggest that LPS is not a critical factor in bacteria driven DC-mediated Th1 development, in support of previous reports (Smits et al., 2004).

Coherent with results from DC cytokine analysis, the cytokine profile of T cells co-incubated with MoDCs primed by Gram-negative bacteria was markedly different from that of T cells activated by MoDCs treated with the Gram-positive *L. rhamnosus*. Again *L. rhamnosus* resulted in lower levels of most of the cytokines measured, a reduction in the pro-inflammatory

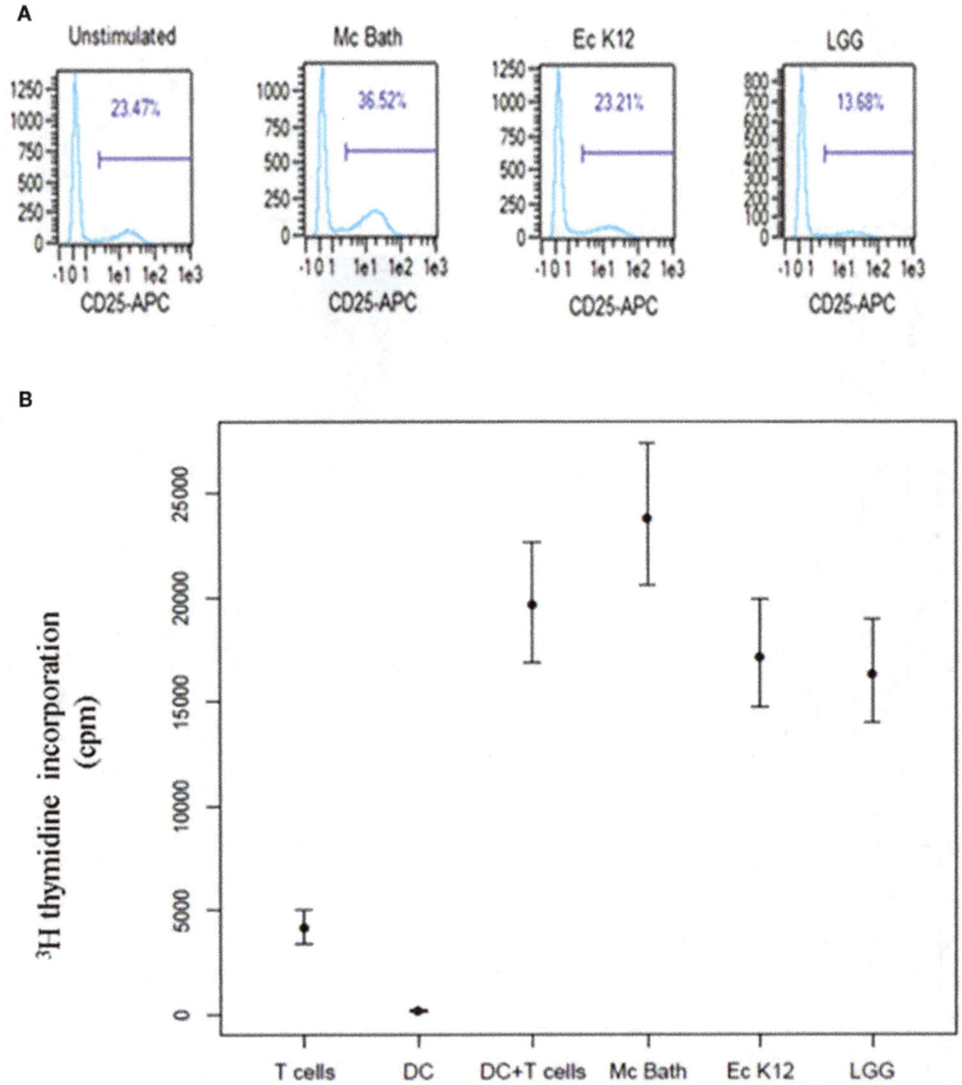

FIGURE 5 | *M. capsulatus* primed MoDCs efficiently induce T cell activation and proliferation. (A) Immature MoDCs were primed by UV inactivated bacteria for 24 h in a ratio of 1:100 (DC: bacteria). Primed MoDCs were co-incubated with allogenic T cells in the presence of IL-2. After 5 days of co-culture cells were harvested, stained for CD4 and CD25 surface protein and analyzed by flow cytometry. Cells were gated on CD4-FITC expression and the percentage of $CD4^+$ cells expressing CD25 are shown. Plots represent results from 4 different MoDC/T cell donor combinations. **(B)** MoDCs primed by either UV-inactivated *M. capsulatus* Bath, *E. coli* K12, or *Lactobacillus rhamnosus* GG for 24 h were co-incubated with allogenic T cells from two different donors. After 96 h cells were pulsed by 1 μCi [^{3}H] thymidine. Thymidine incorporation was determined by liquid scintillation counting 18.5 h after pulsing. The amount of incorporated thymidine is reported as counts per minute (cpm). Bars indicate 95% confidence interval on values from 5 different donor combinations.

IL-18 and no increase of IL-1α, IL1-β, IL-6 compared to negative control. Neither did it induce cytokines typically associated with Th17/Th9/Th22 cells (IL-23, IL-17A, IL-21, IL-22, IL-9, TNF-α) compared to a control of T cells stimulated by unprimed DC. The low T cell-levels of cytokines in response to *L. rhamnosus* is in agreement with a previous report showing that *L. rhamnosus*-primed MoDCs induce hyporesponsive T cells in DC-T cell co-cultures (Braat et al., 2004).

In contrast to *L. rhamnosus M. capsulatus* Bath, and *E. coli* K12 induced proinflammatory cytokines IL-6, IL-1β, and IL-1α as well as cytokines associated with generation and maintenance of the Th17 subset (IL-23, IL-17A, IL-21, IL-22), Th22 cytokines (IL-22, TNF-α) and Th9 cytokines (IL-9 and IL-21). However, *M. capsulatus* induced significantly less pro-inflammatory cytokines IL1-α, IL-1β, and IL-6 and anti-inflammatory IL-10. There was no significant difference in the Th1 signature cytokine IFN-γ or Th9 cytokines IL-9 and IL-21. However, significantly less IL-23, IL-17A, and IL-22 was produced in response to *M. capsulatus* than to *E. coli*. The cytokine profile thus indicated that different effector cells dominate in response to the two Gram-negative bacteria. *E. coli* is a stronger inducer of the Th17 subset whereas *M. capsulatus* induce Th1/T9 effector cells over Th17

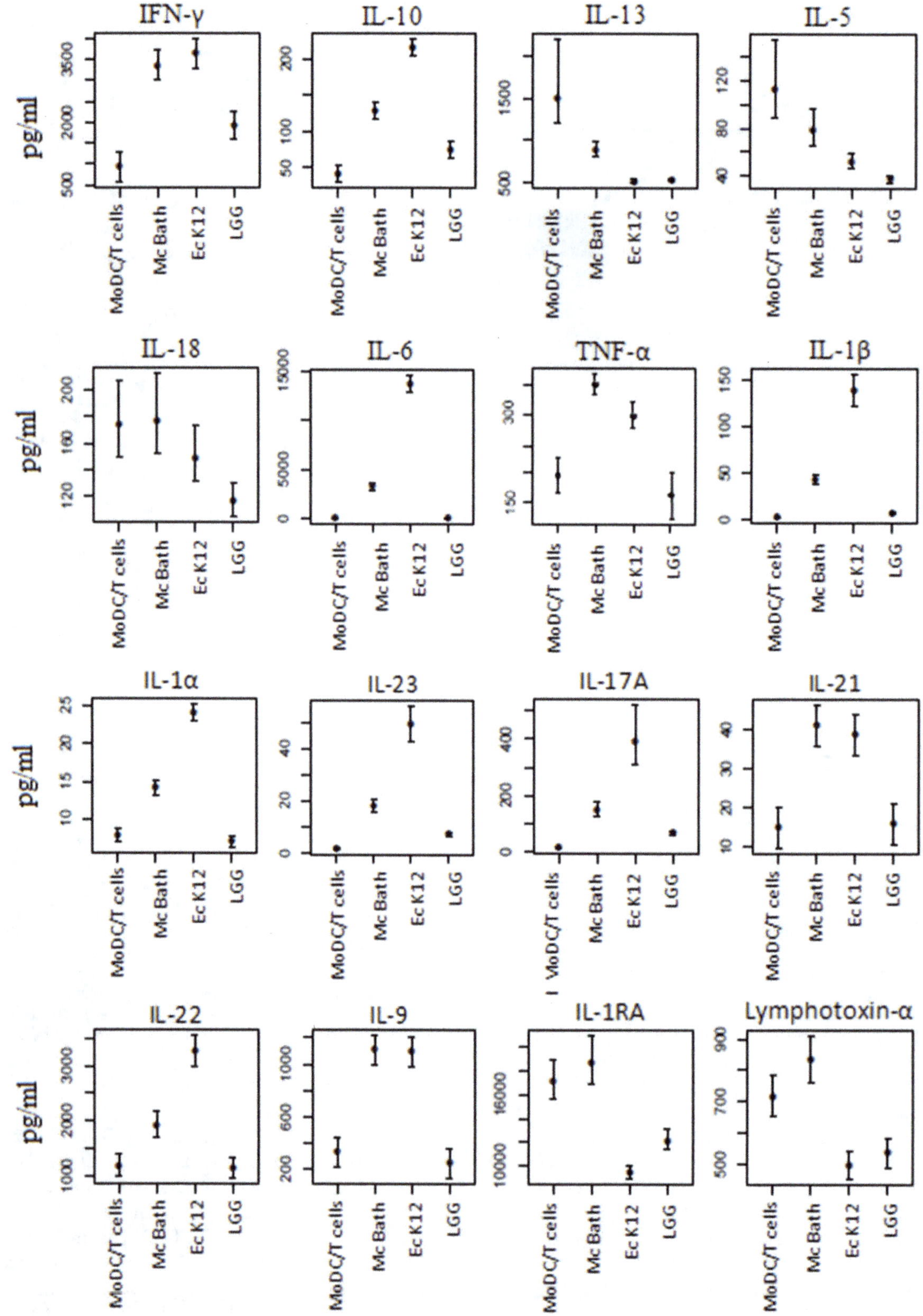

FIGURE 6 | Bacterial stimulation results in different effector T cell profiles. Unprimed MoDCs or MoDCs primed by *M. capsulatus* or control bacteria were co-incubated with allogenic T cells for 5 days. Growth medium was collected and analyzed for cytokines by multiplex immunoassay. Bars represent 95% confidence intervals on cytokine concentrations from 4 donor combinations.

cells *in vitro*. Some probiotics have been reported to induce Foxp3+ regulatory T cells (Kwon et al., 2010). It has been suggested that peripherally-induced Treg develop from naïve, CD4+ cells exposed to antigens under tolerogenic conditions (e.g., by immature DCs with low levels of co-stimulation) with an essential requirement for TGF-β signaling (Marie et al., 2005; Johnston et al., 2016). We did not find detectable levels of TGF-β released from MoDC stimulated by *M. capsulatus*. Neither did we find significantly increased expression of Foxp3 in T cell co-cultures with bacteria stimulated MoDC (data not shown).

E. coli and *L. rhamnosus*, but not *M. capsulatus* Bath, reduced lymphotoxin-α and IL-1RA in culture supernatants. Lymphotoxin-α is important for lymphoid organ development, regulates T cell homing and IgA production in the gut and contributes to shaping the gut microbiome (Ruddle, 2014). The balance between IL-1 and IL-1RA in local tissues plays an important role in the susceptibility and severity of a number of diseases, including IBD (Arend, 2002). For example, significant decrease in the intestinal mucosal IL-1RA/IL-1 ratio has been found in freshly isolated intestinal mucosal cells, and in mucosal biopsies obtained from both Crohn's disease and ulcerative colitis patients as compared to control subjects (Casini-Raggi et al., 1995). The observation that IL-1α and IL-1β is reduced, while IL-1RA is kept high in *M. capsulatus* primed DC-T cell co-cultures is interesting in the light of *M. capsulatus* anti-inflammatory effects in a murine enteritis model (Kleiveland et al., 2013). Screening for cytokine profiles associated with specific T effector cell populations may be a useful first step to identify strains with potential pro- or anti-inflammatory properties e.g., for further mechanistic investigation (Papadimitriou et al., 2015). It is important however to notice the limitations of *in vitro* systems on making *in vivo* predictions. Although the bacteria tested here induced different effects in T cells *in vitro*, caution should be exercised in drawing conclusions both about the direction of T cell polarization by these bacteria and the functional relevance *in vivo*. T cell differentiation occurs in a finely tuned manner dependent on a variety of tissue factors and cytokines, and *in vitro* systems cannot necessarily reflect the complex cytokine environment of the gut. For example, TGF-β a cytokine abundant in the intestines, was not detected in our MoDC supernatants. TGF-β is not only involved in development of Tregs, Th9 and Th17 effector cells, but it also suppresses Th1 and Th2 cell differentiation (Zheng, 2013). TGF-β is produced by $CD103^{+}$ DC (Coombes et al., 2007) a DC subset common in the intestines and is expected to play a prominent role in regulating mucosal immunity (Ruane and Lavelle, 2011). The results of bacterial priming *in vitro* may thus be expected to have different outcomes in an *in vivo* situation. The impact of immune modulatory effects of *M. capsulatus* on DC in maintaining intestinal homeostasis thus remains to be determined (study in preparation).

CONCLUDING REMARKS

Environmental bacteria, although immensely numerous and diverse, have remained largely unexplored for their immunomodulatory properties. Our results demonstrate the direct binding and functional effects of a soil bacterium on human monocyte-derived dendritic cells. The same bacterium has recently been shown to possess anti-inflammatory properties in a murine colitis model. The identification of anti-inflammatory and immunomodulatory properties of this bacterium was serendipitous. In fact, such properties may not be a rare trait of this particular soil bacterium, but rather a common feature of many environmental bacteria. Our study thus emphasizes the need to scrutinize, identify, and understand possible physiological consequences of environmental microbe-host interactions, and we suggests that bacteria from soil and water should receive increased attention for their potential health benefits.

AUTHOR CONTRIBUTIONS

SI contributed to design of the work, acquisition, analysis, and interpretation of data and drafted the work. TL and CK contributed to design of the work, interpretation of data and revising work critically for important intellectual content. RH contributed to data analysis and revising work critically for important intellectual content. MJ contributed to interpretation of data and revising work critically for important intellectual content. All authors approved final version and agreed to be accountable for all aspects of the work.

REFERENCES

Agency USEP (1997). *Escherichia coli K-12 Derivatives Final Risk Assessment - Attachment I.* Biotechnology Program under the Toxic Substances Control Act (TSCA).

Arend, W. P. (2002). The balance between IL-1 and IL-1Ra in disease. *Cytokine Growth Factor Rev.* 13, 323–340. doi: 10.1016/S1359-6101(02)00020-5

Bermudez-Brito, M., Plaza-Diaz, J., Munoz-Quezada, S., Gomez-Llorente, C., and Gil, A. (2012). Probiotic mechanisms of action. *Ann. Nutr. Metab.* 61, 160–174. doi: 10.1159/000342079

Bienenstock, J., Gibson, G., Klaenhammer, T. R., Walker, W. A., and Neish, A. S. (2013). New insights into probiotic mechanisms: a harvest from functional and metagenomic studies. *Gut Microbes* 4, 94–100. doi: 10.4161/gmic.23283

Blattner, F. R., Plunkett, G. III., Bloch, C. A., Perna, N. T., Burland, V., Riley, M., et al. (1997). The complete genome sequence of *Escherichia coli* K-12. *Science* 277, 1453–1462. doi: 10.1126/science.277.5331.1453

Braat, H., van den Brande, J., van Tol, E., Hommes, D., Peppelenbosch, M., and van Deventer, S. (2004). *Lactobacillus rhamnosus* induces peripheral hyporesponsiveness in stimulated CD4+ T cells via modulation of dendritic cell function. *Am. J. Clin. Nutr.* 80, 1618–1625. Available online at: http://ajcn.nutrition.org/content/80/6/1618.long

Brown, E. M., Sadarangani, M., and Finlay, B. B. (2013). The role of the immune system in governing host-microbe interactions in the intestine. *Nat. Immunol.* 14, 660–667. doi: 10.1038/ni.2611

Casadevall, A., and Pirofski, L. A. (2007). Accidental virulence, cryptic pathogenesis, martians, lost hosts, and the pathogenicity of environmental microbes. *Eukaryotic Cell* 6, 2169–2174. doi: 10.1128/EC.00308-07

Casini-Raggi, V., Kam, L., Chong, Y. J., Fiocchi, C., Pizarro, T. T., and Cominelli, F. (1995). Mucosal imbalance of IL-1 and IL-1 receptor antagonist in inflammatory bowel disease. A novel mechanism of chronic intestinal inflammation. *J. Immunol.* 154, 2434–2440.

Coombes, J. L., Siddiqui, K. R., Arancibia-Carcamo, C. V., Hall, J., Sun, C. M., Belkaid, Y., et al. (2007). A functionally specialized population of mucosal CD103^{+} DCs induces Foxp3^{+} regulatory T cells via a TGF-β and retinoic acid-dependent mechanism. *J. Exp. Med.* 204, 1757–1764. doi: 10.1084/jem.20070590

Dalod, M., Chelbi, R., Malissen, B., and Lawrence, T. (2014). Dendritic cell maturation: functional specialization through signaling specificity and transcriptional programming. *EMBO J.* 33, 1104–1116. doi: 10.1002/embj.201488027

Foligne, B., Zoumpopoulou, G., Dewulf, J., Ben Younes, A., Chareyre, F., Sirard, J. C., et al. (2007). A key role of dendritic cells in probiotic functionality. *PLoS ONE* 2:e313. doi: 10.1371/journal.pone.0000313

Hunter, C. A., and Jones, S. A. (2015). IL-6 as a keystone cytokine in health and disease. *Nat. Immunol.* 16, 448–457. doi: 10.1038/ni.3153

Indrelid, S., Mathiesen, G., Jacobsen, M., Lea, T., and Kleiveland, C. R. (2014). Computational and experimental analysis of the secretome of *Methylococcus capsulatus* (Bath). *PLoS ONE* 9:e114476. doi: 10.1371/journal.pone.0114476

Johnston, C. J., Smyth, D. J., Dresser, D. W., and Maizels, R. M. (2016). TGF-β in tolerance, development and regulation of immunity. *Cell. Immunol.* 299, 14–22. doi: 10.1016/j.cellimm.2015.10.006

Kapsenberg, M. L. (2003). Dendritic-cell control of pathogen-driven T-cell polarization. *Nat. Rev. Immunol.* 3, 984–993. doi: 10.1038/nri1246

Kleiveland, C. R., Hult, L. T., Spetalen, S., Kaldhusdal, M., Christofferesen, T. E., Bengtsson, O., et al. (2013). The noncommensal bacterium *Methylococcus capsulatus* (Bath) ameliorates dextran sulfate (Sodium Salt)-Induced Ulcerative Colitis by influencing mechanisms essential for maintenance of the colonic barrier function. *Appl. Environ. Microbiol.* 79, 48–56. doi: 10.1128/AEM.02464-12

Kwon, H. K., Lee, C. G., So, J. S., Chae, C. S., Hwang, J. S., Sahoo, A., et al. (2010). Generation of regulatory dendritic cells and CD4^{+} Foxp3^{+} T cells by probiotics administration suppresses immune disorders. *Proc. Natl. Acad. Sci. U.S.A.* 107, 2159–2164. doi: 10.1073/pnas.0904055107

Lebeer, S., Vanderleyden, J., and De Keersmaecker, S. C. (2010). Host interactions of probiotic bacterial surface molecules: comparison with commensals and pathogens. *Nat. Rev. Microbiol.* 8, 171–184. doi: 10.1038/nrmicro2297

Mann, E. R., Landy, J. D., Bernardo, D., Peake, S. T., Hart, A. L., Al-Hassi, H. O., et al. (2013). Intestinal dendritic cells: their role in intestinal inflammation, manipulation by the gut microbiota and differences between mice and men. *Immunol. Lett.* 150, 30–40. doi: 10.1016/j.imlet.2013.01.007

Marie, J. C., Letterio, J. J., Gavin, M., and Rudensky, A. Y. (2005). TGF-β1 maintains suppressor function and Foxp3 expression in CD4^{+} CD25^{+} regulatory T cells. *J. Exp. Med.* 201, 1061–1067. doi: 10.1084/jem.20042276

Maynard, C. L., and Weaver, C. T. (2008). Diversity in the contribution of interleukin-10 to T-cell-mediated immune regulation. *Immunol. Rev.* 226, 219–233. doi: 10.1111/j.1600-065X.2008.00711.x

Mileti, E., Matteoli, G., Iliev, I. D., and Rescigno, M. (2009). Comparison of the immunomodulatory properties of three probiotic strains of Lactobacilli using complex culture systems: prediction for *in vivo* efficacy. *PLoS ONE* 4:e7056. doi: 10.1371/journal.pone.0007056

Moser, M., and Murphy, K. M. (2000). Dendritic cell regulation of TH1-TH2 development. *Nat. Immunol.* 1, 199–205. doi: 10.1038/79734

Nicholson, J. K., Holmes, E., Kinross, J., Burcelin, R., Gibson, G., Jia, W., et al. (2012). Host-gut microbiota metabolic interactions. *Science* 336, 1262–1267. doi: 10.1126/science.1223813

Papadimitriou, K., Zoumpopoulou, G., Foligne, B., Alexandraki, V., Kazou, M., Pot, B., et al. (2015). Discovering probiotic microorganisms: *in vitro, in vivo*, genetic and omics approaches. *Front. Microbiol.* 6:58. doi: 10.3389/fmicb.2015.00058

Pils, M. C., Bleich, A., Prinz, I., Fasnacht, N., Bollati-Fogolin, M., Schippers, A., et al. (2011). Commensal gut flora reduces susceptibility to experimentally induced colitis via T-cell-derived interleukin-10. *Inflamm. Bowel Dis.* 17, 2038–2046. doi: 10.1002/ibd.21587

Qiu, X., Zhang, M., Yang, X., Hong, N., and Yu, C. (2013). Faecalibacterium prausnitzii upregulates regulatory T cells and anti-inflammatory cytokines in treating TNBS-induced colitis. *J. Crohns. Colitis* 7, e558–e568. doi: 10.1016/j.crohns.2013.04.002

Reis e Sousa, C. (2006). Dendritic cells in a mature age. *Nat. Rev. Immunol.* 6, 476–483. doi: 10.1038/nri1845

Rook, G. A. (2007). The hygiene hypothesis and the increasing prevalence of chronic inflammatory disorders. *Trans. R. Soc. Trop. Med. Hyg.* 101, 1072–1074. doi: 10.1016/j.trstmh.2007.05.014

Rook, G. A. (2010). 99th Dahlem conference on infection, inflammation and chronic inflammatory disorders: darwinian medicine and the 'hygiene' or 'old friends' hypothesis. *Clin. Exp. Immunol.* 160, 70–79. doi: 10.1111/j.1365-2249.2010.04133.x

Rook, G. A., Adams, V., Hunt, J., Palmer, R., Martinelli, R., and Brunet, L. R. (2004). Mycobacteria and other environmental organisms as immunomodulators for immunoregulatory disorders. *Springer Semin. Immunopathol.* 25, 237–255. doi: 10.1007/s00281-003-0148-9

Ruane, D. T., and Lavelle, E. C. (2011). The role of CD103^{+} dendritic cells in the intestinal mucosal immune system. *Front. Immunol.* 2:25. doi: 10.3389/fimmu.2011.00025

Ruddle, N. H. (2014). Lymphotoxin and TNF: how it all began-a tribute to the travelers. *Cytokine Growth Factor Rev.* 25, 83–89. doi: 10.1016/j.cytogfr.2014.02.001

Sang, L. X., Chang, B., Dai, C., Gao, N., Liu, W. X., and Jiang, M. (2014). Heat-killed VSL#3 ameliorates dextran sulfate sodium (DSS)-induced acute experimental colitis in rats. *Int. J. Mol. Sci.* 15, 15–28. doi: 10.3390/ijms15010015

Schreibelt, G., Tel, J., Sliepen, K. H., Benitez-Ribas, D., Figdor, C. G., Adema, G. J., et al. (2010). Toll-like receptor expression and function in human dendritic cell subsets: implications for dendritic cell-based anti-cancer immunotherapy. *Cancer Immunol. Immunother.* 59, 1573–1582. doi: 10.1007/s00262-010-0833-1

Schuijs, M. J., Willart, M. A., Vergote, K., Gras, D., Deswarte, K., Ege, M. J., et al. (2015). Farm dust and endotoxin protect against allergy through A20 induction in lung epithelial cells. *Science* 349, 1106–1110. doi: 10.1126/science.aac6623

Smith, K. A. (1988). Interleukin-2: inception, impact, and implications. *Science* 240, 1169–1176. doi: 10.1126/science.3131876

Smits, H. H., van Beelen, A. J., Hessle, C., Westland, R., de Jong, E., Soeteman, E., et al. (2004). Commensal Gram-negative bacteria prime human dendritic cells for enhanced IL-23 and IL-27 expression and enhanced Th1 development. *Eur. J. Immunol.* 34, 1371–1380. doi: 10.1002/eji.200324815

Sommer, F., and Backhed, F. (2013). The gut microbiota–masters of host development and physiology. *Nat. Rev. Microbiol.* 11, 227–238. doi: 10.1038/nrmicro2974

Souza, E. L., Elian, S. D., Paula, L. M., Garcia, C. C., Vieira, A. T., Teixeira, M. M., et al. (2016). *Escherichia coli* strain Nissle 1917 ameliorates experimental colitis by modulating intestinal permeability, the inflammatory response and clinical signs in a faecal transplantation model. *J. Med. Microbiol.* 65, 201–210. doi: 10.1099/jmm.0.000222

Steinman, R. M. (2012). Decisions about dendritic cells: past, present, and future. *Annu. Rev. Immunol.* 30, 1–22. doi: 10.1146/annurev-immunol-100311-102839

Strachan, D. P. (1989). Hay fever, hygiene, and household size. *BMJ* 299, 1259–1260. doi: 10.1136/bmj.299.6710.1259

Strachan, D. P. (2000). Family size, infection and atopy: the first decade of the "hygiene hypothesis." *Thorax* 55(Suppl. 1), S2–S10. doi: 10.1136/thorax.55.suppl_1.S2

Toumi, R., Soufli, I., Rafa, H., Belkhelfa, M., Biad, A., and Touil-Boukoffa, C. (2014). Probiotic bacteria lactobacillus and bifidobacterium attenuate inflammation in dextran sulfate sodium-induced experimental colitis in mice. *Int. J. Immunopathol. Pharmacol.* 27, 615–627. doi: 10.1177/039463201402700418

Turnbaugh, P. J., Ley, R. E., Hamady, M., Fraser-Liggett, C. M., Knight, R., and Gordon, J. I. (2007). The human microbiome project. *Nature* 449, 804–810. doi: 10.1038/nature06244

Verhasselt, V., Buelens, C., Willems, F., De Groote, D., Haeffner-Cavaillon, N., and Goldman, M. (1997). Bacterial lipopolysaccharide stimulates the production of cytokines and the expression of costimulatory molecules by human peripheral blood dendritic cells: evidence for a soluble CD14-dependent pathway. *J. Immunol.* 158, 2919–2925.

Whittenbury, R., Phillips, K. C., and Wilkinson, J. F. (1970). Enrichment, isolation and some properties of methane-utilizing bacteria. *J. Gen. Microbiol.* 61, 205–218. doi: 10.1099/00221287-61-2-205

Zheng, S. G. (2013). Regulatory T cells vs Th17: differentiation of Th17 versus Treg, are the mutually exclusive? *Am. J. Clin. Exp. Immunol.* 2, 94–106. doi: 10.1007/978-3-0348-0522-3_6

10

Use of Wild Type or Recombinant Lactic Acid Bacteria as an Alternative Treatment for Gastrointestinal Inflammatory Diseases: A Focus on Inflammatory Bowel Diseases and Mucositis

Rodrigo D. De Oliveira Carvalho[1], Fillipe L. R. do Carmo[1], Alberto de Oliveira Junior[1], Philippe Langella[2], Jean-Marc Chatel[2], Luis G. Bermúdez-Humarán[2], Vasco Azevedo[1†] and Marcela S. de Azevedo[1†]*

[1] Federal University of Minas Gerais – Instituto de Ciências Biológicas, Belo Horizonte, Brazil, [2] Micalis Institute, Institut National de la Recherche Agronomique, AgroParisTech, Université Paris-Saclay, Jouy-en-Josas, France

Edited by:
Julio Villena,
Centro de Referencia para Lactobacilos (CONICET), Argentina

Reviewed by:
Maria Guadalupe Vizoso Pinto,
National University of Tucumán, Argentina
Cammie Lesser,
Massachusetts General Hospital, USA

***Correspondence:**
Rodrigo D. De Oliveira Carvalho
rodrigodoc2@gmail.com

†These authors have contributed equally to senior authorship.

The human gastrointestinal tract (GIT) is highly colonized by bacterial communities, which live in a symbiotic relationship with the host in normal conditions. It has been shown that a dysfunctional interaction between the intestinal microbiota and the host immune system, known as dysbiosis, is a very important factor responsible for the development of different inflammatory conditions of the GIT, such as the idiopathic inflammatory bowel diseases (IBD), a complex and multifactorial disorder of the GIT. Dysbiosis has also been implicated in the pathogenesis of other GIT inflammatory diseases such as mucositis usually caused as an adverse effect of chemotherapy. As both diseases have become a great clinical problem, many research groups have been focusing on developing new strategies for the treatment of IBD and mucositis. In this review, we show that lactic acid bacteria (LAB) have been capable in preventing and treating both disorders in animal models, suggesting they may be ready for clinical trials. In addition, we present the most current studies on the use of wild type or genetically engineered LAB strains designed to express anti-inflammatory proteins as a promising strategy in the treatment of IBD and mucositis.

Keywords: inflammatory bowel diseases, mucositis, lactic acid bacteria, *Lactococcus lactis*, genetic engineering

INTRODUCTION

The gastrointestinal tract (GIT) is colonized by a complex community of microorganisms, known as the intestinal microbiota, consisting mainly of bacteria that are classified as indigenous or transient. Symbiotic bacteria, such as short chain fatty acid (SCFA)-producing species from the Lactobacillales order and *Faecalibacterium prausnitzii*, contribute to host metabolism and immune system function while occupying a protected environment rich in nutrients (Hooper and Macpherson, 2010; de Vos and de Vos, 2012; Chang and Lin, 2016). Pathobionts of the GIT, consisting mainly of Proteobacteria such as *Escherichia coli* and *Clostridium difficile*, present a potential risk to the GIT by disrupting the integrity of tissues if, for instance, they are allowed to grow in number (Lebeer et al., 2010; Vangay et al., 2015).

Therefore, the host contains several biological structures that are essential for controlling bacterial overgrowth and invasion. In this context, the mucous layer protecting the intestinal epithelial cells (IECs) plays an important role by restricting the contact of harmful bacteria with host cells (Johansson et al., 2013; Peterson and Artis, 2014). In addition, specialized IEC, such as Paneth cells, secrete several antimicrobial peptides to eliminate microbes that eventually penetrate into the mucus (Salzman et al., 2007; Carlsson et al., 2013). When pathobionts translocate into the intestinal epithelium, the host immune response is activated to eliminate them by producing pro-inflammatory mediators. However, the overproduction of these compounds represents a risk, as they can inflame the tissue, causing intestinal barrier disruption and mucosal dysfunctions in the host (Hidalgo-Cantabrana et al., 2014; Kashyap et al., 2014). Therefore, to maintain intestinal homeostasis, specialized immunological structures, known as the gut-associated lymphoid tissue (GALT), must be able to specifically recognize and eliminate the pathogenic species while tolerating the commensals (Izcue et al., 2009; Carlsson et al., 2013).

Under normal conditions, GALT generates tolerance to commensals mainly through the action of regulatory T (Treg) cells. When the dynamic balance between Treg and activated effector T cells is broken, homeostasis is compromised and may lead to the development of mucosal inflammation in the gut (Strober et al., 2007). In addition to microbiota composition impairment, known as dysbiosis, other factors can influence the proper functioning of the GIT immune system, including individual genetic susceptibility, diet, use of drugs and environmental stress (Ananthakrishnan, 2015). The intersection of these factors may generate an exaggerated pro-inflammatory reaction against the microbiota that causes inflammatory bowel diseases (IBDs), a group of idiopathic and chronic inflammatory conditions of the GIT, which primarily includes ulcerative colitis (CD) and Crohn's disease (UC) (Vangay et al., 2015; Velasquez-Manoff, 2015). In addition, other factors, such as the use of some medications, can also contribute to the breakdown of this immunological tolerance against commensals. It has been reported that chemotherapeutic agents, such as 5-fluoracil, that are widely used in the treatment of advanced solid tumors, may also lead to the development of another inflammatory condition of the GIT known as mucositis, a disease characterized by painful inflammation and ulceration of the mucosal membranes (Soares et al., 2013; Pedroso et al., 2015).

CD and UC are associated with severe intestinal inflammation, and patients have reported gastrointestinal (GI) symptoms such as abdominal pain, diarrhea, rectal bleeding, and weight loss (Lennard-Jones, 1989; Stepaniuk et al., 2015). IBD represent a global health issue, as its incidence has increased in several countries, while safe and efficient therapies are still in development (Molodecky et al., 2012; Ananthakrishnan, 2015). Mucositis induced by 5-FU is of great clinical significance as well, as it might result in cancer therapy being adjusted, affecting a patient's chances of survival (de Vasconcelos Generoso et al., 2015; Antunes et al., 2016). Thus, the scientific community has sought novel therapeutic alternatives to fight both IBD and mucositis. As dysbiosis plays a key role in the pathogenesis of both diseases, the modulation of the patient microbiota via the administration of probiotic bacteria has been proposed.

USE OF PROBIOTIC LACTIC ACID BACTERIA IN THE TREATMENT OF GASTROINTESTINAL INFLAMMATION

Over a century ago, Elie Metchnikoff was the first to propose the rationale for using host-friendly bacteria found in yogurt to manipulate the intestinal microbiome. He also predicted the existence of bacterial translocation, from the intestinal lumen to inner layers of the mucosa and also to systemic organs, and described theories associating the microbiota with intestinal inflammation and other diseases (Mackowiak, 2013). Currently, several research groups have confirmed his hypothesis, demonstrating that the administration of certain bacterial species in several animal models actually provides health benefits to alleviate inflammation, including the containment of inflammatory mediators, stimulation of the immune system and microbiota restoration by competitive exclusion of potentially pathogenic species (Ljungh and Wadström, 2006; Luerce et al., 2014; Quinto et al., 2014; Santos Rocha et al., 2014; Thomas, 2016). These microorganisms are considered to be probiotics, a term defined by the World Health Organization (WHO) as "live microorganisms administered in adequate amounts that confer a beneficial health effect on the host" (FAO/WHO, 2002).

Probiotics are live bacteria and yeasts; however, the majority of strains are gram-positive bacteria belonging to the *Lactobacillus*, *Bifidobacterium*, *Streptococcus*, and *Lactococcus* genera. These genera are included in a diverse group of microorganisms entitled lactic acid bacteria (LAB), as they are able to convert sugars into lactic acid (Holzapfel et al., 1998; Carr et al., 2002). With regards to Gram-negative bacteria, some strains of *E. coli* are also considered to promote health, for instance, *E. coli* Nissle 1917 (EcN1917) was originally isolated from the feces of a soldier during the First World War who did not develop infectious diarrhea during an outbreak of contagious Shigella (Westendorf et al., 2005; Henker et al., 2007).

Although Metchnikoff introduced the concept of probiotics in 1907, some of these microorganisms have been used for centuries to prepare yogurt, sourdough bread, sauerkraut, cucumber pickles and olives, as they are able to produce lactic acid, as previously mentioned (Mackowiak, 2013; Vikhanski, 2016). In the latter half of the 20th century, probiotics have gained visibility as there has been increasing interest in applying them to other areas, such as the pharmaceutical industry. Thus, the selection of new probiotic strains, the development of new food products based on probiotics and freeze-dried probiotic pharmaceutical formulations has increased in importance. There are many studies being conducted that focus on the development of probiotic-based pharmaceutical formulations that can be administered to either the gastrointestinal, nasal, or vaginal mucosa, as well as to the skin of patients (Guglielmetti et al., 2010; Iannitti and Palmieri, 2010; Vicariotto et al., 2012).

The Lactic Acid Bacteria Group

The LAB group includes a heterogeneous group of ubiquitous microorganisms that obtain energy through the conversion of sugars into lactic acid. Morphologically, LAB bacteria can resemble cocci, rods, or bacilli. They are gram-positive microorganisms with a low genomic GC content (54%) and are facultative anaerobes that are non-spore-forming, immotile and do not produce catalase (Stiles and Holzapfel, 1997; Carr et al., 2002). Species of this group can be naturally found in different environments that are rich in nutrients, such as decomposing vegetables and fruits, and even in the oral, urogenital and intestinal tracts of mammals and other animals. They can also be found in several kinds of dairy foods, as some strains are used to produce them (Holzapfel et al., 1998; Liu et al., 2014). LAB species found in the human GIT can be autochthonous as indigenous GI microflora, especially those belonging to the *Lactobacillus* and *Streptococcus* genera, or allochthonous as transients of the GIT, such as *Lactococcus* sp. and some strains of *Lactobacillus* used to produce yogurts. Some species, especially those belonging to the *Streptococcus* genera are pathogenic; however, the vast majority of LAB strains have a positive impact on human health and are generally regarded as safe (GRAS) by the United States Department of Agriculture (USDA) (Felis and Dellaglio, 2007).

After the pioneering work of Elie Metchnikoff, who first suggested that the ingestion of dairy foods produced by LAB fermentation could prevent intestinal infections and promote both health and human longevity, the scientific community is continuously exploring in more detail the positive effects promoted by these bacteria (Johnson and Klaenhammer, 2014; Vikhanski, 2016). Among all LAB species described that exert probiotic effects, *Lactobacillus* spp., *Streptococcus* spp., and *Lactococcus* spp. stand out for use in therapeutic applications for both the treatment and prevention of various intestinal disorders (Majamaa and Isolauri, 1997; Ouwehand et al., 2002; Prescott and Björkstén, 2007; Ohland and MacNaughton, 2010; Luerce et al., 2014; Santos Rocha et al., 2014). This topic has been widely studied, and certain immunological aspects of LAB anti-inflammatory properties have been described.

Effects of Probiotic Lactic Acid Bacteria in Animal Models of Gastrointestinal Inflammation

Lactic acid bacteria probiotic strains can alleviate intestinal inflammation through several mechanisms (**Figure 1**). Accumulating evidence has revealed that probiotic LAB are able to protect the host against potentially pathogenic species that inhabit the GIT of animals, including humans. It seems that lactobacilli strains, such as *L. acidophilus* LA1, can prevent the colonization of the intestine by pathogenic bacteria, such as *Staphylococcus aureus, Salmonella typhimurium*, and *Pseudomonas aeruginosa*, by competitive exclusion (Bernet-Camard et al., 1997; Adolfsson et al., 2004). Apparently, these LAB compete for nutrients and adhesion sites in the intestinal epithelium with these potentially pathogenic bacteria that transit in the GIT and are consequently eliminated. The secretion of lactic acid and bacteriocins (natural antibiotics) by probiotic species has also been implicated in the mechanism of the elimination of pathogens (Ogawa et al., 2001; Moal et al., 2007).

Another manner by which LAB strains may protect the host from pathogen invasion is by boosting the intestinal epithelial barrier. Some LAB microbe-associated molecular pattern (MAMPs) are capable of interacting with epithelial pattern recognition receptors, mainly the Toll-like receptor-2 (TLR2), TLR6 and nod-like receptors (Ren et al., 2016). This activation induces several protective mechanisms that restore tissue damage, such as modulation of the stability of tight junctions (Lebeer et al., 2010; Ohland and MacNaughton, 2010; Villena and Kitazawa, 2014; Bajaj et al., 2015). Species such as *B. infantis*, *L. plantarum*, and *L. casei* have been shown to increase the expression of proteins involved in tight junction barrier function, such as occludins and zonula occludens-1 (ZO-1) (Ewaschuk et al., 2008; Anderson et al., 2010; Eun et al., 2011).

Some *Lactobacillus* strains are capable of increasing the production of other proteins involved in the maintenance of epithelial barrier homeostasis, such as mucin-2 (MUC2), the most abundant glycoprotein in mucus. *In vitro* studies showed that increased MUC2 expression in intestinal epithelial Caco-2 cells blocked the adhesion of pathogenic *E. coli* (Mattar et al., 2002; Mack et al., 2003). Furthermore, an *in vivo* study demonstrated that mice treated with a VSL#3 probiotic-mixture consisting of *S. thermophilus*, four strains of lactobacilli (*L. delbrueckii*, *L. casei*, *L. acidophilus*, and *L. plantarum*) and three species of *Bifidobacterium* (*B. longum*, *B. infantis*, and *B. breve*) for 7 days exhibited an approximate 60-fold increase in the production of MUC2 in treated animals (Gaudier et al., 2005).

Other studies have suggested that some LAB strains are able to induce the secretion of defensins by enterocytes, which are related to the biological control of potentially pathogenic species in the lumen. Administration of certain species of lactobacilli or the VSL#3 probiotic-mixture in mice resulted in an increase in the production of β-defensin-2, which has microbicidal activity against important opportunistic pathogens, such as *P. aeruginosa*, *E. coli*, and *Candida albicans* (Harder et al., 2004; Schlee et al., 2008).

The stimulation of the host immune system and the suppression of pro-inflammatory responses are well-established probiotic effects. One of the major mechanisms of these processes is the stimulation of immunological tolerance to GIT microbiota through an increase in IL-10 secretion and a significant reduction in IFNγ and IL-12 expression. This probiotic effect is caused due to the interaction of "good" bacteria with intestinal dendritic cells that drives the development of T regulatory cells and IgA-producing B cells (Fedorak et al., 2000; Ng et al., 2009). Administration of *B. lactis*, *B. bifidum*, and *B. infantis* in mice previously infected with rotavirus or enterohemorrhagic

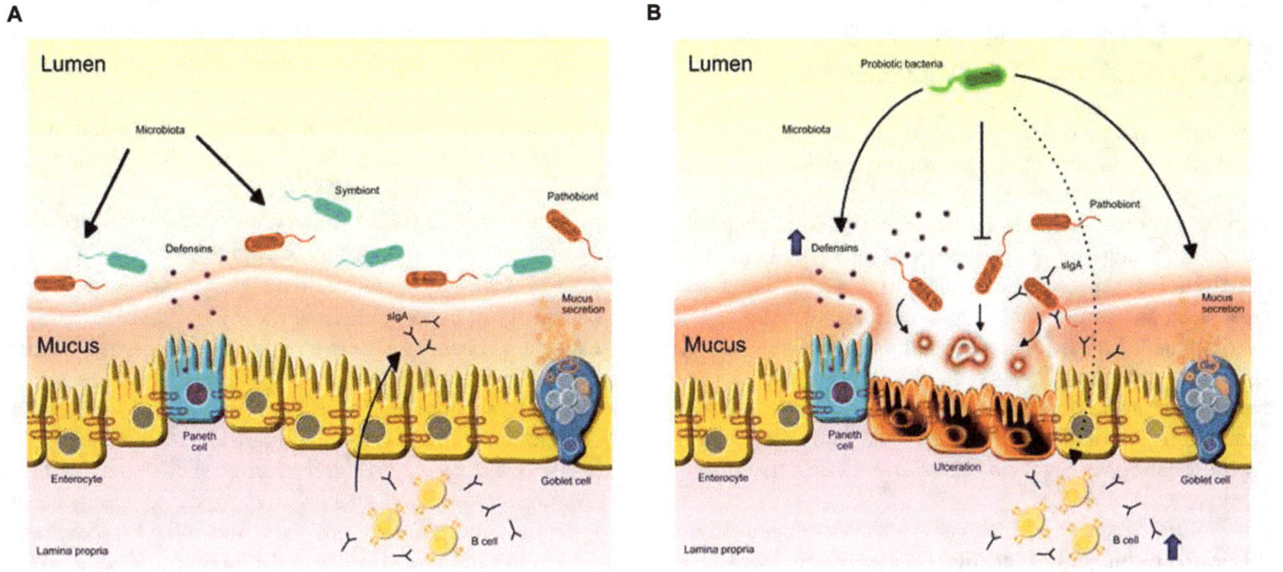

FIGURE 1 | Probiotic LAB anti-inflammatory mechanisms on the intestinal mucosa. (A) Intestinal homeostasis provided by the healthy microbiota role in stimulating ephitelial barrier components such as mucus, Paneth cells activity and eliciting protective immune responses such as IgA. **(B)** The overgrowth of pro-inflammatory mucin-degrading pathobionts induces inflammation in the mucosa. Administration of probiotics prevents inflammatory responses by inhibiting the growth of pathogens directly; increases mucus secretion by goblet cells and the secretion of defensins by Paneth cells; fortificates tight junction stability; stimulates mucosal immunity by inducing IgA production by B cells to the intestinal lumen, limiting harmful microbe adherence and colonization.

E. coli has been shown to increase the titers of specific IgA against the rotavirus (Shu and Gill, 2001; Qiao et al., 2002). For instance, Santos Rocha et al. (2014) showed that the probiotic effect of *L. delbrueckii* strain CNRZ327 was related to an expansion of Treg cells and an increase of total IgA in Dextran sulfate sodium (DSS)-induced colitis in mice. This effect was shown to be enough to prevent inflammation in mice (Santos Rocha et al., 2014). Recently, it was reported that a *Lactococcus lactis* ssp. *lactis* NCDO2118 strain prevented DSS-induced colitis in mice and the protective effect was related to increased IL-10 levels in the colon and the induction of Treg cells in the mesenteric lymph nodes (Luerce et al., 2014). In another study using a similar colitis model, *L. lactis* FC ssp. *cremoris* demonstrated a protective role in treating inflammation in mice, by preventing the NF-kB activation and in decreasing IL-8 expression in epithelial cells (Nishitani et al., 2009).

Lactic acid bacteria have also been studied and has generated promising results, both *in vitro* and *in vivo*, in other models of intestinal inflammation, such as preclinical mucositis models (Tooley et al., 2006; Bowen et al., 2007; Smith et al., 2008; Southcott et al., 2008; Whitford et al., 2009; Tooley et al., 2011; Prisciandaro et al., 2012). *In vitro*, it was observed that IECs previously treated with 5-FU presented reduced levels of cytotoxicity and apoptosis through the inhibition of caspase-3 and caspase-7 when co-cultured with *L. rhamnosus* (Prisciandaro et al., 2012). *In vivo*, *L. fermentum* BR11 administered to mice injected with 5-FU exhibited reduced levels of intestinal inflammation and myeloperoxidase enzyme activity, a marker of eosinophilic inflammation (Smith et al., 2008). In another study, VSL#3 was used in the treatment of mucositis that was induced in rats through the injection of a chemotherapy drug known as irinotecan. The administration of probiotics has been shown to prevent weight loss and reduce diarrhea in these rats. These findings were associated with significant improvement in the integrity of crypts in the jejunum and a reduction in apoptosis levels in both the small and large intestines of irinotecan-treated rats (Bowen et al., 2007). Whitford et al. (2009) compared the efficiency of live *S. thermophilus* TH-4 strain (TH-4), dead TH-4 and TH-4 culture supernatants in rats treated with 5-FU. They showed that live TH-4 significantly reduced disease severity scores as well as crypt fission indices, which is an indicator of longitudinal intestinal growth and stem cell proliferation, suggesting that this strain may be useful for treating diseases characterized by increased crypt fission, such as colorectal carcinoma. However, Tooley et al. (2011) ascertained the effects of live TH-4 on small intestinal damage generated by the injection of methotrexate (MTX), a chemotherapy drug that induces mucositis and tumor progression in tumor-bearing rats. This study verified that although TH-4 did not protect animals from chemotherapy-induced mucositis, the progression of mammary adenocarcinoma was unaffected (Tooley et al., 2011).

The efficacy of cow's milk yogurt containing *L. johnsonii* and sheep's milk yogurt containing *L. bulgaricus* and *S. thermophilus* was assessed in an MTX-induced model of mucositis in rats. It was shown that both types of yogurt reduced intestinal permeability, revealing them to be useful in restoring intestinal barrier function (Southcott et al., 2008).

THE USE OF RECOMBINANT LACTIC ACID BACTERIA FOR THE TREATMENT OF GIT INFLAMMATORY DISEASES

As probiotics have been shown to be capable of acting on many diverse biological processes within the host, they have been experimented with as an alternative therapy against GIT inflammatory disorders. To enhance probiotic properties, research is focusing on the development of genetically modified bacterial strains expressing heterologous proteins of medical interest, such as anti-inflammatory molecules. Recently, the use of recombinant LAB strains with natural probiotic activities have shown promising results in pre-clinical studies as an alternative therapy to treat cancer, obesity, and especially GI tract inflammation (Bermúdez-Humarán et al., 2007; Cortes-Perez et al., 2007; Bahey-El-Din et al., 2010; Bermúdez-Humarán et al., 2013; Wang et al., 2016).

Since 1960, molecular biologists have developed several sophisticated techniques to identify, isolate, and manipulate the genetic components of the bacterial cell. This knowledge enabled the construction of different LAB recombinant strains with increased anti-inflammatory properties. Well-reported examples include the construction of *L. casei*, *L. plantarum*, *S. thermophilus*, and *L. lactis* strains capable of expressing anti-inflammatory molecules, thus increasing the benefitial effects of the above-mentioned strains (**Table 1**) (Han et al., 2006; LeBlanc et al., 2011; Del Carmen et al., 2014). Thus, several studies have focused on the use of recombinant anti-inflammatory LAB as an interesting alternative treatment for GIT inflammatory diseases (de Moreno de LeBlanc et al., 2015; Wang et al., 2016).

Lactic acid bacteria have been proven to successfully express proteins of interest in different cell compartments (in the cytoplasm, anchored to the cell membrane or secreted into the extracellular medium) (Miyoshi et al., 2010; Pontes et al., 2011; Pereira et al., 2014). It has been shown that LAB can be administered orally, making the need for clean needles and syringes unnecessary. In fact, the WHO recommends that immunization or treatment be orally administered due

TABLE 1 | Heterolgous proteins with anti-inflammatory properties produced in different strains of lactic acid bacteria.

Organism	Heterologous protein	Expression system	Inflammatory condition	Anti-inflammatory effects	Reference
L. casei BL23	Superoxide dismutase A from *L. lactis* MG1363	SodA native promoter from *L. lactis* MG1363	Mouse model of DSS-induced colitis	Protection against ROS	Watterlot et al., 2010
L. fermentum I5007	Superoxide dismutase from *B. subtilis*	Constitutive promoter from *L. casei* ATCC334	Mouse model of TNBS-induced colitis	Inhibition of NF-κB pathway	Hou et al., 2014
S. thermophilus CRL807	Superoxide dismutase A from *L. lactis* MG1363	SodA native promoter from *L. lactis* MG1363	Mouse model of TNBS-induced colitis	Reduction of intestinal permeability and histological damage	Del Carmen et al., 2014
L. lactis NCDO2118	Human 15-lipoxygenase-1	XIES	Mouse model of DSS-induced colitis	Decreased IFN-γ and IL-4. Increased IL-10	Carvalho et al., 2016
L. lactis NZ3900	Mouse cathelicidin	NICE	Mouse model of DSS-induced colitis	Reduced tissue damage and MPO activity	Wong et al., 2012
L. lactis NZ9000	Human elafin	NICE	Mouse model of DSS-induced colitis	Inhibition of elastase and proteinase-3	Bermúdez-Humarán et al., 2015
L. lactis NZ9000	Mouse leukocyte protease inhibitor	NICE	Mouse model of DSS-induced colitis	Reduced tissue damage and MPO activity	Bermúdez-Humarán et al., 2015
L. lactis NZ9000	Mouse TGF-β	NICE	Mouse model of DSS-induced colitis	Reduced granulocytes infiltration	Bermúdez-Humarán et al., 2015
L. casei CECT 5276	Human IL-10 combined with 5-aminosalicylic acid (5-ASA)	Lactose inducible promoter	Mouse model of DSS-induced colitis	Inhibition of NF-κB pathway	Qiu et al., 2013
L. lactis MG1363	Mouse IL-10	TREX1	Mouse model of DSS-induced colitis and IL-10 knockout mice	Reduced tissue damage	Steidler et al., 2000
L. lactis MG1363	Mouse IL-10	SICE	Mouse model of DNBS-induced colitis	Reduced tissue damage	Benbouziane et al., 2013
L. lactis AG013	Human IL-10	ThyA native promoter from *L. lactis*	Clinical trial with Crohn's disease patients	No significant improvement comparing to placebo	Steidler et al., 2003
L. lactis NZ9000	Human pancreatitis-associated protein (Reg3A)	NICE	Mouse model of 5-fluoracil – induced intestinal mucositis	Villous architeture preservation and improved Paneth cells activity	Carvalho et al., 2017
L. lactis AG013	Human trefoil factor I	ThyA native promoter from *L. lactis*	Hamsters model of radiation-induced oral mucositis	Reduced clinical scores of oral mucosits	Rottiers et al., 2009
L. lactis AG013	Human trefoil factor I	ThyA native promoter from *L. lactis*	Clinical trial with oral mucositis patients	Reduced the severity and course of radiation-induced oral mucositis	Limaye et al., 2013

to economic, logistical and security reasons. Furthermore, this route offers important advantages over systemic administration, such as reducing side effects, as the molecules are administered locally and have the ability to stimulate the GALT immune responses (Levine and Dougan, 1998; Neutra and Kozlowski, 2006; Bermúdez-Humarán et al., 2011).

The majority of studies in the literature describe the genetic engineering of *L. lactis* because it is the best-characterized member of the LAB group, both physiologically and genetically, and a large number of genetic tools are available for its genetic manipulation. Additional features that make *L. lactis* one of the most extensively studied bacteria are related to its economic importance in cheese production, as it is easy to grow and manipulate and was the first LAB to have its genome completely sequenced (de Vos, 1999; Bolotin et al., 2001; Felis and Dellaglio, 2007; Wells and Mercenier, 2008; Bermúdez-Humarán et al., 2011). In addition, it does not produce endotoxins such as lipopolysaccharide (LPS) and secretes few proteins, facilitating the purification of heterologous proteins. In fact, only the unknown secreted protein of 45 kDa (Usp45) is detectable after sodium dodecyl sulfate polyacrylamide gel electrophoresis (SDS-PAGE) stained with Coomassie brilliant blue (van Asseldonk et al., 1990; Bahey-El-Din et al., 2010).

Lactococcus lactis, the Model Lactic Acid Bacteria for the Expression of Anti-inflammatory Molecules

Properties of *L. lactis*

Lactococcus lactis is a mesophilic, facultative heterofermentative bacterium with an optimum growth temperature of approximately 30°C that is important in dairy industry, especially for cheese production. There are two reported subspecies (ssp.) of *L. lactis*, ssp. *lactis* and ssp. *cremoris*. Both can be found naturally in plants, especially grass. As they are used in the food industry for milk fermentation, both species can also be found in dairy products, such as cheeses, yogurts, and some breads and wines (Carr et al., 2002). *L. lactis* subsp. *cremoris* MG1363 is the most commonly used strain for cloning and protein expression, as it has no plasmids and does not produce any extracellular proteases. In addition, this strain was cataloged by the FDA and the European Food Safety Authority (EFSA) as a safe microorganism (GRAS), non-invasive and non-pathogenic, reinforcing its use as a factory for the production of anti-inflammatory molecules. Although it is considered GRAS, *L. lactis* spp. *lactis* was reported to cause an infection in two individuals who had been diagnosed with cardiac abnormalities. Afterward, they were treated with antibiotics, and the infection was cleared. Both patients did not develop any further infection by *L. lactis* (Mercenier, 1999; Bermúdez-Humarán et al., 2011). As *L. lactis* does not colonize the human GIT, most studies have focused on the beneficial effects of LAB strains in the *Lactobacillus* genus, which is autochthonous. However, recent studies have demonstrated that some allochthonous lactococci strains have anti-inflammatory properties. Ballal et al. (2015) found that *L. lactis* I-1631 prevents colitis in T-bet-/- Rag2-/- mice. Two additional studies have shown that NCDO2118 sub. *lactis* or FC sub. *cremoris* are anti-inflammatory when inoculated in inflamed mice receiving the chemical agent DSS (Nishitani et al., 2009; Luerce et al., 2014). Moreover, *L. lactis*, was used for the treatment of eosinophilic esophagitis in mice. It was demonstrated that the administration of NCC2287 in mice decreased esophageal eosinophilia, which was elicited by epicutaneous sensitization with protein extract from the fungi *Aspergillus fumigatus*, highlighting the beneficial effects of *L. lactis* in another severe inflammatory disease (Holvoet et al., 2016).

As mentioned previously, there are several expression systems available for heterologous protein production in *L. lactis* (Miyoshi et al., 2010). This has allowed the cloning and expression of different heterologous anti-inflammatory proteins by the use of both cloning and expression vectors designed for *L. lactis* (**Table 1**) (Langella and Le Loir, 1999; Le Loir et al., 2005; Bermúdez-Humarán et al., 2011).

Heterologous Protein Expression Systems in *L. lactis*

The first expression systems for use in *Lactococcus lactis* were based on the classic bacterial lactose operon. This operon is activated when the lac promoter is induced in the presence of lactose, while the transcriptional repressor gene (*lacR*) is suppressed in the same condition. Therefore, lactococci strains harboring a plasmid carrying this operon fused to a target gene allow recombinant proteins to be expressed in a tightly controlled fashion (van Rooijen et al., 1992). Wells et al. (1993) improved this system by integrating it with a strong phage promoter that allowed for high levels of heterogous protein production. It consisted of three plasmids containing the lac operon elements and two elements from the T7 bacteriophage found in *E. coli*. In this system, the presence of lactose induces the lac promoter in the first plasmid, promoting expression of the T7 RNA polymerase. Afterward, the T7 RNA polymerase activates expression of the gene of interest controlled by the T7 promoter in the second plasmid. The third plasmid coded for the functional lac operon, allowing the cell to be capable of metabolizing soluble lactose in an artificial medium. This system and other complex systems based on phage promoters have allowed for the strict control of gene expression, although they require many antibiotic resistance markers, making them unsuitable for use in the food and pharmaceutical industry (Wells et al., 1993; Nauta et al., 1996; O'Sullivan, 2001).

In this context, several studies have been carried out to develop safer and more simple vectors. One of the most powerful expression systems already developed for use in the food industry is based on genes involved in the biosynthesis and regulation of the antimicrobial nisin, a peptide naturally secreted by several strains of *Lactococcus lactis*. In brief, the Nisin-Controlled Gene Expression system (NICE) is based on the expression of three genes involved in the production and regulation of the the peptide nisin, which is naturally secreted by various *L. lactis* strains, in a genetically engineered *L. lactis* strain. The *nisR* and *nisK genes* encode a two-component regulatory system (NisRK), which controls the expression of the nisin operon through the activation of signal transduction pathways (Kuipers et al., 1993). The strain used in this system is a genetically modified version of a *L. lactis* MG1363 strain, *L. lactis* NZ9000, in which both *nisR* and *nisK* regulatory genes were inserted into its chromosome. The expression vector contains the nisin promoter P*nisA*, followed by multiple cloning sites (MCSs) for the insertion of heterologous genes coding for anti-inflammatory molecules or antigens (Kuipers et al., 1993; Mierau and Kleerebezem, 2005). Because NICE system expression vectors exist in different versions, heterologous proteins can be expressed in different cellular compartments. In addition to the cytoplasm, recombinant protein can be anchored to the bacterial cell wall by means of a cell wall anchor (CWA) peptide, composed of 30 amino acids located in the carboxy-terminal portion (C-terminus) of the protein. CWA is recognized by the cell anchoring machinery and is usually covalently attached to the peptidoglycan from the cell membrane. Furthermore, recombinant proteins may be coupled with a short (5–30 amino acid long) peptide present at the N-terminus region of the heterologous protein, allowing its translocation across the cell membrane and secretion to the extracellular medium (Le Loir et al., 1994; Piard et al., 1997).

The NICE system has been successfully used to express and address a variety of heterologous proteins of medical and biotechnological interest, and according to some authors, it is considered as one of the best genetic tools already developed for gene cloning and expression in *L. lactis* (Nouaille et al., 2003; Le Loir et al., 2005).

Miyoshi et al. (2004) developed the xylose-inducible expression system (XIES) based on the xylose permease gene promoter (PxylT) from *Lactococcus lactis* NCDO2118. In the presence of glucose, fructose and/or mannose, PxylT was shown to be repressed; otherwise, PxylT is transcriptionally activated by xylose in *Lactococcus lactis* (Miyoshi et al., 2004). Therefore, this system could be successively turned on by adding xylose and turned off by washing the cells and growing them on glucose. The system combines the use of PxylT, the ribosome-binding site (RBS) and the signal peptide (SP) of the lactococcal secreted protein Usp45 and the *Staphylococcus aureus* nuclease gene (*nuc*) as the reporter (Shortle, 1983; Le Loir et al., 1994). This system was successfully used for the production of highlevels of Nuc, which was tested for correct protein targeting in the *Lactococcus lactis* subsp. *lactis* strain NCDO2118. These systems are considered less expensive and safer for laboratory use compared to many available expression methods (de Azevedo et al., 2015).

Most heterologous protein expression systems used in *L. lactis* are based on inducible promoters, which allows for the controlled expression of the protein of interest. In this context, they prevent protein aggregation and degradation within the bacterial cytoplasm. However, the majority of the expression vectors present inherent safety drawbacks due to the necessity to add chemical compounds into the bacterial culture to induce heterologous protein expression prior to *in vivo* administration. Other food grade expression systems that do not require the pre-induction of the cultures to allow the expression of a given recombinant protein have been reported (Derre et al., 1999; Ruiz et al., 2012; Benbouziane et al., 2013). Benbouziane et al. (2013) developed the stress-inducible controlled expression system (SICE), based on the use of the heat shock protein groESL operon promoter (pGroESL) from *L. lactis*, to deliver proteins of health interest *in situ*. Heat-shock proteins play an essential role under different stress conditions such as heat-shock, low pH, UV-irradiation, and salt stress. Indeed, upon administration into the host, recombinant bacteria should find very different conditions from culture conditions and likely suffer different types of stress (Benbouziane et al., 2013). In the case of oral administration, heat stress can be accompanied by an acid stress during passage through the stomach as well as bile stress in the duodenum. SICE system represents an interesting alternative for the treatment of GI inflammatory diseases, since it allows for the local delivery of therapeutic proteins in the GIT during the passage of the bacteria, allowing for the localized action of the protein and thus a greater efficiency. This system is an interesting alternative for proof of concept studies because it does not require the presence of regulatory genes or the pre-induction of the cultures. However, it still presents a bottleneck, since antibiotic resistance markers could be horizontally transferred to harmful microbes in the human GIT in clinical studies. In this context, the scientific community has been trying to develop biological confinement strategies, which are discussed later in this review (Vandermeulen et al., 2011).

Therapeutic Interventions Using Recombinant *L. lactis* Strains to Alleviate GI Inflammation

Since *L. lactis* can be genetically modified to efficiently produce and secrete different anti-inflammatory proteins, recombinant strains of *L. lactis* have been tested in pre-clinical and clinical experimental trials to treat or prevent various human diseases, including intestinal inflammation (**Table 1**) (Steidler et al., 2000; Rochat et al., 2007; LeBlanc et al., 2011; Bermúdez-Humarán et al., 2013; Del Carmen et al., 2014; Carvalho et al., 2016, 2017). The oral administration of *L. lactis* expressing anti-inflammatory proteins is a very interesting strategy to fight GIT inflammation, as this species is non-invasive and allochthonous, as commented on earlier. As it is unable to colonize the GIT, the potential to elicit adverse effects on host microbiota related to its long-term administration is reduced (Nouaille et al., 2003). It has been shown that the oral administration of a recombinant *L. lactis* strain expressing the enzyme SOD, naturally produced by *Bacillus subtilis*, reduced inflammation scores in animals treated with trinitrobenzenesulfonic acid (TNBS). This therapeutic effect was tied to the antioxidant properties of the recombinant SOD (Rochat et al., 2005). Later, the same strain was able to prevent the development of colorectal cancer cells in mice.

In another proof-of-concept study, the anti-inflammatory strain *L. lactis* NCDO 2118 was engineered to produce the oxidative enzyme, 15-lipoxygenase-1 (15-LOX-1), which catalyzes the formation of several anti-inflammatory mediators, such as lipoxins, resolvins and protectins. The 15-LOX-1 produced by *L. lactis* was effective in treating DSS-induced colitis in mice during the remission period and decreased pro-inflammatory cytokines such as IFN-γ and IL-4 while increasing the anti-inflammatory IL-10 (Carvalho et al., 2016). Another strategy has been the use of *L. lactis* to secrete either regulatory cytokines involved in the regulation of inflammation processes, or antibodies that neutralize pro-inflammatory cytokines. *L. lactis* strains able to secrete anti-TNFα antibodies that bind to TNF-α, one of the most important mediators of inflammation, were described (Yoshida and Miyazaki, 2008; Strukelj et al., 2014). It was demonstrated in a DSS-induced colitis mouse model that the oral administration of *L. lactis* expressing murine anti-TNFα showed reduced inflammation, and work by Bermúdez-Humaran and collaborators demonstrated that a recombinant *L. lactis* strain expressing the cytokine TGF-β was able to ameliorate clinical symptoms, such as weight loss and diarrhea in the same DSS model of intestinal inflammation (Yoshida and Miyazaki, 2008; Bermúdez-Humarán et al., 2015). Another strain that is presenting good results in pre-clinical trials expresses IL-10, an anti-inflammatory cytokine capable of suppressing proinflammatory responses of both innate and adaptive immune cells. The effect of the recombinant IL-10 producing *L. lactis* has been tested in several IBD animal models, such as IL-10 knockout mice and TNBS or DSS models (Schotte et al., 2000; Steidler et al., 2000, 2003; Braat et al., 2006; Del Carmen et al., 2014). The recombinant IL-10 producing *L. lactis* strain demonstrated promising results in pre-clinical. Indeed, a large clinical trial using recombinant *L. lactis* secreting the human IL-10 was conducted in patients with Crohn's disease approximately 10 years ago. Its use in humans was allowed by regulatory agencies, such as the Genetically Modified Organisms (GMOs) European Commission, because of a biological containment strategy that was developed. A gene encoding the essential protein thymidylate synthase (ThyA), located on the *L. lactis* chromosome, was exchanged for the human IL-10 gene. Therefore, the strain was only able to survive in the presence of thymine or thymidine that was artificially provided in the culture medium, making *L. lactis*-IL-10 critically dependent on this compound. Inside the human body, the strain could survive and deliver IL-10, since thymine or thymidine is available. Outside of the body, the GMO strain was unable to survive, avoiding its spread into the environment (Steidler et al., 2003). Clinical results showed no significant improvement between patients receiving the IL-10 producing *L. lactis* strain and those who received a placebo (Braat et al., 2006).

Few studies regarding the treatment of mucositis using recombinant *L. lactis* strains expressing therapeutic molecules have been reported. Most pre-clinical studies found in the literature describe the use of purified anti-inflammatory compounds intended to eliminate disease. An example is the systemic administration of either IL-11 or TGF-β regulatory cytokines in patients. The authors noted that this alternative treatment was not able to contain oral mucositis. The possible causes for this failure were linked to an inadequate dosage, route of administration and drug stability (Antin et al., 2002; de Koning et al., 2006). Other clinical studies have tested growth factors that stimulate cell proliferation, thereby maintaining epithelial barrier integrity, such as granulocyte-macrophage colony-stimulating factor (GM-CSF) and epidermal growth factor (EGF). However, their use was associated with an increased risk and progression of tumors (Hong et al., 2009). Rottiers et al. (2009) evaluated the effect of *L. lactis* secreting trefoil factor I (TFF-1), naturally involved in the repair of the epithelial barrier, administered to hamsters with oral mucositis. It was observed that recombinant *L. lactis* was able to reduce mucosal inflammation (Rottiers et al., 2009; Caluwaerts et al., 2010). Furthermore, as undesired reactions were not detected in pre-clinical trials, another genetically modified *L. lactis* strain (AG013), capable of secreting human TFF1, was engineered based on the ThyA biological confinement system. A phase 1 clinical trial was performed in patients with oral mucositis who tolerated the treatment well, and administration of the AG013 strain was shown to be more efficient in ameliorating clinical syntoms than placebo (Limaye et al., 2013). Several molecules with anti-inflammatory properties have sought to be cloned and expressed in *L. lactis*, which has proven to be a safe vehicle for the treatment of GI intestinal disorders. Anti-inflammatory cytokines, anti-oxidant enzymes, epithelial growth factor and especially antimicrobial peptides produced by *L. lactis* are the focus of future research efforts for the development of a possible treatment for GI tract inflammation.

Mammalian Antimicrobial Peptides Produced by *L. lactis* as a Possible Treatment for Intestinal Inflammation

Antimicrobial peptides that are involved in the maintenance of the epithelial barrier could represent an interesting candidate to prevent microbiota-driven inflammatory signaling. Various antimicrobial peptides, such as defensins, cathelicidins and histatins, that are produced by Paneth cells seem to play a critical role in intestinal homeostasis, and their biological activity has been reported to be compromised in IBD patients (Clevers and Bevins, 2013; Peterson and Artis, 2014). Different research groups are investigating whether the administration of these peptides could have a protective effect against intestinal inflammation. In a study conducted by Seo et al. (2012), α-defensin (HD5) and human β-defensin 2 (HBD2), which have been purified from the probiotic *E. coli* Nissle 1917, inhibithed the growth of pathogenic *E. coli*, *S. typhimurium*, or *L. monocytogenes* when co-incubated, *in vitro*, with these bacterial species (Seo et al., 2012).

Another antimicrobial peptide, cathelicidin, was expressed in *L. lactis* and the efficacy of this strain in decreasing intestinal inflammation was evaluated in a DSS murine model. The authors observed a reduced number of bacteria in the feces from animals that received the *L. lactis*-cathelicidin strain, suggesting an anti-microbial effect of the strain. According to the study, these findings were correlated to reduced tissue damage and MPO activity (Wong et al., 2012).

Among the antimicrobial peptides, the C-type lectin, Reg3A has been extensively studied due to its protective effect in the intestines of humans and animals during the inflammation process. This peptide, also known as pancreatitis-associated protein (PAP), belongs to the Reg family, which encodes a diverse group of proteins called secreted C-type lectins that contain a carbohydrate recognition domain (CRD). The Reg3A protein is predominantly produced in the small intestine of mammals, mainly by Paneth cells, where the density of microorganisms is higher (Christa et al., 1996). Several studies revealed that Reg3A exerts a bactericidal activity against Gram-positive bacteria. Furthermore, it appears that its activation in the intestinal mucosa is required to generate a protective response against intestinal microbiota during bacteria-driven inflammatory events (Christa et al., 1999; Malka et al., 2000). In fact, the PAP protective effect in GI inflammation models has been demonstrated for the first time in a DSS-induced colitis rat model. This work used an adenovirus strategy to deliver PAP cDNA into host cells to increase the expression of PAP (Lv et al., 2012). Recently, Breyner et al. (2017, personal communication) have shown that the use of *L. lactis* expressing human PAP could prevent colitis in a DNBS-chemically induced murine model. Interestingly, as it was shown to be useful in the treatment of IBD, another study sought to investigate a protective role of *L. lactis* secreting human PAP in mucositis using the 5-FU-induced intestinal mucositis experimental mouse model. The authors showed that the PAP antimicrobial peptide, cloned into *L. lactis*, has an inhibitory effect against the opportunistic commensal *E. faecalis*. Moreover, *L. lactis* NZ9000 by itself was able to prevent histological damage and reduce neutrophil and eosinophil infiltration in mice injected with 5-FU. In addition, the recombinant lactococci producing PAP improved villous architecture preservation and increased Paneth cell activity in response to 5-FU inflammation (Carvalho et al., 2017).

CONCLUSION

The efficacy of probiotic LAB, especially in the context of using recombinant *L. lactis* strains designed to deliver anti-inflammatory proteins *in situ*, has been demonstrated for treating IBD in many studies in the past decades. Moreover, as highlighted in this review, the same therapeutic approach is being successfully transposed for treating mucositis. Thus, this work reiterates that probiotic LAB, wild type or genetically modified, could also be used as an alternative for treating other GI inflammatory diseases in which dysbiosis has been shown to be implicated. As most of the beneficial effects of recombinant *L. lactis* strains have been demonstrated in proof-of-concept studies, further translational aproaches are needed to make them safe for testing in humans. In this context, biological confinement strategies that prevent recombinant lactococci from escaping into natural ecosystems should be considered.

AUTHOR CONTRIBUTIONS

RC contributed to conception of the work, bibliographic survey, and manuscript writing. FdC contributed to bibliographic survey and drafting or the work. AdO was responsible for creating the figure and contributed to the bibliographic survey. PL was involved in the critical revision of the article. J-MC was involved in the critical revision of the article. LB-H was involved in manuscript correction and drafting of the work. VA contributed to critical revision of the article and conception of the work. MdA contributed to manuscript writing and correction.

REFERENCES

Adolfsson, O., Meydani, S. N., and Russell, R. M. (2004). Yogurt and gut function. *Am. J. Clin. Nutr.* 80, 245–256.

Ananthakrishnan, A. N. (2015). Epidemiology and risk factors for IBD. *Nat. Rev. Gastroenterol. Hepatol.* 12, 205–217. doi: 10.1038/nrgastro.2015.34

Anderson, R. C., Cookson, A. L., McNabb, W. C., Park, Z., McCann, M. J., Kelly, W. J., et al. (2010). Lactobacillus plantarum MB452 enhances the function of the intestinal barrier by increasing the expression levels of genes involved in tight junction formation. *BMC Microbiol.* 10:316. doi: 10.1186/1471-2180-10-316

Antin, J. H., Weisdorf, D., Neuberg, D., Nicklow, R., Clouthier, S., Lee, S. J., et al. (2002). Interleukin-1 blockade does not prevent acute graft-versus-host disease: results of a randomized, double-blind, placebo-controlled trial of interleukin-1 receptor antagonist in allogeneic bone marrow transplantation. *Blood* 100, 3479–3482. doi: 10.1182/blood-2002-03-0985

Antunes, M. M., Leocádio, P. C. L., Teixeira, L. G., Leonel, A. J., Cara, D. C., Menezes, G. B., et al. (2016). Pretreatment with L-citrulline positively affects the mucosal architecture and permeability of the small intestine in a murine mucositis model. *J. Parenter. Enteral. Nutr.* 40, 279–286. doi: 10.1177/0148607114567508

Bahey-El-Din, M., Gahan, C. G., and Griffin, B. T. (2010). *Lactococcus lactis* as a cell factory for delivery of therapeutic proteins. *Curr. Gene Ther.* 10, 34–45. doi: 10.2174/156652310790945557

Bajaj, B. K., Claes, I. J. J., and Lebeer, S. (2015). Functional mechanisms of probiotics. *J. Microbiol. Biotechnol. Food Sci.* 4, 321–327. doi: 10.15414/jmbfs.2015.4.4.321-327

Ballal, S. A., Veiga, P., Fenn, K., Michaud, M., Kim, J. H., Gallini, C. A., et al. (2015). Host lysozyme-mediated lysis of *Lactococcus lactis* facilitates delivery of colitis-attenuating superoxide dismutase to inflamed colons. *Proc. Natl. Acad. Sci. U.S.A.* 112, 7803–7808. doi: 10.1073/pnas.1501897112

Benbouziane, B., Ribelles, P., Aubry, C., Martin, R., Kharrat, P., Riazi, A., et al. (2013). Development of a Stress-Inducible Controlled Expression (SICE) system in *Lactococcus lactis* for the production and delivery of therapeutic molecules at mucosal surfaces. *J. Biotechnol.* 168, 120–129. doi: 10.1016/j.jbiotec.2013.04.019

Bermúdez-Humarán, L. G., Aubry, C., Motta, J.-P., Deraison, C., Steidler, L., Vergnolle, N., et al. (2013). Engineering lactococci and lactobacilli for human health. *Curr. Opin. Microbiol.* 16, 278–283. doi: 10.1016/j.mib.2013.06.002

Bermúdez-Humarán, L. G., Kharrat, P., Chatel, J. M., and Langella, P. (2011). Lactococci and lactobacilli as mucosal delivery vectors for therapeutic proteins and DNA vaccines. *Microb. Cell Fact.* 10(Suppl. 1), S4. doi: 10.1186/1475-2859-10-S1-S4

Bermúdez-Humarán, L. G., Motta, J. P., Aubry, C., Kharrat, P., Rous-Martin, L., Sallenave, J. M., et al. (2015). Serine protease inhibitors protect better than IL-10 and TGF-β anti-inflammatory cytokines against mouse colitis when delivered by recombinant lactococci. *Microb. Cell Fact.* 14, 26. doi: 10.1186/s12934-015-0198-4

Bermúdez-Humarán, L. G., Nouaille, S., Zilberfarb, V., Corthier, G., Gruss, A., Langella, P., et al. (2007). Effects of intranasal administration of a leptin-secreting *Lactococcus lactis* recombinant on food intake, body weight, and immune response of mice. *Appl. Environ. Microbiol.* 73, 5300–5307. doi: 10.1128/AEM.00295-07

Bernet-Camard, M. F., Liévin, V., Brassart, D., Neeser, J. R., Servin, A. L., and Hudault, S. (1997). The human Lactobacillus acidophilus strain LA1 secretes a nonbacteriocin antibacterial substance(s) active *in vitro* and *in vivo*. *Appl. Environ. Microbiol.* 63, 2747–2753.

Bolotin, A., Wincker, P., Mauger, S., Jaillon, O., Malarme, K., Weissenbach, J., et al. (2001). The complete genome sequence of the lactic acid bacterium *Lactococcus lactis* ssp. *lactis* IL1403. *Genome Res.* 11, 731–753. doi: 10.1101/gr.169701

Bowen, J. M., Stringer, A. M., Gibson, R. J., Yeoh, A. S. J., Hannam, S., and Keefe, D. M. (2007). VSL#3 probiotic treatment reduces chemotherapy-induced diarrhea and weight loss. *Cancer Biol. Ther.* 6, 1449–1454. doi: 10.4161/cbt.6.9.4622

Braat, H., Rottiers, P., and Hommes, D. W. (2006). A phase I Trial with transgenic bacteria expressing interleukin-10 in Crohn's disease. *Clin. Gastroenterol. Hepatol.* 4, 754–759. doi: 10.1016/j.cgh.2006.03.028

Caluwaerts, S., Vandenbroucke, K., Steidler, L., Neirynck, S., Vanhoenacker, P., Corveleyn, S., et al. (2010). AG013, a mouth rinse formulation of *Lactococcus lactis* secreting human Trefoil Factor 1, provides a safe and efficacious therapeutic tool for treating oral mucositis. *Oral Oncol.* 46, 564–570. doi: 10.1016/j.oraloncology.2010.04.008

Carlsson, A. H., Yakymenko, O., Olivier, I., Håkansson, F., Postma, E., Keita, ÅV., et al. (2013). *Faecalibacterium prausnitzii* supernatant improves intestinal barrier function in mice DSS colitis. *Scand. J. Gastroenterol.* 48, 1136–1144. doi: 10.3109/00365521.2013.828773

Carr, F. J., Chill, D., and Maida, N. (2002). The lactic acid bacteria: a literature survey. *Crit. Rev. Microbiol.* 28, 281–370. doi: 10.1080/1040-840291046759

Carvalho, R. D. O., Breyner, N., Menezes-Garcia, Z., Rodrigues, N. M., Lemos, L., Maioli, T. U., et al. (2017). Secretion of biologically active pancreatitis-associated protein I (PAP) by genetically modified dairy *Lactococcus lactis* NZ9000 in the prevention of intestinal mucositis. *Microb. Cell Fact.* 16, 27. doi: 10.1186/s12934-017-0624-x

Carvalho, R. D. O., Morais, K., Pereira, V. B., Gomes-Santos, A. C., Luerce, T. D., de Azevedo, M. S. P., et al. (2016). Oral administration of *Lactococcus lactis* expressing recombinant 15-lipoxygenase-1 (15 LOX-1) modulates chemically induced colitis in mice. *Med. Res. Arch.* 4:1. doi: 10.18103/mra.v4i7.612

Chang, C., and Lin, H. (2016). Dysbiosis in gastrointestinal disorders. *Best Pract. Res. Clin. Gastroenterol.* 30, 3–15. doi: 10.1016/j.bpg.2016.02.001

Christa, L., Carnot, F., Simon, M. T., Levavasseur, F., Stinnakre, M. G., Lasserre, C., et al. (1996). HIP/PAP is an adhesive protein expressed in hepatocarcinoma, normal Paneth, and pancreatic cells. *Am. J. Physiol.* 271, G993–G1002.

Christa, L., Simon, M. T., Brezault-bonnet, C., Bonte, E., Carnot, F., Zylberberg, H., et al. (1999). Hepatocarcinoma-intestine-pancreas/pancreatic associated protein (HIP/PAP) is expressed and secreted by proliferating ductules as well as by hepatocarcinoma and cholangiocarcinoma cells. *Am. J. Pathol.* 155, 1525–1533. doi: 10.1016/S0002-9440(10)65468-5

Clevers, H. C., and Bevins, C. L. (2013). Paneth cells: maestros of the small intestinal crypts. *Annu. Rev. Physiol.* 75, 289–311. doi: 10.1146/annurev-physiol-030212-183744

Cortes-Perez, N. G., Ah-Leung, S., Bermúdez-Humarán, L. G., Corthier, G., Wal, J.-M., Langella, P., et al. (2007). Intranasal coadministration of live lactococci producing interleukin-12 and a major cow's milk allergen inhibits allergic reaction in mice. *Clin. Vaccine Immunol.* 14, 226–233. doi: 10.1128/CVI.00299-06

de Azevedo, M., Meijerink, M., Taverne, N., Pereira, V. B., LeBlanc, J. G., Azevedo, V., et al. (2015). Recombinant invasive *Lactococcus lactis* can transfer DNA vaccines either directly to dendritic cells or across an epithelial cell monolayer. *Vaccine* 33, 4807–4812. doi: 10.1016/j.vaccine.2015.07.077

de Koning, B. A., van Dieren, J. M., Lindenbergh-Kortleve, D. J., van der Sluis, M., Matsumoto, T., Yamaguchi, K., et al. (2006). Contributions of mucosal immune cells to methotrexate-induced mucositis. *Int. Immunol.* 18, 941–949. doi: 10.1093/intimm/dxl030

de Moreno de LeBlanc, A., del Carmen, S., Chatel, J.-M., Miyoshi, A., Azevedo, V., Langella, P., et al. (2015). Current review of genetically modified lactic acid bacteria for the prevention and treatment of colitis using murine models. *Gastroenterol. Res. Pract.* 2015:e146972. doi: 10.1155/2015/146972

de Vasconcelos Generoso, V., Rodrigues, N. M., Trindade, L. M., Paiva, N. C., Cardoso, V. N., Carneiro, C. M., et al. (2015). Dietary supplementation with omega-3 fatty acid attenuates 5-fluorouracil induced mucositis in mice. *Lipids Health Dis.* 14:54. doi: 10.1186/s12944-015-0052-z

de Vos, W. M. (1999). Gene expression systems for lactic acid bacteria. *Curr. Opin. Microbiol.* 2, 289–295. doi: 10.1016/S1369-5274(99)80050-2

de Vos, W. M., and de Vos, E. A. (2012). Role of the intestinal microbiome in health and disease: from correlation to causation. *Nutr. Rev.* 70, S45–S56. doi: 10.1111/j.1753-4887.2012.00505.x

Del Carmen, S., de Moreno de LeBlanc, A., Martin, R., Chain, F., Langella, P., Bermúdez-Humarán, L. G., et al. (2014). Genetically engineered immunomodulatory *Streptococcus thermophilus* strains producing antioxidant enzymes exhibit enhanced anti-inflammatory activities. *Appl. Environ. Microbiol.* 80, 869–877. doi: 10.1128/AEM.03296-13

Derre, I., Rapoport, G., and Msadek, T. (1999). CtsR, a novel regulator of stress, and heat shock response, controls clp, and molecular chaperone gene expression in Gram-positive bactéria. *Mol. Microbiol.* 31, 117–131. doi: 10.1046/j.1365-2958.1999.01152.x

Eun, C. S., Kim, Y. S., Han, D. S., Choi, J. H., Lee, A. R., and Park, Y. K. (2011). *Lactobacillus casei* prevents impaired barrier function in intestinal epithelial cells. *APMIS* 119, 49–56. doi: 10.1111/j.1600-0463.2010.02691.x

Ewaschuk, J. B., Diaz, H., Meddings, L., Diederichs, B., Dmytrash, A., Backer, J., et al. (2008). Secreted bioactive factors from *Bifidobacterium infantis* enhance epithelial cell barrier function. *Am. J. Physiol.* 295, G1025–G1034. doi: 10.1152/ajpgi.90227.2008

FAO/WHO (2002). "Guidelines for the evaluation of probiotics in food," in *Proceedings of the Joint FAO/WHO Working Group Meeting*, London, ON.

Fedorak, R. N., Gangl, A., Elson, C. O., Rutgeerts, P., Schreiber, S., Wild, G., et al. (2000). Recombinant human interleukin 10 in the treatment of patients with mild tomoderately active Crohn's disease. The interleukin 10 inflammatory bowel disease cooperative study group. *Gastroenterology* 119, 1473–1482. doi: 10.1053/gast.2000.20229

Felis, G. E., and Dellaglio, F. (2007). Taxonomy of lactobacilli and bifidobacteria. *Curr. Issues Intest. Microbiol* 8, 44–61.

Gaudier, E., Michel, C., Segain, J.-P., Cherbut, C., and Hoebler, C. (2005). The VSL# 3 probiotic mixture modifies microflora but does not heal chronic dextran-sodium sulfate–induced colitis or reinforce the mucus barrier in mice. *J. Nutr.* 135, 2753–2761.

Guglielmetti, S., Taverniti, V., Minuzzo, M., Arioli, S., Stuknyte, M., Karp, M., et al. (2010). Oral bacteria as potential probiotics for the pharyngeal mucosa. *Appl. Environ. Microbiol.* 76, 3948–3958. doi: 10.1128/AEM.00109-10

Han, W., Mercenier, A., Ait-Belgnaoui, A., Pavan, S., Lamine, F., van Swam, I. I., et al. (2006). Improvement of an experimental colitis in rats by lactic acid bacteria producing superoxide dismutase. *Inflamm. Bowel Dis.* 12, 1044–1052. doi: 10.1097/01.mib.0000235101.09231.9e

Harder, J., Meyer-Hoffert, U., Wehkamp, K., Schwichtenberg, L., and Schröder, J.-M. (2004). Differential gene induction of human β-defensins (hBD-1, -2, -3, and -4) in keratinocytes is inhibited by retinoic acid. *J. Investig. Dermatol.* 123, 522–529. doi: 10.1111/j.0022-202X.2004.23234.x

Henker, J., Laass, M., Blokhin, B. M., Bolbot, Y. K., Maydannik, V. G., Elze, M., et al. (2007). The probiotic *Escherichia coli* strain Nissle 1917 (EcN) stops acute diarrhoea in infants and toddlers. *Eur. J. Pediatr.* 166, 311–318. doi: 10.1007/s00431-007-0419-x

Hidalgo-Cantabrana, C., Nikolic, M., López, P., Suárez, A., Miljkovic, M., Kojic, M., et al. (2014). Exopolysaccharide-producing *Bifidobacterium animalis* subsp. *lactis* strains and their polymers elicit different responses on immune cells from blood and gut associated lymphoid tissue. *Anaerobe* 26, 24–30. doi: 10.1016/j.anaerobe.2014.01.003

Holvoet, S., Doucet-Ladevèze, R., Perrot, M., Barretto, C., Nutten, S., and Blanchard, C. (2016). Beneficial effect of *Lactococcus lactis* NCC 2287 in a murine model of eosinophilic esophagitis. *Allergy* 71, 1753–1761. doi: 10.1111/all.12951

Holzapfel, W. H., Haberer, P., Snel, J., Schillinger, U., and Huis in't Veld, J. H. (1998). Overview of gut flora and probiotics. *Int. J. Food Microbiol.* 41, 85–101. doi: 10.1016/S0168-1605(98)00044-0

Hong, J. P., Lee, S.-W., Song, S. Y., Ahn, S. D., Shin, S. S., Choi, E. K., et al. (2009). Recombinant human epidermal growth factor treatment of radiation-induced severe oral mucositis in patients with head and neck malignancies. *Eur. J. Cancer Care* 18, 636–641. doi: 10.1111/j.1365-2354.2008.00971.x

Hooper, L. V. E., and Macpherson, A. J. (2010). Immune adaptations that maintain homeostasis with the intestinal microbiota. *Nat. Rev. Immunol.* 10, 159–169. doi: 10.1038/nri2710

Hou, C. L., Zhang, J., Liu, X. T., Liu, H., Zeng, X. F., and Qiao, S. Y. (2014). Superoxide dismutase recombinant *Lactobacillus fermentum* ameliorates intestinal oxidative stress through inhibiting NF-κB activation in a trinitrobenzene sulphonic acid-induced colitis mouse model. *J. Appl. Microbiol.* 116, 1621–1631. doi: 10.1111/jam.12461

Iannitti, T., and Palmieri, B. (2010). Therapeutical use of probiotic formulations in clinical practice. *Clin. Nutr.* 29, 701–725. doi: 10.1016/j.clnu.2010.05.004

Izcue, A., Coombes, J. L., and Powrie, F. (2009). Regulatory lymphocytes and intestinal inflammation. *Annu. Rev. Immunol.* 27, 313–338. doi: 10.1146/annurev.immunol.021908.132657

Johansson, M. E. V., Sjövall, H., and Hansson, G. C. (2013). The gastrointestinal mucus system in health and disease. *Nat. Rev. Gastroenterol. Hepatol.* 10, 352–361. doi: 10.1038/nrgastro.2013.35

Johnson, B. R., and Klaenhammer, T. R. (2014). Impact of genomics on the field of probiotic research: historical perspectives to modern paradigms. *Antonie Van Leeuwenhoek* 106, 141–156. doi: 10.1007/s10482-014-0171-y

Kashyap, D. R., Rompca, A., Gaballa, A., Helmann, J. D., Chan, J., Chang, C. J., et al. (2014). Peptidoglycan recognition proteins kill bacteria by inducing oxidative, thiol, and metal stress. *PLoS Pathog.* 10:e1004280. doi: 10.1371/journal.ppat.1004280

Kuipers, O. P., Beerthuyzen, M. M., Siezen, R. J., and De Vos, W. M. (1993). Characterization of the nisin gene cluster nisABTCIPR of *Lactococcus lactis*. Requirement of expression of the nisA and nisI genes for development of immunity. *Eur. J. Biochem.* 216, 281–291. doi: 10.1111/j.1432-1033.1993.tb18143.x

Langella, P., and Le Loir, Y. (1999). Heterologous protein secretion in *Lactococcus lactis*: a novel antigen delivery system. *Braz. J. Med. Biol. Res.* 32, 191–198. doi: 10.1590/S0100-879X1999000200007

Le Loir, Y., Azevedo, V., Oliveira, S. C., Freitas, D. A., Miyoshi, A., Bermúdez-Humarán, L. G., et al. (2005). Protein secretion in *Lactococcus lactis*: an efficient way to increase the overall heterologous protein production. *Microb. Cell Fact.* 4, 2.

Le Loir, Y., Gruss, A., Ehrlich, S. D., and Langella, P. (1994). Direct screening of recombinants in gram-positive bacteria using the secreted staphylococcal nuclease as a reporter. *J. Bacteriol.* 176, 5135–5139. doi: 10.1128/jb.176.16.5135-5139.1994

Lebeer, S., Vanderleyden, J., and De Keersmaecker, S. C. J. (2010). Host interactions of probiotic bacterial surface molecules: comparison with commensals and pathogens. *Nat. Rev. Microbiol.* 8, 171–184. doi: 10.1038/nrmicro2297

LeBlanc, J. G., del Carmen, S., Miyoshi, A., Azevedo, V., Sesma, F., Langella, P., et al. (2011). Use of superoxide dismutase and catalase producing lactic acid bacteria in TNBS induced Crohn's disease in mice. *J. Biotechnol.* 151, 287–293. doi: 10.1016/j.jbiotec.2010.11.008

Lennard-Jones, J. E. (1989). Classification of inflammatory Bowel disease. *Scand. J. Gastroenterol.* 24, 2–6. doi: 10.3109/00365528909091339

Levine, M. M., and Dougan, G. (1998). Optimism over vaccines administered via mucosal surfaces. *Lancet* 351, 1375–1376. doi: 10.1016/S0140-6736(05)79439-3

Limaye, S. A., Haddad, R. I., Cilli, F., Sonis, S. T., Colevas, A. D., Brennan, M. T., et al. (2013). Phase 1b, multicenter, single blinded, placebo-controlled, sequential dose escalation study to assess the safety and tolerability of topically applied AG013 in subjects with locally advanced head and neck cancer receiving induction chemotherapy. *Cancer* 119, 4268–4276. doi: 10.1002/cncr.28365

Liu, W., Pang, H., Zhang, H., and Cai, Y. (2014). "Biodiversity of lactic acid bacteria," in *Lactic Acid Bacteria*, eds H. Zhang and Y. Cai (Berlin: Springer), 103–203.

Ljungh, A., and Wadström, T. (2006). Lactic acid bacteria as probiotics. *Curr. Issues Intest. Microbiol.* 7, 73–89.

Luerce, T. D., Gomes-Santos, A. C., Rocha, C. S., Moreira, T. G., Cruz, D. N., Lemos, L., et al. (2014). Anti-inflammatory effects of *Lactococcus lactis* NCDO 2118 during the remission period of chemically induced colitis. *Gut Pathog.* 6:33. doi: 10.1186/1757-4749-6-33

Lv, Y., Yang, X., Huo, Y., Tian, H., Li, S., Yin, Y., et al. (2012). Adenovirus-mediated hepatocarcinoma-intestine-pancreas/pancreatitis-associated protein suppresses dextran sulfate sodium-induced acute ulcerative colitis in rats. *Inflamm. Bowel Dis.* 18, 1950–1960. doi: 10.1002/ibd.22887

Mack, D. R., Ahrne, S., Hyde, L., Wei, S., and Hollingsworth, M. A. (2003). Extracellular MUC3 mucin secretion follows adherence of *Lactobacillus* strains to intestinal epithelial cells *in vitro*. *Gut* 52, 827–833. doi: 10.1136/gut.52.6.827

Mackowiak, P. A. (2013). Recycling metchnikoff: probiotics, the intestinal microbiome and the quest for long life. *Front. Public Health* 1:52. doi: 10.3389/fpubh.2013.00052

Majamaa, H., and Isolauri, E. (1997). Probiotics: a novel approach in the management of food allergy. *J. Allergy Clin. Immunol.* 2, 179–185. doi: 10.1016/S0091-6749(97)70093-9

Malka, D., Vasseur, D., Bodeker, H., Ortiz, E. M., Dusetti, N. J., Verrando, P., et al. (2000). Tumor necrosis factor triggers antiapoptotic mechanisms in rat pancreatic cells through pancreatitis-associated protein I activation. *Gastroenterology* 119, 816–828. doi: 10.1053/gast.2000.16491

Mattar, A., Teitelbaum, D. H., Drongowski, R., Yongyi, F., Harmon, C., and Coran, A. (2002). Probiotics up-regulate MUC-2 mucin gene expression in a Caco-2 cell-culture model. *Pediatr. Surg. Int.* 18, 586–590. doi: 10.1007/s00383-002-0855-7

Mercenier, A. (1999). "Lactic acid bacteria as live vaccines," in *Probiotics: A Critical Review*, ed. G. Tannock (Wymondham: Horizon Scientific Press), 113–127.

Mierau, I., and Kleerebezem, M. (2005). 10 years of the nisin-controlled gene expression system (NICE) in *Lactococcus lactis*. *Appl. Microbiol. Biotechnol.* 68, 705–717. doi: 10.1007/s00253-005-0107-6

Miyoshi, A., Bermúdez-Humarán, L., Azevedo, M. P. D., Langella, P., and Azevedo, V. (2010). "Lactic acid bacteria as live vectors: heterologous protein production and delivery systems," in *Biotechnology of Lactic Acid Bacteria Novel Applications*, eds F. Mozzi, R. Raya, and G. Vignolo (Ames, IA: Blackwell Publishing), 9. doi: 10.1002/9780813820866.ch9

Miyoshi, A., Jamet, E., Commissaire, J., Renault, P., Langella, P., and Azevedo, V. (2004). A xylose-inducible expression system for *Lactococcus lactis*. *FEMS Microbiol. Lett.* 239, 205–212. doi: 10.1016/j.femsle.2004.08.018

Moal, V. L.-L., Sarrazin-Davila, L. E., and Servin, A. L. (2007). An experimental study and a randomized, double-blind, placebo-controlled clinical trial to evaluate the antisecretory activity of *Lactobacillus acidophilus* strain LB against nonrotavirus diarrhea. *Pediatrics* 120:e795-803. doi: 10.1542/peds.2006--2930

Molodecky, N. A., Soon, I. S., Rabi, D. M., Ghali, W. A., Ferris, M., Chernoff, G., et al. (2012). Increasing incidence and prevalence of the inflammatory bowel diseases with time, based on systematic review. *Gastroenterology* 142, 46–54.e42; quiz e30. doi: 10.1053/j.gastro.2011.10.001

Nauta, A., van Sinderen, D., Karsens, H., Smit, E., Venema, G., and Kok, J. (1996). Inducible gene expression mediated by a repressor-operator system isolated from *Lactococcus lactis* bacteriophage r1t. *Mol. Microbiol.* 19, 1331–1341. doi: 10.1111/j.1365-2958.1996.tb02477.x

Neutra, M. R., and Kozlowski, P. A. (2006). Mucosal vaccines: the promise and the challenge. *Nat. Rev. Immunol.* 6, 148–158. doi: 10.1038/nri1777

Ng, S. C., Hart, A. L., Kamm, M. A., Stagg, A. J., and Knight, S. C. (2009). Mechanisms of action of probiotics: recent advances. *Inflamm. Bowel Dis.* 15, 300–310. doi: 10.1002/ibd.20602

Nishitani, Y., Tanoue, T., Yamada, K., Ishida, T., Yoshida, M., Azuma, T., et al. (2009). *Lactococcus lactis* subsp. *cremoris* FC alleviates symptoms of colitis induced by dextran sulfate sodium in mice. *Int. Immunopharmacol.* 9, 1444–1451. doi: 10.1016/j.intimp.2009.08.018

Nouaille, S., Ribeiro, L. A., Miyoshi, A., Pontes, D., Le Loir, Y., Oliveira, S. C., et al. (2003). Heterologous protein production and delivery systems for *Lactococcus lactis*. *Genet. Mol. Res.* 31, 102–111.

Ogawa, J., Matsumura, K., Kishino, S., Omura, Y., and Shimizu, S. (2001). Conjugated linoleic acid accumulation via 10-hydroxy-12-octadecaenoic acid during microaerobic transformation of linoleic acid by *Lactobacillus acidophilus*. *Appl. Environ. Microbiol.* 67, 1246–1252. doi: 10.1128/AEM.67.3.1246-1252.2001

Ohland, C. L., and MacNaughton, W. K. (2010). Probiotic bacteria and intestinal epithelial barrier function. *Am. J. Physiol. Gastrointest. Liver Physiol.* 298, G807–G819. doi: 10.1152/ajpgi.00243.2009

O'Sullivan, D. J. (2001). Screening of intestinal microflora for effective probiotic bacteria. *J. Agric. Food Chem.* 49, 1751–1760. doi: 10.1021/jf0012244

Ouwehand, A. C., Salminen, S., and Isolauri, E. (2002). Probiotics: an overview of beneficial effects. *Antonie Van Leeuwenhoek* 82, 279–289. doi: 10.1023/A:1020620607611

Pedroso, S. H. S. P., Vieira, A. T., Bastos, R. W., Oliveira, J. S., Cartelle, C. T., Arantes, R. M. E., et al. (2015). Evaluation of mucositis induced by irinotecan after microbial colonization in germ-free mice. *Microbiology* 161, 1950–1960. doi: 10.1099/mic.0.000149

Pereira, V. B., Saraiva, T. D. L., Souza, B. M., Zurita-Turk, M., Azevedo, M. S. P., Castro, C. P. D., et al. (2014). Development of a new DNA vaccine based on mycobacterial ESAT-6 antigen delivered by recombinant invasive *Lactococcus lactis* FnBPA+. *Appl. Microbiol. Biotechnol.* 99, 1817–1826. doi: 10.1007/s00253-014-6285-3

Peterson, L. W., and Artis, D. (2014). Intestinal epithelial cells: regulators of barrier function and immune homeostasis. *Nat. Rev. Immunol.* 14, 141–153. doi: 10.1038/nri3608

Piard, J. C., Hautefort, I., Fischetti, V. A., Ehrlich, S. D., Fons, M., and Gruss, A. (1997). Cell wall anchoring of the *Streptococcus pyogenes* M6 protein in various lactic acid bacteria. *J. Bacteriol.* 179, 3068–3072. doi: 10.1128/jb.179.9.3068-3072.1997

Pontes, D. S., de Azevedo, M. S. P., Chatel, J.-M., Langella, P., Azevedo, V., and Miyoshi, A. (2011). *Lactococcus lactis* as a live vector: heterologous protein production and DNA delivery systems. *Protein Expr. Purif.* 79, 165–175. doi: 10.1016/j.pep.2011.06.005

Prescott, S. L., and Björkstén, B. (2007). Probiotics for the prevention or treatment of allergic diseases. *J. Allergy Clin. Immunol.* 120, 255–262. doi: 10.1016/j.jaci.2007.04.027

Prisciandaro, L. D., Geier, M. S., Chua, A. E., Butler, R. N., Cummins, A. G., Sander, G. R., et al. (2012). Probiotic factors partially prevent changes to caspases 3 and 7 activation and transepithelial electrical resistance in a model of 5-fluorouracil-induced epithelial cell damage. *Support Care Cancer* 20, 3205–3210. doi: 10.1007/s00520-012-1446-3

Qiao, H., Duffy, L. C., Griffiths, E., Dryja, D., Leavens, A., Rossman, J., et al. (2002). Immune responses in rhesus rotavirus-challenged Balb/c mice treated with bifidobacteria and prebiotic supplements. *Pediatr. Res.* 51, 750–755. doi: 10.1203/00006450-200206000-00015

Qiu, Z. B., Chen, J., Chen, J. J., Rong, L., Ding, W. Q., Yang, H. J., et al. (2013). Effect of recombinant *Lactobacillus casei* expressing interleukin-10 in dextran sulfate sodium-induced colitis mice. *J. Dig. Dis.* 14, 76–83. doi: 10.1111/1751-2980.12006

Quinto, E. J., Jiménez, P., Caro, I., Tejero, J., Mateo, J., and Girbés, T. (2014). Probiotic lactic acid bacteria: a review. *Food Nutr. Sci.* 5, 1765–1775. doi: 10.4236/fns.2014.518190

Ren, C., Zhang, Q., de Haan, B. J., Zhang, H., Faas, M. M., and de Vos, P. (2016). Identification of TLR2/TLR6 signalling lactic acid bacteria for supporting immune regulation. *Sci. Rep.* 6:34561. doi: 10.1038/srep34561

Rochat, T., Bermúdez-Humarán, L., Gratadoux, J. J., Fourage, C., Hoebler, C., Corthier, G., et al. (2007). Anti-inflammatory effects of *Lactobacillus casei* BL23 producing or not a manganese-dependant catalase on DSS-induced colitis in mice. *Microb. Cell Fact.* 6:22. doi: 10.1186/1475-2859-6-22

Rochat, T., Miyoshi, A., Gratadoux, J. J., Duwat, P., Sourice, S., Azevedo, V., et al. (2005). High-level resistance to oxidative stress in *Lactococcus lactis* conferred by *Bacillus subtilis* catalase KatE. *Microbiology* 151, 3011–3018. doi: 10.1099/mic.0.27861-0

Rottiers, P., Caluwaerts, S., Steidler, L., Vandenbroucke, K., Watkins, B., Sonis, S., et al. (2009). Effect of a mouth rinse formulation with human trefoil factor 1-secreting *Lactococcus lactis* in experimental oral mucositis in hamsters. *J. Clin. Oncol.* 27:e14570.

Ruiz, P., Alvarez-Martin, B., Mayo, C. G., de los Reyes-Gavilan, M., and Gueimonde, A. (2012). Controlled gene expression in bifidobacteria by use of a bile-responsive element. *Appl. Environ. Microbiol.* 78, 581–585. doi: 10.1128/AEM.06611-11

Salzman, N. H., Underwood, M. A., and Bevins, C. L. (2007). Paneth cells, defensins, and the commensal microbiota: a hypothesis on intimate interplay at the intestinal mucosa. *Semin. Immunol.* 19, 70–83. doi: 10.1016/j.smim.2007.04.002

Santos Rocha, C., Gomes-Santos, A. C., Garcias Moreira, T., de Azevedo, M., Diniz Luerce, T., Mariadassou, M., et al. (2014). Local and systemic immune mechanisms underlying the anti-colitis effects of the dairy *Bacterium Lactobacillus* delbrueckii. *PLoS ONE* 9:e85923. doi: 10.1371/journal.pone.0085923

Schlee, M., Harder, J., Köten, B., Stange, E. F., Wehkamp, J., and Fellermann, K. (2008). Probiotic lactobacilli and VSL#3 induce enterocyte β-defensin 2. *Clin. Exp. Immunol.* 151, 528–535. doi: 10.1111/j.1365-2249.2007.03587.x

Schotte, L., Steidler, L., Vandekerckhove, J., and Remaut, E. (2000). Secretion of biologically active murine interleukin-10 by *Lactococcus lactis*. *Enzyme Microb. Technol.* 27, 761–765. doi: 10.1016/S0141-0229(00)00297-0

Seo, E., Weibel, S., Wehkamp, J., and Oelschlaeger, T. A. (2012). Construction of recombinant *E. coli* Nissle 1917 (EcN) strains for the expression and secretion of defensins. *Int. J. Med. Microbiol.* 302, 276–287. doi: 10.1016/j.ijmm.2012.05.002

Shortle, D. (1983). A genetic system for analysis of staphylococcal nuclease. *Gene* 22, 181–189. doi: 10.1016/0378-1119(83)90102-6

Shu, Q., and Gill, H. S. (2001). A dietary probiotic (*Bifidobacterium lactis* HN019) reduces the severity of *Escherichia coli* O157:H7 infection in mice. *Med. Microbiol. Immunol.* 189, 147–152. doi: 10.1007/s430-001-8021-9

Smith, C. L., Geier, M. S., Yazbeck, R., Torres, D. M., Butler, R. N., and Howarth, G. S. (2008). *Lactobacillus fermentum* BR11 and fructo-oligosaccharide partially reduce jejunal inflammation in a model of intestinal mucositis in rats. *Nutr. Cancer* 60, 757–767. doi: 10.1080/01635580802192841

Soares, P. M. G., Mota, J. M. S. C., Souza, E. P., Justino, P. F. C., Franco, A. X., Cunha, F. Q., et al. (2013). Inflammatory intestinal damage induced by 5-fluorouracil requires IL-4. *Cytokine* 61, 46–49. doi: 10.1016/j.cyto.2012.10.003

Southcott, E., Tooley, K. L., Howarth, G. S., Davidson, G. P., and Butler, R. N. (2008). Yoghurts containing probiotics reduce disruption of the small intestinal barrier in methotrexate-treated rats. *Dig. Dis. Sci.* 53, 1837–1841. doi: 10.1007/s10620-008-0275-1

Steidler, L., Hans, W., Schotte, L., Neirynck, S., Obermeier, F., Falk, W., et al. (2000). Treatment of murine colitis by *Lactococcus lactis* secreting interleukin-10. *Science* 289, 1352–1355. doi: 10.1126/science.289.5483.1352

Steidler, L., Neirynck, S., Huyghebaert, N., Snoeck, V., Vermeire, A., Goddeeris, B., et al. (2003). Biological containment of genetically modified *Lactococcus lactis* for intestinal delivery of human interleukin 10. *Nat. Biotechnol.* 21, 785–789. doi: 10.1038/nbt840

Stepaniuk, P., Bernstein, C. N., Targownik, L. E., and Singh, H. (2015). Characterization of inflammatory bowel disease in elderly patients: a review of epidemiology, current practices and outcomes of current management strategies. *Can. J. Gastroenterol. Hepatol.* 29, 327–333. doi: 10.1155/2015/136960

Stiles, M. E., and Holzapfel, W. H. (1997). Lactic acid bacteria of foods and their current taxonomy. *Int. J. Food Microbiol.* 36, 1–29. doi: 10.1016/S0168-1605(96)01233-0

Strober, W., Fuss, I., and Mannon, P. (2007). The fundamental basis of inflammatory bowel disease. *J. Clin. Invest.* 117, 514–521. doi: 10.1172/JCI30587

Strukelj, B., Perse, M., Ravnikar, M., Lunder, M., Cerar, A., and Berlec, A. (2014). Improvement in treatment of experimental colitis in mice by using recombinant *Lactococcus lactis* with surface-displayed affibody against TNFα (THER4P.889). *J. Immunol.* 192, 137.1–137.1.

Thomas, H. (2016). IBD: Probiotics for IBD: a need for histamine? *Nat. Rev. Gastroenterol. Hepatol.* 13, 62–63. doi: 10.1038/nrgastro.2016.2

Tooley, K. L., Howarth, G. S., Lymn, K. A., Lawrence, A., and Butler, R. N. (2006). Oral ingestion of streptococcus thermophilus diminishes severity of small intestinal mucositis in methotrexate treated rats. *Cancer Biol. Ther.* 5, 593–600. doi: 10.4161/cbt.5.6.2659

Tooley, K. L., Howarth, G. S., Lymn, K. A., Lawrence, A., and Butler, R. N. (2011). Oral ingestion of *Streptococcus thermophilus* does not affect mucositis severity or tumor progression in the tumor-bearing rat. *Cancer Biol. Ther.* 12, 131–138. doi: 10.4161/cbt.12.2.15720

van Asseldonk, M., Rutten, G., Oteman, M., Siezen, R. J., De Vos, W. M., and Simons, G. (1990). Cloning of usp45, a gene encoding a secreted protein from *Lactococcus lactis* subsp. *lactis* MG1363. *Gene* 95, 155–160. doi: 10.1016/0378-1119(90)90428-T

van Rooijen, R. J., Gasson, M. J., and de Vos, W. M. (1992). Characterization of the *Lactococcus lactis* lactose operon promoter: contribution of flanking sequences and LacR repressor to promoter activity. *J. Bacteriol.* 174, 2273–2280. doi: 10.1128/jb.174.7.2273-2280.1992

Vandermeulen, G., Marie, C., Scherman, D., and Préat, V. (2011). New generation of plasmid backbones devoid of antibiotic resistance marker for gene therapy trials. *Mol. Ther.* 19, 1942–1949. doi: 10.1038/mt.2011.182

Vangay, P., Ward, T., Gerber, J. S., and Knights, D. (2015). Antibiotics, pediatric dysbiosis, and disease. *Cell Host Microbe* 17, 553–564. doi: 10.1016/j.chom.2015.04.006

Velasquez-Manoff, M. (2015). Gut microbiome: the peacekeepers. *Nature* 518, S3–S11. doi: 10.1038/518S3a

Vicariotto, F., Del Piano, M., Mogna, L., and Mogna, G. (2012). Effectiveness of the association of 2 probiotic strains formulated in a slow release vaginal product, in women affected by vulvovaginal candidiasis: a pilot study. *J. Clin. Gastroenterol.* 46, S73–S80. doi: 10.1097/MCG.0b013e3182684d71

Vikhanski, L. (2016). *Immunity: How Elie Metchnikoff Changed the Course of Modern Medicine.* Chicago, IL: Chicago Review Press.

Villena, J., and Kitazawa, H. (2014). Modulation of intestinal TLR4-inflammatory signaling pathways by probiotic microorganisms: lessons learned from *Lactobacillus jensenii* TL2937. *Front. Immunol.* 4:512. doi: 10.3389/fimmu.2013.00512

Wang, M., Gao, Z., Zhang, Y., and Pan, L. (2016). Lactic acid bacteria as mucosal delivery vehicles: a realistic therapeutic option. *Appl. Microbiol. Biotechnol.* 100, 5691–5701. doi: 10.1007/s00253-016-7557-x

Watterlot, L., Rochat, T., Sokol, H., Cherbuy, C., Bouloufa, I., Lefèvre, F., et al. (2010). Intragastric administration of a superoxide dismutase-producing recombinant *Lactobacillus casei* BL23 strain attenuates DSS colitis in mice. *Int. J. Food Microbiol.* 144, 35–41. doi: 10.1016/j.ijfoodmicro.2010.03.037

Wells, J. M., and Mercenier, A. (2008). Mucosal delivery of therapeutic and prophylactic molecules using lactic acid bacteria. *Nat. Rev. Microbiol.* 6, 349–362. doi: 10.1038/nrmicro1840

Wells, J. M., Wilson, P. W., Norton, P. M., Gasson, M. J., and Le PageR, W. (1993). *Lactococcus lactis*: high-level expression of tetanus toxin fragment C and protection against lethal challenge. *Mol. Microbiol.* 8, 1155–1162. doi: 10.1111/j.1365-2958.1993.tb01660.x

Westendorf, A. M., Gunzer, F., Deppenmeier, S., Tapadar, D., Hunger, J. K., Schmidt, M. A., et al. (2005). Intestinal immunity of *Escherichia coli* NISSLE 1917: a safe carrier for therapeutic molecules. *FEMS Immunol. Med. Microbiol.* 43, 373–384. doi: 10.1016/j.femsim.2004.10.023

Whitford, E. J., Cummins, A. G., Butler, R. N., Prisciandaro, L. D., Fauser, J. K., Yazbeck, R., et al. (2009). Effects of *Streptococcus thermophilus* TH-4 on intestinal mucositis induced by the chemotherapeutic agent, 5-Fluorouracil (5-FU). *Cancer Biol. Ther.* 8, 505–511. doi: 10.4161/cbt.8.6.7594

Wong, C. C. M., Zhang, L., Li, Z. J., Wu, W. K. K., Ren, S. X., Chen, Y. C., et al. (2012). Protective effects of cathelicidin-encoding *Lactococcus lactis* in murine ulcerative colitis. *J. Gastroenterol. Hepatol.* 27, 1205–1212. doi: 10.1111/j.1440-1746.2012.07158.x

Yoshida, H., and Miyazaki, Y. (2008). Regulation of immune responses by interleukin-27. *Immunol. Rev.* 226, 234–247. doi: 10.1111/j.1600-065X.2008.00710.x

11

Serine-Rich Repeat Adhesins Contribute to *Streptococcus gordonii*-Induced Maturation of Human Dendritic Cells

Eun Byeol Ko[1], Sun Kyung Kim[1], Ho Seong Seo[2], Cheol-Heui Yun[3] and Seung Hyun Han[1]*

[1] Department of Oral Microbiology and Immunology, DRI, and BK21 Plus Program, School of Dentistry, Seoul National University, Seoul, South Korea, [2] Biotechnology Research Division, Korea Atomic Energy Research Institute, Jeongeup, South Korea, [3] Department of Agricultural Biotechnology and Research Institute for Agriculture and Life Sciences, Seoul National University, Seoul, South Korea

Edited by:
Julio Villena,
Reference Centre for Lactobacilli (CERELA-CONICET), Argentina

Reviewed by:
Hans-Gerhard Burgert,
University of Warwick, UK
Haruki Kitazawa,
Tohoku University, Japan

***Correspondence:**
Seung Hyun Han
shhan-mi@snu.ac.kr

Dendritic cells (DCs) play a pivotal role in the induction of immunity by recognition, capture, process, and presentation of antigens from infectious microbes. *Streptococcus gordonii* is able to cause life-threatening systemic diseases such as infective endocarditis. Serine-rich repeat (SRR) glycoproteins of *S. gordonii* are sialic acid-binding adhesins mediating the bacterial adherence to the host and the development of infective endocarditis. Thus, the SRR adhesins are potentially involved in the bacterial adherence to DCs and the maturation and activation of DCs required for the induction of immunity to *S. gordonii*. Here, we investigated the phenotypic and functional changes of human monocyte-derived DCs treated with wild-type *S. gordonii* or the SRR adhesin-deficient mutant. The mutant poorly bound to DCs and only weakly increased the expression of CD83, CD86, MHC class II, and PD-L1 on DCs compared with the wild-type. In addition, the mutant induced lower levels of TNF-α, IL-6, and IL-12 than the wild-type in DCs. When DCs sensitized with the mutant were co-cultured with autologous T cells, they induced weaker proliferation and activation of T cells than DCs stimulated with the wild-type. Blockade of SRR adhesin with 3′-sialyllactose markedly reduced *S. gordonii* binding and internalization, causing attenuation of the bacterial immunostimulatory potency in DC maturation. Collectively, our results suggest that SRR adhesins of *S. gordonii* are important for maturation and activation of DCs.

Keywords: *Streptococcus gordonii*, serine-rich repeat adhesins, dendritic cells, maturation, T cell activation

INTRODUCTION

Streptococcus gordonii is a Gram-positive facultative anaerobic bacterium belonging to the viridans group of oral streptococci (Loo et al., 2000). Although *S. gordonii* is a part of the normal flora in the oral cavity, it is able to cause various infectious diseases such as septic arthritis (Yombi et al., 2012) and life-threatening infective endocarditis with high mortality (Keane et al., 2010) through systemic spread following tooth extraction, brushing, or flossing (Forner et al., 2006). Upon entering the bloodstream, *S. gordonii* preferentially binds to human platelets, causing their aggregation, facilitating bacterial colonization in the endocardium and heart valves and resulting in endocarditis (Takahashi et al., 2006). Previous studies have shown that oral streptococci associated with endocarditis promote rapid differentiation of monocytes into mature dendritic cells (DCs) (Hahn et al., 2005) and *S. gordonii* induces the secretion of cytokines including TNF-α, IL-6, and IL-12 in DCs (Corinti et al., 1999), implying the importance of DCs in the disease development and immune responses.

Bacterial adherence is an important step for microbial pathogenesis (Moschioni et al., 2010). As one of the initial colonizers of dental biofilms, *S. gordonii* abundantly expresses diverse adhesins that mediate its binding to host tissues. *S. gordonii* utilizes serine-rich repeat (SRR) adhesins, antigen I/II family proteins, cell-surface fibrillar proteins, and amylase-binding proteins to bind to human platelets and monocytes (Takahashi et al., 2004; Urano-Tashiro et al., 2012). Among them, SRR adhesins play an important role in the development of infective endocarditis (Xiong et al., 2008; Jakubovics et al., 2009). *S. gordonii* adheres to sialic acids on platelets or erythrocytes through SRR adhesins in injured heart valves, exacerbating inflammatory responses by promoting deposition of bacterium-platelet-fibrin complexes and recruiting inflammatory immune cells in tissues (Yajima et al., 2008).

Serine-rich repeat adhesins are sialoglycan-binding glycoproteins expressed on the surface of Gram-positive bacteria. They consist of conserved domains including an N-terminal signal peptide, a short SRR region, a ligand-binding basic region (BR) (Jakubovics et al., 2009), a long SRR region, and a C-terminal cell wall-anchoring domain (Bensing et al., 2016). Although the domains are conserved, BRs are highly divergent in amino acid sequence conferring the binding specificity to their cognate ligand (Takamatsu et al., 2005). For instance, Hsa and GspB, which are homologous SRR adhesins expressed on *S. gordonii* CH1 and M99 strains, respectively, have different BR structures with distinct binding ability: Hsa binds to both 3′-sialyllactose and sialyl-T antigen, whereas GspB binds only to sialyl-T antigen (Urano-Tashiro et al., 2016).

Dendritic cells are antigen-presenting cells that link the innate and adaptive immune responses (Steinman, 2006). Under infectious conditions, DCs exert various functions as sentinels; they recognize, phagocytose, and process infecting microbes to present the microbial epitopes to naïve T lymphocytes (Kapsenberg, 2003). Upon sensing antigens, DCs upregulate the expression of MHC proteins and co-stimulatory molecules such as CD40, CD80, and CD86. DCs also produce cytokines such as TNF-α, IL-6, and IL-12p70 that result in activation and differentiation of T lymphocytes. Mature DCs can migrate to draining lymph nodes to present antigens to T lymphocytes and induce antigen-specific adaptive immune responses (Mempel et al., 2004).

Serine-rich repeat adhesins of *S. gordonii* are important for this microbe to bind to host cells. This interaction appears to be critical in bacterial infection and host immunity. In the present study, we investigated the role of *S. gordonii* SRR adhesins, Hsa and GspB, in maturation and activation of human DCs treated with wild-type *S. gordonii* and SRR adhesin-deficient mutant strains.

MATERIALS AND METHODS

Reagents and Chemicals

Ficoll-Paque PLUS was obtained from GE Healthcare (Uppsala, Sweden). Penicillin-streptomycin solution and RPMI-1640 were purchased from Hyclone (Logan, UT, USA). Fetal bovine serum (FBS) was purchased from GIBCO (Grand Island, NY, USA). Recombinant human granulocyte macrophage-colony stimulating factor (GM-CSF) and IL-4 were purchased from R&D Systems (Minneapolis, MN, USA) and CreaGene (Sungnam, Korea), respectively. Anti-human CD14 magnetic particles and anti-human CD3 magnetic particles were purchased from BD Biosciences (San Diego, CA, USA). Dimethyl sulfoxide, Red Blood Cell Lysis Buffer, and cytochalasin D were purchased from Sigma–Aldrich (St. Louis, MO, USA). 5-(and-6)-Carboxyfluorescein diacetate succinimidyl ester (CFDA-SE) was obtained from Molecular Probes (Eugene, OR, USA). PE-labeled anti-human CD83, APC-labeled anti-human CD86, APC-labeled anti-human PD-L1, and APC-labeled anti-human CD25 antibodies were purchased from BioLegend (San Diego, CA, USA). FITC-labeled anti-human HLA-DR, DP, and DQ antibodies for MHC class II were obtained from BD Biosciences. All isotype-matched antibodies were obtained from BioLegend or BD Biosciences. Enzyme-linked immunosorbent assay (ELISA) kits for measuring the concentrations of TNF-α, IL-12p70, and IL-6 were purchased from BioLegend. Todd Hewitt broth was obtained from MB Cell (Seoul, South Korea). Bacto^{TM} yeast extract and Bacto^{TM} agar were purchased from BD Biosciences (Sparks, MD, USA). 3′-Sialyllactose (3′SL) was purchased from Cayman Chemical Company (Ann Arbor, MI, USA).

Generation of Human Monocyte-Derived DCs

All experiments using human blood were conducted under approval of the Institutional Review Board at Seoul National University, South Korea. The Korean Red Cross provided blood from healthy human donors after obtaining informed consent. Peripheral blood mononuclear cells (PBMCs) were isolated using Ficoll-Paque PLUS, as previously described (Kim et al., 2013). PBMCs were then incubated with CD14 magnetic beads for 30 min at room temperature, followed by separation in a magnetic field to isolate CD14^{+} monocytes. The purified CD14^{+} monocytes were suspended in RPMI-1640 supplemented with 10% FBS, 1% penicillin-streptomycin solution, 5 ng/ml GM-CSF, and 10 ng/ml IL-4 and were seeded in 60-mm cell culture dishes at a density of 2×10^6 cells/ml. The monocytes were cultured for 5 days to differentiate into immature DCs. Culture media supplemented with GM-CSF and IL-4 was changed every 3 days.

Bacteria and Culture Conditions

Wild-type *S. gordonii* CH1 and M99 strains, the Hsa-deficient mutant strain PS798, and the GspB-deficient mutant strain PS846 were kindly provided by Dr. Paul M. Sullam (University of California at San Francisco). The mutants were generated by double cross-over recombination, as described previously

(Bensing et al., 2004; Xiong et al., 2008). All bacteria were cultured in TH media containing 0.5% yeast extract until mid-log phase at 37°C. The mutant strains grew comparably well *in vitro* (data not shown). Bacterial cells were harvested by centrifugation at 8,000 rpm for 10 min at 37°C and were washed with PBS. To prepare stocks of wild-type *S. gordonii* and mutant strains, the bacterial pellet was suspended in 50% glycerol THY media to 5×10^8 CFU/ml and stored at −80°C in a freezer.

Analysis of Bacterial Adherence and Internalization

To label *S. gordonii* with CFSE, the bacterial pellet was suspended in 1 ml PBS containing 10 μM CFDA-SE and incubated for 15 min at 37°C. The bacterial cells were then washed with PBS. Immature DCs (5×10^4 cells) were incubated with either CFSE-labeled wild-type *S. gordonii* or SRR adhesin-deficient mutant strains at 5×10^5, 5×10^6, or 5×10^7 CFU in 50 μl PBS for 1 h at 4°C or 37°C, respectively. Flow cytometry (FACSCalibur, BD Biosciences) was used to measure bacterial binding at 4°C and internalization at 37°C. All cytometric data were analyzed using FlowJo software (TreeStar, San Carlos, CA, USA).

Analysis of DC Phenotypes

Immature DCs (2.5×10^5 cells/ml) were stimulated with either wild-type *S. gordonii* or SRR adhesin-deficient mutant (1×10^6 CFU/ml) in the presence of GM-CSF (2.5 ng/ml) and IL-4 (5 ng/ml). After 1 h, gentamycin (200 μg/ml) was added to the culture to prevent the bacterial growth and the DCs were further incubated for 23 h. The DCs were stained with fluorochrome-conjugated monoclonal antibodies specific to CD83, CD86, MHC class II, and PD-L1 for 30 min on ice and washed with PBS. The mean fluorescence intensity (MFI) of DCs was analyzed by FACSCalibur, and all flow cytometry data were analyzed by FlowJo software.

Quantification of Cytokines

Immature DCs (2.5×10^5 cells/ml) were stimulated with either wild-type *S. gordonii* or an SRR adhesin-deficient mutant (1×10^6 CFU/ml) in the presence of GM-CSF and IL-4. To kill *S. gordonii*, gentamicin was added to the DCs, and cells were further incubated for 23 h. Concentrations of TNF-α, IL-12p70, and IL-6 in the culture supernatants were measured by ELISA kits, as described previously (Lee et al., 2015).

Co-culture of DCs with Autologous T Lymphocytes

Immature DCs (2.5×10^5 cells/ml) were stimulated with either wild-type *S. gordonii* or an SRR adhesin-deficient mutant (1×10^6 CFU/ml) in the presence of GM-CSF and IL-4. After 1 h, DCs were treated with gentamycin to kill *S. gordonii* and were further incubated for another 15 h. To isolate $CD3^+$ T lymphocytes, PBMCs were incubated with anti-human CD3 magnetic particles for 30 min at room temperature. $CD3^+$ cells were isolated by positive selection according to the manufacturer's instruction. To label isolated $CD3^+$ T lymphocytes with CFSE, the cells were incubated in RPMI-1640 supplemented with 10% FBS, 1% penicillin-streptomycin solution, and 10 μM CFDA-SE for 15 min at 37°C and then washed with PBS. The CFSE-labeled autologous $CD3^+$ T lymphocytes (5×10^4 cells) were mixed with *S. gordonii*-stimulated DCs (5×10^4 cells) for 4 days, and the cells were stained with anti-human CD25 antibody. The proliferative activity and activation marker expression of cells were subsequently analyzed by flow cytometry.

Statistical Analysis

The statistical difference between experimental groups and the control group was analyzed by Student's *t*-test. *P*-values less than 0.05 were considered statistically significant. Results are indicated as mean of triplicated measurements ± standard error of the mean (SEM).

RESULTS

SRR Adhesin-Deficient *S. gordonii* Exhibits Attenuated Binding and Internalization to DCs Compared to the Wild-Type Strain

Bacterial binding and internalization are important processes for DCs to initiate immune responses (Kapsenberg, 2003). The role of SRR adhesins of *S. gordonii* was examined, with focus on Hsa for the CH1 strain and GspB for the M99 strain. Bacterial adherence to DCs was studied at 4°C, while internalization was examined at 37°C. Hsa-deficient *S. gordonii* exhibited attenuated binding and internalizing abilities compared to the wild-type (**Figures 1A,C**). Likewise, GspB-deficient *S. gordonii* more weakly bound and internalized to the DCs than did the wild-type (**Figures 1B,D**). The results indicate that SRR adhesins Hsa and GspB are crucial for the adherence and internalization of *S. gordonii* to DCs.

SRR Adhesin-Deficient *S. gordonii* More Weakly Increases the Expression of Phenotypic Maturation Markers on DCs than Does the Wild-Type Strain

Upon sensing microbial antigens, DCs upregulate a number of molecules such as CD83, CD86, MHC proteins, PD-L1, and PD-L2 to induce an antigen-specific adaptive immune response (Kapsenberg, 2003). To examine the roles of *S. gordonii* Hsa and GspB in inducing phenotypic maturation of DCs, the expression of CD83, CD86, MHC class II, and PD-L1 on DCs upon stimulation with either wild-type *S. gordonii* or an SRR adhesin-deficient mutant was compared. Both wild-type *S. gordonii* CH1 and M99 markedly induced the expression of CD83 (**Figures 2A,E** and Supplementary Figures 1A,E, 2A,E), CD86 (**Figures 2B,F** and Supplementary Figures 1B,F, 2B,F), MHC class II (**Figures 2C,G** and Supplementary Figures 1C,G, 2C,G), and PD-L1 (**Figures 2D,H** and Supplementary Figures 1D,H, 2D,H). However, stimulation with the SRR adhesin-deficient mutant showed lower potency

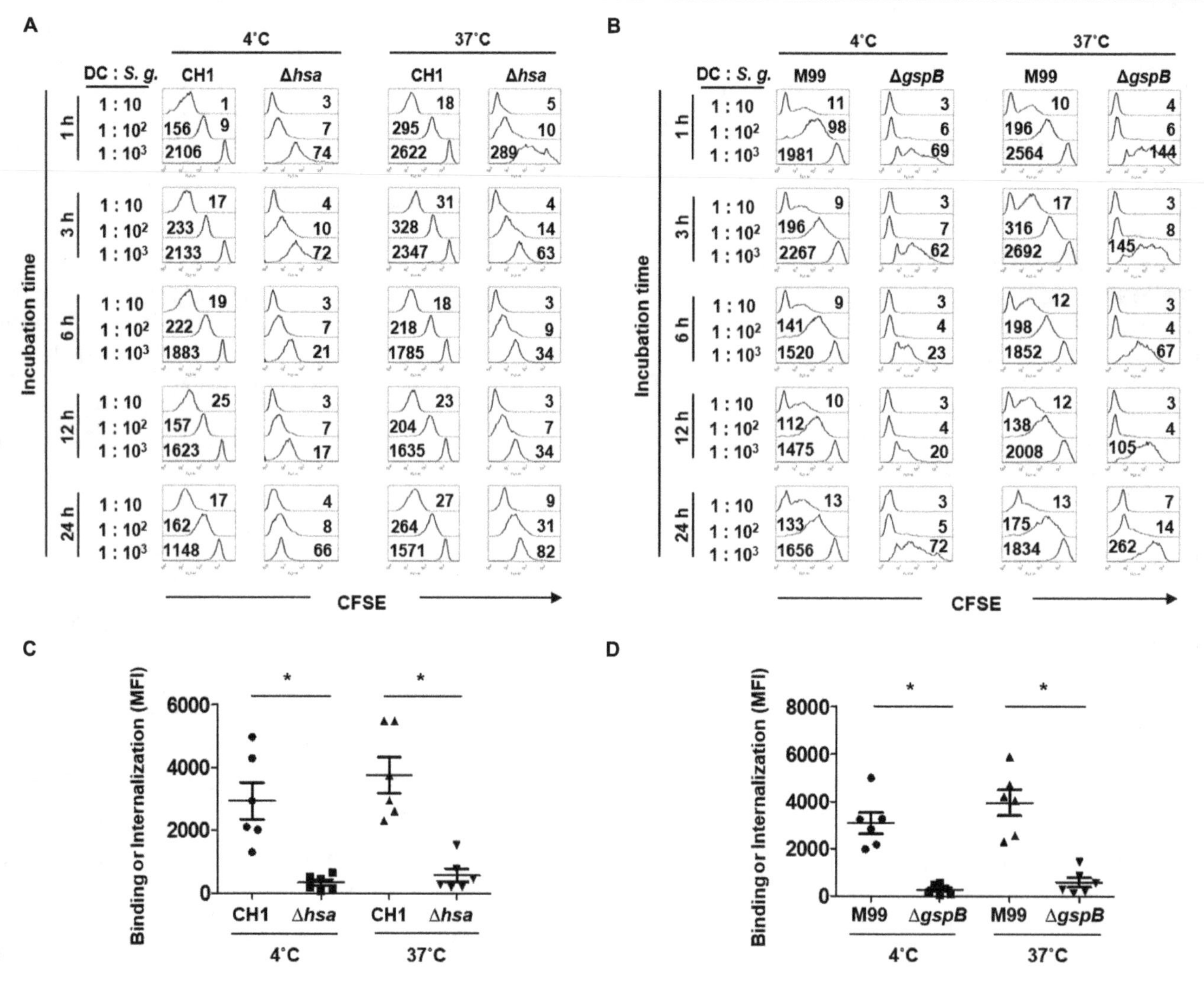

FIGURE 1 | Serine-rich repeat (SRR) adhesin-deficient *Streptococcus gordonii* exhibits attenuated binding and internalization to dendritic cells (DCs). Immature DCs (5×10^4 cells) were co-cultured with CFSE-labeled *S. gordonii* CH1 and M99 strains or their SRR adhesin-deficient mutants (Δ*hsa* for CH1 strain and Δ*gspB* for M99 strain) at 1–10, 10^2, or 10^3 at 4°C (for binding) and 37°C (for internalization). At 1 h after the treatment, gentamycin (200 μg/ml) was added to prevent the bacterial growth followed by incubation for additional 2, 5, 11, or 23 h. Then, the binding and internalization of **(A)** *S. gordonii* CH1 strain and **(B)** M99 strain to DCs were analyzed by flow cytometry. Immature DCs (5×10^4 cells) were co-cultured with CFSE-labeled *S. gordonii* CH1 and M99 strains or their SRR adhesin-deficient mutants (Δ*hsa* for CH1 strain and Δ*gspB* for M99 strain) at 1–10^2 at 4°C (for binding) or 37°C (for internalization) for 1 h. The numbers on the histograms indicate the mean fluorescence intensity (MFI). Binding and internalization of **(C)** *S. gordonii* CH1 strain and **(D)** M99 strain to DCs were analyzed by flow cytometry. Graphs of dot plot represent the mean MFI ± SEM from six independent experiments. Asterisk (*) indicates statistical significance ($P < 0.05$).

in inducing those molecules (**Figures 2A–H** and Supplementary Figures 1A–H, 2A–H). These results indicate that Hsa and GspB of *S. gordonii* contribute to the expression of activation markers on DCs.

SRR Adhesin-Deficient *S. gordonii* Induces Cytokine Production Less Potently than the Wild-Type Bacteria

When DCs are activated, they express cytokines such as IL-12, IL-10, and TNF-α to mediate inflammatory responses and the activation and differentiation of other immune cells including T lymphocytes (Kapsenberg, 2003). Thus, we next examined cytokine production of DCs induced by stimulation with wild-type *S. gordonii* or SRR adhesin-deficient mutants. DCs stimulated with Hsa-deficient mutant (**Figures 3A–C**) or GspB-deficient mutant (**Figures 3D–F**) resulted in significantly lower production of IL-12p70, TNF-α, and IL-6 in the Hsa-deficient CH1 strain as compared to wild-type. Similarly, a substantially lower secretion of these cytokines was also seen in the GspB-deficient mutant as compared to the M99 WT strain. Neither *S. gordonii* CH1 nor M99 strains induced IL-10 production in DCs (data not shown). These results suggest that SRR adhesins play an important role in *S. gordonii*-induced inflammatory cytokine production by DCs.

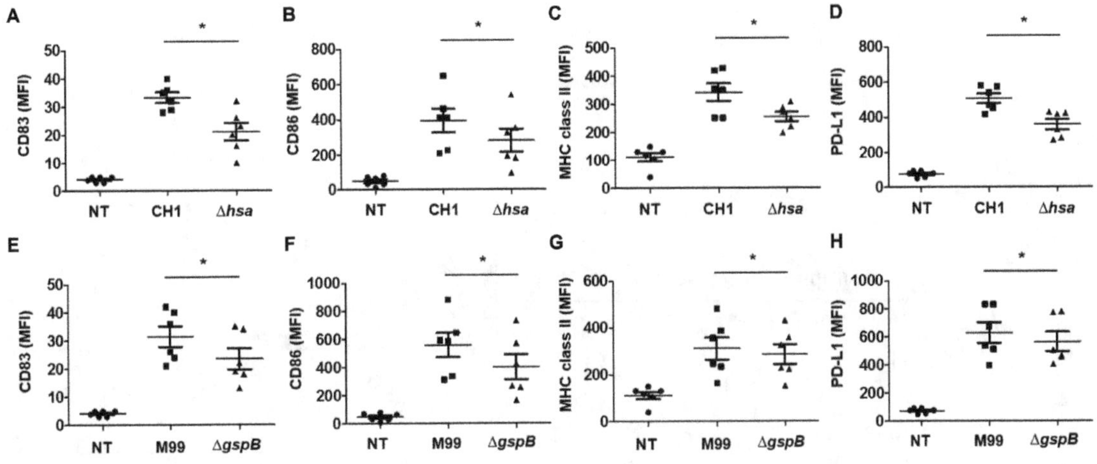

FIGURE 2 | Serine-rich repeat adhesin-deficient *S. gordonii* weakly induces phenotypic maturation of DCs. Immature DCs (2.5×10^5 cells/ml) were stimulated with various concentrations of *S. gordonii* CH1 and M99 strains or their SRR adhesin-deficient strains at 1×10^6 CFU/ml for 24 h. Expression of **(A,E)** CD83, **(B,F)** CD86, **(C,G)** MHC class II, and **(D,H)** PD-L1 on DCs was analyzed by flow cytometry. Graphs of dot plot represent the mean MFI ± SEM from six independent experiments. Asterisk (*) indicates statistical significance ($P < 0.05$). NT, non-treatment.

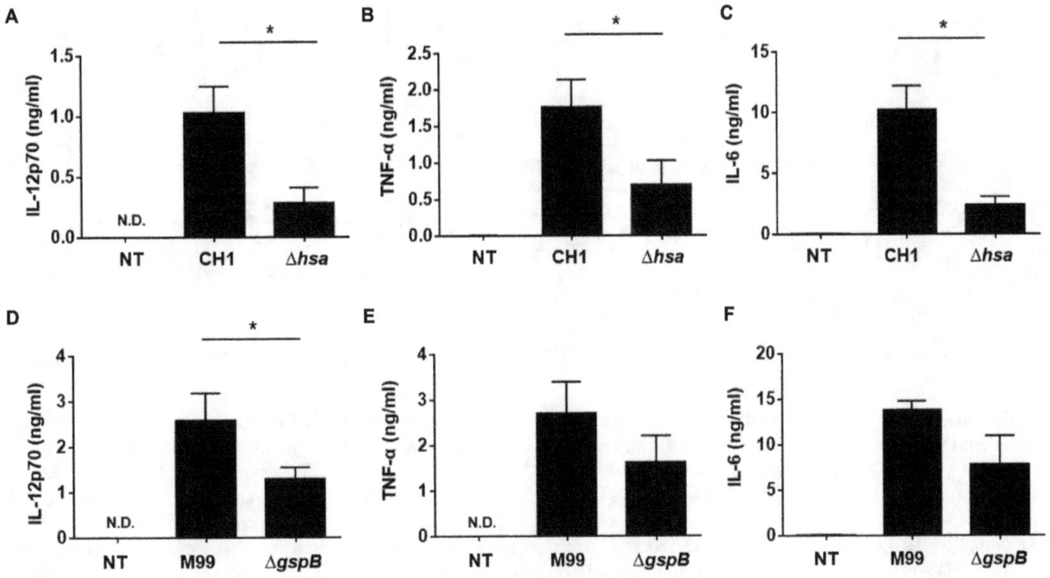

FIGURE 3 | Serine-rich repeat adhesin-deficient *S. gordonii* more weakly induces DC cytokine production than wild-type *S. gordonii*. Immature DCs (2.5×10^5 cells/ml) were stimulated with *S. gordonii* CH1 and M99 strains or their SRR adhesin-deficient strains at 1×10^6 CFU/ml for 24 h. The levels of **(A,D)** IL-12p70, **(B,E)** TNF-α, and **(C,F)** IL-6 in the culture media were measured by ELISA. Concentrations of cytokines are indicated as mean value ± SEM from three independent experiments. Statistical difference between experimental groups was analyzed by Student's *t*-test. *P*-values less than 0.05 were considered statistically significant and are indicated by asterisks (*). N.D., not detected; NT, non-treatment.

DCs Stimulated with SRR Adhesin-Deficient *S. gordonii* More Weakly Induce Proliferation and Activation of Autologous T Cells than DCs Stimulated with Wild-Type *S. gordonii*

Functionally mature DCs exhibit increased expression of MHC proteins, co-stimulatory molecules, and cytokines required for adequate activation of T lymphocytes (Kapsenberg, 2003). To examine the effect of *S. gordonii* SRR adhesins on the T cell-activating capacity of DCs, the proliferative activity and activation marker expression of T lymphocytes were examined through DCs sensitized with wild-type *S. gordonii* or SRR adhesin-deficient mutants. The results showed that Hsa-deficient mutant-sensitized DCs induced proliferation and CD25 expression of T lymphocytes less potently than DCs sensitized with wild-type *S. gordonii* (**Figure 4A**). Likewise, T lymphocytes

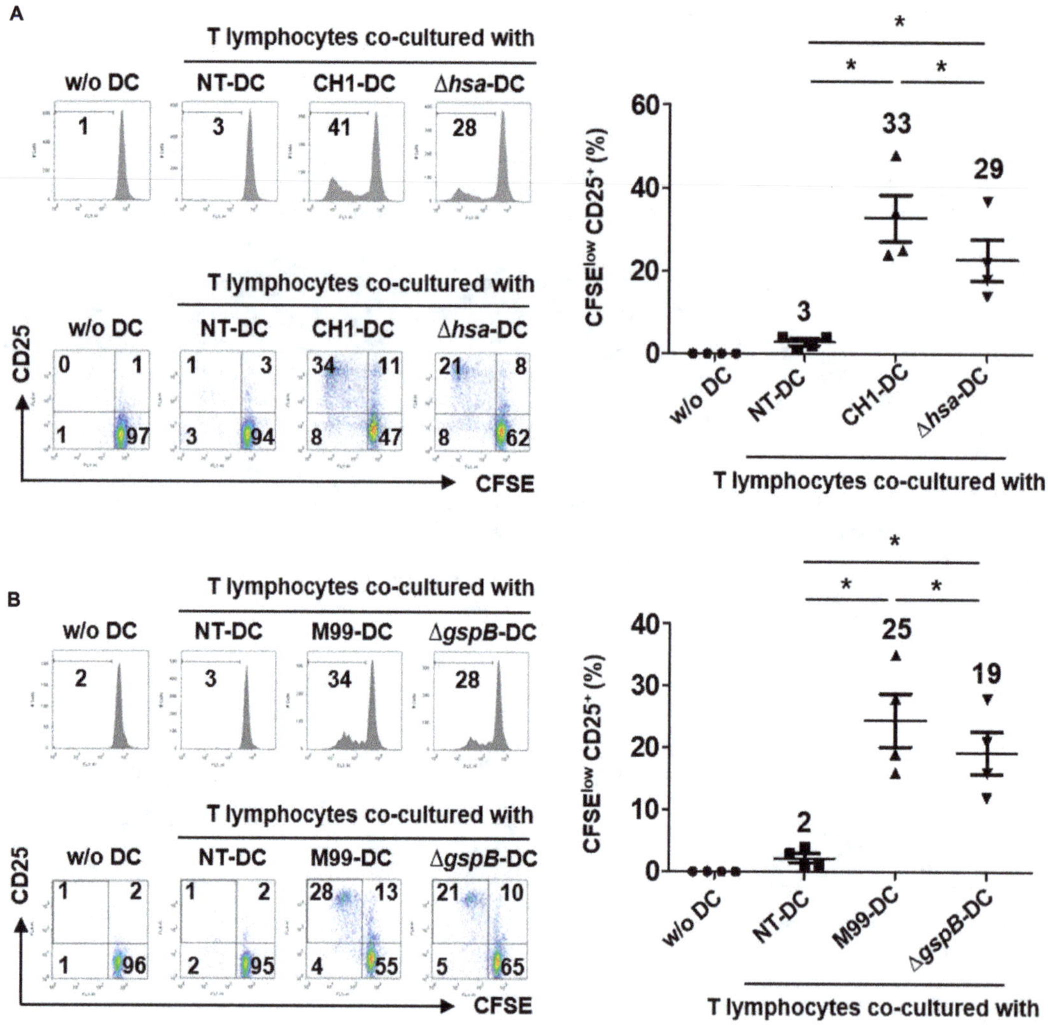

FIGURE 4 | Dendritic cells stimulated with SRR adhesin-deficient *S. gordonii* more weakly induce proliferation and activation of autologous T cells than DCs stimulated with wild-type *S. gordonii*. Immature DCs (2.5×10^5 cells/ml) were stimulated with *S. gordonii* CH1 and M99 strains or their SRR adhesin-deficient strains at 1×10^6 CFU/ml for 16 h. DCs were co-cultured with CFSE-labeled autologous T lymphocytes (2.5×10^5 cells/ml) for 5 days. **(A,B)** Proliferation and CD25 expression of T lymphocytes induced by **(A)** DCs sensitized with *S. gordonii* CH1 strain or its mutant and **(B)** DCs sensitized with *S. gordonii* M99 strain or its mutant were examined by flow cytometry. The numbers in each histogram and quadrant indicate the percentage. Histograms represent the proliferation level of T lymphocytes determined by reduced CFSE fluorescence intensity. Graphs of dot plot indicate the mean values of CFSE^{low} CD25^{+} ± SEM from four independent experiments and the actual mean values are on top of each group. Asterisk (*) indicates statistical significance ($P < 0.05$). NT, non-treatment.

exhibited weakened proliferative activity and activation marker expression in response to GspB-deficient mutant-sensitized DCs (**Figure 4B**). Taken together, these results indicate that Hsa and GspB contribute to DC-mediated immune activation of T lymphocytes by *S. gordonii.*

Blockade of SRR Adhesins Abolishes *S. gordonii* Binding and Internalization to DCs and Attenuates Immunostimulating Potency

Hsa, the SRR adhesion of *S. gordonii* CH1 strain, specifically bind to 3′SL (Urano-Tashiro et al., 2016). In order to further examine the role of Hsa in the bacterial interaction with DCs, *S. gordonii* CH1 strain pretreated with 3′SL (named CH1-SL) was treated with DCs followed by analysis of the bacterial adherence to DCs and phenotypic and functional maturation of DCs. CH1-SL showed marked attenuation in binding and internalizing DCs (**Figure 5A**). In addition, pretreatment with 3′SL abolished the immunostimulatory potency of *S. gordonii.* DCs stimulated with CH1-SL exhibited lower expression of maturation markers such as CD86, MHC class II, and PD-L1 than DCs stimulated with unpretreated *S. gordonii* (**Figure 5B**). Furthermore, stimulation with CH1-SL diminished the production of IL-12p70, TNF-α, and IL-6 by DCs (**Figure 5C**). When CH1-SL-sensitized DCs were co-cultured with autologous T lymphocytes, proliferation and activation of T lymphocytes were more weakly induced than with DCs sensitized by unpretreated *S. gordonii*

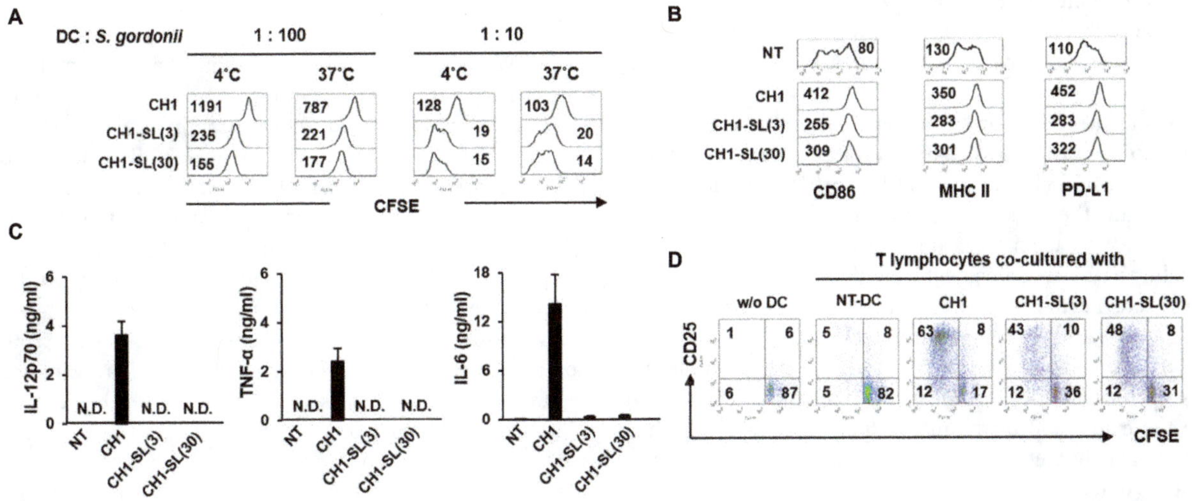

FIGURE 5 | Blockade of SRR adhesins abolishes *S. gordonii* binding and internalization to DCs and attenuates the immunostimulating potency of bacterium in DCs. *S. gordonii* CH1 (6.7×10^6 CFU/ml) was pretreated with 3′-sialyllactose (3 and 30 μM) for 1 h at room temperature to block bacterial Hsa and was washed with PBS. **(A)** Immature DCs (5×10^4 cells) were incubated in the absence or presence of 3′-sialyllactose-pretreated *S. gordonii* (5×10^5 and 5×10^6 CFU) in 50 μl PBS for 1 h at 4 and 37°C, respectively. Bacterial binding (4°C) and internalization (37°C) to DCs were analyzed by flow cytometry. The numbers on the histogram indicate the MFI of DCs. **(B,C)** Immature DCs (2.5×10^5 cells/ml) were either untreated or stimulated with 3′-sialyllactose-pretreated *S. gordonii* (1×10^6 CFU/ml) for 24 h. **(B)** Expression of CD86, MHC II, and PD-L1 on DCs was analyzed by flow cytometry. The numbers on the histogram indicate the MFI of DCs. **(C)** Concentrations of IL-12p70, TNF-α, and IL-6 in DC culture supernatants were measured by ELISA. **(D)** *S. gordonii*-sensitized DCs (5×10^4 cells) were co-cultured with autologous $CD3^+$ T lymphocytes (5×10^4 cells) for 4 days. Proliferative activity and CD25 expression of T lymphocytes were analyzed by flow cytometry. The numbers in each quadrant indicate the percentage of T lymphocytes. Results are representative of two similar experiments. N.D., not detected; NT, non-treatment; CH1, *S. gordonii* CH1 unpretreated with 3′-sialyllactose; CH1-SL(3), *S. gordonii* CH1 pretreated with 3 μM 3′-sialyllactose; CH1-SL(30), *S. gordonii* CH1 pretreated with 30 μM 3′-sialyllactose.

(**Figure 5D**). These results suggest that Hsa is a primary target molecule mediating *S. gordonii* binding and internalization to DCs and the immunostimulatory potency of the bacteria in DC maturation.

DISCUSSION

Streptococcus gordonii SRR adhesins, Hsa and GspB, are important not only for bacterial adhesion to host cells, but also for activation of host immune responses. Here, we demonstrated that *S. gordonii* lacking SRR adhesins showed marked reduction in DC maturation, production of inflammatory cytokines, and T cell-activating ability compared to wild-type *S. gordonii*. These results suggest that SRR adhesins Hsa and GspB are major surface molecules that are responsible for *S. gordonii*-induced DC maturation and activation.

Intact *S. gordonii* appears to induce the maturation and activation of human DCs, which is coincident with previous findings that phenotypic maturation and cytokine production take place in murine and human DCs stimulated with *S. gordonii* (Corinti et al., 1999; Mayer et al., 2009). On the other hand, IL-10 was hardly induced in human DCs treated with *S. gordonii* while other cytokines such as TNF-α, IL-6, and IL-12 were substantially increased under the same condition. Interestingly, however, previous reports demonstrated IL-10 induction in human DCs treated with *S. gordonii* (Corinti et al., 1999, 2001). Some possible explanations for this discrepancy can be made. One might be the difference in the intrinsic property of DCs originated from blood of humans with different ethnic backgrounds. Another might be the difference in the experimental conditions used for the preparation of DCs such as the separation method of DC precursors, the concentration of GM-CSF and IL-4, and the culture media composition containing supplementary ingredients. The third one might be the difference in the bacteria-to-DC ratio. The previous report demonstrated no induction of IL-10 at *S. gordonii*-to-DC ratio of 1:1 while a small amount of IL-10 (<100 pg/ml) at 10:1 (Corinti et al., 1999). Another study showed that *S. gordonii*-to-DC ratio of 50:1 was comparable to *S. typhi*-to-DC ratio of 1:1 for the induction of IL-10 at the similar extent, implying the low potentcy of *S. gordonii* to induce IL-10 in DCs (Corinti et al., 2001). Therefore, our results showing no IL-10 induction could be due to the difference in the intrinsic property of DCs derived from different ethnic background, the experimental method, and/or the use of low *S. gordonii*-to-DC ratio at 4:1.

We used SRR adhesin-deficient mutant strains to demonstrate that SRR adhesins Hsa and GspB contribute to *S. gordonii*-induced DC maturation and activation. This is in line with previous findings that *S. gordonii* binding to human monocytes via Hsa promoted their differentiation into DCs (Urano-Tashiro et al., 2012). Interestingly, other surface adhesins of *S. gordonii* are also involved in the activation of innate immune cells. SspA and SspB, famous adhesins of *S. gordonii*, are the best examples for the induction of cytokines in epithelial cells and DCs (Andrian et al., 2012). We suggest that the SRR adhesins of *S. gordonii* are not only involved in bacterial adherence, but also actively contribute to the induction of innate immunity by maturation and activation of DCs.

Although SRR-deficient *S. gordonii* showed a decreased augmentation on the expression of maturation markers including CD83, CD86, MHC class II, and PD-L1, in comparison with the wild-type strain, the difference between the wild-type and mutant appears to vary in each marker. It is likely due to the difference in the signaling pathways coincident with differential induction and turn-over rate. Furthermore, the more bacteria were treated, the less difference was observed in their expression. It may be because *S. gordonii* also possesses other immunostimulatory molecules such as lipoprotein and LTA in the cell wall that are known to involve the expression of the maturation markers on the host immune cells (Chan et al., 2007; Cho et al., 2013). On the other hand, it is notable that the loss of Hsa in *S. gordonii* CH1 strain was more dramatic than the loss of GspB in *S. gordonii* M99 strain in the phenotypic and functional maturation of DCs. The differential profiles of DC maturation might be due to the difference in the ligand-binding BR structure and glycan specificity between GspB and Hsa (Bensing et al., 2016) as demonstrated by the previous study that Hsa binds to both 3′SL and sialyl-T antigen, whereas GspB binds only to sialyl-T antigen (Urano-Tashiro et al., 2016).

Accumulating reports suggest that *S. gordonii* exhibit similar properties with regard to binding and internalization in various cell types, including monocytes, macrophages, erythrocytes, and platelets (Kerrigan et al., 2007; Urano-Tashiro et al., 2008). For example, *S. gordonii* binds to membrane glycoprotein Ibα on human platelets through bacterial Hsa or GspB, and the lack of GspB decreased platelet binding of the *S. gordonii* M99 strain by approximately 70% (Takamatsu et al., 2005; Xiong et al., 2008). Concordant with previous reports, the current results also showed that *S. gordonii* lacking Hsa or GspB was not efficiently adhered or internalized to DCs, leading to insufficient maturation and activation of DCs. These results support the hypothesis that SRR adhesins Hsa and GspB are important for the interaction of *S. gordonii* and DCs, which stimulate innate immunity mediated through DCs.

Serine-rich repeat adhesins were reported to bind to sialic acids of host cells, contributing to the pathogenesis of *S. gordonii* (Urano-Tashiro et al., 2008). Indeed, *S. gordonii* CH1 exhibited markedly attenuated binding and internalizing ability to DCs in the presence of 3′SL, which might interfere with the interaction of the bacterial Hsa with sialylated motifs on DCs. Moreover, the bacteria pretreated with 3′SL showed weakened induction of maturation, cytokine production, and T cell-activating ability of DCs. Interestingly, the inhibitory effect of 3′SL was dramatic on the induction of cytokine production in comparison with that of phenotypic marker expression. Those differential effects could be due to the distinct intracellular signal transduction pathways required for the expression of cytokines and co-stimulatory receptors. For example, the expression of co-stimulatory receptors including CD80 and CD86 was highly induced by lipopolysaccharide without induction of TNF-α or IL-12 in MyD88-deficient DCs (Kaisho et al., 2001). Therefore, we speculate that the bacterial interaction through SRR with DCs could predominantly participate in the stimulation of signaling pathways for the induction of cytokines rather than phenotypic markers in DCs.

Bacterial binding and internalization are important steps for DC maturation. Many previous studies have reported that a blockade of bacterial adherence and internalization to DCs attenuated the phenotypic and functional activation of DCs. One study showed that clinically isolated Group A Streptococcus did not induce maturation of DCs when binding and/or internalization was perturbed by bacterial hyaluronic acid capsular polysaccharides (Cortes and Wessels, 2009). In addition, encapsulated *Klebsiella pneumoniae* hardly induced DC maturation because a thick capsule layer on the bacterial surface hindered its phagocytosis by Evrard et al. (2010). Consistent with these reports, our findings showed that SRR adhesin-deficient *S. gordonii* mutant strains had weak binding and internalizing abilities. This consequently induced phenotypic and functional activation of DCs to a lesser extent. Furthermore, the inhibition of bacterial internalization with cytochalasin D abrogated *S. gordonii*-induced maturation and activation of DCs (data not shown). Therefore, Hsa- or GspB-mediated binding and internalization of *S. gordonii* to DCs could be the important step for DC maturation and activation.

Although oral streptococci are considered normal flora of the human oral cavity, some have recently been suggested as etiologic agents for systemic diseases including infective endocarditis and osteomyelitis (Li et al., 2000). It is important to understand the exact pathogenic mechanisms of oral bacteria and to characterize their major virulence factors in order to develop preventive and therapeutic agents against *S. gordonii* infection. Because DCs are the primary sentinel cells used to monitor infections and bridge innate and adaptive immunity for host protection, the SRR adhesins of *S. gordonii* might be major immunomodulatory molecules. Further studies are needed to identify the DC receptors that specifically bind to Hsa and GspB and elucidate downstream signal pathways to activate DCs. The results suggest that the SRR adhesins of *S. gordonii* are major virulence factors involved in bacterial adherence to the host and also trigger DC maturation and activation.

AUTHOR CONTRIBUTIONS

SH conceived the idea and contributed to the discussion of the results followed by writing and reviewing the manuscript. SH, EBK, and SK designed the experiments, performed the experiments, and/or interpreted the data. HS and C-HY provided critical comments and contributed to the discussion of the results followed by writing and reviewing the manuscript.

ACKNOWLEDGMENTS

This work was supported by grants from the National Research Foundation of Korea, which is funded by the

Korean government (MISIP) (2015M2A2A6A01044894 and 2015R1A2A1A15055453) and the Korea Health Technology R&D Project through the Korea Health Industry Development Institute (KHIDI), which is funded by the Ministry of Health & Welfare (HI14C0469), South Korea.

REFERENCES

Andrian, E., Qi, G., Wang, J., Halperin, S. A., and Lee, S. F. (2012). Role of surface proteins SspA and SspB of *Streptococcus gordonii* in innate immunity. *Microbiology* 158, 2099–2106. doi: 10.1099/mic.0.058073-0

Bensing, B. A., Khedri, Z., Deng, L., Yu, H., Prakobphol, A., Fisher, S. J., et al. (2016). Novel aspects of sialoglycan recognition by the Siglec-like domains of streptococcal SRR glycoproteins. *Glycobiology* 26, 1222–1234. doi: 10.1093/glycob/cww042

Bensing, B. A., Lopez, J. A., and Sullam, P. M. (2004). The *Streptococcus gordonii* surface proteins GspB and Hsa mediate binding to sialylated carbohydrate epitopes on the platelet membrane glycoprotein Ibalpha. *Infect. Immun.* 72, 6528–6537. doi: 10.1128/IAI.72.11.6528-6537.2004

Chan, K. G., Mayer, M., Davis, E. M., Halperin, S. A., Lin, T. J., and Lee, S. F. (2007). Role of D-alanylation of *Streptococcus gordonii* lipoteichoic acid in innate and adaptive immunity. *Infect. Immun.* 75, 3033–3042. doi: 10.1128/IAI.01549-06

Cho, K., Arimoto, T., Igarashi, T., and Yamamoto, M. (2013). Involvement of lipoprotein PpiA of *Streptococcus gordonii* in evasion of phagocytosis by macrophages. *Mol. Oral. Microbiol.* 28, 379–391. doi: 10.1111/omi.12031

Corinti, S., Albanesi, C., la Sala, A., Pastore, S., and Girolomoni, G. (2001). Regulatory activity of autocrine IL-10 on dendritic cell functions. *J. Immunol.* 166, 4312–4318. doi: 10.4049/jimmunol.166.7.4312

Corinti, S., Medaglini, D., Cavani, A., Rescigno, M., Pozzi, G., Ricciardi-Castagnoli, P., et al. (1999). Human dendritic cells very efficiently present a heterologous antigen expressed on the surface of recombinant gram-positive bacteria to CD4+ T lymphocytes. *J. Immunol.* 163, 3029–3036.

Cortes, G., and Wessels, M. R. (2009). Inhibition of dendritic cell maturation by group A *Streptococcus. J. Infect. Dis.* 200, 1152–1161. doi: 10.1086/605696

Evrard, B., Balestrino, D., Dosgilbert, A., Bouya-Gachancard, J. L., Charbonnel, N., Forestier, C., et al. (2010). Roles of capsule and lipopolysaccharide O antigen in interactions of human monocyte-derived dendritic cells and *Klebsiella pneumoniae. Infect. Immun.* 78, 210–219. doi: 10.1128/IAI.00864-09

Forner, L., Larsen, T., Kilian, M., and Holmstrup, P. (2006). Incidence of bacteremia after chewing, tooth brushing and scaling in individuals with periodontal inflammation. *J. Clin. Periodontol.* 33, 401–407. doi: 10.1111/j.1600-051X.2006.00924.x

Hahn, C. L., Schenkein, H. A., and Tew, J. G. (2005). Endocarditis-associated oral streptococci promote rapid differentiation of monocytes into mature dendritic cells. *Infect. Immun.* 73, 5015–5021. doi: 10.1128/IAI.73.8.5015-5021.2005

Jakubovics, N. S., Brittan, J. L., Dutton, L. C., and Jenkinson, H. F. (2009). Multiple adhesin proteins on the cell surface of *Streptococcus gordonii* are involved in adhesion to human fibronectin. *Microbiology* 155, 3572–3580. doi: 10.1099/mic.0.032078-0

Kaisho, T., Takeuchi, O., Kawai, T., Hoshino, K., and Akira, S. (2001). Endotoxin-induced maturation of MyD88-deficient dendritic cells. *J. Immunol.* 166, 5688–5694. doi: 10.4049/jimmunol.166.9.5688

Kapsenberg, M. L. (2003). Dendritic-cell control of pathogen-driven T-cell polarization. *Nat. Rev. Immunol.* 3, 984–993. doi: 10.1038/nri1246

Keane, C., Petersen, H., Reynolds, K., Newman, D. K., Cox, D., Jenkinson, H. F., et al. (2010). Mechanism of outside-in {alpha}IIb{beta}3-mediated activation of human platelets by the colonizing Bacterium, *Streptococcus gordonii. Arterioscler. Thromb. Vasc. Biol.* 30, 2408–2415. doi: 10.1161/ATVBAHA.110.216515

Kerrigan, S. W., Jakubovics, N. S., Keane, C., Maguire, P., Wynne, K., Jenkinson, H. F., et al. (2007). Role of *Streptococcus gordonii* surface proteins SspA/SspB and Hsa in platelet function. *Infect. Immun.* 75, 5740–5747. doi: 10.1128/IAI.00909-07

Kim, S. K., Yun, C. H., and Han, S. H. (2013). Enhanced anti-cancer activity of human dendritic cells sensitized with gamma-irradiation-induced apoptotic colon cancer cells. *Cancer Lett.* 335, 278–288. doi: 10.1016/j.canlet.2013.02.038

Lee, J. Y., Lee, B. H., and Lee, J. Y. (2015). Gambogic acid disrupts toll-like receptor4 activation by blocking lipopolysaccharides binding to myeloid differentiation factor 2. *Toxicol. Res.* 31, 11–16. doi: 10.5487/TR.2015.31.1.011

Li, X., Kolltveit, K. M., Tronstad, L., and Olsen, I. (2000). Systemic diseases caused by oral infection. *Clin. Microbiol. Rev.* 13, 547–558. doi: 10.1128/CMR.13.4.547-558.2000

Loo, C. Y., Corliss, D. A., and Ganeshkumar, N. (2000). *Streptococcus gordonii* biofilm formation: identification of genes that code for biofilm phenotypes. *J. Bacteriol.* 182, 1374–1382. doi: 10.1128/JB.182.5.1374-1382.2000

Mayer, M. L., Phillips, C. M., Townsend, R. A., Halperin, S. A., and Lee, S. F. (2009). Differential activation of dendritic cells by Toll-like receptor agonists isolated from the Gram-positive vaccine vector *Streptococcus gordonii. Scand. J. Immunol.* 69, 351–356. doi: 10.1111/j.1365-3083.2009.02232.x

Mempel, T. R., Henrickson, S. E., and Von Andrian, U. H. (2004). T-cell priming by dendritic cells in lymph nodes occurs in three distinct phases. *Nature* 427, 154–159. doi: 10.1038/nature02238

Moschioni, M., Pansegrau, W., and Barocchi, M. A. (2010). Adhesion determinants of the *Streptococcus* species. *Microb. Biotechnol.* 3, 370–388. doi: 10.1111/j.1751-7915.2009.00138.x

Steinman, R. M. (2006). Linking innate to adaptive immunity through dendritic cells. *Novartis Found. Symp.* 279, 101–109. doi: 10.1002/9780470035399.ch9

Takahashi, Y., Takashima, E., Shimazu, K., Yagishita, H., Aoba, T., and Konishi, K. (2006). Contribution of sialic acid-binding adhesin to pathogenesis of experimental endocarditis caused by *Streptococcus gordonii* DL1. *Infect. Immun.* 74, 740–743. doi: 10.1128/IAI.74.1.740-743.2006

Takahashi, Y., Yajima, A., Cisar, J. O., and Konishi, K. (2004). Functional analysis of the *Streptococcus gordonii* DL1 sialic acid-binding adhesin and its essential role in bacterial binding to platelets. *Infect. Immun.* 72, 3876–3882. doi: 10.1128/IAI.72.7.3876-3882.2004

Takamatsu, D., Bensing, B. A., Cheng, H., Jarvis, G. A., Siboo, I. R., Lopez, J. A., et al. (2005). Binding of the *Streptococcus gordonii* surface glycoproteins GspB and Hsa to specific carbohydrate structures on platelet membrane glycoprotein Ibalpha. *Mol. Microbiol.* 58, 380–392. doi: 10.1111/j.1365-2958.2005.04830.x

Urano-Tashiro, Y., Takahashi, Y., Oguchi, R., and Konishi, K. (2016). Two arginine residues of *Streptococcus gordonii* sialic acid-binding adhesin Hsa are essential for interaction to host cell receptors. *PLoS ONE* 11:e0154098. doi: 10.1371/journal.pone.0154098

Urano-Tashiro, Y., Yajima, A., Takahashi, Y., and Konishi, K. (2012). *Streptococcus gordonii* promotes rapid differentiation of monocytes into dendritic cells through interaction with the sialic acid-binding adhesin. *Odontology* 100, 144–148. doi: 10.1007/s10266-011-0044-z

Urano-Tashiro, Y., Yajima, A., Takashima, E., Takahashi, Y., and Konishi, K. (2008). Binding of the *Streptococcus gordonii* DL1 surface protein Hsa to the host cell membrane glycoproteins CD11b, CD43, and CD50. *Infect. Immun.* 76, 4686–4691. doi: 10.1128/IAI.00238-08

Xiong, Y. Q., Bensing, B. A., Bayer, A. S., Chambers, H. F., and Sullam, P. M. (2008). Role of the serine-rich surface glycoprotein GspB of *Streptococcus gordonii* in the pathogenesis of infective endocarditis. *Microb. Pathog.* 45, 297–301. doi: 10.1016/j.micpath.2008.06.004

Yajima, A., Urano-Tashiro, Y., Shimazu, K., Takashima, E., Takahashi, Y., and Konishi, K. (2008). Hsa, an adhesin of *Streptococcus gordonii* DL1, binds to alpha2-3-linked sialic acid on glycophorin A of the erythrocyte membrane. *Microbiol. Immunol.* 52, 69–77. doi: 10.1111/j.1348-0421.2008.00015.x

Yombi, J., Belkhir, L., Jonckheere, S., Wilmes, D., Cornu, O., Vandercam, B., et al. (2012). *Streptococcus gordonii* septic arthritis: two cases and review of literature. *BMC Infect. Dis.* 12:215. doi: 10.1186/1471-2334-12-215

12

Supplementation with *Lactobacillus plantarum* WCFS1 Prevents Decline of Mucus Barrier in Colon of Accelerated Aging *Ercc1*$^{-/\Delta 7}$ Mice

Adriaan A. van Beek[1,2,3†], Bruno Sovran[2,4], Floor Hugenholtz[2,5], Ben Meijer[1], Joanne A. Hoogerland[1], Violeta Mihailova[1], Corine van der Ploeg[1], Clara Belzer[2,5], Mark V. Boekschoten[2,6], Jan H. J. Hoeijmakers[7,8], Wilbert P. Vermeij[7], Paul de Vos[2,9], Jerry M. Wells[2,4], Pieter J. M. Leenen[10], Claudio Nicoletti[3,11], Rudi W. Hendriks[12] and Huub F. J. Savelkoul[1,2]*

[1] Cell Biology and Immunology Group, Wageningen University, Wageningen, Netherlands, [2] Top Institute Food and Nutrition, Wageningen, Netherlands, [3] Gut Health and Food Safety, Institute of Food Research, Norwich, UK, [4] Host Microbe Interactomics, Wageningen University, Wageningen, Netherlands, [5] Laboratory of Microbiology, Wageningen University, Wageningen, Netherlands, [6] Human Nutrition, Wageningen University, Wageningen, Netherlands, [7] Department of Molecular Genetics, Erasmus University Medical Center, Rotterdam, Netherlands, [8] CECAD Forschungszentrum, Universität zu Köln, Köln, Germany, [9] University of Groningen, Groningen, Netherlands, [10] Department of Immunology, Erasmus University Medical Center, Rotterdam, Netherlands, [11] Department of Experimental and Clinical Medicine, University of Florence, Florence, Italy, [12] Department of Pulmonary Medicine, Erasmus University Medical Center, Rotterdam, Netherlands

Edited by:
Julio Villena,
CERELA-CONICET, Argentina

Reviewed by:
Jennelle Maree Kyd,
Swinburne University of Technology, Australia
Susana Salva,
CERELA-CONICET, Argentina

***Correspondence:**
Huub F. J. Savelkoul
huub.savelkoul@wur.nl

Although it is clear that probiotics improve intestinal barrier function, little is known about the effects of probiotics on the aging intestine. We investigated effects of 10-week bacterial supplementation of *Lactobacillus plantarum* WCFS1, *Lactobacillus casei* BL23, or *Bifidobacterium breve* DSM20213 on gut barrier and immunity in 16-week-old accelerated aging *Ercc1*$^{-/\Delta 7}$ mice, which have a median lifespan of ~20 weeks, and their wild-type littermates. The colonic barrier in *Ercc1*$^{-/\Delta 7}$ mice was characterized by a thin (< 10 μm) mucus layer. *L. plantarum* prevented this decline in mucus integrity in *Ercc1*$^{-/\Delta 7}$ mice, whereas *B. breve* exacerbated it. Bacterial supplementations affected the expression of immune-related genes, including Toll-like receptor 4. Regulatory T cell frequencies were increased in the mesenteric lymph nodes of *L. plantarum*- and *L. casei*-treated *Ercc1*$^{-/\Delta 7}$ mice. *L. plantarum*- and *L. casei*-treated *Ercc1*$^{-/\Delta 7}$ mice showed increased specific antibody production in a T cell-dependent immune response *in vivo*. By contrast, the effects of bacterial supplementation on wild-type control mice were negligible. Thus, supplementation with *L. plantarum* – but not with *L. casei* and *B. breve* – prevented the decline in the mucus barrier in *Ercc1*$^{-/\Delta 7}$ mice. Our data indicate that age is an important factor influencing beneficial or detrimental effects of candidate probiotics. These findings also highlight the need for caution in translating beneficial effects of probiotics observed in young animals or humans to the elderly.

INTRODUCTION

Aging is accompanied by multiple age-related diseases (1), posing a major burden to public health care (2). With age, a decline in the regenerative potential of tissues due to stem cell exhaustion occurs (3). Turnover in epithelial cells is rapid, and mounting evidence indicates that intestinal stem cells are compromised with aging (4). For example, a crucial component of the intestinal barrier is mucus secreted by goblet cells (5). The Muc2 glycoprotein regulates immunity by inducing tolerogenic signals in mucosal dendritic cells (6) and is important in host–microbe interactions (7). Thus, changes in mucus quantity and integrity influence immunity (6, 8).

Aging is accompanied by the development of a low-grade inflammation ("inflammaging"), which is characterized by elevated IL-6 and TNF serum levels in elderly (9). Involution of the thymus and the bone marrow (BM) leads to decreased T and B cell production (10, 11). By contrast, the production of myeloid cells is enhanced with aging, characterized by a progressive increase of neutrophil frequencies in the circulation (12).

Probiotics are defined as live bacteria that confer health benefits to the host, for example, by competing with pathogens, enhancing intestinal barrier function, and regulating immunity (13, 14). They might, therefore, prevent some of the undesired age-related intestinal barrier and immune effects. Probiotic supplementation of elderly subjects led to changes in fecal microbiota composition (15–17), and affected the distribution and function of NK cells, macrophages, granulocytes, and T cells in the circulation (18, 19). Supplementation of aged mice with *Lactobacillus paracasei* resulted in increased IgG2a serum titers after antigenic challenge (20). Middle-aged mice that were supplemented with *Bifidobacterium animalis* showed decreased colon permeability, extended lifespan, and improved quality of life (21). Besides these studies, little is known about how exposure to probiotics impacts on the aging intestinal barrier and immune system. Moreover, it is unknown whether the beneficial effects of probiotics are age dependent.

In this report, we have used an accelerated aging mouse model to evaluate the effects of candidate probiotics in aging. Based on a variety of histological, functional, metabolomic, and proteomic data, it has been concluded that *Ercc1*$^{-/\Delta7}$ mice resemble normal murine aging (22). Recently, we have shown that the immune system of *Ercc1*$^{-/\Delta7}$ mice resembles the immune system of aged WT mice. For instance, we showed a similar decrease in B cell precursors and naïve T cells, and a similar increase in memory T cells and regulatory T cells (23). The ERCC1 protein is involved in multiple DNA repair pathways. *Ercc1*$^{-/\Delta7}$ mice (median lifespan ~20 weeks) are deficient for fully functional ERCC1 protein. The expression of ERCC1-XPF (excision repair cross-complementation group 1-xeroderma pigmentosum group F) DNA repair endonuclease is reduced to ~5% compared with *Ercc1*$^{+/+}$ mice. Moreover, the residual ERCC1-XPF protein present is expressed from a truncated allele, and lacks the last seven amino acids. A reduction of ERCC1 protein activity leads to increased accumulation of DNA damage and, hence, results in an accelerated aging phenotype (24, 25).

The aim of this study was to investigate the potential of supplementation with candidate probiotic strains to ameliorate the effects of aging on the intestinal barrier and the immune system. Previously, probiotic activity was documented for *Lactobacillus plantarum* WCFS1 (26–28), *Lactobacillus casei* BL23 (29, 30), and relatives of *Bifidobacterium breve* DSM20213 (31). We selected these strains on the basis of induced IL-10/TNF ratios in young and aged immune cells *in vitro* (32). The three strains can be classified as potential pro-inflammatory (*L. plantarum*), regulatory (*L. casei*), or anti-inflammatory (*B. breve*), based on low, intermediate, or high IL-10/TNF ratios, respectively.

For this study, we supplemented 6-week-old *Ercc1*$^{+/+}$ mice and *Ercc1*$^{-/\Delta7}$ mice with *L. plantarum*, *L. casei*, or *B. breve* for 10 weeks. Mucus barrier, microbiota composition, and gene regulation in the colon were analyzed, as well as the distribution of immune cells in various mucosal and peripheral lymphoid organs. We determined immune competence by antigenic challenge.

MATERIALS AND METHODS

Mice

The generation and characterization of *Ercc1*$^{+/\Delta7}$ and *Ercc1*$^{-/+}$ mice has been previously described (25). *Ercc1*$^{-/\Delta7}$ mice were obtained by crossing *Ercc1*$^{+/\Delta7}$ with *Ercc1*$^{-/+}$ mice of pure C57Bl6/J and FVB backgrounds to yield *Ercc1*$^{-/\Delta7}$ with an F1 C57Bl6J/FVB hybrid background. Genotyping was performed as described previously (33). Wild-type littermates (C57Bl6J/FVB F1) were used as controls. Four-month-old and 18-month-old C57Bl6/J mice were purchased from Harlan (Horst, The Netherlands; only used in **Figure 1**).

Animals were housed in individual ventilated cages under SPF conditions. Experiments were performed in accordance with the Principles of Laboratory Animal Care and with Dutch legislation. This study was carried out in accordance with the recommendations of the Dutch Ethical Committee of Wageningen that approved the work. Blood was taken from mice being sacrificed, and serum was frozen in −80°C for later use. After mice ($n = 4$–6) were sacrificed, feces from colon was collected and snap-frozen. Distal ileum and proximal colon sections were isolated and fixed in Carnoy or snap-frozen in liquid nitrogen. BM, thymus, spleen, mesenteric lymph nodes (MLN), and Peyer's patches (PPs) were isolated.

Bacterial Cultures and Supplementation

L. plantarum WCFS1, *L. casei* BL23, and *B. breve* DSM20213 were grown on MRS medium (Merck, Darmstadt, Germany) until stationary phase, frozen in glycerol, and stored in −80°C until use. Upon use, bacteria were thawed and 10× diluted in NaHCO3/PBS buffer. Around 2×10^8 CFU in 200 μL were administered to mice by gavage, three times per week. Treatment of mice started at 6 weeks of age until 1 day before sacrifice at 16 weeks or until death.

Histology and Fluorescence *In Situ* Hybridization

Carnoy-fixed proximal colon sections were embedded in paraffin. Paraffin sections (5 μm) were attached to poly-L-lysine-coated glass slides (Thermo Scientific, Germany). After overnight

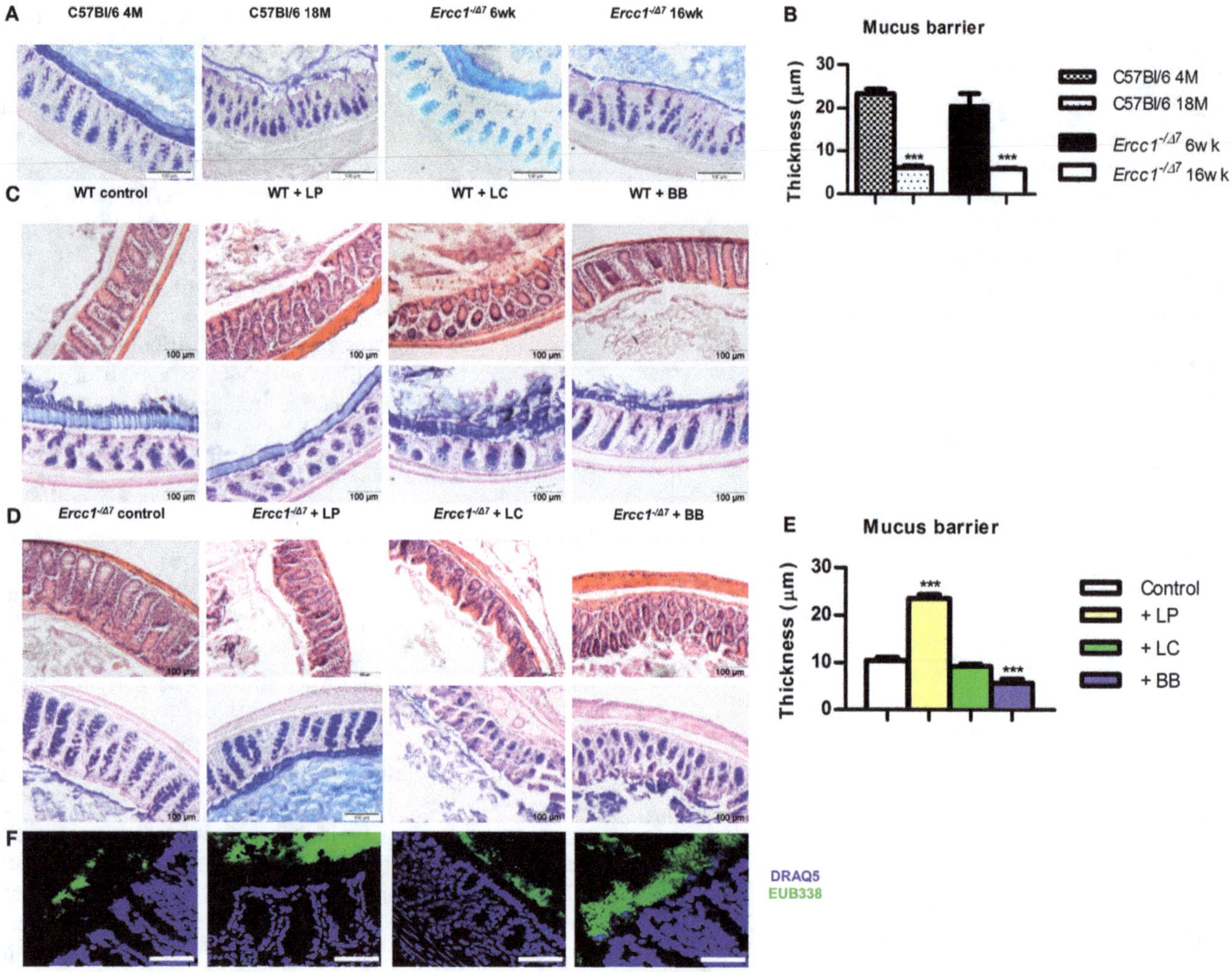

FIGURE 1 | Treatment with *L. plantarum* prevented the age-related decline in colonic mucus barrier of accelerated aging *Ercc1*$^{-/\Delta7}$ mice. **(A)** Representative pictures of proximal colon stained with PAS/Alcian Blue of 4-month-old (4 M) or 18-month-old (18 M) WT mice and 6-week-old (6 weeks) or 16-week-old (16 weeks) *Ercc1*$^{-/\Delta7}$ mice. **(B)** Quantitative measurement of mucus thickness in young and old WT and *Ercc1*$^{-/\Delta}$ mice by ImageJ. **(C)** Representative pictures of proximal colon stained with H&E or PAS/Alcian Blue of *Ercc1*$^{+/+}$ mice supplemented with control treatment, *L. plantarum* WCFS1 (LP), *L. casei* BL23 (LC), or *B. breve* DSM20213 (BB). **(D)** Representative pictures of proximal colon stained with H&E and PAS/Alcian Blue of *Ercc1*$^{-/\Delta7}$ mice supplemented with control treatment, LP, LC, or BB. **(E)** Quantitative measurement of mucus thickness in *Ercc1*$^{-/\Delta7}$ mice by ImageJ. **(F)** Fluorescence *in situ* hybridization (FISH) of proximal colon from *Ercc1*$^{-/\Delta7}$ mice. Data represent the mean + SEM from four to six animals per group. ***$p < 0.001$. Scale bars histological pictures: 100 µm; scale bars FISH: 50 µm.

incubation at 37°C, slides were de-waxed and rehydrated. Sections were stained with hematoxylin and eosin (H&E) and PAS/Alcian blue. Mucus layer thickness was measured using ImageJ software (NIH, MD, USA), as previously published (34). For detection of bacteria, tissue sections were used for fluorescence *in situ* hybridization (FISH), as previously published (8).

MIT-Chips/16S Sequencing

Microbiota composition in colonic content was analyzed by Mouse Intestinal Tract Chip (MITChip), as described previously (35). The data were normalized and analyzed using a set of R-based scripts in combination with a custom-designed relational database, which operates under the MySQL database management system. For the microbial profiling, the Robust Probabilistic Averaging signal intensities of 2667 specific probes for the 94 genus-level bacterial groups detected on the MITChip were used (36). Diversity calculations were performed using a microbiome R-script package (https://github.com/microbiome). Multivariate statistics, redundancy analysis (RDA), and principal response curves were performed in Canoco 5.0 and visualized in triplots or a principal response curves plot (37).

RNA Isolation and Transcriptome Analysis

Total RNA was isolated from proximal colon ($n = 3$–6 per group) using the RNeasy kit (Qiagen) with a DNase digestion step according to the manufacturer's protocol. Transcriptome analysis on individual samples was performed as previously described (8). The gene expression datasets were deposited in NCBI's Gene Expression Omnibus (GEO) and are accesible through GEO Series accession number: GSE87368.

General Flow Cytometry Procedures

Single-cell suspensions of BM were obtained by crushing femurs, tibias, iliac crests, and sternum with mortar and pestle. BM cells were then filtered on a 40-μm cell strainer. A proportion of the BM cells was frozen for later use in *in vitro* cultures. Spleen, MLN, PP, thymus, and peritoneal cavity single-cell suspensions were obtained by gently pushing cells through a 40-μm cell strainer with a syringe. All cells were stained for extracellular markers and dead cells were identified with fixable live/dead stain (Ebioscience, San Diego, CA, USA), after which intracellular staining was enabled by fixing and permeabilizing cells with Fix/Perm buffer (Ebioscience) according to manufacturer's instructions. Antibodies used for flow cytometric measurements are listed in Supplementary Table 1 in Data Sheet 1. All flow cytometric measurements were performed on a Canto II flow cytometer (BD Biosciences, Erembodegem, Belgium). FlowJo vX.07 software (Tree Star) was used for data analysis. Gating of all presented immune cell populations was based on single live cells.

Spleen Cell Cultures

Splenic cells were cultured at 10^6 cells/mL for 4 days in the absence or presence of 5 μg/mL concanavalin A (ConA). Proliferation was measured by Ki-67 (Ebioscience). Supernatants were stored at −20°C. After thawing, levels of IL-2, IL-4, IL-6, IL-10, IL-17A, IFN-γ, and TNF were measured with the Cytometric Bead Array Th1/Th2/Th17 Kit (BD Biosciences), according to manufacturer's instructions. Samples were acquired on a Canto II flow cytometer. Data were analyzed using FCAP Array version 3.0 (BD Biosciences) software.

Antibody Titers in Serum

Levels of IgM, IgG1, IgG2a, IgG2b, IgG3, IgE, and IgA were analyzed in serum using ProcartaPlex Mouse Antibody Isotyping Panel kit on the Luminex platform (Affymetrix, Santa Clara, CA, USA) according to the manufacturer's instructions. Data were acquired on a BioPlex 200 (Bio-Rad, Hercules, CA, USA) and analyzed with BioPlex software (version 5.0, Bio-Rad).

In Vivo Immunization and Antibody Detection

Primary and secondary T cell-dependent (TD) immune responses against TNP-KLH were measured 7 days after primary i.p. immunization and 7 days after i.p. booster immunization. The primary immunization was performed at 8 weeks of age (TNP-KLH in alum), booster doses were injected at 12 weeks of age (TNP-KLH in PBS). Total and TNP-specific Ig subclasses were determined by sandwich ELISA as previously described (38).

Statistical Analysis

Values are expressed as mean + SEM. Normal distribution of the data was confirmed using the Kolmogorov–Smirnov test. Statistical comparisons were performed using the two-sided Student's *t*-test. Where non-Gaussian distribution was demonstrated, we applied the non-parametric Mann–Whitney U test. Where no equal variances were observed, we applied the two-sided Student's *t*-test with Welch's correction. Statistical comparisons for lifespan data were performed using the log-rank (Mantel–Cox) test. Statistical comparisons for serum immunoglobulins were performed using two-way ANOVA, with subsequent Bonferroni posttests. Values of $p < 0.05$ were considered to be statistically significant. Values between $p > 0.05$ and $p < 0.10$ were considered as a trend.

RESULTS

The Mucus Layer in the Colon Declines with Age

To assess the mucus barrier in normal and accelerated aging, we compared the proximal colon of 4-month-old (young) with 18-month-old (aged) C57Bl/6 mice, and of 6-week-old (young) with 16-week-old (aged) *Ercc1*$^{-/\Delta7}$ mice. We observed that in aged C57Bl/6 and *Ercc1*$^{-/\Delta7}$ mice, a thinner mucus layer was present, compared with young C57Bl/6 and *Ercc1*$^{-/\Delta7}$ mice (**Figure 1A**). With ImageJ, we measured the thickness of the mucus layer. In young C57Bl/6 and *Ercc1*$^{-/\Delta7}$ mice, a mucus layer of ~20 μm was present, whereas in normal and accelerated aged mice, a significantly thinner mucus layer of less than 10 μm was observed ($p < 0.001$; **Figure 1B**).

Bacterial Supplementations Do Not Change the Mucus Layer in Colon of Young WT Mice

To determine the effects of the three selected bacterial strains in the young intestine, we analyzed proximal colon tissues of WT mice that were treated with *L. plantarum* WCFS1, *L. casei* BL23, or *B. breve* DSM20213 for 10 weeks. No change in tissue integrity (H&E) or mucus layer (PAS/Alcian Blue) was observed in the colon after supplementation with bacterial strains (**Figure 1C**).

Age-Related Decline in the Mucus Barrier is Prevented by Supplementation of *Ercc1*$^{-/\Delta7}$ Mice with *L. plantarum*

Because the mucus layer declines with age, we questioned whether bacterial supplementation of *Ercc1*$^{-/\Delta7}$ mice prevents the decline in mucus barrier. Colon tissue of 10-week treated *Ercc1*$^{-/\Delta7}$ mice was checked for tissue integrity and mucus layer thickness. In contrast to our findings in WT mice, bacterial supplementation had significant effects on tissue integrity and the mucus layer. In *Ercc1*$^{-/\Delta7}$ mice supplemented with *L. plantarum*, the colon showed a thicker mucus layer than their controls (**Figure 1D**). *L. plantarum* supplementation completely prevented age-related decline in the mucus layer compared with controls ($p < 0.001$; **Figure 1E**), resulting in a mucus thickness comparable to young WT mice. Spatial compartmentalization of bacteria in the colon was improved after *L. plantarum* supplementation (**Figure 1F**), as demonstrated by FISH analyses. On the contrary, *Ercc1*$^{-/\Delta7}$ mice supplemented with *L. casei* or *B. breve* showed loss of tissue integrity (**Figure 1D**). No difference in mucus thickness was observed after supplementation with *L. casei* (**Figure 1E**). *B. breve* supplementation resulted in a deteriorated mucus layer and a loss in mucus thickness ($p < 0.001$; **Figure 1E**). *B. breve* supplementation also resulted in less spatial compartmentalization of bacteria in the colon of *Ercc1*$^{-/\Delta 7}$ mice (**Figure 1F**).

Collectively, these data show that *L. plantarum* supplementation improves the mucus layer in the aged (but not young) colon. In addition, supplementation with *L. casei* or *B. breve* exacerbates the age-related decline of mucus barrier in the colon.

Bacterial Supplementation Associated with Minor Alterations in Colonic Microbiota Composition

As we introduced bacteria by bacterial supplementations into the intestinal microbial community, we investigate whether changes in the microbiota composition were underlying the observed changes in the mucus barrier of *Ercc1*$^{-/\Delta 7}$ mice. Microbiota composition was determined by performing 16S rRNA gene microbiota profiles of colonic content. The bacterial supplementations did not significantly alter microbial diversity nor richness (data not shown).

Redundancy analysis showed that 10.1% of the total variability of the gut microbiota can be related to the bacterial supplementations (**Figure 2**). No statistical significance was established. The first ordination axis explained 4.9% of the variability and separated *Ercc1*$^{-/\Delta 7}$ mice supplemented with either of the three bacterial strains from the control *Ercc1*$^{-/\Delta 7}$ mice. The second ordination axis explained 3.6% of the variability but did not result in a separation between groups. The third ordination axis explained an additional 1.6% of the variability (data not shown).

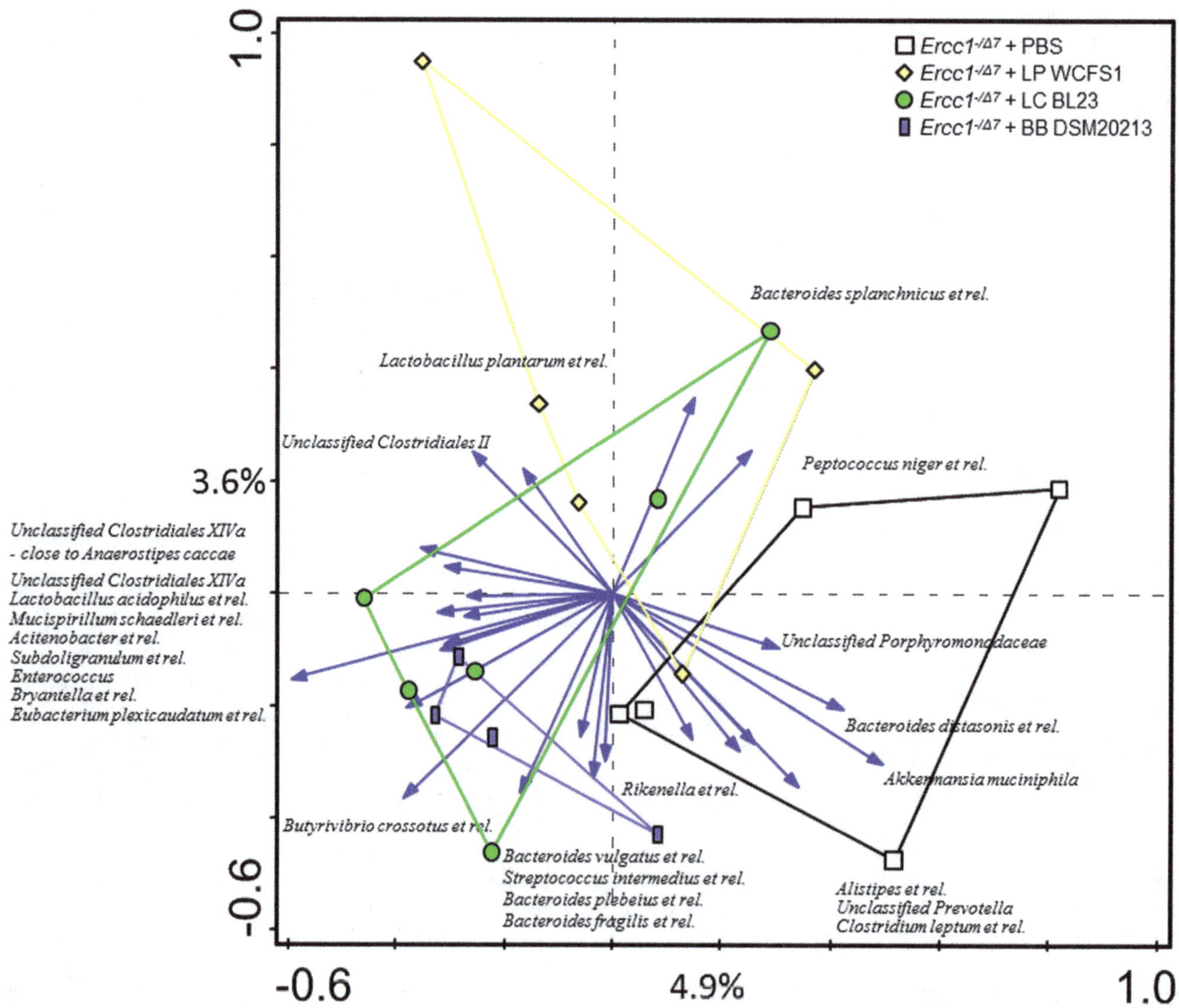

FIGURE 2 | The effect of bacterial supplementations on colonic microbiota composition in *Ercc1*$^{-/\Delta 7}$ mice. Redundancy analysis of the microbial composition after bacterial supplementations, on genus-like level of the MITChip analysis. Mice belonging to control-, LP-, LC-, and BB-treated groups are indicated by white squares, yellow diamonds, green circles, and blue rectangles, respectively. First and second ordination axes are plotted, showing 4.9 and 3.6% of the variability in the dataset, respectively. No significant changes were observed. LP, *L. plantarum* WCFS1; LC, *L. casei* BL23; BB, *B. breve* DSM20213.

To assess whether significant changes in the microbial genus-like bacterial groups existed after different bacterial supplementations in *Ercc1*$^{-/\Delta7}$ mice, we performed the Wilcoxon test. *Subdoligranulum* was higher in mice supplemented with *L. casei* ($p < 0.05$), whereas it tended to be higher in mice supplemented with *B. breve* ($p = 0.05$), as compared with control mice (**Figure 3**). *Akkermansia muciniphila* tended to be less present ($p = 0.06$) in mice supplemented with *L. plantarum* compared with control mice. *Eubacterium plexicaudatum* and a close relative to *Anaerostipes caccae* tended to be higher ($p = 0.06$) in *Ercc1*$^{-/\Delta7}$ mice supplemented with *L. casei*.

These data demonstrate some differences in microbial species between control-treated *Ercc1*$^{-/\Delta7}$ mice and *Ercc1*$^{-/\Delta7}$ mice treated with bacterial supplementations.

Distinct Gene Expression Profiles in Colon after Each Bacterial Supplementation

To understand the mechanisms by which bacterial supplementation changes the mucus barrier, we performed transcriptome analysis on the proximal colon of *Ercc1*$^{-/\Delta7}$ mice. Gene expression microarrays on total proximal colon samples from *Ercc1*$^{-/\Delta7}$ mice treated with bacterial supplementations or control treatment revealed relatively low numbers of differentially expressed genes: 84 by *L. plantarum*, 238 by *L. casei*, and 384 by *B. breve*. Only a few genes were overlapping between two or three different bacterial supplementations, whereas most of the differentially expressed genes were distinctly regulated by one of the treatments (**Figure 4**).

Several growth- and immune-related genes were differentially expressed after bacterial supplementation. Apolipoprotein (APO) A-1, APOA-4, suppressor of cytokine signaling (SOCS) 3, and toll-like receptor (TLR) 4 were upregulated more than 1.2-fold after *L. plantarum* supplementation (Data Sheet 2 in the Supplementary Material). Several immunoglobulin variable genes and TLR13 were upregulated after administration of *L. casei*, whereas defensin 40β was 1.3-fold downregulated. Defensin 24α, amphiregulin, and keratinocyte growth factor 7 (FGF7) were upregulated more than 1.4-fold after administration of *B. breve*, while TLR6, TLR7, and CCL3 (MIP-1α) were more than 1.2-fold downregulated (Data Sheet 2 in the Supplementary Material). Remarkably, we found no significant up- or downregulation in any mucin.

Bacterial Supplementation Alters Growth- and Immune-Related Pathways in Colon

Because we found relatively low numbers of differentially expressed genes, we applied a gene set enrichment analysis (GSEA) (39) to gain insight into the regulated pathways by bacterial supplementations. Upstream regulators that can explain the observed changes in gene expression were identified using Ingenuity Upstream Regulator Analysis.

Gene set enrichment analysis revealed that *L. plantarum* supplementation significantly enhanced several processes involved in growth and cell cycle, and immunity (Supplementary Table 2 in Data Sheet 1), such as "Type II Interferon Signaling," "VIP pathway," and "IL8/CXCR1 pathway." Interestingly, in the top-10

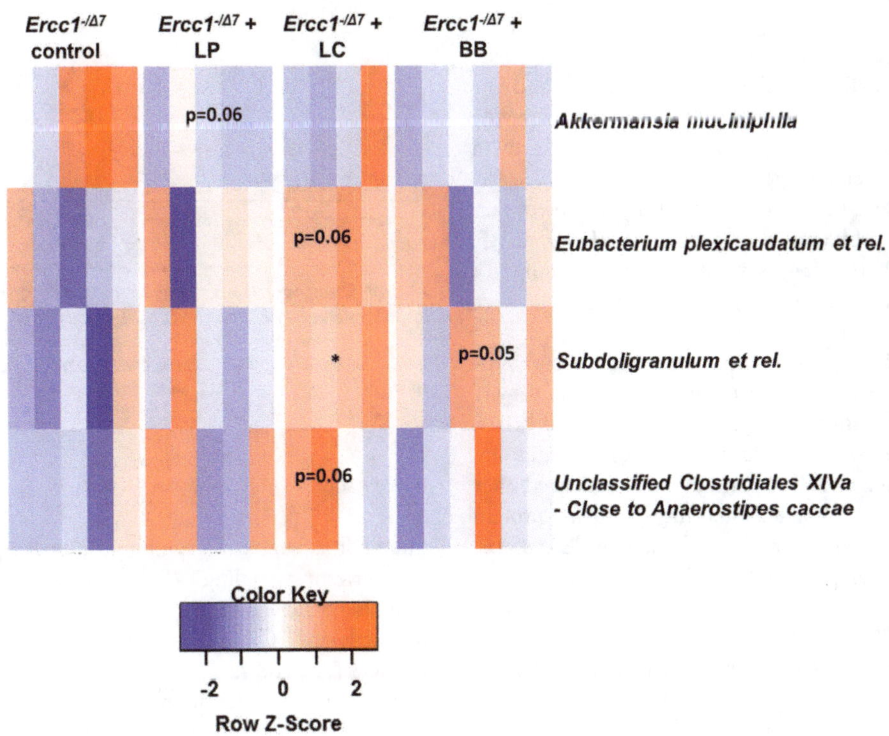

FIGURE 3 | Bacterial supplementation induced changes in bacterial taxa in the colon of *Ercc1*$^{-/\Delta7}$ mice. Wilcoxon tests comparing mice treated with bacterial strains with control group. Data represent $n = 4$–6 mice per group. $^*p < 0.05$.

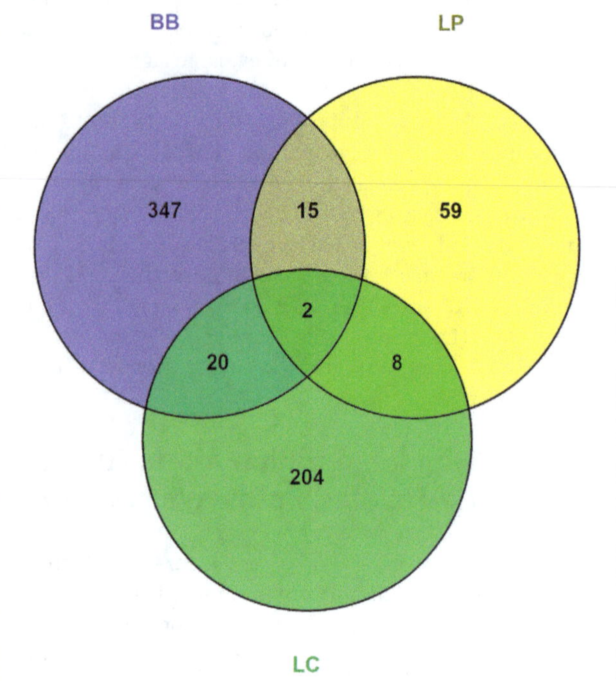

FIGURE 4 | Venn diagrams of differentially regulated genes in colon of *Ercc1*$^{-/\Delta 7}$ mice after bacterial supplementations. Total number of genes altered in the proximal colon of *Ercc1*$^{-/\Delta 7}$ mice treated with *L. plantarum* WCFS1 (LP), *L. casei* BL23 (LC), or *B. breve* DSM20213 (BB) compared with control-treated *Ercc1*$^{-/\Delta 7}$ mice. Venn diagram of the total number of genes upregulated and downregulated in the proximal colon of *Ercc1*$^{-/\Delta 7}$ mice treated with LP, BB, or LC ($p < 0.05$ and >1.2-fold difference).

of upregulated pathways, three pathways were linked to DNA repair: the "Fanconi Pathway," "ATRBRCA pathway," and the "Fanconi anemia pathway." Several growth factors were activated after *L. plantarum* supplementation: leptin, epidermal growth factor (EGF), platelet-derived growth factor (PDGF) BB, early growth response protein (EGR) 1, and insulin-like growth factor (IGF) 1 (**Table 1**). Inflammatory cytokines (IFN-γ, IL-1β, IL-4, TNF) and CD40L (CD154) were activated in colon of mice supplemented with *L. plantarum*, compared with colon of mice supplemented with control treatment.

Lactobacillus casei supplementation enhanced several processes involved in growth and cell cycle, like "Mitotic G1-G1 S Phases," "DNA replication," "Synthesis of DNA," and "G1 S transition" (Supplementary Table 2 in Data Sheet 1). In addition, the "NOD-like receptor signaling pathway" was enhanced after *L. casei* supplementation, as well as and the "Unfolded protein response" (UPR), indicated endoplasmatic reticulum (ER) stress. Upstream regulators resistin-like β (RTNLB; activated) and GATA3 (inhibited) were regulated in the colon of mice supplemented with *L. casei* (**Table 1**).

Several metabolic pathways were enhanced in colon of *B. breve*-supplemented mice (Supplementary Table 2 in Data Sheet 1). Of note, "Protein folding" was upregulated. In contrast to *L. plantarum* and *L. casei* supplementation, *B. breve* supplementation significantly inhibited several processes involved in immunity, such as "IL2 STAT5 pathway," "Immunoregulatory interactions between lymphoid/non-lymphoid cells," "Type II Interferon signaling," "IL4 2 pathway," and "IL6 7 pathway" (Supplementary Table 3 in Data Sheet 1). *B. breve* supplementation activated EGF and inhibited fibroblast growth factor (FGF) 2. IgG, GATA2, and IL-2-inducible T cell kinase (ITK) were inhibited in colon of mice supplemented with *B. breve*. In line with GSEA, IFN-γ was inhibited as well after *B. breve* supplementation.

These data indicate that immune pathways in the colon are enhanced by *L. plantarum* and *L. casei*, but are inhibited by *B. breve* supplementation.

TABLE 1 | Activation *z*-scores of upstream regulators in proximal colon of *Ercc1*$^{-/\Delta 7}$ mice after bacterial supplementations *L. plantarum* WCFS1 (LP), *L. casei* BL23 (LC), or *B. breve* DSM20213 (BB) as determined by Ingenuity.

Upstream regulator	LP	LC	BB
Leptin	2.41		
EGF	2.36		3.36
IL4	2.18		
IFN-γ	2.00		−1.35
PDGF BB	2.00		1.15
P38 MAPK	1.97		
CD40L	1.96		
Palmitic acid	1.96		
EGR1	1.95		
IGF1	1.82		
IL1β	1.77		
Ethanol	1.76		
CREB1	1.55		
CREBBP	1.54		
TNF	1.53		
KLF4		2.04	
Resistin-like β		2.00	
PML		−1.73	
miR-4800-5p		−1.98	
GATA3		−1.98	
MTOR		−2.00	
miR-4455		−2.22	
ADCYAP1			2.60
EDN1			2.17
WNT3A			2.16
VIP			1.95
FGF2			1.74
GLI1			1.63
miR-6967-5p			−1.58
Klra7 (includes others)			−1.87
IgG			−1.89
EZH2			−1.96
GATA2			−2.00
ANXA7			−2.00
miR-4707-5p			−2.16
ITK			−2.19
miR-4459			−2.63

Upstream regulators involved in growth and cell cycle are highlighted in blue; upstream regulators involved in immunity are highlighted in orange. Cut-off values for activation z-score ≥1.5 or ≤−1.5 combined with $p < 0.05$. Activated in blue, inhibited in red. ADCYAP, adenylate cyclase activating polypeptide; ANX, annexin; CREB(BP), cAMP-responsive element (binding protein); EDN, endothelin; EGF, epidermal growth factor; EGR, early growth response protein; EHZ, enhancer of zeste homolog; FGF, fibroblast growth factor; GLI, glioma-associated oncogene family zinc finger; IFN, interferon; IGF, insulin-like growth factor; ITK, IL-2-inducible T cell kinase; KLF, Kruppel-like factor; Klra, killer cell lectin-like receptor, subfamily A; LEP, leptin; MTOR, mechanistic target of rapamycin; PDGF, platelet-derived growth factor; PML, promyelocytic leukemia protein; RETNLB, resistin-like β; TNF, tumor necrosis factor; VIP, vasoactive intestinal peptide; WNT, wingless-type MMTV integration site family.

L. plantarum and *L. casei* Supplementation Induce Regulatory T Cells in MLN

Based on the regulation of immune genes by bacterial supplementations, we tested whether the distribution of immune cells was altered in mucosal immune organs of *Ercc1*$^{-/\Delta 7}$ mice.

First, we evaluated changes in distribution of immune cells in PPs and MLN. B cell frequencies were reduced in PP and MLN ($p < 0.05$) after *L. casei* supplementation in *Ercc1*$^{-/\Delta 7}$ mice (**Figure 5A**). By contrast, frequencies of T cells were increased in PP ($p < 0.01$) and MLN ($p < 0.05$; **Figure 5B**). The frequencies of regulatory T (Treg) cells in MLN were increased after *L. plantarum* and *L. casei* supplementation ($p < 0.05$; **Figures 5C,D**). No changes in distribution of B and T cells were observed upon bacterial supplementation in WT mice, except for a tendency to decreased Treg cells after *L. casei* supplementation ($p = 0.09$; Supplementary Figure 1 in Data Sheet 1).

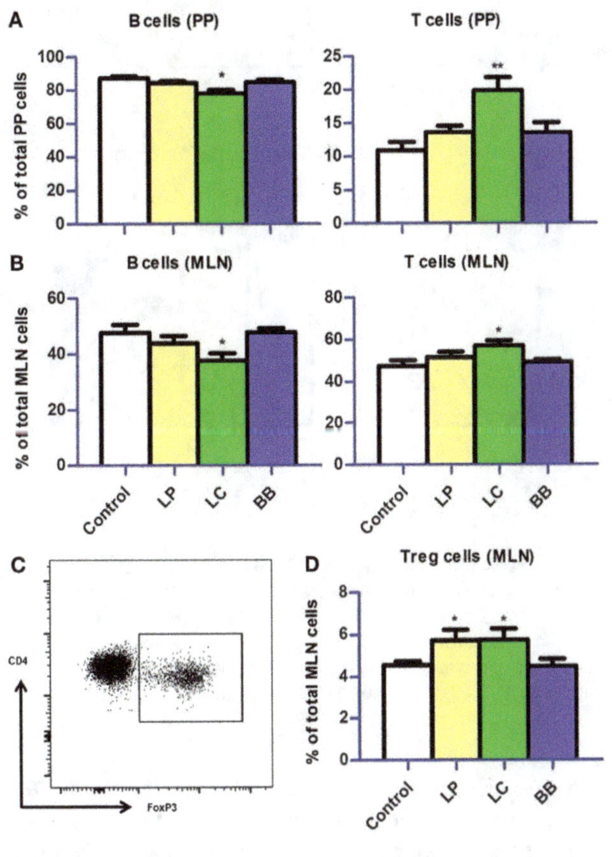

FIGURE 5 | Distribution of B cells and T cells in Peyer's patches (PP) and mesenteric lymph nodes (MLN) upon bacterial supplementation in *Ercc1*$^{-/\Delta 7}$ mice. **(A,B)** Mean frequencies of B and T cells in PP and MLN were determined by flow cytometry. B cells were defined as CD19$^+$, T cells were defined as CD3$^+$. **(C)** Flow cytometric analysis of CD3$^+$CD4$^+$CD8$^-$ regulatory T (Treg) cells in MLN. **(D)** Mean frequencies of Treg cells in MLN. Data represent the mean + SEM from four to six animals per group. LP, *L. plantarum* WCFS1; LC, *L. casei* BL23; BB, *B. breve* DSM20213. $^*p < 0.05$; $^{**}p < 0.01$.

L. casei Elevates Systemic Inflammatory Markers

Next, we assessed distribution of immune cells in the spleen. We noted that the relative spleen weight increased after *L. casei* supplementation in *Ercc1*$^{-/\Delta 7}$ mice (Supplementary Figure 2A in Data Sheet 1). Absolute numbers of spleen cells were not affected by bacterial supplementations (data not shown). Splenic B cell frequencies tended to be decreased after *L. casei* supplementation ($p = 0.06$; **Figure 6A**), but no changes in T cell frequencies were observed (**Figure 6B**). Treg cell frequencies in the spleen were increased after *L. casei* supplementation in *Ercc1*$^{-/\Delta 7}$ mice ($p < 0.05$; **Figure 6C**).

Increased frequencies of CD11b$^+$Ly6G$^-$CD68$^+$Ly6C^{hi} monocytes ($p < 0.01$; **Figures 6D,E**) and a tendency to increased frequencies of CD11b$^+$CD68^{int}Ly6C^{int}Ly6G$^+$ neutrophils were observed after *L. casei* supplementation ($p = 0.07$; **Figure 6F**). In addition, the proportions of CD3$^+$CD4$^+$RORγt$^+$ Th17 cells (Supplementary Figure 2B in Data Sheet 1) were increased after *L. casei* supplementation ($p < 0.05$; **Figure 6G**). A 4-day culture of splenocytes stimulated with concanavalin A (ConA), also showed increased IL-17A production ($p < 0.01$; **Figure 6H**) and a decreased T cell proliferation in splenocytes derived from *L. casei*-treated mice ($p < 0.01$; **Figure 6I**). None of these changes were observed in *Ercc1*$^{-/\Delta 7}$ mice treated with *L. plantarum* or *B. breve*, and in WT mice treated with each of the bacterial supplementations (Supplementary Figure 3 in Data Sheet 1). These data suggest that *L. casei*, in contrast to *L. plantarum* and *B. breve*, raises several inflammatory markers in *Ercc1*$^{-/\Delta 7}$ mice.

Lymphocyte and Myeloid Development Affected after *L. plantarum* or *L. casei* Supplementation

We subsequently investigated the development of B cells and myeloid cells in BM and of T cells in thymus of *Ercc1*$^{-/\Delta 7}$ mice, as the observed changes in cell distribution in PP, MLN, and spleen might be explained by an altered migration or production. Absolute numbers in the BM were unchanged after bacterial supplementation (data not shown). In the BM, we observed significantly higher Lin$^-$CD117^{hi}CD11c$^-$CD135$^-$CD16/32$^+$ granulocyte-monocyte precursor (GMP), CD11b$^+$Ly6G$^+$ neutrophil, and Ly6C^{hi}CD31$^-$ monocyte frequencies after *L. casei* supplementation (**Figures 7A–C**). Frequencies of total CD19$^+$CD45R$^+$ B-lineage cells were decreased after *L. plantarum* ($p < 0.05$) and *L. casei* supplementation ($p < 0.001$), but not after *B. breve* supplementation (**Figure 7D**). We observed a reduction in all B-lineage subsets, except pro-B cells, after *L. casei* and *L. plantarum* supplementation (data not shown). In thymus, only *L. casei* supplementation caused changes in cell distribution, with significantly reduced CD3$^-$CD4$^+$CD8$^+$ double-positive (DP) cell numbers (**Figures 7E–H**).

In WT mice, we found no effect of bacterial supplementations on distribution of immune cells in BM or thymus, except for B-lineage cells after *L. plantarum* and *L. casei* supplementation (Supplementary Figure 4 in Data Sheet 1).

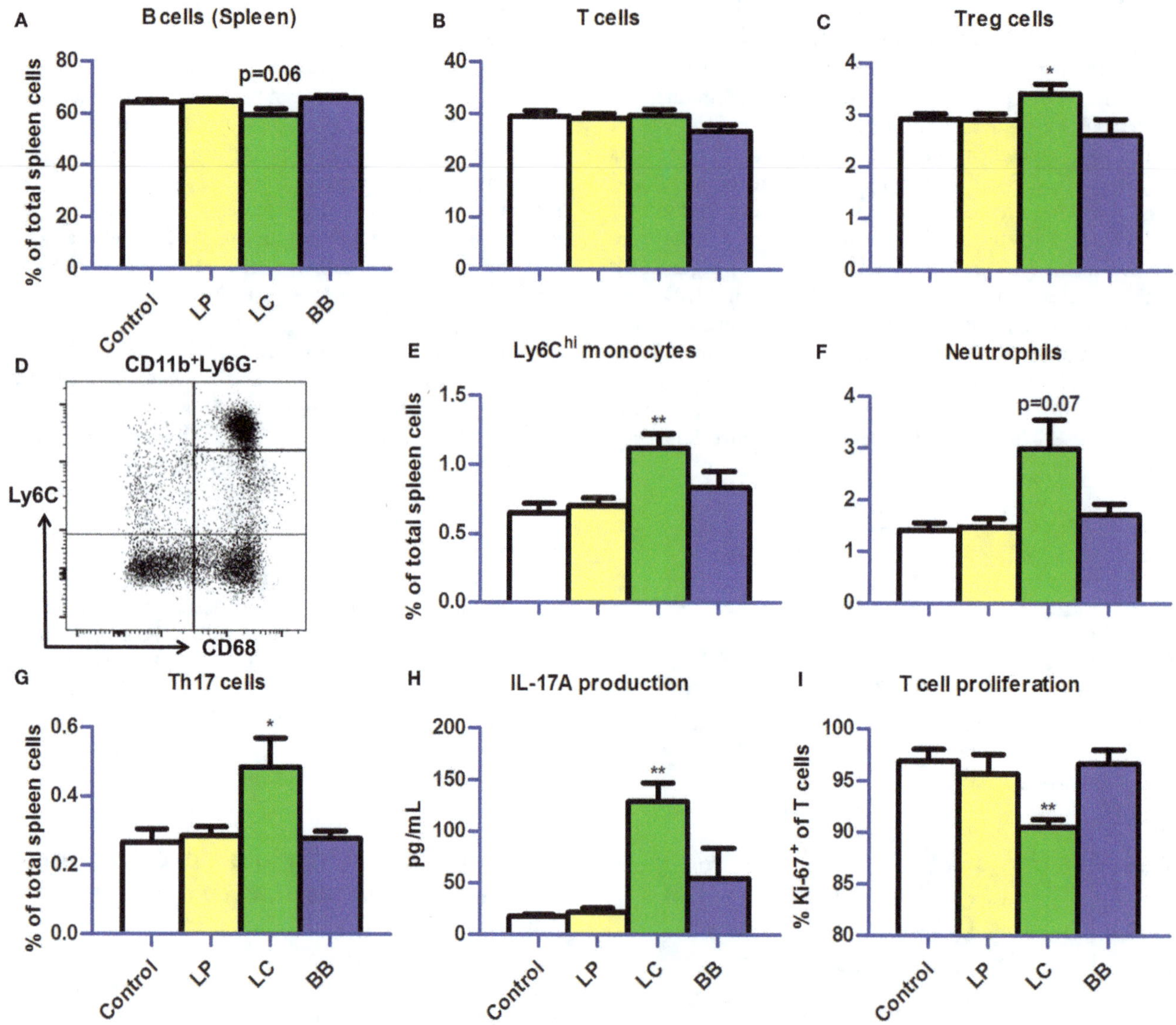

FIGURE 6 | ***L. casei* supplementation of *Ercc1*$^{-/\Delta7}$ mice raised inflammatory markers in spleen. (A,B)** Mean frequencies of B and T cells in spleen were determined by flow cytometry. B cells were defined as CD19$^+$, T cells were defined as CD3$^+$. **(C)** Mean frequencies of Treg cells in spleen. **(D)** Flow cytometric analysis of splenic monocytes. CD11b$^+$Ly6G$^-$CD68$^+$ cells were divided in Ly6C^{hi}, Ly6C^{int}, and Ly6C^{lo} monocytes. **(E–G)** Mean frequencies of Ly6C^{hi} monocytes, neutrophils, and CD3$^+$CD4$^+$CD8$^-$Rorγt$^+$ Th17 cells were determined by flow cytometry. **(H)** Mean concentration of IL-17A production by splenocytes stimulated with ConA for 4 days, as determined by Cytometric Bead Array. **(I)** Mean proliferating T cells (Ki-67$^+$) in splenocyte culture stimulated with ConA for 4 days, as determined by flow cytometry. Data represent the mean + SEM from four to six animals per group. *$p < 0.05$; **$p < 0.01$. LP, *L. plantarum* WCFS1; LC, *L. casei* BL23; BB, *B. breve* DSM20213.

Bacterial Supplementations Do Not Alter Lifespan of *Ercc1*$^{-/\Delta7}$ Mice

The accelerated aging of *Ercc1*$^{-/\Delta7}$ mice enabled us to assess the potential life-extending properties of the bacterial strains. No significant change in lifespan of *Ercc1*$^{-/\Delta7}$ mice was observed after lifelong supplementation with *L. plantarum* or *L. casei* (Supplementary Figure 5 in Data Sheet 1).

L. casei Supplementation Increases IgG Serum Titers

Because *L. casei* supplementation led to decreased B cell proportions in several immune organs of *Ercc1*$^{-/\Delta7}$ mice, we tested whether serum antibody titers in *Ercc1*$^{-/\Delta7}$ mice were altered. Total IgG1 and IgG2b (but not IgG2a, IgG3, IgE, and IgA) titers were significantly increased after *L. casei* supplementation (**Figure 8**). *L. plantarum* and *B. breve* supplementation did not significantly change titers of any Ig subclass.

Immune Competence Improved by *L. casei* and *L. plantarum* Supplementation

To test whether changes in immune cell distribution also impact immune competence, we analyzed the B cell response of *Ercc1*$^{-/\Delta7}$ mice to the T cell-dependent antigen TNP-KLH. Specific anti-TNP-KLH Ig titers of the three tested isotype classes (IgM, IgG1,

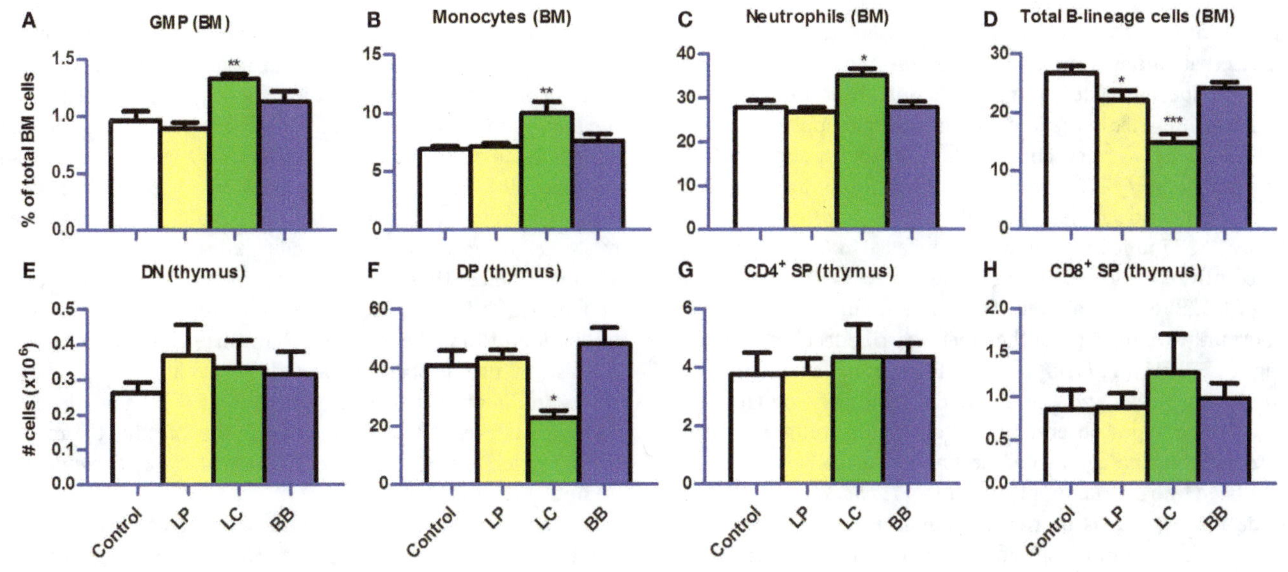

FIGURE 7 | *L. casei* or *L. plantarum* supplementation altered myeloid and lymphoid development in bone marrow and thymus of *Ercc1*$^{-/\Delta7}$ mice. **(A–D)** Mean frequencies in bone marrow (BM) were determined by flow cytometry. Granulocyte–monocyte precursors (GMP) were defined as Lin$^-$CD117^{hi}CD11c$^-$CD135$^-$CD16/32$^+$, neutrophils as CD11b$^+$Ly6G$^+$, monocytes as Ly6C^{hi}CD31$^-$, and B-lineage cells as CD19$^+$CD45R$^+$. **(E–H)** Mean absolute numbers were determined by cell counts and flow cytometry. Double-negative (DN) cells were defined as CD3$^-$CD4$^-$CD8$^-$, double-positive (DP) cells as CD3$^-$CD4$^+$CD8$^+$, CD4$^+$ single-positive (SP) as CD3$^+$CD4$^+$CD8$^-$, and CD8$^+$ SP as CD3$^+$CD4$^-$CD8$^+$. Data represent the mean + SEM from four to six animals per group. $^*p < 0.05$; $^{**}p < 0.01$; $^{***}p < 0.001$. LP, *L. plantarum* WCFS1; LC, *L. casei* BL23; BB, *B. breve* DSM20213.

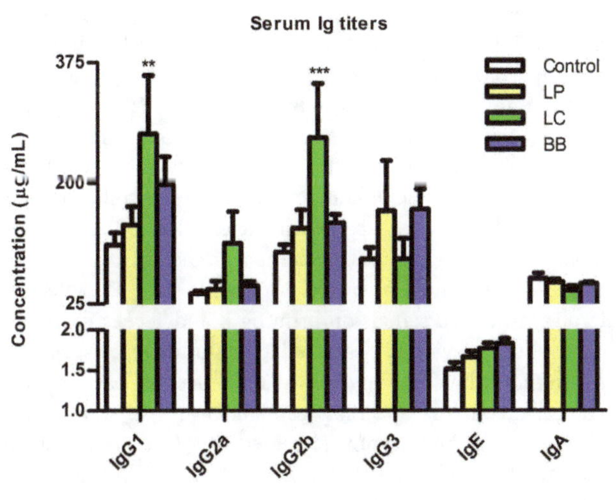

FIGURE 8 | *L. casei* supplementation increased IgG1 and IgG2b titers in *Ercc1*$^{-/\Delta7}$ mice. Mean titers of IgG1, IgG2a, IgG2b, IgG3, IgE, and IgA in serum, as determined by Luminex. Data represent the mean + SEM from three to six animals per group. $^{**}p < 0.01$; $^{***}p < 0.001$. LP = *L. plantarum* WCFS1; LC = *L. casei* BL23; BB = *B. breve* DSM20213.

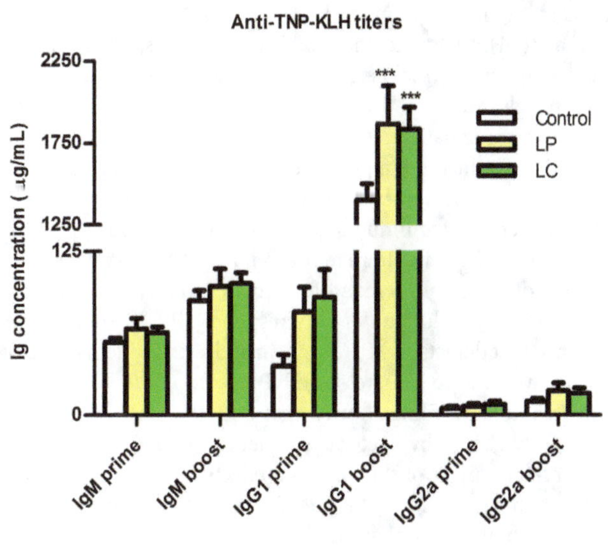

FIGURE 9 | Supplementation of *L. plantarum* and *L. casei* increased specific anti-TNP-KLH antibody responses of *Ercc1*$^{-/\Delta7}$ mice. Mean TNP-specific IgM, IgG1, and IgG2a concentrations in serum were determined by ELISA, 7 days after primary immunization (prime, age 9 weeks), or 7 days after booster immunization (boost, age 13 weeks). Data represent the mean + SEM of 6–12 animals per group. $^{***}p < 0.001$. LP, *L. plantarum* WCFS1; LC, *L. casei* BL23.

IgG2a) after primary and booster immunization were consistently higher after *L. plantarum* and *L. casei* supplementation (**Figure 9**). In particular, IgG1 titers after booster immunization increased in both *L. plantarum*- and *L. casei*-supplemented mice compared with control-treated mice ($p < 0.001$).

From these findings, we conclude that *L. plantarum* and *L. casei* enhance T cell-dependent B cell responses in *Ercc1*$^{-/\Delta7}$ mice.

DISCUSSION

The effects of bacterial supplementations on the intestinal barrier and cellular parameters of immunity were studied in fast aging

$Ercc1^{-/\Delta7}$ mice. We observed that the mucus layer in the colon declines with age and that bacterial supplementation may prevent or exacerbate the age-related decline in the mucus layer, dependent on the specific bacterial strain. Additionally, we demonstrated a marked difference in the response to bacterial supplementations between $Ercc1^{-/\Delta7}$ mice and WT mice. Finally, supplementation with *L. casei* BL23 profoundly changed the distribution of immune cells and supplementation with *L. plantarum* WCFS1 or *L. casei* BL23 improved immune competence in $Ercc1^{-/\Delta7}$ mice.

Recently, we showed the age-related decline in mucus barrier of C57Bl/6 mice as well (Sovran et al., unpublished data). Importantly, we report that the mucus barrier declines with age, in aged C57Bl/6 and $Ercc1^{-/\Delta7}$ mice (**Figure 1**). This finding adds another age-related phenotype to the wide spectrum of age-related phenotypes observed in $Ercc1^{-/\Delta7}$ mice (40). Moreover, we report that the age-related decline in mucus barrier can be modulated by bacterial supplementation. *L. plantarum* prevented the decline in mucus barrier. *L. plantarum* is able to bind to mucus with a mannose-specific adhesin, which is described as a potential probiotic feature (41). In total, *L. plantarum* harbors four mucus-binding proteins (42). Based on the improved spatial compartmentalization of bacteria after *L. plantarum* supplementation, we postulate that *L. plantarum* adheres to the mucus. In addition, we found that *L. plantarum* supplementation tended to decrease the abundance of *Akkermansia muciniphila* (**Figure 3**), which is known as a mucus degrader (43). Thus, it would be conceivable that mucus degradation is decreased after *L. plantarum* supplementation. By contrast, *B. breve* is known as a mucus degrader (44), and could, therefore, be directly responsible for the decrease in mucus thickness in the colon of *B. breve*-treated mice. Interestingly, several pathways involved in protein folding and the UPR were upregulated after *L. casei* and *B. breve* supplementation (Data Sheet 2 in the Supplementary Material). A high demand for synthesis of secretory proteins (such as mucins) induces ER stress, which in turn induces the UPR (45). The close proximity of bacteria to the epithelium in *L. casei*- and *B. breve*-treated mice might induce a high demand for mucin production and secretion, leading to induction of ER stress and UPR. There is indeed evidence that defects in MUC2 mucin and a subsequent defective mucus layer lead to ER stress and UPR (46).

Microbiota profiling showed that only few microbial species are slightly altered by bacterial supplementation (**Figures 2** and **3**). Therefore, most of the observed effects in the mucus barrier and immune system may be directly linked to the supplementation of each of the bacterial strains.

We found that the different bacterial strains elicited characteristically different responses in gene regulation in the colon (**Figure 4**). *L. plantarum* is known for its moderately pro-inflammatory profile, and relatively high IL-10 induction, when tested in human PBMC cultures (28, 47). In line with these studies, several upstream regulators predicted to be activated after *L. plantarum* supplementation included the inflammatory cytokines IFN-γ, IL-1β, IL-4, and TNF. The association between increased activation of inflammatory cytokines and the improved integrity of the colon after *L. plantarum* supplementation raises the possibility that it might be beneficial to locally increase inflammatory cytokine levels. This suggestion is corroborated by the absence of activation of these inflammatory cytokines after *L. casei* or *B. breve* supplementation, which did not improve or exacerbate the age-related decline in mucus integrity. A "tonic" level of constitutive TLR activation by commensal bacteria was previously shown to be crucial in the recovery from DSS-induced epithelial damage due to the role of NF-κB in epithelial repair processes (48). This notion that "physiological pro-inflammatory signals" is required for intestinal homeostasis is also supported by studies using epithelium-specific iκB kinase-γ (or NEMO) ablation in mice. These mice develop spontaneous colitis due to the failure of NF-κB to induce epithelial repair and steady-state production of innate effector mechanisms in the intestine (49). TLR2 signaling has been implicated in tight junction regulation *in vivo* and *in vitro* (13). Thus, it is possible that aged mice have sub-optimal level of TLR stimulation in the intestine to promote innate barrier defenses and that this is enhanced by *L. plantarum*, but not by *L. casei* and *B. breve*.

Remarkably, none of the significantly regulated genes were directly linked to mucus production. However, while performing Upstream Regulator Analysis, growth factors, such as EGF, IGF1, and EGR1, were predicted to be activated after *L. plantarum* supplementation. Together, these findings may indicate that mucus production by goblet cells is not directly enhanced, but is part of general epithelial integrity, supported by a number of growth factors.

Because many regulated genes involved immune-related genes, we additionally analyzed the makeup of the immune system after bacterial supplementation. Whereas supplementation with *B. breve* exacerbated the age-related decline in mucus barrier in colon, it did not cause any changes in mucosal or systemic immunity (**Figures 5–8**). Oppositely, *L. casei* supplementation caused various signs of inflammation, such as Ly6C^{hi} monocyte and neutrophil influx and production in spleen and BM, respectively. These inflammatory signs were coincided with the general decrease in B cell frequencies (also in the BM) and double-positive thymocytes. There is evidence that neutrophils in the BM are primed by microbial ligands (50). The effects of microbiota-derived signals on priming B and T cells in the BM have not been previously described. Our study suggests an, up to now, unknown link between microbiota, intestinal barrier, and B and T cell precursors. Specific precursor stages (i.e., small resting pre-B cells) were significantly decreased after *L. casei* supplementation, and to a lesser extent after *L. plantarum* supplementation. In the case of *L. plantarum* supplementation, we suggest that improved intestinal barrier function might alter circulating microbiota-derived products, such as peptidoglycan (PGN) and lipopolysaccharide (LPS). For instance, hematopoietic stem cells are damaged after chronic exposure to LPS (51). Interestingly, the decrease in small resting pre-B cells after *L. casei* supplementation (and to lesser extent by *L. plantarum*) was the only finding that could be reproduced in WT mice supplemented with these bacterial strains (Supplementary Figure 4 in Data Sheet 1). This may indicate that the effect of *L. casei* and *L. plantarum* supplementation on B cell development is independent of age.

A previous study showed lifespan extension after *B. animalis* supplementation (21). Therefore, we performed a lifespan study for *L. plantarum* and *L. casei*, which indicated that neither of them is shortening or extending lifespan (Supplementary Figure 5 in Data Sheet 1).

Surprisingly, anti-TNP-KLH IgG1 titers in serum increased not only after *L. plantarum* but also after *L. casei* supplementation (**Figure 9**). This increase suggests that a demise in B cell development and B cell distribution does not necessarily translate into impaired B cell function. Previously, it has been shown that antigen-specific antibody titers can be enhanced by probiotic supplementation in aged mice (20), but data on B cell development are lacking.

The effects of the candidate probiotic strains were pronounced on the mucus barrier in the colon of *Ercc1*$^{-/\Delta7}$ mice compared with WT mice. It has been shown in previous studies that strains, such as *L. casei* and *B. breve*, have beneficial effects on immunological parameters and intestinal barrier function in young mice (29–31). In our hands, *L. casei* and *B. breve* had no effect on mucus barrier or systemic immunity in young WT mice (except for the above-discussed finding on B cell development). A severe deteriorating effect, however, was observed on the mucus barrier or systemic immunity in *Ercc1*$^{-/\Delta7}$ mice. These findings highlight the need for caution in translating beneficial effects of probiotics observed in young animals or humans to the elderly.

Our study has a number of limitations. We observed remarkable changes in the mucus layer, but could not pinpoint a single gene that is directly linked to the mucus layer. Furthermore, we did not include commercially available probiotic bacterial strains, such as *Lactobacillus rhamnosus* GG, or a non-probiotic bacterial strain. Nevertheless, our study reveals a previously unknown effect of age on the mucus barrier. We also show that it is possible to modulate this age-related decline in the mucus barrier by supplementation of bacterial strains, with coinciding effects on systemic immunity. More research is warranted to elucidate the interplay between bacteria, the aged gut epithelium, and the immune system.

Our data provide evidence that a comprehensive analysis of the intestinal barrier and immunity are needed in order to evaluate how bacterial supplementation contributes to the restoration of the age-related decline in intestinal barrier. A positive finding was that probiotic strains, such as *L. plantarum*, might contribute to maintenance of intestinal integrity by preventing age-related deterioration of the colonic mucus layer.

AUTHOR CONTRIBUTIONS

AB, BS, JHH, WV, PV, JW, PL, CN, RH, and HS conceived the study. AB, BS, FH, BM, CB, JAH, VM, CP, and MB performed the experiments. AB wrote the manuscript. BS, FH, BM, CB, JAH, JHH, WV, PV, JW, PL, CN, RH, and HS contributed to the revisions of the draft manuscripts.

ACKNOWLEDGMENTS

Authors thank Steven Aalvink, Marjolein de Jong-de Bruijn, and Jenny Jansen for technical help. We acknowledge the excellent help of all animal caretakers.

SUPPLEMENTARY MATERIAL

The Supplementary Material for this article can be found online at http://journal.frontiersin.org/article/10.3389/fimmu.2016.00408

DATA SHEET 1

SUPPLEMENTARY TABLE 1 | Used antibodies in flow cytometry.

SUPPLEMENTARY TABLE 2 | Top-10 biological processes upregulated (as determined with GSEA) by bacterial supplementations in proximal colon of *Ercc1*$^{-/\Delta7}$ mice treated with *L. plantarum* WCFS1 (LP), *L. casei* BL23 (LC), or *B. breve* DSM20213 (BB).

SUPPLEMENTARY TABLE 3 | Top-10 biological processes downregulated (as determined with GSEA) by bacterial supplementations in proximal colon of *Ercc1*$^{-/\Delta7}$ mice treated with *L. plantarum* WCFS1 (LP), *L. casei* BL23 (LC), or *B. breve* DSM20213 (BB).

SUPPLEMENTARY FIGURE 1 | Distribution of B cells and T cells in Peyer's patches and mesenteric lymph nodes not changed upon bacterial supplementation in *Ercc1*$^{+/+}$ mice. (A/B) Mean frequencies were determined by flow cytometry. B cells were defined as CD19$^+$, T cells were defined as CD3$^+$. **(C)** Mean frequencies of CD3$^+$CD4$^+$CD8$^-$FoxP3$^+$ regulatory T (Treg) cells in MLN. Data represent the mean + SEM from four to six animals per group. LP, *L. plantarum* WCFS1; LC, *L. casei* BL23; BB, *B. breve* DSM20213.

SUPPLEMENTARY FIGURE 2 | Increased relative spleen weight after *L. casei* supplementation of *Ercc1*$^{-/\Delta7}$ mice. (A) Spleen weights relative to body weight. Data represent mean spleen weights + SEM of four to six animals per group. **(B)** Flow cytometric analysis of splenic Th17 cells. CD3$^+$CD4$^+$CD8$^-$ cells were gated for RORγt and FSC (forward scatter).

SUPPLEMENTARY FIGURE 3 | Bacterial supplementation of *Ercc1*$^{+/+}$ mice did not change splenic parameters. (A) Mean frequencies of Treg cells in spleen. **(B–D)** Mean frequencies of Ly6C^{hi} monocytes, neutrophils, and CD3$^+$CD4$^+$CD8$^-$Rorγt$^+$ Th17 cells were determined by flow cytometry. **(E)** Mean concentration of IL-17A production by splenocytes stimulated with ConA for 4 days, as determined by Cytometric Bead Array. **(F)** Mean proliferating T cells (Ki-67$^+$) in splenocyte culture stimulated with ConA for 4 days, as determined by flow cytometry. Data represent the mean + SEM from four to six animals per group. LP, *L. plantarum* WCFS1; LC, *L. casei* BL23; BB, *B. breve* DSM20213.

SUPPLEMENTARY FIGURE 4 | *L. casei* supplementation altered B cell development in bone marrow of *Ercc1*$^{+/+}$ mice. (A–E) Mean frequencies in bone marrow (BM) were determined by flow cytometry. Granulocyte–monocyte precursors (GMP) were defined as Lin$^-$CD117^{hi}CD11c$^-$CD135$^-$CD16/32$^+$, neutrophils as CD11b$^+$Ly6G$^+$, monocytes as Ly6C^{hi}CD31$^-$, B-lineage cells as CD19$^+$CD45R$^+$, and small resting pre-B cells as sIgκ/λ$^-$cIgM$^+$CD2$^+$. **(F)** Mean absolute numbers were determined by cell counts and flow cytometry. Double-positive (DP) cells were defined as CD3$^-$CD4$^+$CD8$^+$. Data represent the mean + SEM from four to six animals per group. $^*p<0.05$. LP, *L. plantarum* WCFS1; LC, *L. casei* BL23; BB, *B. breve* DSM20213.

SUPPLEMENTARY FIGURE 5 | Bacterial supplementations did not change lifespan of *Ercc1*$^{-/\Delta7}$ mice. Data represent 11–12 animals per group (with an additional 6 animals per group censored at 16 weeks). LP, *L. plantarum* WCFS1; LC, *L. casei* BL23.

DATA SHEET 2 | Total file with differentially expressed genes after bacterial supplementations.

REFERENCES

1. CDC. *The State of Aging and Health in America 2013*. Atlanta, GA: (2013). Available from: http://www.cdc.gov/aging/pdf/state-aging-health-in-america-2013.pdf
2. Lozano R, Naghavi M, Foreman K, Lim S, Shibuya K, Aboyans V, et al. Global and regional mortality from 235 causes of death for 20 age groups in 1990 and 2010: a systematic analysis for the Global Burden of Disease Study 2010. *Lancet* (2013) 380(9859):2095–128. doi:10.1016/S0140-6736(12)61728-0
3. López-Otín C, Blasco MA, Partridge L, Serrano M, Kroemer G. The hallmarks of aging. *Cell* (2013) 153(6):1194–217. doi:10.1016/j.cell.2013.05.039
4. Man AL, Gicheva N, Nicoletti C. The impact of ageing on the intestinal epithelial barrier and immune system. *Cell Immunol* (2014) 289(1):112–8. doi:10.1016/j.cellimm.2014.04.001
5. Johansson ME, Ambort D, Pelaseyed T, Schütte A, Gustafsson JK, Ermund A, et al. Composition and functional role of the mucus layers in the intestine. *Cell Mol Life Sci* (2011) 68(22):3635–41. doi:10.1007/s00018-011-0822-3
6. Shan M, Gentile M, Yeiser JR, Walland AC, Bornstein VU, Chen K, et al. Mucus enhances gut homeostasis and oral tolerance by delivering immunoregulatory signals. *Science* (2013) 342(6157):447–53. doi:10.1126/science.1237910
7. Johansson ME, Larsson JMH, Hansson GC. The two mucus layers of colon are organized by the MUC2 mucin, whereas the outer layer is a legislator of host-microbial interactions. *Proc Natl Acad Sci U S A* (2011) 108(Suppl 1):4659–65. doi:10.1073/pnas.1006451107
8. Sovran B, Loonen LM, Lu P, Hugenholtz F, Belzer C, Stolte EH, et al. IL-22-STAT3 pathway plays a key role in the maintenance of ileal homeostasis in mice lacking secreted mucus barrier. *Inflamm Bowel Dis* (2015) 21(3):531–42. doi:10.1097/MIB.0000000000000319
9. Franceschi C, Bonafè M, Valensin S, Olivieri F, de Luca M, Ottaviani E, et al. Inflamm-aging: an evolutionary perspective on immunosenescence. *Ann N Y Acad Sci* (2000) 908(1):244–54. doi:10.1111/j.1749-6632.2000.tb06651.x
10. Min H, Montecino-Rodriguez E, Dorshkind K. Effects of aging on the common lymphoid progenitor to pro-B cell transition. *J Immunol* (2006) 176(2):1007–12. doi:10.4049/jimmunol.176.2.1007
11. George AJ, Ritter MA. Thymic involution with ageing: obsolescence or good housekeeping? *Immunol Today* (1996) 17(6):267–72. doi:10.1016/0167-5699(96)80543-3
12. Valiathan R, Ashman M, Asthana D. Effects of ageing on the immune system: infants to elderly. *Scand J Immunol* (2016) 83(4):255–66. doi:10.1111/sji.12413
13. Karczewski J, Troost FJ, Konings I, Dekker J, Kleerebezem M, Brummer R-JM, et al. Regulation of human epithelial tight junction proteins by *Lactobacillus plantarum* in vivo and protective effects on the epithelial barrier. *Am J Physiol Gastrointest Liver Physiol* (2010) 298(6):G851–9. doi:10.1152/ajpgi.00327.2009
14. Sherman PM, Ossa JC, Johnson-Henry K. Unraveling mechanisms of action of probiotics. *Nutr Clin Pract* (2009) 24(1):10–4. doi:10.1177/0884533608329231
15. Akatsu H, Iwabuchi N, Xiao J-Z, Matsuyama Z, Kurihara R, Okuda K, et al. Clinical effects of probiotic *Bifidobacterium longum* BB536 on immune function and intestinal microbiota in elderly patients receiving enteral tube feeding. *J Parenter Enteral Nutr* (2012) 37(5):631–40. doi:10.1177/0148607112467819
16. Spaiser SJ, Culpepper T, Nieves C Jr, Ukhanova M, Mai V, Percival SS, et al. *Lactobacillus gasseri* KS-13, *Bifidobacterium bifidum* G9-1, and *Bifidobacterium longum* MM-2 ingestion induces a less inflammatory cytokine profile and a potentially beneficial shift in gut microbiota in older adults: a randomized, double-blind, placebo-controlled, crossover study. *J Am Coll Nutr* (2015) 34(6):459–69. doi:10.1080/07315724.2014.983249
17. Rampelli S, Candela M, Severgnini M, Biagi E, Turroni S, Roselli M, et al. A probiotics-containing biscuit modulates the intestinal microbiota in the elderly. *J Nutr Health Aging* (2013) 17(2):166–72. doi:10.1007/s12603-012-0372-x
18. Gill H, Rutherfurd K, Cross M. Dietary probiotic supplementation enhances natural killer cell activity in the elderly: an investigation of age-related immunological changes. *J Clin Immunol* (2001) 21(4):264–71. doi:10.1023/A:1010979225018
19. Gill HS, Rutherfurd KJ, Cross ML, Gopal PK. Enhancement of immunity in the elderly by dietary supplementation with the probiotic *Bifidobacterium lactis* HN019. *Am J Clin Nutr* (2001) 74(6):833–9.
20. Vidal K, Benyacoub J, Moser M, Sanchez-Garcia J, Serrant P, Segura-Roggero I, et al. Effect of *Lactobacillus paracasei* NCC2461 on antigen-specific T-cell mediated immune responses in aged mice. *Rejuvenation Res* (2008) 11(5):957–64. doi:10.1089/rej.2008.0780
21. Matsumoto M, Kurihara S, Kibe R, Ashida H, Benno Y. Longevity in mice is promoted by probiotic-induced suppression of colonic senescence dependent on upregulation of gut bacterial polyamine production. *PLoS One* (2011) 6(8):e23652. doi:10.1371/journal.pone.0023652
22. Gurkar AU, Niedernhofer LJ. Comparison of mice with accelerated aging caused by distinct mechanisms. *Exp Gerontol* (2015) 68:43–50. doi:10.1016/j.exger.2015.01.045
23. van Beek AA, Hugenholtz F, Meijer B, Sovran B, Perdijk O, Vermeij WP, et al. Tryptophan restriction arrests B cell development and enhances microbial diversity in WT and prematurely aging Ercc1−/Δ7 mice. *J Leukoc Biol* (2016). doi:10.1189/jlb.1HI0216-062RR
24. Dollé ME, Kuiper RV, Roodbergen M, Robinson J, de Vlugt S, Wijnhoven SW, et al. Broad segmental progeroid changes in short-lived Ercc1−/Δ7 mice. *Pathobiol Aging Age Relat Dis* (2011) 1:7219. doi:10.3402/pba.v1i0.7219
25. Weeda G, Donker I, de Wit J, Morreau H, Janssens R, Vissers C, et al. Disruption of mouse ERCC1 results in a novel repair syndrome with growth failure, nuclear abnormalities and senescence. *Curr Biol* (1997) 7(6):427–39. doi:10.1016/S0960-9822(06)00190-4
26. Ivanovic N, Minic R, Dimitrijevic L, Skodric SR, Zivkovic I, Djordjevic B. *Lactobacillus rhamnosus* LA68 and *Lactobacillus plantarum* WCFS1 differently influence metabolic and immunological parameters in high fat diet-induced hypercholesterolemia and hepatic steatosis. *Food Funct* (2015) 6:558–65. doi:10.1039/c4fo00843j
27. Meijerink M, Wells JM, Taverne N, Zeeuw Brouwer ML, Hilhorst B, Venema K, et al. Immunomodulatory effects of potential probiotics in a mouse peanut sensitization model. *FEMS Immunol Med Microbiol* (2012) 65(3):488–96. doi:10.1111/j.1574-695X.2012.00981.x
28. Snel J, Vissers Y, Smit B, Jongen J, Van der Meulen E, Zwijsen R, et al. Strain-specific immunomodulatory effects of *Lactobacillus plantarum* strains on birch-pollen-allergic subjects out of season. *Clin Exp Allergy* (2011) 41(2):232–42. doi:10.1111/j.1365-2222.2010.03650.x
29. Foligne B, Nutten S, Grangette C, Dennin V, Goudercourt D, Poiret S, et al. Correlation between in vitro and in vivo immunomodulatory properties of lactic acid bacteria. *World J Gastroenterol* (2007) 13(2):236–43. doi:10.3748/wjg.v13.i2.236
30. Bäuerl C, Pérez-Martínez G, Yan F, Polk DB, Monedero V. Functional analysis of the p40 and p75 proteins from *Lactobacillus casei* BL23. *J Mol Microbiol Biotechnol* (2010) 19(4):231–41. doi:10.1159/000322233
31. Hougee S, Vriesema A, Wijering S, Knippels L, Folkerts G, Nijkamp F, et al. Oral treatment with probiotics reduces allergic symptoms in ovalbumin-sensitized mice: a bacterial strain comparative study. *Int Arch Allergy Immunol* (2009) 151(2):107–17. doi:10.1159/000236000
32. Van Beek AA, Hoogerland JA, Belzer C, De Vos P, De Vos W, Savelkoul HF, et al. Interaction of mouse splenocytes and macrophages with bacterial strains in vivo: the effect of age in the immune response. *Benef Microbes* (2016) 7(2):275–87. doi:10.3920/BM2015.0094
33. Cho JS, Kook SH, Robinson AR, Niedernhofer LJ, Lee BC. Cell autonomous and nonautonomous mechanisms drive hematopoietic stem/progenitor cell loss in the absence of DNA repair. *Stem Cells* (2013) 31(3):511–25. doi:10.1002/stem.1261
34. Sovran B, Lu P, Loonen LM, Hugenholtz F, Belzer C, Stolte EH, et al. Identification of commensal species positively correlated with early stress responses to a compromised mucus barrier. *Inflamm Bowel Dis* (2016) 22(4):826–40. doi:10.1097/MIB.0000000000000688
35. Rajilić-Stojanović M, Heilig HG, Molenaar D, Kajander K, Surakka A, Smidt H, et al. Development and application of the human intestinal tract chip, a phylogenetic microarray: analysis of universally conserved phylotypes in the abundant microbiota of young and elderly adults. *Environ Microbiol* (2009) 11(7):1736–51. doi:10.1111/j.1462-2920.2009.01900.x
36. Lahti L, Elo LL, Aittokallio T, Kaski S. Probabilistic analysis of probe reliability in differential gene expression studies with short oligonucleotide arrays. *IEEE/ACM Trans Comput Biol Bioinform* (2011) 8(1):217–25. doi:10.1109/TCBB.2009.38

37. Braak CJF, Šmilauer P. *CANOCO Reference Manual and User's Guide: Software for Ordination (Version 5.0)*. Ithaca: Biometris (2012).
38. van Loo PF, Dingjan GM, Maas A, Hendriks RW. Surrogate-light-chain silencing is not critical for the limitation of pre-B cell expansion but is for the termination of constitutive signaling. *Immunity* (2007) 27(3):468–80. doi:10.1016/j.immuni.2007.07.018
39. Subramanian A, Tamayo P, Mootha VK, Mukherjee S, Ebert BL, Gillette MA, et al. Gene set enrichment analysis: a knowledge-based approach for interpreting genome-wide expression profiles. *Proc Natl Acad Sci U S A* (2005) 102(43):15545–50. doi:10.1073/pnas.0506580102
40. Vermeij WP, Hoeijmakers J, Pothof J. Genome integrity in aging: human syndromes, mouse models, and therapeutic options. *Annu Rev Pharmacol Toxicol* (2016) 56(11):427–45. doi:10.1146/annurev-pharmtox-010814-124316
41. Pretzer G, Snel J, Molenaar D, Wiersma A, Bron PA, Lambert J, et al. Biodiversity-based identification and functional characterization of the mannose-specific adhesin of *Lactobacillus plantarum*. *J Bacteriol* (2005) 187(17):6128–36. doi:10.1128/JB.187.17.6128-6136.2005
42. Boekhorst J, Helmer Q, Kleerebezem M, Siezen RJ. Comparative analysis of proteins with a mucus-binding domain found exclusively in lactic acid bacteria. *Microbiology* (2006) 152(1):273–80. doi:10.1099/mic.0.28415-0
43. Derrien M, Vaughan EE, Plugge CM, de Vos WM. *Akkermansia muciniphila* gen. nov., sp. nov., a human intestinal mucin-degrading bacterium. *Int J Syst Evol Microbiol* (2004) 54(5):1469–76. doi:10.1099/ijs.0.02873-0
44. Rokhsefat S, Lin A, Comelli EM. Mucin–microbiota interaction during post-natal maturation of the intestinal ecosystem: clinical implications. *Dig Dis Sci* (2016) 61(6):1473–86. doi:10.1007/s10620-016-4032-6
45. Hetz C. The unfolded protein response: controlling cell fate decisions under ER stress and beyond. *Nat Rev Mol Cell Biol* (2012) 13(2):89–102. doi:10.1038/nrm3270
46. Heazlewood CK, Cook MC, Eri R, Price GR, Tauro SB, Taupin D, et al. Aberrant mucin assembly in mice causes endoplasmic reticulum stress and spontaneous inflammation resembling ulcerative colitis. *PLoS Med* (2008) 5(3):e54. doi:10.1371/journal.pmed.0050054
47. van Hemert S, Meijerink M, Molenaar D, Bron PA, de Vos P, Kleerebezem M, et al. Identification of *Lactobacillus plantarum* genes modulating the cytokine response of human peripheral blood mononuclear cells. *BMC Microbiol* (2010) 10(1):293. doi:10.1186/1471-2180-10-293
48. Rakoff-Nahoum S, Paglino J, Eslami-Varzaneh F, Edberg S, Medzhitov R. Recognition of commensal microflora by toll-like receptors is required for intestinal homeostasis. *Cell* (2004) 118(2):229–41. doi:10.1016/j.cell.2004.07.002
49. Nenci A, Becker C, Wullaert A, Gareus R, van Loo G, Danese S, et al. Epithelial NEMO links innate immunity to chronic intestinal inflammation. *Nature* (2007) 446(7135):557–61. doi:10.1038/nature05698
50. Clarke TB, Davis KM, Lysenko ES, Zhou AY, Yu Y, Weiser JN. Recognition of peptidoglycan from the microbiota by Nod1 enhances systemic innate immunity. *Nat Med* (2010) 16(2):228–31. doi:10.1038/nm.2087
51. Esplin BL, Shimazu T, Welner RS, Garrett KP, Nie L, Zhang Q, et al. Chronic exposure to a TLR ligand injures hematopoietic stem cells. *J Immunol* (2011) 186(9):5367–75. doi:10.4049/jimmunol.1003438

13

Peptidoglycan from Immunobiotic *Lactobacillus rhamnosus* Improves Resistance of Infant Mice to Respiratory Syncytial Viral Infection and Secondary Pneumococcal Pneumonia

Patricia Clua[1,2†], Paulraj Kanmani[3,4†], Hortensia Zelaya[1,5], Asuka Tada[3], A. K. M. Humayun Kober[3,4], Susana Salva[1,2], Susana Alvarez[1,2,5], Haruki Kitazawa[3,4] and Julio Villena[1,2,3]**

[1] Immunobiotics Research Group, Tucuman, Argentina, [2] Laboratory of Immunobiotechnology, Reference Centre for Lactobacilli (CERELA-CONICET), Tucuman, Argentina, [3] Food and Feed Immunology Group, Laboratory of Animal Products Chemistry, Graduate School of Agricultural Science, Tohoku University, Sendai, Japan, [4] Livestock Immunology Unit, International Education and Research Center for Food and Agricultural Immunology (CFAI), Graduate School of Agricultural Science, Tohoku University, Sendai, Japan, [5] Institute of Applied Biochemistry, National University of Tucumán, Tucuman, Argentina

Edited by:
Hao Shen,
Perelman School of Medicine,
United States

Reviewed by:
Mariela Segura,
Université de Montréal, Canada
Yan Wang,
University of Pennsylvania,
United States

***Correspondence:**
Haruki Kitazawa
haruki.kitazawa.c7@tohoku.ac.jp;
Julio Villena
jcvillena@cerela.org.ar

†These authors have contributed equally to this work.

Several research works have demonstrated that beneficial microbes with the capacity to modulate the mucosal immune system (immunobiotics) are an interesting alternative to improve the outcome of bacterial and viral respiratory infections. Among the immunobiotic strains with the capacity to beneficially modulate respiratory immunity, *Lactobacillus rhamnosus* CRL1505 has outstanding properties. Although we have significantly advanced in demonstrating the capacity of *L. rhamnosus* CRL1505 to improve resistance against respiratory infections as well as in the cellular and molecular mechanisms involved in its beneficial activities, the potential protective ability of this strain or its immunomodulatory cellular fractions in the context of a secondary bacterial pneumonia has not been addressed before. In this work, we demonstrated that the nasal priming with non-viable *L. rhamnosus* CRL1505 or its purified peptidoglycan differentially modulated the respiratory innate antiviral immune response triggered by toll-like receptor 3 activation in infant mice, improving the resistance to primary respiratory syncytial virus (RSV) infection, and secondary pneumococcal pneumonia. In association with the protection against RSV-pneumococcal superinfection, we found that peptidoglycan from *L. rhamnosus* CRL1505 significantly improved lung $CD3^+CD4^+IFN\text{-}\gamma^+$, and $CD3^+CD4^+IL\text{-}10^+$ T cells as well as $CD11c^+SiglecF^+IFN\text{-}\beta^+$ alveolar macrophages with the consequent increases of IFN-γ, IL-10, and IFN-β in the respiratory tract. Our results also showed that the increase of these three cytokines is necessary to achieve protection against respiratory superinfection since each of them are involved in different aspect of the secondary pneumococcal pneumonia that have to be controlled in order to reduce the severity of the infectious disease: lung pneumococcal colonization, bacteremia, and inflammatory-mediated lung tissue injury.

Keywords: immunobiotics, peptidoglycan, toll-like receptor 3, viral immunity, *Streptococcus pneumoniae*, respiratory syncytial virus

INTRODUCTION

Respiratory viral attack often result in mild to moderate infection; however, life-threatening disease can occur in high-risk populations such as infants, elderly, and immunocompromised hosts. Moreover, secondary bacterial pneumonia is an important complication responsible for high morbidity and mortality during epidemic and pandemic viral respiratory infections in infants and children (1–3). It was demonstrated that secondary bacterial respiratory infections are caused primarily by *Streptococcus pneumoniae*. The majority of the clinical observations and experiments in animal models have focused in post-influenza pneumococcal pneumonia (4). In fact, numerous studies have investigated how primary influenza virus (IFV) infection enhances the susceptibility to secondary pneumococcal disease, by increasing bacterial attachment and colonization, disrupting epithelial barriers, and altering the innate immune response in the respiratory tract (3). Although IFV and *S. pneumoniae* interaction has been extensively studied because of its great impact in the severity of respiratory infections, other viruses like the Respiratory Syncytial Virus (RSV) have been associated to an increased susceptibility to secondary pneumococcal pneumonia.

Clinical and epidemiologic data suggest that RSV is linked to increases in the frequency (5) and severity (6) of pneumococcal disease. It was also demonstrated that mice infected with RSV before pneumococcal challenge as well as mice infected with both respiratory pathogens simultaneously showed enhanced lung alterations and elevated levels of bacteremia (7, 8). Mechanisms underlying pneumococcal superinfection include RSV-induced local destruction of the epithelium and respiratory ciliary dyskinesia that impairs mucociliary clearance in the airways (8). Elevated pneumococcal adherence to the respiratory tract epithelium is also considered one of the mechanisms facilitating *S. pneumoniae* infection. It was reported that intercellular adhesion molecule 1 (ICAM-1), carcinoembryonic adhesion molecule 1 (CEACAM1), and platelet activating factor receptor (PAF) are upregulated by RSV infection in respiratory epithelial cells, which are molecules used by pneumococci for colonization (9). Moreover, *in vitro* experiments with HEp-2 cells (human nasopharyngeal), A549 cells (pneumocyte type II), or human airway epithelial cell primary cultures showed that RSV virions enhance pneumococcal adherence through the expression of the viral G protein in epithelial surfaces that serve as an adhesion molecule for pneumococci (7, 8, 10). Surprisingly, transcriptomic analysis performed by Smith et al. (8) showed that the direct interaction between RSV and *S. pneumoniae* alters bacterial gene expression. The work demonstrated that the pneumococcal penicillin-binding protein 1a binds RSV G protein and that this interaction alters *S. pneumoniae* transcriptome increasing the expression of the virulence factors pneumolysin and neuraminidase A/B. These results indicate that complex interactions exist between RSV, *S. pneumoniae*, and host, which must be fully characterized in order to reduce the severity and mortality of respiratory superinfections caused by these pathogens.

During the last years, several research works have demonstrated that beneficial microbes with the capacity to modulate the mucosal immune system (immunobiotics) are a potential alternative to improve the outcome of bacterial (11) and viral (12) respiratory infections. Among the immunobiotic strains with the capacity of beneficially modulate respiratory immunity, our research group has demonstrated that *Lactobacillus rhamnosus* CRL1505 has outstanding properties. Nasal priming with *L. rhamnosus* CRL1505 is able to significantly increase the resistance against the respiratory pathogens *S. pneumoniae*, IFV, or RSV (13–15). We have also reported that immunobiotic *L. rhamnosus* CRL1505 is able to differentially regulate the levels and kinetics of respiratory inflammatory cells and cytokines in mice after activation of Toll-like receptor 3 (TLR3) by the nasal administration of poly(I:C), or after the challenge with RSV or IFV (13, 14). This beneficial regulation of virus-triggered inflammatory response in the respiratory tract by the CRL1505 strain correlated with a significant reduction in lung damage and improved survival of infected mice (13, 14). Of interest, we have demonstrated that viability of the immunobiotic strain is not necessary to achieve the protective effect. In fact, protection against RSV or *S. pneumoniae* infections can be improved by nasal administration of non-viable *L. rhamnosus* CRL1505 (13) or its peptidoglycan (15), respectively. Although we have significantly advanced in demonstrating the capacity of *L. rhamnosus* CRL1505 to improve resistance against respiratory infections as well as in the cellular and molecular mechanisms involved in its beneficial activities (12), the potential protective ability of this strain or its immunomodulatory cellular fractions in the context of a secondary bacterial pneumonia has not been addressed before.

We hypothesized that the effect of immunobiotics or their immunomodulatory cellular fractions in the respiratory antiviral innate immune response could beneficially influence the resistance to secondary bacterial infections. Therefore, in the present study, we investigated how the exposure of infant mice to the nasal priming with non-viable *L. rhamnosus* CRL1505 or its peptidoglycan influences the respiratory innate immune response triggered by TLR3 activation, the susceptibility to primary RSV infection, and the resistance to secondary pneumococcal pneumonia. We demonstrated that peptidoglycan from immunobiotic *L. rhamnosus* CRL1505 improves respiratory antiviral innate immune response, reduces bacterial transmigration across the lung, and limits pulmonary inflammatory damage caused by *S. pneumoniae* after the challenge with poly(I:C) or the infection with RSV.

MATERIALS AND METHODS

Microorganisms and Peptidoglycan

Lactobacillus rhamnosus CRL1505 was obtained from the CERELA culture collection (Chacabuco 145, San Miguel de Tucumán, Argentina). The culture was kept freeze-dried. For experiments the culture was rehydrated using a medium containing 15 g of peptone, 10 g tryptone, and 5 g of meat extract in 1 l of distilled water, pH 7. Then, lactobacilli were cultured for 12 h at 37°C (final log phase) in Man–Rogosa–Sharpe broth (MRS, Oxoid). The bacteria were harvested by centrifugation at 3,000 × *g* for 10 min, washed three times with sterile 0.01 mol/l phosphate buffer saline (PBS, pH 7.2), and resuspended in sterile PBS. Non-viable *L. rhamnosus* CRL1505 (HK1505) was obtained as described previously (13). Bacteria were killed by tyndallization in a water bath at 80°C for 30 min, and the lack of bacterial growth was confirmed using MRS agar plates. Peptidoglycan from *L. rhamnosus* CRL1505 (PG1505) was obtained as described previously (15). Briefly, the bacterium was grown in MRS broth for 18 h at 37°C, washed three times with sterile PBS, and lyophilized. Lactobacilli were resuspended in sterile water (0.1 g/ml) and lysed by sonication in an Ultrasonic Homogenizer (Cole Parmer) with cycles of 2.5 min and amplitude of 70%. The cell wall obtained was delipidated by successive refluxing with methanol, methanol–chloroform (1:1), and chloroform. The delipidated preparation was resuspended in Tris–HCl buffer 50 μM (pH 7.5) and treated with bovine pancreatic DNAse I (Sigma) (50 μg/ml) and ribonuclease A (Sigma) (100 μg/ml) at 37°C, 4 h. Finally, cell wall was treated with 50% hydrogen chloride at 4°C for 20 h. The PG1505 obtained was washed with sterile water, adjusted to pH 7.2, and lyophilized until use.

Animals and Feeding Procedures

Infant (3-week-old) BALB/c mice were obtained from the closed colony kept at CERELA (San Miguel de Tucumán, Argentina). They were housed in plastic cages at room temperature. Mice were housed individually during the experiments and the assays for each parameter studied were performed in 5–6 mice per group for each time point. HK1505 was nasally administered to infant mice for 2 consecutive days at a dose of 10^8 cells/mouse/day in 50 μl of PBS (13). PG1505 was nasally administered to infant mice for 2 consecutive days at a dose of 8 μg/ml, in 50 μl of PBS (15). Anesthesia was not necessary for HK1505 or PG1505 administration since mice did not show any sing of discomfort. The treated groups and the untreated control group were fed a conventional balanced diet *ad libitum*. This study was carried out in strict accordance with the recommendations in the Guide for the Care and Use of Laboratory Animals of the Guidelines for Animal Experimentation of CERELA and all efforts were made to minimize suffering.

Intranasal Administration of Poly(I:C)

Administration of the viral pathogen molecular pattern poly(I:C) was performed on day 3, after the 2-day treatments with HK1505 or PG1505 as shown in **Figure 1A**. Mice were lightly anesthetized and 100 μl of PBS, containing 250 μg poly(I:C) (equivalent to 10 mg/kg body weight), was administered dropwise, *via* the nares (13, 16, 17). Control animals received 100 μl of PBS. Mice received three doses of poly(I:C) or PBS with 24 h rest period between each administration.

RSV Infection

Human RSV strain A2 was grown in Vero cells as described previously (13, 16). Briefly, Vero cells were infected with RSV at

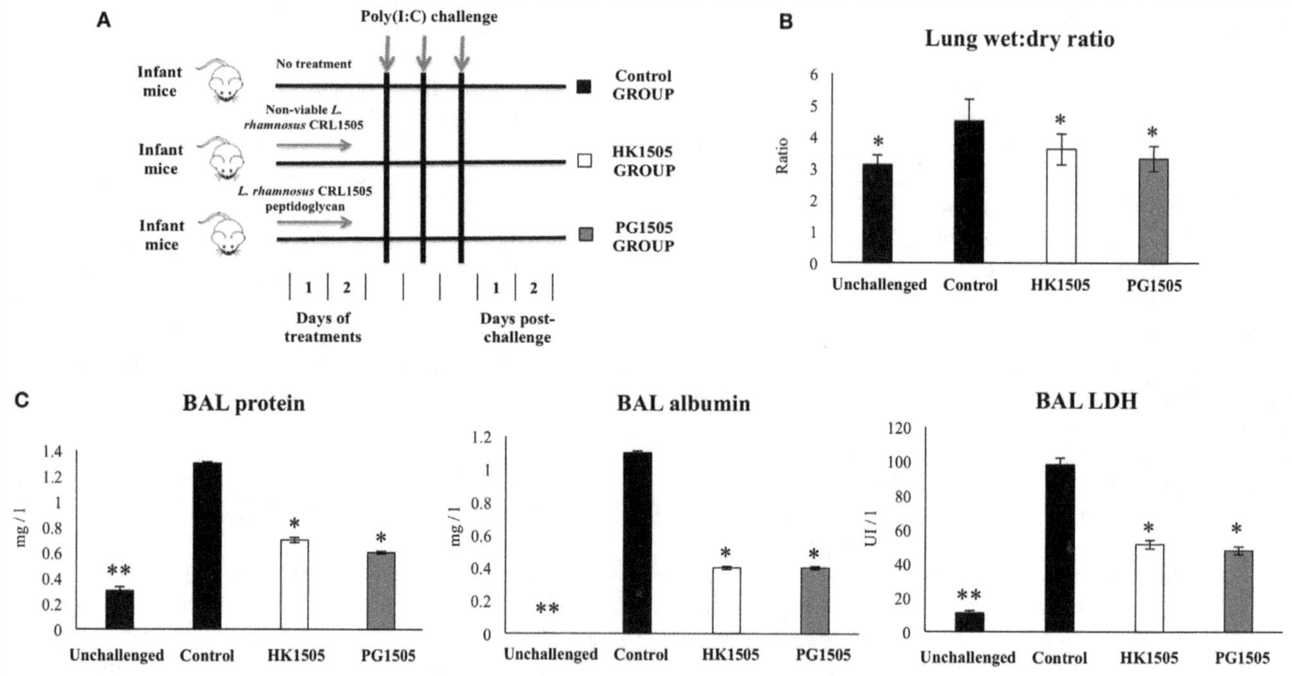

FIGURE 1 | Effect of non-viable *Lactobacillus rhamnosus* CRL1505 (HK1505) and its peptidoglycan (PG1505) on lung tissue damage induced by the nasal administration of the viral pathogen-associated molecular pattern poly(I:C). Infant mice were nasally primed with HK1505 or PG1505 during two consecutive days and then challenged with three once-daily doses of poly(I:C) **(A)**. Non-treated infant mice challenged with poly(I:C) were used as controls. 2 days after the last poly(I:C) administration lung wet:dry weight ratio **(B)**, lactate dehydrogenase (LDH) activity and, albumin and protein concentrations in bronchoalveolar lavages (BAL) **(C)** were determined. The results represent data from three independent experiments. Significant differences between treated and control groups, $^*P < 0.05$, $^{**}P < 0.05$.

a multiplicity of infection of 1 in 5 ml of Dulbecco's modified Eagle's medium (DMEM). Cells were infected for 3 h at 37°C, 5% CO_2. After infection, 7 ml of DMEM with 10% fetal bovine serum (Sigma, Tokyo, Japan), 0.1% penicillin–streptomycin (Pen/Strep) (Sigma, Tokyo, Japan), and 0.001% ciprofloxacin (Bayer) was added to the flask, and cells were incubated until extensive syncytium formation was detected. Then, Vero cells were scraped and sonicated three times, 5 s per time, at 25 W on ice. Cell debris was removed by centrifugation at 700 g for 10 min at 4°C. Virus supernatant was sucrose density gradient purified and stored in 30% sucrose at −80°C. For *in vivo* infection, mice were lightly anesthetized with isoflurane and intranasally challenged with 3.1×10^6 PFU of RSV (13, 16). Viral challenge was performed on day 3, after the 2-day treatments with HK1505 or PG1505. Lung RSV titers and tissue damage were evaluated during 5 days after viral infection.

For the evaluation of viral infection, the RSV immunoplaque assay was performed as described previously (13, 16). In brief, lung tissue was removed from infant mice and stored in 30% sucrose for plaque assay. Lungs were homogenized using a pellet pestle and centrifuged at $2{,}600 \times g$ for 10 min at 4°C to clarify supernatant. Serial dilutions of lung tissue-clarified supernatants were added into fresh Vero cells monolayers, and incubated at 37°C, 5% CO_2 for 3 h. All samples were run in triplicate. After incubation and removal of supernatant, 1 ml of fresh DMEM medium containing 10% FBS, 0.1% Pen/Strep, and 0.001% ciprofloxacin was added to monolayers. When extensive syncytia developed, monolayers were fixed with 1 ml of ice-cold acetone:methanol (60:40). Then, well were treated with primary RSV anti-F (clones 131-2A; Chemicon) and anti-G (Mouse monoclonal [8C5 (9B6)] to RSV glycoprotein, Abcam) antibodies for 2 h, followed by secondary horseradish peroxidase anti-mouse immunoglobulin antibody (Anti-mouse IgG, HRP-linked Antibody #7076, Cell signaling Technology) for 1 h. Plates washed twice with PBS containing 0.5% Tween 20 (Sigma) after each antibody incubation step. Individual plaques were developed using a DAB substrate kit (ab64238, Abcam) following manufacture's specifications. Results were expressed as log10 PFU/g of lung.

S. pneumoniae Secondary Infection

Streptococcus pneumoniae serotype 6B (ANLIS, Argentina) was obtained from the respiratory tract of a patient from the Children's Hospital, Tucuman, Argentina. Pneumococci were grown on blood agar for 18 h. Colonies were suspended in Todd Hewitt broth (Oxoid), incubated overnight at 37°C, harvested, and washed with sterile PBS. Cell density was adjusted to 4×10^7 CFU/ml.

Challenge with pneumococci was performed 1, 3, and 5 days after the last administration of poly(I:C) (data not shown), and a higher susceptibility to bacterial infection was found when the challenge was performed 5 days after TLR3 activation. In addition, several published articles performed bacterial infection 5–7 days after respiratory viral challenge considering that viral load and cytokine environment are different in the earlier and later stages of viral infection (4, 18). Then, challenge with pneumococci was also performed 5 days after the infection with RSV. HK1505- and PG1505-treated as well as control infant mice were challenged intranasally with the pathogen by dripping 25 µl of inoculums containing 10^3, 10^4, 10^6, or 10^7 CFU (log phase) in PBS into each nostril.

Treated and control mice were sacrificed 2 days after *S. pneumoniae* infection. Lungs were excised, weighed, and homogenized in sterile peptone water. Homogenates were diluted appropriately, plated in duplicate on blood agar and incubated for 18 h at 37°C. *S. pneumoniae* was identified by standard techniques and the results were expressed as log of CFU/g of lung. Bacteremia was monitored by blood samples obtained by cardiac puncture which were plated on blood agar. Results were reported as negative or positive hemocultures.

Blocking Experiments

In order to evaluate the role of IFN-β, IFN-γ, and IL-10 in the immunoprotective effect of HK1505 and PG1505, anti-IFN-β, anti-IFN-γ, and anti-IL-10 receptor (IL-10R) blocking antibodies were used (16). Different groups of mice were nasally primed with HK1505 or PG1505 for 2 days and then challenged with poly(I:C) for 3 days as described above. On days 2 and 4 after poly(I:C) challenge, mice were nasally treated with 50 µg of purified IFN-β (LEAF™ Purified anti-mouse IFN-β antibody, #519202 BioLegend), purified anti-IFN-γ (LEAF™ Purified anti-mouse IFN-γ antibody, #505706 BioLegend), or anti-IL-10R (LEAF™ Purified anti-mouse IL-10R antibody, #112708, BioLegend, Tokyo, Japan) antibodies or 250 µg isotype control antibodies (LEAF™ Purified Rat IgG1, Isotype Ctrl, BioLegend). Twelve hours later mice were challenged with *S. pneumoniae* (Figure S1 in Supplementary Material). The efficiency of blocking antibodies was determined by evaluating serum and respiratory concentration of IFN-β, IFN-γ, or IL-10 12 h after the last administration.

Lung Injury Parameters

Bronchoalveolar lavages (BAL) samples were obtained as described previously (13, 16). Briefly, the trachea was exposed and intubated with a catheter, and two sequential lavages were performed in each mouse by injecting sterile PBS. The recovered fluid was centrifuged for 10 min at $900 \times g$; and frozen at −70°C for subsequent analyses.

Protein and albumin content, a measure to quantitate increased permeability of the bronchoalveolar–capillarity barrier, and lactate dehydrogenase (LDH) activity, an indicator of general cytotoxicity, were determined in the acellular BAL fluid. Protein content was measured by the bicinchoninic (BCA) protein assay (Pierce Biotechnology Inc., Rockford, IL, USA). Albumin content was determined colorimetrically based on albumin binding to bromcresol green using an albumin diagnostic kit (Wiener Lab, Buenos Aires, Argentina). LDH activity, expressed as units per liter of BAL fluid, was determined by measuring the formation of the reduced form of nicotinamide adenine dinucleotide using the Wiener reagents and procedures (Wiener Lab). Lung wet:dry weight ratio was measured as previously described (13, 17). Wet:dry weight ratio was calculated as an index of intrapulmonary fluid accumulation, without correction for blood content.

Histopathological examination was also performed in order to further evaluate tissue damage. Lungs were aseptically removed, fixed in 4% formalin, and embedded in histowax (Leica Microsystems). Histopathological assessment was performed on

5-μm tissue sections stained with hematoxylin–eosin. At least four tissue sections from various areas of the lung of each mouse in all experimental groups were examined.

Cytokine Concentrations in Serum and BAL

Tumor necrosis factor (TNF)-α (Mouse TNF-alpha Quantikine enzyme-linked immunosorbent assay (ELISA) Kit, sensitivity: 7.2 pg/ml), interferon (IFN)-α (Mouse IFN-alpha ELISA Kit, sensitivity: 12.5 pg/ml), IFN-β (Mouse IFN-beta ELISA Kit, sensitivity: 15.5 pg/ml), IFN-γ (Mouse IFN-gamma Quantikine ELISA Kit, sensitivity: 2 pg/ml), interleukin (IL)-6 (Mouse IL-6 Quantikine ELISA Kit, sensitivity: 1.8 pg/ml), IL-8 (Mouse IL-8 Quantikine ELISA Kit, sensitivity: 2 pg/ml), IL-10 (Mouse IL-10 Quantikine ELISA Kit, sensitivity: 5.2 pg/ml), and monocyte chemoattractant protein (MCP)-1 (Mouse/Rat CCL2/JE/MCP-1 Quantikine ELISA Kit, sensitivity: 2 pg/ml) concentrations in serum and BAL were measured with commercially available ELISA technique kits following the manufacturer's recommendations (R&D Systems, MN, USA).

Lung Cells Preparation and Flow Cytometry Studies

Single lung cells from mice were prepared as previously described (13, 17). Lungs were removed, finely minced, and incubated for 90 min with 300 U of collagenase (Yakult Honsha Co., Tokyo, Japan) in 15 ml of RPMI 1640 medium (Sigma, Tokyo, Japan). To dissociate the tissue into single cells, collagenase-treated minced lungs were gently tapped into a plastic dish. After removal of debris, erythrocytes were depleted by hypotonic lysis. The cells were washed with RPMI medium supplemented with 100 U/ml of penicillin and 100 mg/ml of streptomycin and then resuspended in a medium supplemented with 10% heat-inactivated fetal calf serum. Cells were counted using Trypan Blue exclusion and then resuspended at an appropriate concentration of 5×10^6 cells/ml.

Lung cell suspensions were pre-incubated with anti-mouse CD32/CD16 monoclonal antibody (Fc block) for 15 min at 4°C. Cells were incubated in the antibody mixes for 30 min at 4°C and washed with FACS buffer. Then, cells were stained with fluorochrome-conjugated antibodies against CD3, CD4, CD8, CD11c, CD11b, CD103, MHC-II, IFN-γ, IL-10, sialic acid-binding immunoglobulin-like lectin F (SiglecF) (BD Bioscience), IFN-β, and CD45 (eBioscience). Cells were then acquired on a BD FACSCalibur™ flow cytometer (BD Biosciences) and data were analyzed with FlowJo software (TreeStar). The total number of cells in each population was determined by multiplying the percentages of subsets within a series of marker negative or positive gates by the total cell number determined for each tissue (13, 17).

Statistical Analysis

Experiments were performed in triplicate and results were expressed as mean ± SD. After verification of the normal distribution of data, 2-way ANOVA was used. Tukey's test (for pairwise comparisons of the means) was used to test for differences between the groups. Differences were considered significant at $P < 0.05$.

RESULTS

Nasally Administered Peptidoglycan from *L. rhamnosus* CRL1505 Reduces Poly(I:C)-Induced Lung Injuries

We have previously demonstrated that nasal administration of non-viable *L. rhamnosus* CRL1505 (HK1505) reduced lung injuries triggered by TLR3 activation (13). Here, we aimed to evaluate the effect of the nasal priming with the peptidoglycan from *L. rhamnosus* CRL1505 (PG1505) on the immune response triggered by the viral pathogen-associated molecular pattern poly(I:C) and compare it with the effect induced by HK1505. For this purpose, infant mice were treated with PG1505 and then challenged with poly(I:C) as shown in the experimental protocol of **Figure 1A**. HK1505 treatment was used as a positive control. Lung injury was studied on day 2 post-challenge as we described previously (13, 17). An altered lung wet:dry weight ratio (**Figure 1B**), as well as increased levels of LDH activity and protein and albumin concentrations (**Figure 1C**) were found in BAL samples of poly(I:C)-treated infant mice, indicating local cellular damage and impairment of the alveolar-capillary barrier. Nasally administered HK1505 or PG1505 did not induce significant changes in the BAL biochemical parameters evaluated before poly(I:C) administration (data not shown). Both, HK1505 or PG1505 significantly diminished wet:dry weight ratio and the three biochemical parameters evaluated in BAL after poly(I:C) challenge (**Figure 1**). HK1505 and PG1505 were equally effective to reduce the lung alterations induced by TLR3 activation.

Nasally Administered Peptidoglycan from *L. rhamnosus* CRL1505 Beneficially Modulates Immune Response Triggered by Poly(I:C) Challenge

In order to evaluate the effect of HK1505 and PG1505 in the respiratory immune system of infant mice, we first determined the levels of different cytokines in BAL before poly(I:C) administration (**Figure 2**). Both, HL1505 and PG1505 treatments significantly increased the levels of BAL IFN-α, IFN-β, IFN-γ, IL-10, and IL-6. BAL concentrations of IFN-α in HK1505 mice and IL-6 in PG1505 mice were higher than the other experimental groups. No significant differences were found when the levels of TNF-α, MCP-1, and IL-8 of control mice were compared with mice receiving HK1505 or PG1505 (**Figure 2**). The treatments were also able to increase serum IFN-α, IFN-β, IFN-γ, IL-10, and IL-6, being both HK1505 and PG1505 equally effective to achieve this effect (Figure S2 in Supplementary Material). No differences were found in the levels of serum TNF-α, MCP-1, or IL-8 when comparing HK1505 and PG1505 with controls. We also evaluated the changes induced by nasally administered HK1505 and PG1505 in lung immune cells using flow cytometry. Nasal priming with HK1505 and PG1505 enhanced the number of $CD3^+CD4^+IFN\text{-}\gamma^+$ and $CD3^+CD4^+IL\text{-}10^+$ T cells in lungs

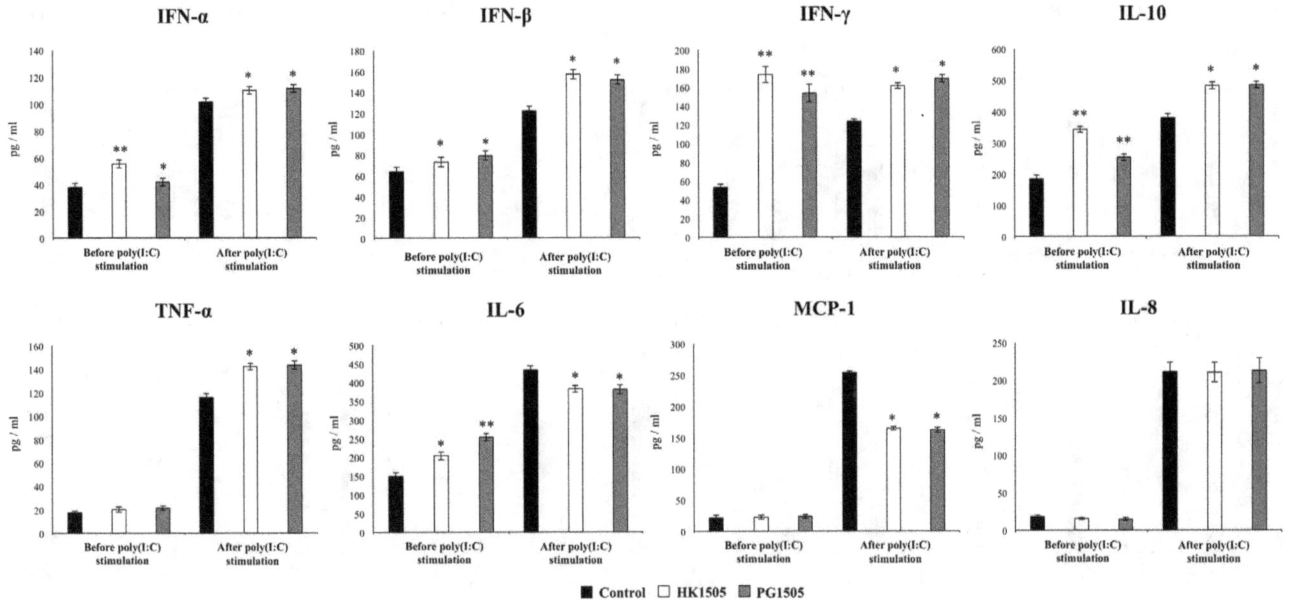

FIGURE 2 | Effect of non-viable *Lactobacillus rhamnosus* CRL1505 (HK1505) and its peptidoglycan (PG1505) on respiratory cytokines before and after the nasal administration of the viral pathogen-associated molecular pattern poly(I:C). Infant mice were nasally primed with HK1505 or PG1505 during two consecutive days and then challenged with three once-daily doses of poly(I:C). Non-treated infant mice challenged with poly(I:C) were used as controls. Before and 2 days after poly(I:C) administration, the levels of tumor necrosis factor (TNF)-α, interferon (IFN)-α, IFN-β, IFN-γ, interleukin (IL)-6, IL-8, IL-10, and monocyte chemoattractant protein-1 (MCP-1) were determined in bronchoalveolar lavages. The results represent data from three independent experiments. Significant differences between treated and control groups, *$P < 0.05$.

while no effect was observed for $CD3^+CD8^+IFN\text{-}\gamma^+$ T cells when compared to controls (**Figure 3**). In addition, three population of antigen presenting cells were studied in lungs: myeloid DCs ($MHC\text{-}II^+CD11c^+CD11b^{low}CD103^+$ and $MHC\text{-}II^+CD11c^+CD11b^{high}CD103^-$ cells) and alveolar macrophages ($CD45^+MHC\text{-}II^-CD11c^+SiglecF^+$). HK1505 and PG1505 significantly increased the number of both lung $CD11c^+CD11b^{low}CD103^+$ and $CD11c^+CD11b^{high}CD103^-$ DCs, while no quantitative changes were detected in $CD45^+CD11c^-SiglecF^+$ macrophages (**Figure 3**) or $CD45^+Gr1^+$neutrophils (data not shown).

The respiratory immune response triggered by poly(I:C) in infant mice and the effect of the nasal priming with HK1505 and PG1505 in that response were next studied. As we described previously (13, 17), the nasal administration of poly(I:C) significantly increased respiratory levels of type I IFNs (IFN-α, IFN-β), IFN-γ, and pro-inflammatory cytokines and chemokines (TNF-α, IL-6, MCP-1, IL-8) in BAL of infant mice (**Figure 2**). Both HK1505 and PG1505 treatments significantly increased the levels of BAL IFN-α, IFN-β, IFN-γ, and TNF-α while they diminished the concentration of IL-6 and MCP-1 (**Figure 2**). In addition, IL-8 was not modified in HK1505 or PG1505 groups when compared to control mice (**Figure 2**). Poly(I:C) stimulation also induced an increase in the respiratory levels of IL-10 that were significantly higher in HK1505- or PG1505-treated mice when compared to controls (**Figure 2**). Lung immune cells populations were also evaluated in poly(I:C)-challenged mice (**Figure 3**). Poly(I:C) administration increased the numbers of $CD3^+CD4^+IFN\text{-}\gamma^+$, $CD3^+CD4^+IL\text{-}10^+$, $CD3^+CD8^+IFN\text{-}\gamma^+$ T cells, and myeloid DCs ($MHC\text{-}II^+CD11c^+CD11b^{low}CD103^+$ and $MHC\text{-}II^+CD11c^+CD11b^{high}CD103^-$ cells) in lungs as we described previously (13, 17). In addition, we also observed an increase in alveolar macrophages ($CD45^+CD11c^+SiglecF^+$) and neutrophils ($CD45^+Gr1^+$) after the challenge with poly(I:C) when compared to basal levels (**Figure 3**). Nasal priming with HK1505 or PG1505 increased the numbers of lung $CD3^+CD4^+IFN\text{-}\gamma^+$, and $CD3^+CD4^+IL\text{-}10^+$ T cells as well as $MHC\text{-}II^+CD11c^+CD103^+$ and $MHC\text{-}II^+CD11c^+CD11b^{high}$ DCs (**Figure 3**). No significant modification of the numbers of lung $CD3^+CD8^+IFN\text{-}\gamma^+$ T cells or $CD45^+CD11c^+SiglecF^+$ macrophages (**Figure 3**) were observed after HK1505 or PG1505 treatments when compared to controls. Significantly reduced numbers of neutrophils in BAL and lung were found in HK1505- or PG1505-treated mice when compared to controls (**Figure 3**).

Nasally Administered Peptidoglycan from *L. rhamnosus* CRL1505 Improves Resistance against RSV Infection

We next evaluated whether the changes induced by PG1505 in the respiratory immune system affected the outcome of RSV infection in infant mice as described previously for HK1505 (13). Therefore, infant mice were treated with HK1505 or PG1505 by the nasal route and then challenged with 10^6 PFU of RSV (13, 16). Evaluation of viral loads of infected mice showed that RSV was present in lungs of all the experimental groups during the 5 days studied (**Figure 4A**). However, significantly lower viral titers were found in mice treated with HK1505 or PG1505 when compared to controls, being both treatments equally effective to reduce

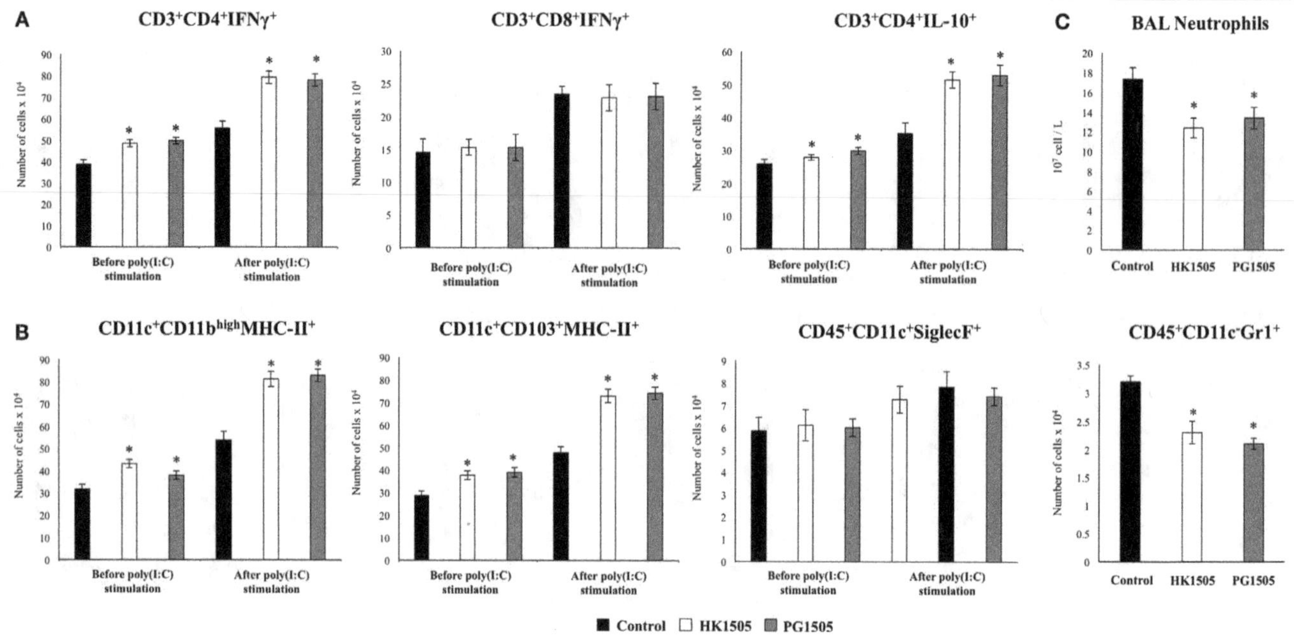

FIGURE 3 | Effect of non-viable *Lactobacillus rhamnosus* CRL1505 (HK1505) and its peptidoglycan (PG1505) on respiratory immune cell populations before and after the nasal administration of the viral pathogen-associated molecular pattern poly(I:C). Infant mice were nasally primed with HK1505 or PG1505 during two consecutive days and then challenged with three once-daily doses of poly(I:C). Non-treated infant mice challenged with poly(I:C) were used as controls. Before and 2 days after poly(I:C) administration, the numbers of lung T cells **(A)** including CD3⁺CD4⁺IFN-γ⁺, CD3⁺CD4⁺IL-10⁺, and CD3⁺CD8⁺IFN-γ⁺ T lymphocytes, as well as antigen presenting cells **(B)** including MHC-II⁺CD11c⁺CD11b^{low}CD103⁺ and MHC-II⁺CD11c⁺CD11b^{high}CD103⁻ dendritic cells, and CD45⁺CD11c⁺SiglecF⁺ alveolar macrophages were determined by flow cytometry. In addition, bronchoalveolar lavages (BAL) neutrophils and lung CD45⁺CD11c⁻Gr1⁺ cells **(C)** were determined. The results represent data from three independent experiments. Significant differences between treated and control groups, *$P < 0.05$.

RSV replication in the respiratory tract. Moreover, HK1505 and PG1505 significantly improved the body weight gain during RSV infection when compared to controls (**Figure 4B**). The markers of lung tissue damage in RSV-infected mice showed that the viral infection induced a significant cellular damage and alveolar–capillary barrier alterations (**Figure 4C**). Both, BAL LDH and albumin concentrations were significantly lower in infant mice previously treated with HK1505 or PG1505 than in RSV-challenged control mice (**Figure 4C**).

Nasally Administered Non-Viable *L. rhamnosus* CRL1505 and Its Peptidoglycan Improve Resistance to Secondary Pneumococcal Pneumonia after Poly(I:C) Treatment

As mentioned before, respiratory viral infections increase the susceptibly of secondary bacterial pneumonia in infants. Taking into consideration the beneficial effects of nasal HK1505 (13) or PG1505 on the respiratory antiviral innate immune response, we next addressed whether these treatments where able to increase the resistance of infant mice to secondary pneumococcal pneumonia. For this purpose, we first performed comparative studies of secondary pneumococcal infection in Swiss albino and BALB/c mice that are naturally susceptible and resistant to pneumococci, respectively. We found that BALB/c mice, which are highly susceptible to poly(I:C) and RSV, were a better animal model for studying poly(I:C)-pneumococcal or RSV-pneumococcal infection than Swiss albino mice (data not shown). In line with our findings, some works have established that BALB/c mice are suitable for studying poly(I:C)-induced respiratory damage and RSV-bacterial infections. Stark et al. (19) demonstrated that exposure of BALB/c mice to RSV significantly decreased *S. pneumoniae*, *Staphylococcus aureus*, or *Pseudomonas aeruginosa* clearance. In addition, the work showed that the effect of RSV infection on bacterial clearance was dependent on the mouse genetic background by performing experiments with C57BL/6J and FVBN/J mice, which are relatively resistant and susceptible to RSV infection respectively. C57BL/6J mice showed a modest change in pneumococcal clearance following RSV challenge, whereas FVBN/J mice showed a decrease in pneumococcal clearance following RSV.

As shown in the experimental protocol illustrated in **Figure 5A**, mice were nasally primed with HK1505 or PG1505, stimulated with poly(I:C), and 5 days after the last poly(I:C) administration challenged with the respiratory bacterial pathogen *S. pneumoniae*. Pneumococcal colonization and bacteremia as well as lung tissue damage were evaluated on day 2 post-pneumococcal challenge. Two doses (10^3 and 10^4 cells) of *S. pneumoniae* were evaluated. Pneumococci were detected in lungs (**Figure 5B**) and blood (**Figure 5C**) of control infant mice for the two doses of the respiratory pathogen. HK1505 significantly reduced lung bacterial cell counts and the dissemination of *S. pneumoniae* into the blood in infant mice infected with

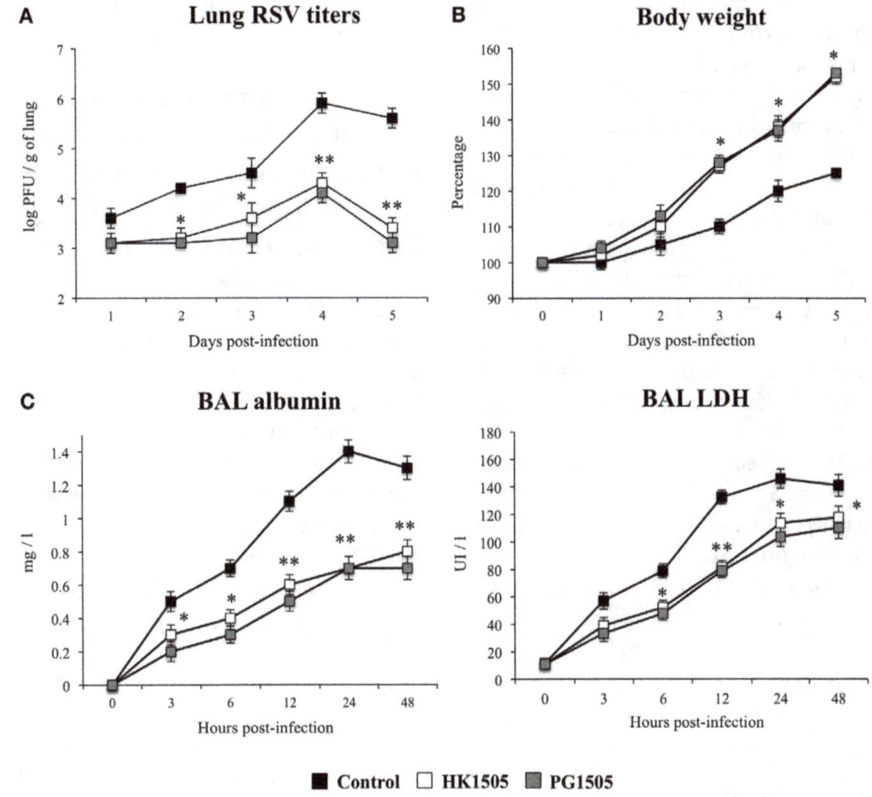

FIGURE 4 | Effect of non-viable *Lactobacillus rhamnosus* CRL1505 (HK1505) and its peptidoglycan (PG1505) on the resistance to primary Respiratory Syncytial Virus (RSV) infection. Infant mice were nasally primed with HK1505 or PG1505 during two consecutive days and then challenged with RSV. Non-treated infant mice challenged with the viral pathogen were used as controls. Lung RSV titers **(A)**, changes in body weight **(B)**, and lactate dehydrogenase (LDH) activity and albumin concentrations in bronchoalveolar lavages (BAL) **(C)** were evaluated on different time points after the viral challenge. The results represent data from three independent experiments. Significant differences between treated and control groups $^{*}P < 0.05$, $^{**}P < 0.01$.

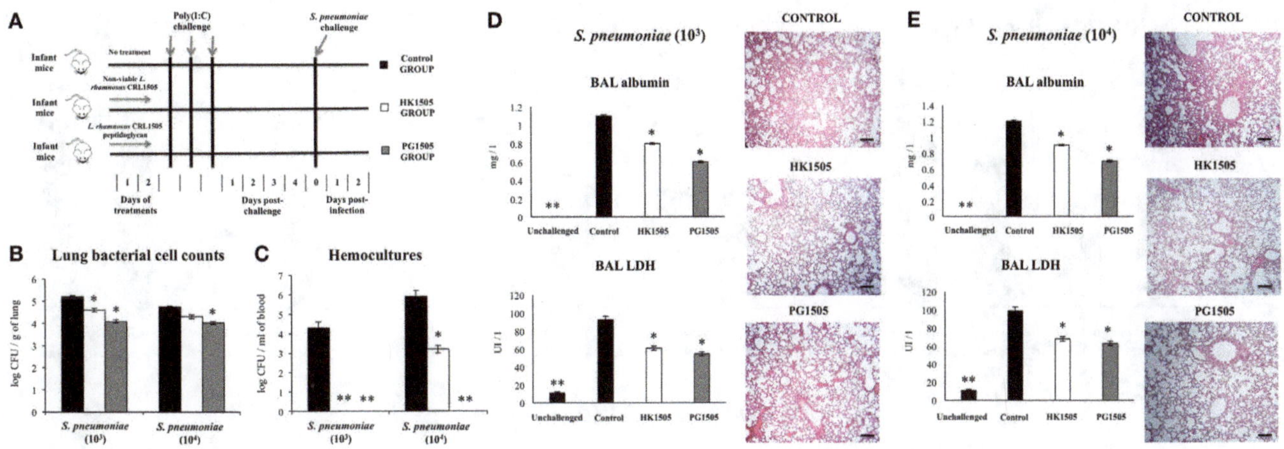

FIGURE 5 | Effect of non-viable *Lactobacillus rhamnosus* CRL1505 (HK1505) and its peptidoglycan (PG1505) on the resistance to secondary pneumococcal pneumonia after the nasal administration of the viral pathogen-associated molecular pattern poly(I:C). Infant mice were nasally primed with HK1505 or PG1505 during two consecutive days, challenged with three once-daily doses of poly(I:C) and, infected with two different doses of *Streptococcus pneumoniae* 5 days after the last poly(I:C) administration **(A)**. Non-treated infant mice stimulated with poly(I:C) and challenged with *S. pneumoniae* were used as controls. Lung bacterial cells counts **(B)**, hemocultures **(C)**, lactate dehydrogenase (LDH) activity and albumin concentrations in bronchoalveolar lavages (BAL) **(D,E)**, and lung histopathological examination **(D,E)** were determined on day 2 post-pneumococcal challenge. Scale bar = 100 μm. The results represent data from three independent experiments. Significant differences between treated and control groups, $^{*}P < 0.05$, $^{**}P < 0.01$.

10^3 pneumococcal cells while no significant differences in these parameters were found in animals infected with 10^4 pneumococcal cells (**Figure 5**). Interestingly, PG1505 significantly reduced lung bacterial cell counts and the dissemination of the respiratory pathogen into the blood in infant mice infected with both 10^3 and 10^4 pneumococcal cells (**Figures 5B,C**). Evaluation of lung tissue injury showed that secondary pneumococcal pneumonia induced a significant cellular damage and alveolar–capillary barrier alterations as demonstrated by the significant higher levels of BAL LDH and albumin when compared to basal levels (**Figures 5D,E**). Lung histological examination revealed inflammatory cell recruitment around alveoli and blood vessels, focal hemorrhage, and a significant reduction of gas exchange spaces (**Figures 5D,E**). Biochemical markers and histology also showed that lung tissue injuries were comparable in mice infected with both 10^3 and 10^4 pneumococcal cells. BAL LDH and albumin concentrations were significantly lower in infant mice treated with HK1505 or PG1505 when compared to controls for both 10^3 and 10^4 pneumococcal cells (**Figures 5D,E**). Moreover, lung histology of HK1505- or PG1505-treated mice showed a significant reduction in the alterations of gas exchange spaces, hemorrhage, and inflammatory cells infiltration.

Nasally Administered Non-Viable *L. rhamnosus* CRL1505 and Its Peptidoglycan Differentially Modulate the Immune Response Triggered by Secondary Pneumococcal Pneumonia

Our previous results indicate that IFN-β, IFN-γ, and IL-10 are involved in the immunoregulatory effects of nasally administered immunobiotics (12). Moreover, as we described in **Figure 2**, the levels of these three cytokines were significantly increased in the respiratory tract of HK1505- or PG1505-treated mice. Therefore, we aimed to investigate the levels of IFN-β, IFN-γ, and IL-10 before (day 0) and after (day 2) the infection with *S. pneumoniae* as indicated in the experimental protocol of **Figure 5A**. The three cytokines were increased in HK1505 and PG1505 groups indicating that their elevated levels persisted up to 5 days of the last poly(I:C) administration (**Figure 6A**). Pneumococcal challenge

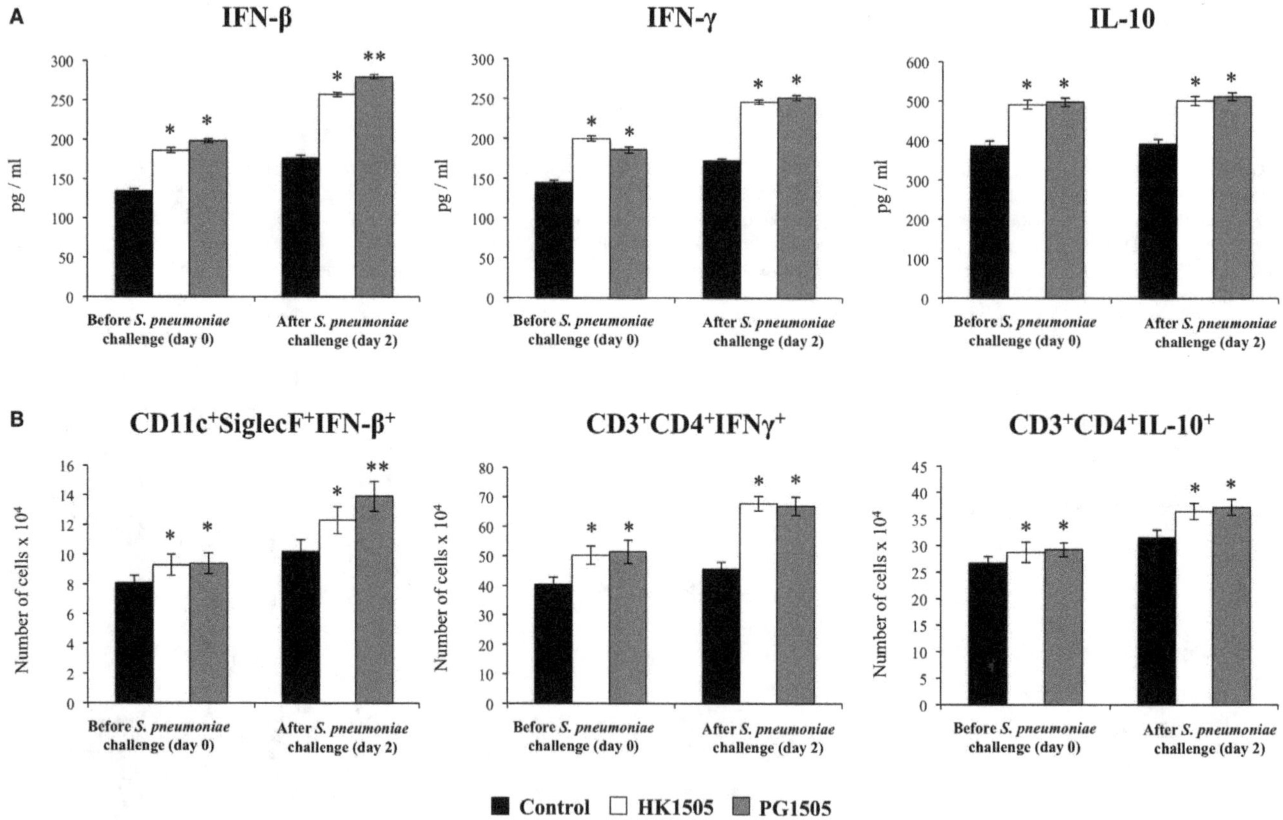

FIGURE 6 | Effect of non-viable *Lactobacillus rhamnosus* CRL1505 (HK1505) and its peptidoglycan (PG1505) on the respiratory immune response to secondary pneumococcal pneumonia after the nasal administration of the viral pathogen-associated molecular pattern poly(I:C). Infant mice were nasally primed with HK1505 or PG1505 during two consecutive days, challenged with three once-daily doses of poly(I:C) and, infected with two different doses of *Streptococcus pneumoniae* 5 days after the last poly(I:C) administration. Non-treated infant mice stimulated with poly(I:C) and challenged with *S. pneumoniae* were used as controls. The levels of interferon (IFN)-β, IFN-γ, and interleukin (IL)-10 in bronchoalveolar lavages **(A)**, as well as the numbers of lung $CD3^+CD4^+IFN\text{-}\gamma^+$, and $CD3^+CD4^+IL\text{-}10^+$ T cells and $CD45^+CD11c^+SiglecF^+$ alveolar macrophages **(B)** were determined before (day 0) and after (day 2) pneumococcal challenge. The results represent data from three independent experiments. Significant differences between treated and control groups, $^*P < 0.05$, $^{**}P < 0.01$.

further increase BAL IFN-β, IFN-γ, and IL-10 that were higher in HK1505- or PG1505-treated mice when compared to controls (**Figure 6A**). We also investigated the potential source of these cytokines within the immune cell populations of lungs. As we described previously, we found that IFN-γ and IL-10 were mainly produced by CD4$^+$ T cells. In this work, we also demonstrated that IFN-β was mainly produced by alveolar macrophages and the CD45$^-$ population of lung (probably respiratory epithelial cells) (data not shown). Similar to the results of cytokines' levels, we found that lung CD3$^+$CD4$^+$IFN-γ$^+$, and CD3$^+$CD4$^+$IL-10$^+$ T cells as well as CD11c$^+$SiglecF$^+$IFN-β$^+$ macrophages were significantly increased before and after the infection with *S. pneumoniae* in HK1505- or PG1505-treated mice when compared to control animals (**Figure 6B**). Of interest, both CD11c$^+$SiglecF$^+$IFN-β$^+$ macrophages and BAL IFN-β levels were higher in the PG1505 group than in HK1505 mice (**Figure 6**).

In order to further evaluate the role of IFN-β, IFN-γ, and IL-10 in the immunoregulatory effect of HK1505 and PG1505 during secondary pneumococcal infection we used blocking anti-IFN-β, anti-IFN-γ, and anti-IL-10R antibodies as described in the experimental protocol of Figure S2 in Supplementary Material. Treatment of mice with anti-IFN-β significantly abolished the capacity of HK1505 and PG1505 to avoid pneumococcal dissemination into the blood although it had no effect on lung bacterial cell counts (**Figure 7A**). In addition, the ability of HK1505 and PG1505 to protect against pulmonary damage was lost with anti-IFN-β antibodies administration (**Figure 7D**). Treatment with anti-IFN-γ significantly abolished the capacity of HK1505 and PG1505 to reduce lung bacterial cell counts and had no effect on bacteremia (**Figure 7B**) or in the protection against lung tissue damage (**Figure 7E**). On the other hand, administration of anti-IL-10R to infant mice significantly abolished the capacity of HK1505 and PG1505 to reduce lung tissue injuries (**Figure 7F**), while they did not affect lung pneumococcal colonization or dissemination into the blood (**Figure 7C**).

Nasally Administered Non-Viable *L. rhamnosus* CRL1505 and Its Peptidoglycan Improve Resistance to Secondary Pneumococcal Pneumonia after RSV Infection

Finally, we aimed to evaluate whether HK1505 or PG1505 treatments were able to protect against secondary pneumococcal pneumonia after the infection of infant mice with RSV. For this purpose, mice were nasally primed with HK1505 or PG1505, infected with RSV, and 5 days after the infection they were challenged with 10^3 cells of *S. pneumoniae*. Similar to the experiments performed with poly(I:C), pneumococcal colonization and bacteremia were evaluated on day 2 post-pneumococcal challenge. In addition, RSV titers as well as lung tissue damage were studied before (day 0) and after (day 2) the infection with *S. pneumoniae* (**Figure 8**). RSV was detected in the lungs of infected infant mice before and after pneumococcal infection (**Figure 8A**). In addition, pneumococci were detected in lungs (**Figure 8B**) and blood (**Figure 8C**) of control infant mice. Both, HK1505 and PG1506 significantly reduced RSV titers as well as lung bacterial cell counts and the dissemination of *S. pneumoniae* into the blood (**Figures 8A–C**), which was in line with the improved survival of HK1505- and PG1506-treated mice when compared to controls (**Figure 8D**). Of interest, PG1505 was more effective than HK1505 to diminish lung bacterial cell counts. When lung injury was studied, it was observed that the secondary pneumococcal pneumonia induced a significant increase of the BAL biochemical parameters that evaluate cellular damage and alveolar–capillary barrier alterations (**Figure 8E**). In addition, histological examination of lungs showed a significant reduction of gas exchange spaces, inflammatory cell recruitment, and focal hemorrhage (**Figure 8F**). HK1505 and PG1505 significantly reduced pulmonary damage as demonstrated by the diminished BAL LDH and albumin concentrations and the lower histological alterations when compared to controls (**Figures 8E,F**).

DISCUSSION

It was established that the mortality associated to respiratory viral infections is not due to the viral infection alone but instead, secondary bacterial pneumonia complicates many severe cases in infected hosts (1–3). Therefore, it is crucial to understand how respiratory viral infections alter the host's respiratory microenvironment and the local innate immunity to benefit the establishment of secondary bacterial infections, in order develop preventive or therapeutic strategies aimed to protect against mortality. Considering the elevated incidence of viral infections and the high frequency of associated secondary bacterial infections that contribute to aggravate the health status, several approaches are been investigated for preventing or treating respiratory superinfections, including antibiotics and immunomodulatory drugs (20). To our knowledge, no study has evaluated the potential protective ability of immunobiotics or their immunomodulatory cellular fractions in the context of a secondary bacterial pneumonia. Therefore, we demonstrated here for the first time, that the nasal priming with peptidoglycan from the immunobiotic *L. rhamnosus* CRL1505 is able to improve the resistance of infant mice to primary RSV infection and secondary pneumococcal pneumonia.

The first conclusion that can be obtained from the data presented in this work is that peptidoglycan from immunobiotic *L. rhamnosus* CRL1505 preserves the immunomodulatory properties of the viable strain. We have demonstrated previously that the nasal priming with viable *L. rhamnosus* CRL1505 beneficially modulates the respiratory immune response triggered by TLR3 activation and increases the resistance to RSV infection (13). Similar to viable *L. rhamnosus* CRL1505, its purified peptidoglycan administered before the nasal challenge with three once-daily doses of poly(I:C) significantly increased the levels of BAL type I IFNs, especially IFN-β. Thus, PG1505 would enhance the expression of hundreds of IFNs-induced genes that counteract viral replication. This is in line with the improved resistance of PG1505-treated infant mice to the infectious challenge with RSV. Moreover, PG1505 differentially regulated the production of pro- and anti-inflammatory cytokines in response to TLR3 activation which are also important for the generation of an effective respiratory antiviral response. PG1505 improved the

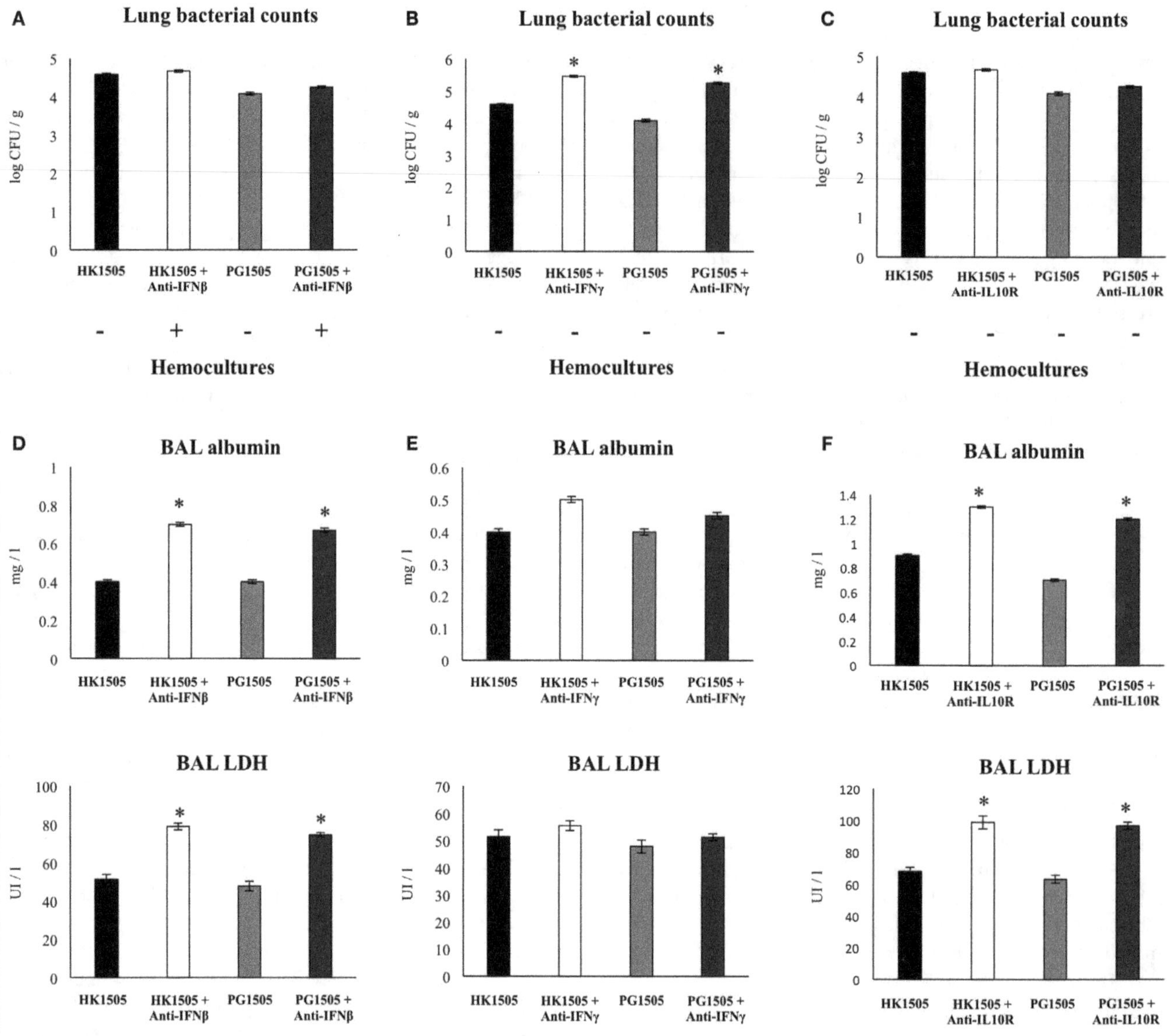

FIGURE 7 | Role of interferon (IFN)-β, IFN-γ, and interleukin (IL)-10 in the immunomodulatory effect of non-viable *Lactobacillus rhamnosus* CRL1505 (HK1505) and its peptidoglycan (PG1505) on the resistance to secondary pneumococcal pneumonia after the nasal administration of the viral pathogen-associated molecular pattern poly(I:C). Infant mice were nasally primed with HK1505 or PG1505 during two consecutive days, and then challenged with three once-daily doses of poly(I:C). On days 2 and 4 after poly(I:C) challenge, mice were nasally treated anti-IFN-β, anti-IFN-γ, or anti-IL-10 receptor (IL-10R) blocking antibodies. Control HK1505 and PG1505 received isotype control antibodies. Twelve hours later mice were challenged with *Streptococcus pneumoniae*. Lung bacterial cells counts and hemocultures **(A–C)**, as well as lactate dehydrogenase (LDH) activity and albumin concentrations in bronchoalveolar lavages (BAL) **(D–F)** were determined on day 2 post-pneumococcal challenge. The results represent data from three independent experiments. Significant differences between treated and control groups, $^{*}P < 0.05$.

production of some cytokines (TNF-α, IL-10) while it reduced the levels of other pro-inflammatory factors (IL-6, MIP-1) indicating that the inflammatory response was differentially modulated. In fact, PG1505-treated mice showed an improved capacity to control RSV replication in the respiratory tract and a reduced inflammatory damage in the lung tissue. Resembling the effect of viable *L. rhamnosus* CRL1505 (13), PG1505 improved the numbers of $CD3^+CD4^+IFN\text{-}\gamma^+$, $MHC\text{-}II^+CD11b^{low}CD103^+$, and $MHC\text{-}II^+CD11b^{high}CD103^-$ DCs as well as the respiratory levels of IFN-γ indicating the generation of a Th1 response, that is also involved in the immune protection against respiratory viral attack. These results indicate that peptidoglycan is a key bacterial component involved in the immunomodulatory and antiviral capacity of the immunobiotic strain *L. rhamnosus* CRL1505.

An important finding of this work is that both HK1505 and PG1505 were able to differentially modulate the response of infant mice to the secondary pneumococcal pneumonia produced after the challenge with poly(I:C) or RSV. Slight but still significant reduction of pneumococcal cell counts were found in the lungs of HK1505- or PG1505-treated mice when compared

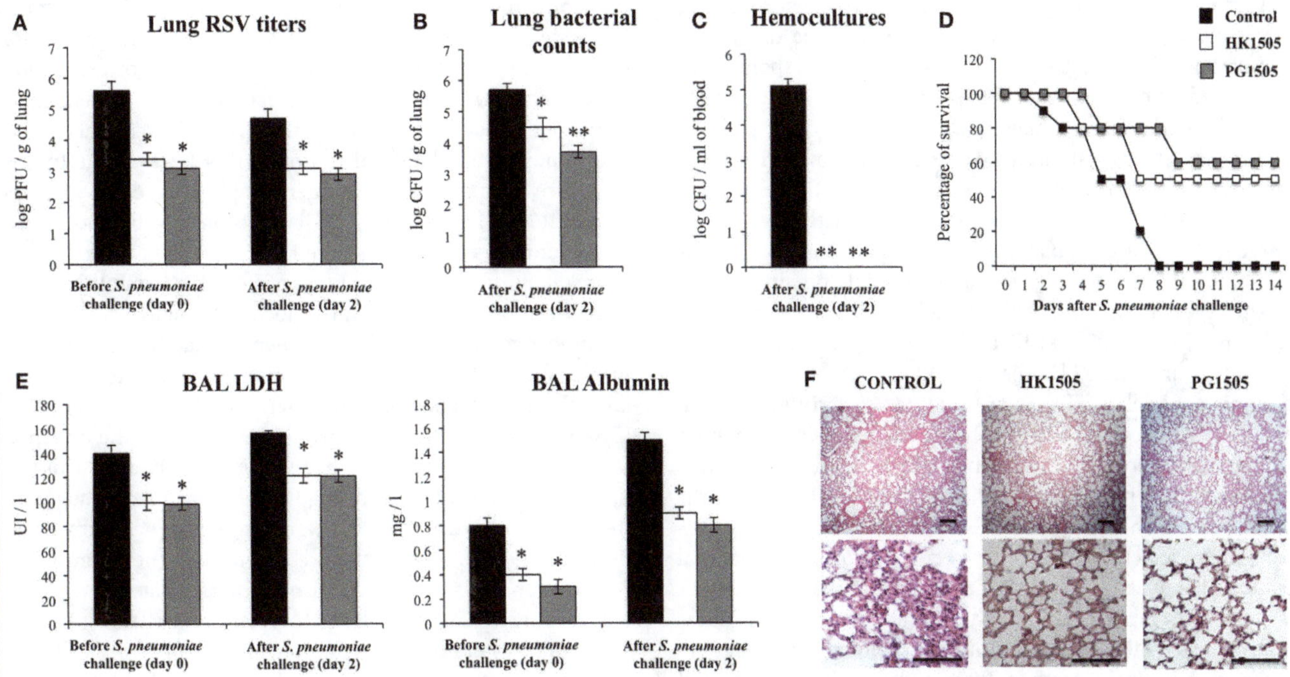

FIGURE 8 | Effect of non-viable *Lactobacillus rhamnosus* CRL1505 (HK1505) and its peptidoglycan (PG1505) on the resistance to secondary pneumococcal pneumonia after the primary infection with Respiratory Syncytial Virus (RSV). Infant mice were nasally primed with HK1505 or PG1505 during two consecutive days, challenged with RSV and, infected with *Streptococcus pneumoniae* 5 days after the viral infection. Non-treated infant mice infected with RSV and challenged with *S. pneumoniae* were used as controls. Lung RSV titers **(A)**, lung bacterial cells counts **(B)**, hemocultures **(C)**, survival **(D)**, lactate dehydrogenase (LDH) activity, and albumin concentrations in bronchoalveolar lavages (BAL) **(E)**, and lung histopathological examination **(F)** were determined on day 2 post-pneumococcal challenge. Scale bar = 100 μm. The results represent data from three independent experiments. Significant differences between treated and control groups, **$P < 0.05$, **$P < 0.01$.

to controls. The effect of HK1505 and PG1505 in reducing lung pneumococcal cell counts was modest compared with our own previous studies. We had reported that the nasal administration of viable *Lactococcus lactis* NZ9000 to adult and infant mice reduced in more than 2 log *S. pneumoniae* cell counts in lungs (21). In addition, non-viable *L. casei* CRL431 (22), and non-viable *L. rhamnosus* CRL1505 or its peptidoglycan (15) allowed to immunocopromised malnourished mice to completely eliminate *S. pneumoniae* from lungs. Moreover, HK1505 and PG1505 evaluated in an infant mice model of primary pneumococcal infection also reduced in more than 2 log *S. pneumoniae* cell counts in lungs when compared to untreated controls (data not shown). Then, immunobiotics and their cellular fractions would be more efficient to improve resistance to primary than secondary pneumococcal pneumonia.

Despite the modest results obtained by measuring the burden of the pathogen in the respiratory tract, PG1505 treatment was able to significantly reduce lung tissue damage and bacterial dissemination into the blood stream. These findings are of importance because studies in clinical trials (5, 6) and animal models of RSV-*S. pneumoniae* superinfection (7, 8) showed that enhanced lung injuries and elevated levels of bacteremia are critical factors that determine the severity of infection and the rate of mortality. In fact, PG1505-treated infant mice showed a significant improvement of survival after superinfection with RSV and *S. pneumoniae*. As mentioned before, several modifications induced by respiratory viruses are involved in facilitating *S. pneumoniae* infection, including the destruction of the respiratory epithelium, ciliary dyskinesia, enhancement of adhesion factors, and alterations of the immune response (7–10). In relation to immunopathology, it was reported that sequential infection with RSV and *S. pneumoniae* induced a significantly greater inflammation with high levels of infiltrated neutrophils and elevated levels of pro-inflammatory factors in the lung compared with mice that were inoculated with each pathogen separately (19). It is possible to speculate that the protective effect of PG1505 would be exerted at different levels. (a) The improvement of antiviral response and the consequent reduction of RSV titers in the lung, would contribute to the reduction of respiratory epithelium damage. (b) A reduction *S. pneumoniae* adhesion by diminishing the expression of RSV G protein and adhesion molecules in respiratory epithelial cells. In relation to this point, although we have not evaluated the impact of PG1505 in the expression of adhesion molecules in the respiratory tract, our recent transcriptomic studies evaluating the effect of *L. rhamnosus* CRL1505 in poly(I:C) challenged intestinal epithelial cells showed that the immunobiotic strain is able to differentially modulate the expression of several adhesion molecules including selectins E and L as well as ICAM-1, and EPCAM (23). Therefore, evaluating the effect of PG1505 on the expression of relevant adhesion molecules in respiratory epithelial cells is an interesting topic for future investigations. (c) The differential modulation of the respiratory innate immune response that allow a reduction of RSV and *S. pneumoniae* replication with minimal inflammatory damage of lung tissue.

Our results suggest that pneumococcal growth in lungs, dissemination into blood, and inflammatory tissue damage are events which are not strictly coupled with each other. Moreover, they are regulated by different factors during the development of secondary pneumococcal pneumonia as became evident when experiment with blocking anti-IFN-β, anti-IFN-γ, and anti-IL-10R antibodies were performed. In line with our results, Damjanovic et al. (24) demonstrated in a mice model of IFV-*S. pneumoniae* superinfection that uncontrolled bacterial outgrowth and excessive inflammation are not strictly coupled events, and that both are contributors to deleterious lung immunopathology and death. In fact, the work reported that the use of a bacteriostatic antibiotic effectively improved clinical outcome by controlling pneumococcal replication but it failed to significantly diminish pulmonary immunopathology. On the other hand, the use of dexamethasone slightly reduced immunopathology while it had no impact on bacterial clearance. Interestingly, administration of dexamethasone in combination the bacteriostatic antibiotic significantly improved pulmonary immunopathology, bacterial elimination, and most importantly the survival of infected mice (24). All these results together suggest that effective intervention strategies for respiratory superinfections need to involve an efficient control of pathogens growth and aberrant host inflammatory responses.

We found that at least three cytokines are involved in the immunomodulatory protective effect of HK1505 and PG1505 in the respiratory superinfection: IL-10, IFN-β, and IFN-γ. Our results indicated that IL-10 was involved in the protection against inflammatory damage while IFN-γ participated in the reduction of pneumococcal growth in the lungs. This is in line with our previous findings demonstrating that the protection of infant mice against poly(I:C) or RSV challenge induced by viable *L. rhamnosus* CRL1505 was dependent of both IL-10 and IFN-γ (16). Moreover, as observed for viable *L. rhamnosus* CRL1505 (16), both HK1505 and PG1505 improved the numbers of $CD3^+CD4^+IFN\text{-}\gamma^+$, and $CD3^+CD4^+IL\text{-}10^+$ T cells in the lungs of infant mice. These immune cell populations remained significantly elevated when compared to controls after pneumococcal challenge, indicating their participation in the protection against secondary bacterial pneumonia.

In addition, we showed that IFN-β was involved in the protection against lung tissue injury as well in the control of pneumococcal dissemination into the blood. The lung epithelial–endothelial layer is an important barrier in pneumococcal pathogenesis, since its alteration results in serious complications such as bacteremia and meningitis that are associated with high mortality. Some works have demonstrated an important role of IFN-β in the control of pneumococcal infection and invasiveness. Studies in IFNAR1 or IFN-β knockout mice showed that the abolishment of the IFN-β-IFNAR1 pathway increased nasopharyngeal carriage and enhanced mortality upon pneumococcal infection (25, 26). It was also demonstrated by LeMessurier et al. (27) that IFN-β increase the expression of tight junction proteins and reduce PAF receptor expression, which correlates with diminished pneumococcal invasion and transmigration of pulmonary epithelial and endothelial cells. In addition, intranasal administration of IFN-β was found to protect mice against the development of pneumococcal systemic disease (27). The role of IFN-β in secondary pneumococcal pneumonia has been also studied. No significant differences in *S. pneumoniae* counts in the lungs of $IFNAR1^{-/-}$ and $IFNAR1^{+/+}$ mice were observed after pneumococcal challenge. However, pneumococci were observed earlier and at higher numbers in blood samples of $IFNAR1^{-/-}$ mice compared to wild-type animals (27). We demonstrated here that the improvement of IFN-β by PG1505 treatment would be related to the enhancement of $CD11c^+SiglecF^+IFN\text{-}\beta^+$ alveolar macrophages. This is in line with studies demonstrating that alveolar macrophages are the main producers of type I IFNs during pulmonary viral infections (28, 29). However, it should be noted that the primary type I IFN response is mediated not only by alveolar macrophages but also by epithelial cells of the respiratory tract (25, 27). Therefore, respiratory epithelial cells may represent promising cellular target for future mechanistic studies in order to explain the protective effect of PG1505.

Our results demonstrated that the modulation of the three cytokines (IFN-β, IFN-γ, and IL-10) are necessary to achieve protection against secondary pneumococcal pneumonia. Therefore, an appropriate balance between pro- and anti-inflammatory factors would be necessary in order to obtain full protection without affecting lung structure and function. In line with this statement, some works have demonstrated that the excessive production of one particular cytokine have negative consequences in the outcome of respiratory infections. It was showed that excessive production of IFN-β during viral infection induce impaired neutrophils responses due to inadequate production of neutrophil chemoattractants (30). Although neutrophils infiltration has been linked to lung tissue damage, the phagocytic and bactericidal activities of these cells are necessary for the initial control of pneumococci. In addition, it was observed that neutralization of IFN-γ in IFV-infected mice considerably diminished bacterial susceptibility and improved survival after secondary pneumococcal pneumonia (31). This effect was explained by the inhibition of bacterial phagocytosis by the excessive production of IFN-γ. Data obtained from mice infected with IFV and *S. pneumoniae* demonstrated that the exaggerated production of IL-10 was associated with increased pneumococcal colonization and enhanced mortality (32). The work showed that the treatment of mice with blocking anti-IL-10 antibodies before secondary pneumococcal infection resulted in reduced bacterial cell counts in lungs and prolonged survival (32). Moreover, it can be anticipated that other cytokines are involved in susceptibility to secondary bacterial respiratory infections. In this regard, recent findings of Chen et al. (33) demonstrated that the anti-inflammatory cytokine IL-35 contributes to the decreased resistance to secondary pneumococcal pneumonia. The work reported that IFV infection induced a high expression of IL-35 in the respiratory tract and that secondary pneumococcal infection leaded to a synergistic production of this cytokine. Lung enhancement of IL-35 inhibited the early immune response against *S. pneumoniae*.

In summary, we demonstrated that the nasal priming with peptidoglycan from *L. rhamnosus* CRL1505 differentially modulates the respiratory innate antiviral immune response triggered by TLR3 activation in infant mice, improving the resistance to primary RSV infection, and secondary pneumococcal pneumonia. In association with the protection against RSV-pneumococcal superinfection, we found that peptidoglycan from *L. rhamnosus* CRL1505 significantly improved lung $CD3^+CD4^+IFN\text{-}\gamma^+$, and $CD3^+CD4^+IL\text{-}10^+$ T cells as well as $CD11c^+SiglecF^+IFN\text{-}\beta^+$ alveolar macrophages with the consequent increases of IFN-γ, IL-10, and IFN-β in the respiratory tract. Our results also demonstrated that the increase of the three cytokines is necessary to reduce the severity of the respiratory superinfection since each of them are involved in different aspect of the secondary pneumococcal pneumonia that have to be controlled in order to reduce the severity of the infectious disease: lung pneumococcal colonization, bacteremia, and inflammatory-mediated lung tissue injury. The findings of this work will lead us in new directions to explore the molecular mechanisms *via* which peptidoglycan from *L. rhamnosus* CRL1505 interacts with immune and non-immune cells of the respiratory tract and to investigate whether its immunomodulatory properties are unique or common to peptidoglycans of other immunobiotic strains with antiviral capabilities.

ETHICS STATEMENT

This study was carried out in strict accordance with the recommendations in the Guide for the Care and Use of Laboratory Animals of the Guidelines for Animal Experimentation of CERELA and all efforts were made to minimize suffering.

AUTHOR CONTRIBUTIONS

SA, HK, and JV designed the study and wrote the manuscript. PC, PK, HZ, AT, AK, and SS did the laboratory work. PC, PK, SS, and JV performed statistical analysis. SS, SA, HK, and JV contributed to data analysis and interpretation. All authors read and approved the manuscript.

SUPPLEMENTARY MATERIAL

The Supplementary Material for this article can be found online at http://journal.frontiersin.org/article/10.3389/fimmu.2017.00948/full#supplementary-material.

FIGURE S1 | Role of interferon (IFN)-β, IFN-γ, and interleukin (IL)-10 in the immunomodulatory effect of non-viable *Lactobacillus rhamnosus* CRL1505 (HK1505) and its peptidoglycan (PG1505) on the resistance to secondary pneumococcal pneumonia after the nasal administration of the viral pathogen-associated molecular pattern poly(I:C). Infant mice were nasally primed with HK1505 or PG1505 during two consecutive days, and then challenged with three once-daily doses of poly(I:C). On days 2 and 4 after poly(I:C) challenge, mice were nasally treated anti-IFN-β, anti-IFN-γ, or anti-IL-10 receptor blocking antibodies. Control HK1505 and PG1505 received isotype control antibodies. Twelve hours later mice were challenged with *Streptococcus pneumoniae*.

FIGURE S2 | Effect of non-viable *Lactobacillus rhamnosus* CRL1505 (HK1505) and its peptidoglycan (PG1505) on blood cytokines. HK1505 or PG1505 were nasally administered to infant mice during two consecutive days. Non-treated infant mice were used as controls. Levels of tumor necrosis factor (TNF)-α, interferon (IFN)-α, IFN-β, IFN-γ, interleukin (IL)-6, IL-8, IL-10, and monocyte chemoattractant protein-1 (MCP-1) were determined in bronchoalveolar lavages (BAL) **(A)** and serum **(B)**. The results represent data from three independent experiments. Significant differences between treated and control groups, $^*P < 0.05$, $^{**}P < 0.01$.

REFERENCES

1. Liu L, Johnson HL, Cousens S, Perin J, Scott S, Lawn JE, et al. Global, regional, and national causes of child mortality: an updated systematic analysis for 2010 with time trends since 2000. *Lancet* (2012) 379:2151–61. doi:10.1016/S0140-6736(12)60560-1
2. Muscedere J, Ofner M, Kumar A, Long J, Lamontagne F, Cook D, et al. The occurrence and impact of bacterial organisms complicating critical care illness associated with 2009 influenza A (H1N1) infection. *Chest* (2013) 144:39–47. doi:10.1378/chest.12-1861
3. Bosch AA, Biesbroek G, Trzcinski K, Sanders EA, Bogaert D. Viral and bacterial interactions in the upper respiratory tract. *PLoS Pathog* (2013) 9(1):e1003057. doi:10.1371/journal.ppat.1003057
4. Rynda-Apple A, Robinson KM, Alcorn JF. Influenza and bacterial superinfection: illuminating the immunologic mechanisms of disease. *Infect Immun* (2015) 83(10):3764–70. doi:10.1128/IAI.00298-15
5. Weinberger DM, Givon-Lavi N, Shemer-Avni Y, Bar-Ziv J, Alonso WJ, Greenberg D, et al. Influence of pneumococcal vaccines and respiratory syncytial virus on alveolar pneumonia, Israel. *Emerg Infect Dis* (2013) 19:1084–91. doi:10.3201/eid1907.121625
6. Cebey-López M, Pardo-Seco J, Gómez-Carballa A, Martinón-Torres N, Martinón-Sánchez JM, Justicia-Grande A, et al. Bacteremia in children hospitalized with respiratory syncytial virus infection. *PLoS One* (2016) 11(2):e0146599. doi:10.1371/journal.pone.0146599
7. Hament JM, Aerts PC, Fleer A, van Dijk H, Harmsen T, Kimpen JL, et al. Direct binding of respiratory syncytial virus to pneumococci: a phenomenon that enhances both pneumococcal adherence to human epithelial cells and pneumococcal invasiveness in a murine model. *Pediatr Res* (2005) 58(6):1198–203. doi:10.1203/01.pdr.0000188699.55279.1b
8. Smith CM, Sandrini S, Datta S, Freestone P, Shafeeq S, Radhakrishnan P, et al. Respiratory syncytial virus increases the virulence of *Streptococcus pneumoniae* by binding to penicillin binding protein 1a: a new paradigm in respiratory infection. *Am J Respir Crit Care Med* (2014) 190(2):196–207. doi:10.1164/rccm.201311-2110OC
9. Avadhanula V, Rodriguez CA, Devincenzo JP, Wang Y, Webby RJ, Ulett GC, et al. Respiratory viruses augment the adhesion of bacterial pathogens to respiratory epithelium in a viral species and cell type-dependent manner. *J Virol* (2006) 80:1629–36. doi:10.1128/JVI.80.4.1629-1636.2006
10. Avadhanula V, Wang Y, Portner A, Adderson E. Nontypeable *Haemophilus influenzae* and *Streptococcus pneumoniae* bind respiratory syncytial virus glycoprotein. *J Med Microbiol* (2007) 56:1133–7. doi:10.1099/jmm.0.47086-0
11. Villena J, Oliveira ML, Ferreira P, Salva S, Alvarez S. Lactic acid bacteria in the prevention of pneumococcal respiratory infection: future opportunities and challenges. *Int Immunopharmacol* (2011) 11:1633–45. doi:10.1016/j.intimp.2011.06.004
12. Zelaya H, Alvarez S, Kitazawa H, Villena J. Respiratory antiviral immunity and immunobiotics: beneficial effects on inflammation-coagulation interaction during influenza virus infection. *Front Immunol* (2016) 7:633. doi:10.3389/fimmu.2016.00633
13. Tomosada Y, Chiba E, Zelaya H, Takahashi T, Tsukida K, Kitazawa H, et al. Nasally administered *Lactobacillus rhamnosus* strains differentially modulate respiratory antiviral immune responses and induce protection against respiratory syncytial virus infection. *BMC Immunol* (2013) 14:40. doi:10.1186/1471-2172-14-40
14. Zelaya H, Tada A, Vizoso-Pinto MG, Salva S, Kanmani P, Agüero G, et al. Nasal priming with immunobiotic *Lactobacillus rhamnosus* modulates

inflammation-coagulation interactions and reduces influenza virus-associated pulmonary damage. *Inflamm Res* (2015) 64(8):589–602. doi:10.1007/s00011-015-0837-6
15. Kolling Y, Salva S, Villena J, Marranzino G, Alvarez S. Non-viable immunobiotic *Lactobacillus rhamnosus* CRL1505 and its peptidoglycan improve systemic and respiratory innate immune response during recovery of immunocompromised-malnourished mice. *Int Immunopharmacol* (2015) 25(2):474–84. doi:10.1016/j.intimp.2015.02.006
16. Chiba E, Tomosada Y, Vizoso-Pinto MG, Salva S, Takahashi T, Tsukida K, et al. Immunobiotic *Lactobacillus rhamnosus* improves resistance of infant mice against respiratory syncytial virus infection. *Int Immunopharmacol* (2013) 17(2):373–82. doi:10.1016/j.intimp.2013.06.024
17. Villena J, Chiba E, Tomosada Y, Salva S, Marranzino G, Kitazawa H, et al. Orally administered *Lactobacillus rhamnosus* modulates the respiratory immune response triggered by the viral pathogen-associated molecular pattern poly(I:C). *BMC Immunol* (2012) 13:53. doi:10.1186/1471-2172-13-53
18. Reppe K, Radünzel P, Dietert K, Tschernig T, Wolff T, Hammerschmidt S, et al. Pulmonary immunostimulation with MALP-2 in influenza virus-infected mice increases survival after pneumococcal superinfection. *Infect Immun* (2015) 83(12):4617. doi:10.1128/IAI.00948-15
19. Stark JM, Stark MA, Colasurdo GN, LeVine AM. Decreased bacterial clearance from the lungs of mice following primary respiratory syncytial virus infection. *J Med Virol* (2006) 78:829–38. doi:10.1002/jmv.20631
20. Robinson KM, Kolls JK, Alcorn JF. The immunology of influenza virus-associated bacterial pneumonia. *Curr Opin Immunol* (2015) 34:59–67. doi:10.1016/j.coi.2015.02.002
21. Medina M, Villena J, Salva S, Vintiñi E, Langella P, Alvarez S. Nasal administration of *Lactococcus lactis* improves the local and systemic immune responses against *Streptococcus pneumonia*. *Microbiol Immunol* (2008) 52:399–409. doi:10.1111/j.1348-0421.2008.00050.x
22. Villena J, Barbieri NP, Salva S, Herrera HM, Alvarez S. Nasal treatment with *Lactobacillus casei* enhances immunty against pneumococcal challenge in malnourished mice. *Microbiol Immunol* (2009) 53:636–46. doi:10.1111/j.1348-0421.2009.00171.x
23. Albarracin L, Kobayashi H, Iida H, Sato N, Nochi T, Aso H, et al. Transcriptomic analysis of the innate antiviral immune response in porcine intestinal epithelial cells: influence of immunobiotic lactobacilli. *Front Immunol* (2017) 8:57. doi:10.3389/fimmu.2017.00057
24. Damjanovic D, Lai R, Jeyanathan M, Hogaboam CM, Xing Z. Marked improvement of severe lung immunopathology by influenza-associated pneumococcal superinfection requires the control of both bacterial replication and host immune responses. *Am J Pathol* (2013) 183(3):868–80. doi:10.1016/j.ajpath.2013.05.016
25. Parker D, Martin FJ, Soong G, Harfenist BS, Aguilar JL, Ratner AJ, et al. *Streptococcus pneumoniae* DNA initiates type I interferon signaling in the respiratory tract. *MBio* (2011) 2:e00016–11. doi:10.1128/mBio.00016-11
26. Mancuso G, Midiri A, Biondo C, Beninati C, Zummo S, Galbo R, et al. Type I IFN signaling is crucial for host resistance against different species of pathogenic bacteria. *J Immunol* (2007) 178:3126–33. doi:10.4049/jimmunol.178.5.3126
27. LeMessurier KS, Häcker H, Chi L, Tuomanen E, Redecke V. Type I interferon protects against pneumococcal invasive disease by inhibiting bacterial transmigration across the lung. *PLoS Pathog* (2013) 9(11):e1003727. doi:10.1371/journal.ppat.1003727
28. Kumagai Y, Takeuchi O, Kato H, Kumar H, Matsui K, Morii E, et al. Alveolar macrophages are the primary interferon-alpha producer in pulmonary infection with RNA viruses. *Immunity* (2007) 27(2):240–52. doi:10.1016/j.immuni.2007.07.013
29. Divangahi M, King IL, Pernet E. Alveolar macrophages and type I IFN in airway homeostasis and immunity. *Trends Immunol* (2015) 36(5):307–14. doi:10.1016/j.it.2015.03.005
30. Shahangian A, Chow EK, Tian X, Kang JR, Ghaffari A, Liu SY, et al. Type I IFNs mediate development of postinfluenza bacterial pneumonia in mice. *J Clin Invest* (2009) 119(7):1910–20. doi:10.1172/JCI35412
31. Sun K, Metzger DW. Inhibition of pulmonary antibacterial defense by interferon-gamma during recovery from influenza infection. *Nat Med* (2008) 14:558–64. doi:10.1038/nm1765
32. van der Sluijs KF, van Elden LJR, Nijhuis M, Schuurman R, Pater JM, Florquin S, et al. IL-10 is an important mediator of the enhanced susceptibility to pneumococcal pneumonia after influenza infection. *J Immunol* (2004) 172:7603–9. doi:10.4049/jimmunol.172.12.7603
33. Chen Y, Wang CJ, Lin SH, Zhang M, Li SY, Xu F. Interleukin-35 is upregulated in response to influenza virus infection and secondary bacterial pneumonia. *Cytokine* (2016) 81:23–7. doi:10.1016/j.cyto.2016.01.016

14

Local Treatment with Lactate Prevents Intestinal Inflammation in the TNBS-Induced Colitis Model

*Carolina Iraporda[1], David E. Romanin[2], Ana A. Bengoa[1], Agustina J. Errea[2], Delphine Cayet[3], Benoit Foligné[3], Jean-Claude Sirard[3], Graciela L. Garrote[1], Analía G. Abraham[1,4] and Martín Rumbo[2]**

[1] Centro de Investigación y Desarrollo en Criotecnología de Alimentos (CIDCA, UNLP-CONICET-CIC.PBA), La Plata, Argentina, [2] Instituto de Estudios Inmunológicos y Fisopatológicos (IIFP, UNLP-CONICET), La Plata, Argentina, [3] CNRS, INSERM, CHU Lille, Institut Pasteur de Lille, U1019 – UMR 8204 – CIIL – Center for Infection and Immunity of Lille, University of Lille, Lille, France, [4] Área Bioquímica y Control de Alimentos, Facultad de Ciencias Exactas, UNLP, La Plata, Argentina

Edited by:
Julio Villena,
Reference Centre for Lactobacilli (CERELA-CONICET), Argentina

Reviewed by:
Angelica Thomaz Vieira,
Universidade Federal de Minas Gerais, Brazil
Paulraj Kanmani,
Tohoku University, Japan

***Correspondence:**
Martín Rumbo
rumbo.martin@gmail.com

Lactate has long been considered as a metabolic by-product of cells. Recently, this view has been changed by the observation that lactate can act as a signaling molecule and regulates critical functions of the immune system. We previously identified lactate as the component responsible for the modulation of innate immune epithelial response of fermented milk supernatants *in vitro*. We have also shown that lactate downregulates proinflammatory responses of macrophages and dendritic cells. So far, *in vivo* effects of lactate on intestinal inflammation have not been reported. We evaluated the effect of intrarectal administration of lactate in a murine model of colitis induced by 2,4,6-trinitrobenzenesulfonic acid (TNBS). The increase in lactate concentration in colon promoted protective effects against TNBS-induced colitis preventing histopathological damage, as well as bacterial translocation and rise of IL-6 levels in serum. Using intestinal epithelial reporter cells, we found that flagellin treatment induced reporter gene expression, which was abrogated by lactate treatment as well as by glycolysis inhibitors. Furthermore, lactate treatment modulated glucose uptake, indicating that high levels of extracellular lactate can impair metabolic reprograming induced by proinflammatory activation. These results suggest that lactate could be a potential beneficial microbiota metabolite and may constitute an overlooked effector with modulatory properties.

Keywords: innate immunity, lactate, TNBS-induced colitis, flagellin, immunomodulation

INTRODUCTION

Inflammatory bowel disease (IBD) involves a group of chronic, inflammatory disorders of the gastrointestinal tract, including Crohn's disease and ulcerative colitis, affecting people of all ages including the pediatric population. The etiology of IBD is still unknown but is thought to be due to a combination of genetic, microbial, immunological, and environmental factors that result in an abnormal and excessive immune response against commensal microbiota (1). The intestinal microbiota profoundly regulates the host immune function under physiological conditions and is likely the most important environmental factor in IBD as the target of the inflammatory response (2).

Dysbiosis or a lack of specific bacteria with anti-inflammatory properties may be responsible for gut inflammation (3–6). Although the molecular mechanisms of host–microbiota interactions are still not fully elucidated, manipulation of microbiota by probiotics or prebiotics is becoming increasingly recognized as a therapeutic option, for the treatment of the dysfunction or inflammation of the intestinal tract (7). The metabolic output of the modification of gut microbiota is the production of different profiles of short chain fatty acids (SCFA) such as butyrate, propionate, and acetate, and these metabolites are of relevance in the modulation of key signaling pathways involved in the inflammation of the gastrointestinal mucosa (7–9).

The impact of probiotic bacteria on intestinal health with the aim to prevent IBD or improve its treatment has been studied (10–12), as well as it has been shown that metabolites present in the supernatants of fermented dairy products can exert a protective effect *ex vivo* on intestinal mucosa exposed to inflammatory insults (13).

Lactate is the main metabolite of many fermented products and can also be generated *in situ* on the intestinal mucosa. Although lactate has been known to biochemists for over 200 years, it has been considered as a mere intermediate of carbon metabolite with specific organoleptic/antimicrobial properties rather than a bioactive molecule. Recently, lactate has been rediscovered as an active signaling metabolite in multiple fields of biology and medicine (14). Lactate mediates signaling pathways on several cell types, including production of pro- and anti-inflammatory mediators by T cells and macrophages and migratory changes and metabolic adaptation in T cells, endothelial cells, and neurons. Intracellular lactate can directly bind to proteins, influence the redox state *via* the lactate dehydrogenase reaction, stabilize hypoxia inducible factor-1, induce reactive oxygen species, and act as an inhibitor of glucose breakdown (15). The occurrence of these effects might depend on the cell type. Hoque et al. (16) demonstrated that administration of lactate reduced inflammation and organ injury in mice with immune hepatitis (16). Moreover, besides immunomodulation, Okada et al. (17) showed that luminal lactate-stimulated enterocyte proliferation in a murine model of hunger feedback, contributing to maintain intestinal barrier function (17). We have recently shown that lactate abrogates TLR and IL-1β dependent NF-κB activation of intestinal epithelial cells (18) and can regulate critical functions of several key players of the immune system such as macrophages and dendritic cells (19). In order to determine if the immunomodulatory capacity of lactate operates *in vivo*, the present work evaluated the effect of lactate in innate-driven murine model of colitis.

MATERIALS AND METHODS

Chemicals and Reagents

Different chemical reagents used 2,4,6-trinitrobenzenesulfonic acid (TNBS), 2 deoxyglucose (2DO), sodium oxamate, sodium 3-bromopyruvate (3BrPA) were purchased to Sigma Chemicals. DL-lactic acid (J. T. Baker) was employed. Flagellin was purified from *Salmonella*, detoxified, and controlled as previously described (20). Other proinflammatory stimulators, such as human interleukin-1β (IL-1β) and tumor necrosis factor (TNF), were purchased from R&D Systems (Minneapolis, MN, USA).

Animals

Male BALB/c AnN, 6 weeks old mice with weight over 20 g were purchased from Faculty of Science Veterinary from National University of La Plata, Argentina. The animals kept in polypropylene cages were maintained under standard conditions. The experimental protocols were approved by the Animal Ethics Committee of Faculty of Exact Sciences, National University of La Plata, Argentina (Approval No 011-01-15). Before conducting experiments, animals were acclimatized to animal facility conditions for 7 days.

Treatment and Induction of Experimental Colitis Using TNBS

Procedure was performed as previously described (21). Briefly, mice randomly divided into four groups were instilled with PBS (200 μL) (two groups) and with lactate solution in PBS 200 mM (200 μL) (two groups) by intrarectal route. Two hours post-administration, experimental colitis was induced by intrarectal instillation of 0.5 mg TNBS (SIGMA-Aldrich, USA) in ethanol 50% (v/v). Control animals were instilled with ethanol 50% (v/v) in distilled water. Enemas were gently instilled through a polyurethane catheter (18 G) inserted into the colon 4 cm proximally to the anal verge, and mice were held thereafter in a head-down position for 30 s. The weight of each mouse was determined and blood sampled at the beginning of the experiment and at 24 and 48 h. After 48 h, animals were sacrificed by cervical dislocation; colon tissues were collected for histological analysis (hematoxylin and eosin staining); and livers were aseptically taken to determine microbial translocation.

Serum IL-6 Determination

Blood was collected by submandibular bleeding and serum was isolated. Serum IL-6 determination was performed using BD Bioscience OptEIATM Mouse IL-6 ELISA Kit (Franklin Lakes, NJ, USA), according to manufacturer instructions.

Assessment of Colonic Epithelial Damage and Inflammation

Histopathological damage was determined following the criteria described previously (21). This system records two separate scores evaluating epithelial damage and infiltration. Briefly, the epithelial damage was scored as 0 for none, 1 for a minimal loss of goblet cells, 2 for extensive loss of goblet cells, 3 for a minimal loss of crypts and extensive loss of goblet cells, and 4 points for extensive loss of crypts; the infiltration was scored as 0 for none, 1 for an infiltrate around crypts bases, 2 for an infiltrate in *muscularis mucosa*, 3 for extensive infiltrate in *muscularis mucosa* with edema, and 4 points for the infiltration of submucosa. Preparations were assessed double blind, and the histopathological activity index was calculated as the sum of the epithelial damage and the infiltration score, ranging between 0 and 8 points from unaffected to severe colitis.

Microbial Translocation

Portions of liver were aseptically collected and placed in a sterile tube with a volume of BHI broth (Oxoid, England) in order to obtain 1 g organ/10 mL. These suspensions were homogenized, enriched in total viable bacteria by incubation 24 h at 37°C and used to inoculate BHI agar plates. Translocation of bacteria was defined by growth of microorganism on plates after 48–72 h of incubation at 37°C.

Cell Culture and CCL20:LUC Reporter Assay

Caco-2 cells stably transfected with a luciferase reporter construction under the control of the chemokine-ligand-20 (CCL20) promoter (Caco-2-*CCL20:LUC*) have been previously described (20). The cells were routinely grown in Dulbecco's Modified Eagle's Minimum Essential Medium (DMEM, GIBCO BRL Life Technologies, Rockville, MD, USA); supplemented with 15% (v/v) heat-inactivated (30 min, 60°C) fetal-bovine serum (FBS, PAA, GE Healthcare Bio-Sciences Corp., USA), 1% (v/v) non-essential amino acids (GIBCO BRL Life Technologies, Rockville, MD, USA) and the following antibiotics (Parafarm, Saporiti SACIFIA, Buenos Aires, Argentina): penicillin (12 IU/mL), streptomycin (12 μg/mL), and gentamicin (50 μg/mL). Caco-2-*CCL20:LUC* cells were used at 24 h post-confluence after 8 days of culture at subculture passages between 12 and 22 from the original stocks. All experiments were performed in serum-free medium.

Confluent Caco-2-*CCL20:LUC* cells cultured in 48-well plates were treated for 30 min with different concentrations of lactate pH 7.4 or different solutions of glycolysis inhibitors. The cells were then exposed to stimulation by flagellin (1 μg/mL), Il-1β (10 ng/mL), or TNF-α (100 ng/mL), during 6 h at 37°C in an atmosphere of 5% CO_2—95% air. A basal condition without any treatment was included as a control lacking stimulation; while flagellin, TNF-α, or IL1-β was added to cell that did not receive any treatment as control of 100% of induction of the proinflammatory response. The cells were next lysed with lysis Buffer (Promega, Madison, WI, USA), and luciferase activity was evaluated using the Luciferase Assay Kit (Promega, Madison, WI, USA) following manufacturer's instructions and measured in a luminometer (Luminoskan TL Plus). Luminescence was normalized to the stimulated control cells and expressed as a percentage of the normalized average luminescence (% normalized luciferase activity) ± SD from at least three independent experiments.

Cytotoxicity Assay

As a method of assessing treatment-induced cytotoxicity, mitochondrial activity was evaluated employing commercial kit CellTiter 96® AQueous One Solution Cell Proliferation Assay (Promega, Madison, WI, USA) following manufacturer's instruction.

Glucose Consumption by Epithelial Cells against TLR5 Agonist Stimulation

Confluent Caco-2/TC-7 epithelial cells cultured in 48-well plates were incubated at 37°C, in controlled atmosphere 5% CO_2 in DMEM containing initially 2 g/L glucose. Glucose uptake was determined in the culture medium employing a commercial enzymatic kit (Wiener lab, Rosario, Argentina). Samples were taken after 3, 6, 15, and 24 h of incubation either in basal condition, stimulated with flagellin with and without lactate 100 mM in the culture medium.

Statistical Analysis

The results are expressed as mean ± SD. Data analysis was performed using Graph Pad Prism version 5.01 for Windows (GraphPad Software, CA, USA). Analyses of variance followed by Dunnet Test or Bonferroni Test were applied. A p-value <0.05 indicated a significant difference.

RESULTS

Lactate Treatment Prevents Tissue Inflammation, Early IL-6 Production, and Bacterial Translocation in a TNBS-Induced Colitis Model

To address the *in vivo* immunomodulatory capacity of lactate, we evaluated the capacity to protect mice from colitis induced by intrarectal administration of TNBS. During the experiment, we compared the development of TNBS-induced colitis in mice that received intrarectal administration of lactate 200 mM or PBS as control. Such administration guaranteed lactate contact with intestinal cells exposed to the TNBS. The intrarectal administration of PBS or lactate followed by vehicle administration did not induce any significant changes of animal weight. In contrast, the rectal administration of TNBS causes progressive weight loss reaching up to 15% of the initial weight at 48 h. In both TNBS-treated groups (PBS/TNBS and Lactate/TNBS), a significant weight loss was observed (Figure S1 in Supplementary Material). Although the differences were not significant, the weight loss was lower in lactate/TNBS than in PBS/TNBS (10 versus 15%). Histological features of colitis were observed in the PBS/TNBS group as determined by epithelial damage, loss of goblet cells, edema, and infiltration of immune cells, leading to a pathology index of 4.67 ± 2.33 (**Figure 1**). In contrast, the group of mice pretreated with lactate (lactate/TNBS) showed significant protection from TNBS-induced inflammation, with lack of epithelial damage and minimal edema. Indeed, the histological sections were similar to the control groups that did not receive TNBS (PBS/vehicle and lactate/vehicle). The histopathology index of 1.40 ± 0.54 was significantly different from that of PBS/TNBS group ($p = 0.039$) (**Figures 1A,B**). This was in concordance with a clear better behavior of lactate-treated animals, indicating that lactate treatment prevents intestinal inflammation in the TNBS colitis model.

Inflammation is associated with the production of various inflammatory mediators, primarily cytokines that are key players in the innate and adaptive immune responses. Levels of circulating IL-6 were determined in the different experimental groups before and 24 or 48 h after instillation (**Figure 2**). IL-6 levels were significantly increased 24 h after treatment with TNBS in control group but decreased to the baseline at 48 h. In contrast, lactate treatment abolished the production of circulating IL-6 at

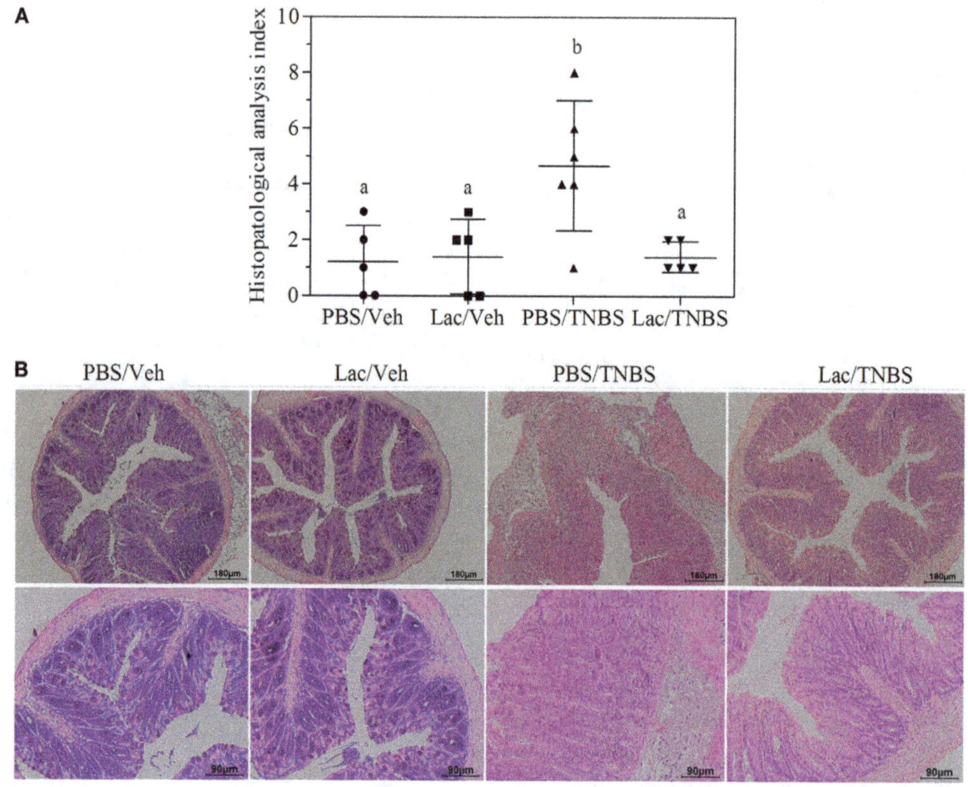

FIGURE 1 | Rectal administration of lactate protects animals against damage in TNBS acute colitis model. Mice were treated with lactate or PBS (i.r.) 2 h before TNBS or vehicle instillation and 48 h afterward tissue was collected for histopathological analysis. In all cases, groups of at least five mice were used. Results from a representative experiment out of five are shown. **(A)** Histopathological activity index assigned to different experimental groups. Different letter indicates significant differences with $p < 0.05$. **(B)** Photomicrograph of H&E-stained cross section (×100 top line and ×200 bottom line) of distal colon of a representative mouse of each experimental groups.

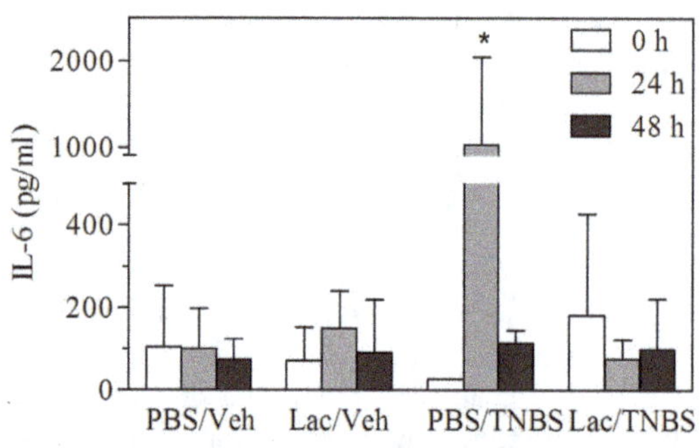

FIGURE 2 | Rectal administration of lactate protects animals against early IL-6 production. Serum was obtained from animals treated as in **Figure 1,** and levels of IL-6 were measured by ELISA. Serum levels of IL-6 (pg/ml) (□) before (▒) 24 h (■) 48 h, after TNBS or vehicle administration. Results from a representative experiment out of five are shown, expressed as the mean ± SD, *indicates significant difference with $p < 0.05$ respect to its corresponding control.

24 h, resulting in levels similar to control group. These results indicate that lactate pretreatment also prevents systemic alteration induced by TNBS treatment.

2,4,6-trinitrobenzenesulfonic acid is known to disrupt the mucosal barrier function by interacting with surface-active phospholipids of the colonic mucosa, a process that is evidenced by microbial translocation. We assessed the disruption by measuring the presence of bacteria into the liver. Our data demonstrated bacterial translocation four out of six animals in the PBS/TNBS group (**Table 1**). On the contrary, we did not find any bacteria in liver of animals pretreated with lactate and exposed to TNBS. These results were similar to the groups of mice that received vehicle (PBS/vehicle and lactate/vehicle) and did not experimented disruption of the mucosal barrier. Overall, our results show that luminal lactate could prevent bacterial translocation and reduce tissue inflammation induced by TNBS.

Lactate Downregulates Proinflammatory Response in Intestinal Epithelial Cells and Induces Metabolic Changes

In order to unravel the mechanisms of the anti-inflammatory effect of lactate in mice, an *in vitro* assay in the intestinal epithelial cell line Caco-2-*CCL20:LUC* that enables the monitoring of proinflammatory activation was used. In concordance to previous reports, pretreatment of Caco-2-*CCL20:LUC* cells with lactate produced a significant decrease of luciferase activity induced by various proinflammatory stimuli, i.e., flagellin (the TLR5 agonist), the cytokines IL1-β, and TNF (**Figure 3A**). In all stimulation conditions, a similar pattern of downregulation of the proinflammatory signaling was observed. For instance, exposure to concentrations of lactate of 5 mM or higher elicited a significant decrease of IL1-β-induced activation. These inhibitory effects of lactate were increased in a dose-dependent manner.

We have previously observed that lactate treatment abrogates enhanced glycolysis in TLR-stimulated macrophages, which correlates with its activity as modulator of innate response (22), Caco-2-*CCL20:LUC* reporter cell line was utilized to evaluate if the effects of lactate on epithelial cells could be related to metabolic changes.

TABLE 1 | Microbial translocation to liver observed 48 h after 2,4,6-trinitrobenzenesulfonic acid (TNBS)-induced colitis.

Treatment	Animals with positive translocation/total animals in the group
PBS/VEH	0/5
LAC/VEH	0/5
PBS/TNBS	4/6
LAC/TNBS	0/5

Results from a representative experiment out of five are shown.

Treatment of cells during 6 h with glycolysis inhibitors such as 2DO or 3BrPA (competitive inhibitors of hexokinase) and oxamate (inhibitor of lactate dehydrogenase) in different concentrations did not affect luciferase activity in non-stimulated condition. Luciferase activity induced by flagellin was significantly lower in cells pretreated with glycolysis inhibitors, and this effect was dose-dependent (**Figures 3B–D**). Cell viability was not affected by 6 h incubation with glycolysis inhibitors, showing an enzymatic activity on MTT reduction over 85% in all cases (not shown).

We observed that Caco-2 intestinal epithelial cells decreased their rate of glucose consumption in the presence of lactate either in basal as well as with flagellin conditions. This could be associated with an inhibition of glycolysis in presence of lactate (**Figure 4**). Overall, these results indicate that lactate modulation of epithelial response, correlates with its capacity to alter glycolytic activity, which alters the capacity to trigger the effectors of innate response activation.

DISCUSSION

Although the etiology of IBD is still unknown, increasing evidence shows that IBD may involve in genetically susceptible individuals a dysregulation of their immune response to resident microbiota (23). It is now widely accepted that a misbalanced gut ecosystem also plays an important role other pathologies of the gastrointestinal tract (24).

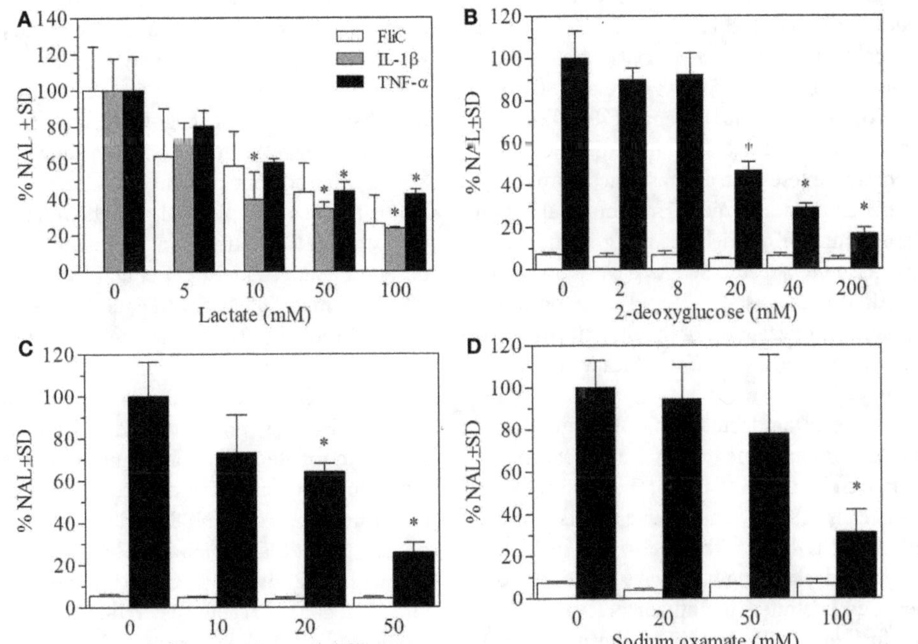

FIGURE 3 | Lactate pretreatment as well as glycolysis inhibition leads to downregulation of inflammatory response in Caco-2-*CCL20:LUC* cells. Reporter cells were stimulated with IL1-β (10 ng/mL), tumor necrosis factor (TNF)-α (100 ng/mL), or flagellin (1 μg/mL), after pretreatment with different concentrations of lactate. **(A)** Results are expressed as normalized luciferase activity, using the levels of stimulated cells in absence of lactate as 100% of activation. The Caco-2-*CCL20:LUC* cells pretreated with solutions of glycolysis inhibitors **(B)** 2DG (mM) **(C)** 3-bromopyruvate (μm) **(D)** Oxamate (mM). Results shown are the mean and SEM from independent triplicates. Results from a typical experiment out of at least three are depicted. □ Non-stimulated and ■ stimulated Flic. *Indicates a significant difference from the cells without treatment and stimulated with flagellin, IL-1β, and TNF-α, respectively, with $p < 0.05$.

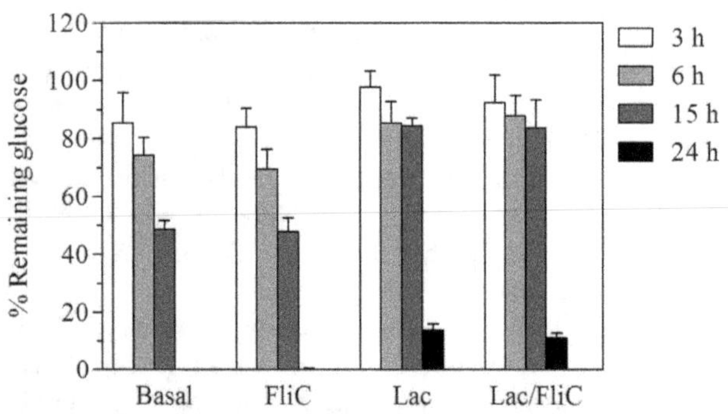

FIGURE 4 | Lactate treatment decreases glucose uptake of Caco-2/TC-7 cells either in basal as well as stimulated conditions. Percentage of glucose remaining in culture medium of Caco-2/TC-7 cells either with lactate 100 mM or not, non-stimulated and stimulated with flagellin (1 μg/mL), incubated for (□) 3, (■) 6, (■) 15, and (■) 24 h.

Several therapeutic strategies proposed to reduce the symptoms of IBD are based on the use of anti-inflammatory drugs (such as corticoids, 5-aminosalicylic acid, and anti-TNF-α antibodies), all having marked long-term side effects. Other proposed treatments are based on microbiota-based dietary interventions, either by the use of probiotics or prebiotics (25). Therapeutic administration of probiotic species such as *Bifidobacterium* spp., *Lactobacillus* spp., or *Propionibacterium* has been shown to have protective effects on IBD models through the production of anti-inflammatory metabolites (26, 27). Almost two decades ago, proof of concept in clinical studies demonstrated the efficacy of SCFAs-based treatments in IBD, specifically in ulcerative colitis, treating the inflamed region using a mixture of SCFAs (acetate 80 mM, butyrate 40 mM and propionate 30 mM) enemas (28–30). In the recent years, therapeutic strategies related to intestinal SCFAs to manage IBDs have renewed interest based on studies from either animal models or intestinal metabolomic/microbiota analysis on patients. Interventions in animal models resulting in increased exposure of intestinal tissue to specific SCFAs have shown protective effects in intestinal mucosa (31, 32) and new combined interventions with pharmaceuticals and oral SCFAs formulated to be released in large intestine have shown efficacy in patient management (33).

We have previously shown that lactate can downregulate the proinflammatory responses of immune cells such as macrophages and dendritic cells, as well as those of mucosal structural cells like intestinal epithelial cells (18, 19). The diverse effects of lactic acid on various immune cells suggest that lactic acid or lactate may influence widely used signaling pathways. Indeed, both molecules have been demonstrated to influence several MAP kinases, NFkB signaling, or the PI3K/AKT pathway (15, 34). Aiming to analyze effects of lactate on inflammation *in vivo*, in a proof of concept experimental design, we found that pretreatment with lactate 200 mM modulates the epithelial damage and infiltration induced by TNBS. This effect was not observed when lactate 200 mM was administered in drinking water, on account of low lactate levels measured in distal colon (not shown). This reduced content could be due to either intestinal absorption by enterocytes, lactate consumption by microbiota, or both. To have protective effect, lactate luminal levels should be high, such as those reached by intrarectal administration. TNBS i.r. administration has been used as model for innate-driven intestinal inflammation due to epithelial damage and increased access of microbial-derived molecules to the immune cells in the lamina propria compartment (35). The use of the TNBS model that produce an acute local activation of inflammatory response allowed us to evaluate the local effect of lactate after a short term exposure, upon i.r intervention. Due to experimental design, contribution of microbiota, other fermentation metabolites, or other microbial products to the anti-inflammatory effect is expected to be low, indicating that is lactate the main responsible for the modulation observed.

Using different strategies, several authors showed that prevention of inflammation in the TNBS model is usually correlated with lower bacterial translocation from the gut to mesenteric lymph nodes and systemic compartment (36–40). In coincidence with these results, we have shown that lactate administration protects against microbial translocation to the liver in animals treated with TNBS and the increase in lactate concentration in colon alleviates TNBS-induced colitis. Furthermore, lactate treatment also prevented serum rise of levels of IL6 (**Figure 2**), in coincidence with our previous observations that lactate pretreatment abrogates NFkB activation and proinflammatory gene expression such as IL12, IL1β, or IL6 (18, 19). Some proinflammatory cytokines that may be modulated in this way, such as IL1b and IL18, have also the capacity to trigger epithelial renewal and reinforce barrier function (41). Nevertheless, in our system, the overall effect of lactate is to promote tissue protection as appreciated by hystopathological analysis (**Figure 1**).

There are several possible non-mutually exclusive mechanisms that may explain the capacity of lactate to prevent inflammation in our model. We have recently shown that lactate, as other SCFAs, may prevent TLR-mediated activation of macrophage and dendritic cells (19). Several reports indicate that the blockage of macrophage activation can modulate colonic inflammation in different acute models; Du et al. (42) have shown that targeting intestinal macrophages with gadolinium chloride block colitis in a TNBS model (42). Furthermore, several treatments targeting intestinal macrophage activation, using miRNAs or modulation of specific GPCRs, can also modulate colitis in TNBS model (43, 44). Besides, previous studies have shown that lactate can modulate innate activation of intestinal epithelial cells (18, 19). Since epithelial cells can also contribute to the amplification of inflammation in the TNBS model, this could be another possible cellular target that explains the bioactive properties of lactate. In line with this possibility, Cheng et al. have shown that targeting intestinal epithelial cells may reduce colitis in IBD models (45).

Beyond the cellular target of lactate, there are also several mechanisms that may account for its activity. We have recently shown that lactate impairs macrophage metabolic reprograming after LPS activation in a GPR81-independent manner (22), which has also been associated with blunting the proinflammatory cytokine response (46). In accordance with these results, Selleri et al. (47) have shown that local increase of lactate in the environment of mesenchymal stromal cells shifts macrophage M1 activation toward the less inflammatory M2 (47). Colegio et al. (48) have shown also the blunting of M1 macrophage activation in the solid tumor environment due to high lactate production of Warburg metabolism of tumor cells (48). Kreutz and colleagues have shown that increase in extracellular lactate of macrophages impair proinflammatory activation by altering its capacity to rise its glycolitic flux, effect that is enhanced at low pH (34, 49). Inhibition of lactate efflux from macrophages blocks LPS-driven activation by a mechanism also associated to impairment of glycolytic reprograming of macrophage upon activation (50).

Metabolic reprograming upon proinflammatory activation of myeloid cells implicates enhanced glycolysis with low respiratory rate (51). In the case of macrophages, this implies high rate of urea cycle intermediates for the production of NO from arginine (46) and production of lipid metabolites from citrate. In the case of dendritic cells, metabolic reprograming supplies carbon from glycolysis to lipid metabolites, mainly to allow expansion of endoplasmic reticulum in order to facilitate antigen presentation (52). Although it is not clear that the extent of metabolic reprograming takes place in epithelial cells upon TLR activation, there are some reports that show similarities on macrophage and epithelial cell response to mediators of metabolic reprograming (53). Our results indicate that blocking of glycolysis impairs flagellin-induced CCL20 transcriptional activation observed in our reporter system (**Figure 3**). Furthermore, we observed less consumption of glucose in the presence of extracellular lactate (**Figure 4**). These results are consistent with the necessity of enhancement of glycolysis rate in epithelial cells for a full functional TLR response, as is the case of macrophages.

Although our experimental design was first aimed to confirm the bioactive properties of lactate observed *in vitro* in a preclinical model, it opens the possibility of using lactate in local treatments to modulate inflammation. Furthermore, it can be considered that local production of lactate by probiotic microorganisms that attach to the intestinal epithelium may also contribute to their protective capacity in inflammatory situations (14), providing alternative cues for selection of microorganisms to be used as complement in the management of IBDs.

CONCLUSION

Results shown here were conclusive in relation to the effect of lactate at local level in a model of acute intestinal inflammation, contributing to a decrease in epithelial damage, signs of inflammation, and the secretion of proinflammatory cytokine IL-6, presenting a first approximation *in vivo* about the role of lactate in preventing intestinal inflammation.

Although several possibilities remain to be considered to explain the cellular and molecular mechanisms responsible for the observed effect, a correlation between impairment of glycolysis and proinflammatory activation of epithelial cells was observed, in coincidence with previous works in macrophages.

These results suggest that lactate could be a potential beneficial microbiota metabolite and may contribute to health-promoting properties on the intestinal mucosa.

AUTHOR CONTRIBUTIONS

CI performed experimental work, participated in the study design and conception and manuscript writing. AB, DR, AE, and DC performed experimental work, participated in study design. BF performed experimental work, participated in study design and manuscript writing. J-CS participated in study design, funding, and manuscript writing. GG, AA, and MR participated in study design and conception, funding, and manuscript writing.

ACKNOWLEDGMENTS

CI and AB are fellows of Argentina National Research Council (CONICET), DR, AE, AA, GG, and MR are members of Scientific Career of CONICET. DC, J-CS, and BF are supported by the Institut Pasteur de Lille, the University of Lille, CNRS and Inserm. Work was supported by grants from CONICET, Agencia Nacional de Promoción Científica y Tecnológica (ANPCYT) and ECOS A12B03 grant of the National Ministry of Science, Technology and Innovation (MINCYT-Argentina).

SUPPLEMENTARY MATERIAL

The Supplementary Material for this article can be found online at http://journal.frontiersin.org/article/10.3389/fimmu.2016.00651/full#supplementary-material.

FIGURE S1 | Intrarectal administration of lactate protects animals against weight loss in 2,4,6-trinitrobenzenesulfonic acid (TNBS) acute colitis model. Weight variation after 24 and 48 h of TNBS-induced colitis (% of initial weight). In all cases, groups of at least five mice were used. Results from a representative experiment out of five are shown. Different letter indicates significant differences with $p < 0.05$.

REFERENCES

1. Wallace KL, Zheng LB, Kanazawa Y, Shih DQ. Immunopathology of inflammatory bowel disease. *World J Gastroenterol* (2014) 20:6–21. doi:10.3748/wjg.v20.i1.6
2. Round JL, Mazmanian SK. The gut microbiota shapes intestinal immune responses during health and disease. *Nat Rev Immunol* (2009) 9:313–23. doi:10.1038/nri2515
3. Sokol H, Pigneur B, Watterlot L, Lakhdari O, Bermudez-Humaran LG, Gratadoux JJ, et al. *Faecalibacterium prausnitzii* is an anti-inflammatory commensal bacterium identified by gut microbiota analysis of Crohn disease patients. *Proc Natl Acad Sci U S A* (2008) 105:16731–6. doi:10.1073/pnas.0804812105
4. Kang S, Denman SE, Morrison M, Yu Z, Dore J, Leclerc M, et al. Dysbiosis of fecal microbiota in Crohn's disease patients as revealed by a custom phylogenetic microarray. *Inflamm Bowel Dis* (2010) 16:2034–42. doi:10.1002/ibd.21319
5. Morgan XC, Tickle TL, Sokol H, Gevers D, Devaney KL, Ward DV, et al. Dysfunction of the intestinal microbiome in inflammatory bowel disease and treatment. *Genome Biol* (2012) 13:R79. doi:10.1186/gb-2012-13-9-r79
6. Eeckhaut V, Machiels K, Perrier C, Romero C, Maes S, Flahou B, et al. Butyricicoccus pullicaecorum in inflammatory bowel disease. *Gut* (2013) 62:1745–52. doi:10.1136/gutjnl-2012-303611
7. Kanauchi O, Andoh A, Mitsuyama K. Effects of the modulation of microbiota on the gastrointestinal immune system and bowel function. *J Agric Food Chem* (2013) 61:9977–83. doi:10.1021/jf402441f

8. Maslowski KM, Mackay CR. Diet, gut microbiota and immune responses. *Nat Immunol* (2011) 12:5–9. doi:10.1038/ni0111-5
9. Koh A, De Vadder F, Kovatcheva-Datchary P, Backhed F. From dietary fiber to host physiology: short-chain fatty acids as key bacterial metabolites. *Cell* (2016) 165:1332–45. doi:10.1016/j.cell.2016.05.041
10. Minocha A. Probiotics for preventive health. *Nutr Clin Pract* (2009) 24:227–41. doi:10.1177/0884533608331177
11. Martin R, Miquel S, Ulmer J, Kechaou N, Langella P, Bermudez-Humaran LG. Role of commensal and probiotic bacteria in human health: a focus on inflammatory bowel disease. *Microb Cell Fact* (2013) 12:71. doi:10.1186/1475-2859-12-71
12. Foligne B, Parayre S, Cheddani R, Famelart MH, Madec MN, Ple C, et al. Immunomodulation properties of multi-species fermented milks. *Food Microbiol* (2016) 53:60–9. doi:10.1016/j.fm.2015.04.002
13. Tsilingiri K, Barbosa T, Penna G, Caprioli F, Sonzogni A, Viale G, et al. Probiotic and postbiotic activity in health and disease: comparison on a novel polarised ex-vivo organ culture model. *Gut* (2012) 61:1007–15. doi:10.1136/gutjnl-2011-300971
14. Garrote GL, Abraham AG, Rumbo M. Is lactate an undervalued functional component of fermented food products? *Front Microbiol* (2015) 6:629. doi:10.3389/fmicb.2015.00629
15. Haas R, Cucchi D, Smith J, Pucino V, Macdougall CE, Mauro C. Intermediates of metabolism: from bystanders to signalling molecules. *Trends Biochem Sci* (2016) 41:460–71. doi:10.1016/j.tibs.2016.02.003
16. Hoque R, Farooq A, Ghani A, Gorelick F, Mehal WZ. Lactate reduces liver and pancreatic injury in Toll-like receptor- and inflammasome-mediated inflammation via GPR81-mediated suppression of innate immunity. *Gastroenterology* (2014) 146:1763–74. doi:10.1053/j.gastro.2014.03.014
17. Okada T, Fukuda S, Hase K, Nishiumi S, Izumi Y, Yoshida M, et al. Microbiota-derived lactate accelerates colon epithelial cell turnover in starvation-refed mice. *Nat Commun* (2013) 4:1654. doi:10.1038/ncomms2668
18. Iraporda C, Romanin D, Rumbo M, Garrote G, Abraham A. The role of lactate in the immunomodulatory properties of kefir non bacterial fraction. *Food Res Int* (2014) 62:247–53. doi:10.1016/j.foodres.2014.03.003
19. Iraporda C, Errea A, Romanin DE, Cayet D, Pereyra E, Pignataro O, et al. Lactate and short chain fatty acids produced by microbial fermentation downregulate proinflammatory responses in intestinal epithelial cells and myeloid cells. *Immunobiology* (2015) 220:1161–9. doi:10.1016/j.imbio.2015.06.004
20. Nempont C, Cayet D, Rumbo M, Bompard C, Villeret V, Sirard JC. Deletion of flagellin's hypervariable region abrogates antibody-mediated neutralization and systemic activation of TLR5-dependent immunity. *J Immunol* (2008) 181:2036–43. doi:10.4049/jimmunol.181.3.2036
21. Romanin DE, Llopis S, Genoves S, Martorell P, Ramon VD, Garrote GL, et al. Probiotic yeast *Kluyveromyces marxianus* CIDCA 8154 shows anti-inflammatory and anti-oxidative stress properties in in vivo models. *Benef Microbes* (2015) 7:83–93. doi:10.3920/BM2015.0066
22. Errea A, Cayet D, Marchetti P, Tang C, Kluza J, Offermanns S, et al. Lactate inhibits the pro-inflammatory response and metabolic reprogramming in murine macrophages in a GPR81-independent manner. *PLoS One* (2016) 11:e0163694. doi:10.1371/journal.pone.0163694
23. Baker PI, Love DR, Ferguson LR. Role of gut microbiota in Crohn's disease. *Expert Rev Gastroenterol Hepatol* (2009) 3:535–46. doi:10.1586/egh.09.47
24. Bennet SM, Ohman L, Simren M. Gut microbiota as potential orchestrators of irritable bowel syndrome. *Gut Liver* (2015) 9:318–31. doi:10.5009/gnl14344
25. Breton J, Ple C, Guerin-Deremaux L, Pot B, Lefranc-Millot C, Wils D, et al. Intrinsic immunomodulatory effects of low-digestible carbohydrates selectively extend their anti-inflammatory prebiotic potentials. *Biomed Res Int* (2015) 2015:13. doi:10.1155/2015/162398
26. van Baarlen P, Wells JM, Kleerebezem M. Regulation of intestinal homeostasis and immunity with probiotic lactobacilli. *Trends Immunol* (2013) 34:208–15. doi:10.1016/j.it.2013.01.005
27. Ple C, Breton J, Richoux R, Nurdin M, Deutsch SM, Falentin H, et al. Combining selected immunomodulatory *Propionibacterium freudenreichii* and *Lactobacillus delbrueckii* strains: reverse engineering development of an anti-inflammatory cheese. *Mol Nutr Food Res* (2016) 60:935–48. doi:10.1002/mnfr.201500580
28. Vernia P, Marcheggiano A, Caprilli R, Frieri G, Corrao G, Valpiani D, et al. Short-chain fatty acid topical treatment in distal ulcerative colitis. *Aliment Pharmacol Ther* (1995) 9:309–13. doi:10.1111/j.1365-2036.1995.tb00386.x
29. Scheppach W. Treatment of distal ulcerative colitis with short-chain fatty acid enemas. A placebo-controlled trial. German-Austrian SCFA study group. *Dig Dis Sci* (1996) 41:2254–9.
30. Breuer RI, Soergel KH, Lashner BA, Christ ML, Hanauer SB, Vanagunas A, et al. Short chain fatty acid rectal irrigation for left-sided ulcerative colitis: a randomised, placebo controlled trial. *Gut* (1997) 40:485–91. doi:10.1136/gut.40.4.485
31. Komiyama Y, Andoh A, Fujiwara D, Ohmae H, Araki Y, Fujiyama Y, et al. New prebiotics from rice bran ameliorate inflammation in murine colitis models through the modulation of intestinal homeostasis and the mucosal immune system. *Scand J Gastroenterol* (2011) 46:40–52. doi:10.3109/00365521.2010.513062
32. Vieira EL, Leonel AJ, Sad AP, Beltrao NR, Costa TF, Ferreira TM, et al. Oral administration of sodium butyrate attenuates inflammation and mucosal lesion in experimental acute ulcerative colitis. *J Nutr Biochem* (2012) 23:430–6. doi:10.1016/j.jnutbio.2011.01.007
33. Assisi RF, GISDI Study Group. Combined butyric acid/mesalazine treatment in ulcerative colitis with mild-moderate activity. Results of a multicentre pilot study. *Minerva Gastroenterol Dietol* (2008) 54:231–8.
34. Peter K, Rehli M, Singer K, Renner-Sattler K, Kreutz M. Lactic acid delays the inflammatory response of human monocytes. *Biochem Biophys Res Commun* (2015) 457:412–8. doi:10.1016/j.bbrc.2015.01.005
35. Antoniou E, Margonis GA, Angelou A, Pikouli A, Argiri P, Karavokyros I, et al. The TNBS-induced colitis animal model: an overview. *Ann Med Surg (Lond)* (2016) 11:9–15. doi:10.1016/j.amsu.2016.07.019
36. Fiorucci S, Distrutti E, Mencarelli A, Barbanti M, Palazzini E, Morelli A. Inhibition of intestinal bacterial translocation with rifaximin modulates lamina propria monocytic cells reactivity and protects against inflammation in a rodent model of colitis. *Digestion* (2002) 66:246–56. doi:10.1159/000068362
37. Daniel C, Poiret S, Goudercourt D, Dennin V, Leyer G, Pot B. Selecting lactic acid bacteria for their safety and functionality by use of a mouse colitis model. *Appl Environ Microbiol* (2006) 72:5799–805. doi:10.1128/AEM.00109-06
38. Akcan A, Kucuk C, Sozuer E, Esel D, Akyildiz H, Akgun H, et al. Melatonin reduces bacterial translocation and apoptosis in trinitrobenzene sulphonic acid-induced colitis of rats. *World J Gastroenterol* (2008) 14:918–24. doi:10.3748/wjg.14.1222
39. Halaclar B, Agac Ay A, Akcan AC, Ay A, Oz B, Arslan E. Effects of glucagon-like peptide-2 on bacterial translocation in rat models of colitis. *Turk J Gastroenterol* (2012) 23:691–8. doi:10.4318/tjg.2012.0468
40. Martinez-Moya P, Ortega-Gonzalez M, Gonzalez R, Anzola A, Ocon B, Hernandez-Chirlaque C, et al. Exogenous alkaline phosphatase treatment complements endogenous enzyme protection in colonic inflammation and reduces bacterial translocation in rats. *Pharmacol Res* (2012) 66:144–53. doi:10.1016/j.phrs.2012.04.006
41. Lissner D, Siegmund B. The multifaceted role of the inflammasome in inflammatory bowel diseases. *ScientificWorldJournal* (2011) 11:1536–47. doi:10.1100/tsw.2011.139
42. Du C, Wang P, Yu Y, Chen F, Liu J, Li Y. Gadolinium chloride improves the course of TNBS and DSS-induced colitis through protecting against colonic mucosal inflammation. *Sci Rep* (2014) 4:6096. doi:10.1038/srep06096
43. Huang Z, Ma J, Chen M, Jiang H, Fu Y, Gan J, et al. Dual TNF-alpha/IL-12p40 interference as a strategy to protect against colitis based on miR-16 precursors with macrophage targeting vectors. *Mol Ther* (2015) 23:1611–21. doi:10.1038/mt.2015.111
44. Stancic A, Jandl K, Hasenohrl C, Reichmann F, Marsche G, Schuligoi R, et al. The GPR55 antagonist CID16020046 protects against intestinal inflammation. *Neurogastroenterol Motil* (2015) 27:1432–45. doi:10.1111/nmo.12639
45. Cheng X, Zhang X, Su J, Zhang Y, Zhou W, Zhou J, et al. miR-19b downregulates intestinal SOCS3 to reduce intestinal inflammation in Crohn's disease. *Sci Rep* (2015) 5:10397. doi:10.1038/srep10397
46. Jha AK, Huang SC, Sergushichev A, Lampropoulou V, Ivanova Y, Loginicheva E, et al. Network integration of parallel metabolic and transcriptional data reveals metabolic modules that regulate macrophage polarization. *Immunity* (2015) 42:419–30. doi:10.1016/j.immuni.2015.02.005

47. Selleri S, Bifsha P, Civini S, Pacelli C, Dieng MM, Lemieux W, et al. Human mesenchymal stromal cell-secreted lactate induces M2-macrophage differentiation by metabolic reprogramming. *Oncotarget* (2016) 7:30193–210. doi:10.18632/oncotarget.8623
48. Colegio OR, Chu NQ, Szabo AL, Chu T, Rhebergen AM, Jairam V, et al. Functional polarization of tumour-associated macrophages by tumour-derived lactic acid. *Nature* (2014) 513:559–63. doi:10.1038/nature13490
49. Dietl K, Renner K, Dettmer K, Timischl B, Eberhart K, Dorn C, et al. Lactic acid and acidification inhibit TNF secretion and glycolysis of human monocytes. *J Immunol* (2010) 184:1200–9. doi:10.4049/jimmunol.0902584
50. Tan Z, Xie N, Banerjee S, Cui H, Fu M, Thannickal VJ, et al. The monocarboxylate transporter 4 is required for glycolytic reprogramming and inflammatory response in macrophages. *J Biol Chem* (2015) 290:46–55. doi:10.1074/jbc.M114.603589
51. O'Neill LA, Pearce EJ. Immunometabolism governs dendritic cell and macrophage function. *J Exp Med* (2016) 213:15–23. doi:10.1084/jem.20151570
52. Everts B, Amiel E, Huang SC, Smith AM, Chang CH, Lam WY, et al. TLR-driven early glycolytic reprogramming via the kinases TBK1-IKKvarepsilon supports the anabolic demands of dendritic cell activation. *Nat Immunol* (2014) 15:323–32. doi:10.1038/ni.2833
53. Cordes T, Wallace M, Michelucci A, Divakaruni AS, Sapcariu SC, Sousa C, et al. Immunoresponsive gene 1 and itaconate inhibit succinate dehydrogenase to modulate intracellular succinate levels. *J Biol Chem* (2016) 291:14274–84. doi:10.1074/jbc.M115.685792

15

Respiratory Antiviral Immunity and Immunobiotics: Beneficial Effects on Inflammation-Coagulation Interaction during Influenza Virus Infection

Hortensia Zelaya[1,2], Susana Alvarez[1,2,3], Haruki Kitazawa[4,5] and Julio Villena[1,3,4]**

[1] Immunobiotics Research Group, Tucuman, Argentina, [2] Institute of Applied Biochemistry, National University of Tucuman, Tucuman, Argentina, [3] Laboratory of Immunobiotechnology, Reference Centre for Lactobacilli (CERELA-CONICET), Tucuman, Argentina, [4] Food and Feed Immunology Group, Laboratory of Animal Products Chemistry, Graduate School of Agricultural Science, Tohoku University, Sendai, Japan, [5] Livestock Immunology Unit, International Education and Research Center for Food and Agricultural Immunology (CFAI), Graduate School of Agricultural Science, Tohoku University, Sendai, Japan

Edited by:
José Roberto Mineo, Federal University of Uberlandia, Brazil

Reviewed by:
Mirko Trilling, University of Duisburg, Germany
Dina Weilhammer, Lawrence Livermore National Laboratory (DOE), USA

***Correspondence:**
Haruki Kitazawa
haruki.kitazawa.c7@tohoku.ac.jp;
Julio Villena
jcvillena@cerela.org.ar

Influenza virus (IFV) is a major respiratory pathogen of global importance, and the cause of a high degree of morbidity and mortality, especially in high-risk populations such as infants, elderly, and immunocompromised hosts. Given its high capacity to change antigenically, acquired immunity is often not effective to limit IFV infection and therefore vaccination must be constantly redesigned to achieve effective protection. Improvement of respiratory and systemic innate immune mechanisms has been proposed to reduce the incidence and severity of IFV disease. In the last decade, several research works have demonstrated that microbes with the capacity to modulate the mucosal immune system (immunobiotics) are a potential alternative to beneficially modulate the outcome of IFV infection. This review provides an update of the current status on the modulation of respiratory immunity by orally and nasally administered immunobiotics, and their beneficial impact on IFV clearance and inflammatory-mediated lung tissue damage. In particular, we describe the research of our group that investigated the influence of immunobiotics on inflammation–coagulation interactions during IFV infection. Studies have clearly demonstrated that hostile inflammation is accompanied by dysfunctional coagulation in respiratory IFV disease, and our investigations have proved that some immunobiotic strains are able to reduce viral disease severity through their capacity to modulate the immune-coagulative responses in the respiratory tract.

Keywords: immunobiotics, influenza virus, inflammation, coagulation, respiratory immunity

INTRODUCTION

Influenza virus (IFV) is a member of the *Orthomyxoviridae* family that contains a negative-sense, single-stranded, segmented RNA genome protected by a capsid of viral ribonucleoproteins. This virus is categorized into subtypes based on the expression of hemagglutinin (HA) and neuraminidase on the surface of the viral envelope.

Influenza is a highly contagious viral infection that has a substantial impact on global health and IFV is a major respiratory pathogen that causes a high degree of morbidity and mortality, especially in high-risk populations such as infants, elderly, and immunocompromised hosts. Given the high capacity of IFV to change antigenically, acquired immunity is often not effective to limit infection and therefore vaccination must be constantly redesigned to achieve protection. Improvement of respiratory and systemic innate immune mechanisms has been proposed to reduce the incidence and severity of IFV disease.

In the last decade, several research works have demonstrated that microbes with the capacity to modulate the mucosal immune system (immunobiotics) are a potential alternative to beneficially modulate the outcome of IFV infection. This review provides an update of the current status on the modulation of respiratory immunity by orally and nasally administered immunobiotics, and their beneficial impact on IFV clearance and inflammatory-mediated lung tissue damage. In particular, we describe the research of our group that investigated the influence of immunobiotics on inflammation–coagulation interactions during IFV infection. Studies have clearly demonstrated that hostile inflammation is accompanied by dysfunctional coagulation in respiratory IFV disease, and our investigations have proved that some immunobiotic strains are able to reduce viral disease severity through their capacity to modulate the immune-coagulative responses in the respiratory tract.

RESPIRATORY IMMUNE RESPONSE AND IFV

The first barrier that protects the host against IFV infection is the respiratory epithelium through its capacity to recognize the viral attack. When IFV successfully overcomes the respiratory barrier constituted by the mucus layer and the ciliar movement, it mediates its attachment and internalization into respiratory epithelial cells to start its replication (1). During the viral attack, several pathogen-associated molecular patterns (PAMPs) are exposed and recognized by pattern-recognition receptors (PRRs) expressed in respiratory cells (**Figure 1**). It is now well established that the most important PRRs involved in the recognition of IFV are the Toll-like receptor (TLR)-3 and TLR7 and the RNA recognition protein RIG-1 (2). TLR3 is expressed in endosomes and is able to recognize viral double-stranded RNA (dsRNA) that is produced during viral replication; while endosomal TLR7 and cytoplasmic RIG-I recognize single-stranded RNA (ssRNA). RIG-I signals through mitochondrial antiviral signaling protein. The PAMPs–PPRs interaction leads to the activation of several signaling pathways that induce the activation of nuclear factor κB (NF-κB) and interferon (IFN) regulatory factor 3 (IRF3) and the production of type I and III IFNs and inflammatory cytokines (2).

Type I IFNs, especially IFN-β, produced and released during the earlier stages of IFV infection are key to develop an antiviral state in the respiratory tract. It was reported that human bronchial epithelial cells release preformed IFN-β in response to IFV challenge inducing a protective role (3). IFNs produced by infected cells are able to act in a paracrine or autocrine manner activating their receptors (IFNAR) and increasing the expression of hundreds of genes that counteract viral replication. Functional genomic studies have identified several of the IFN-induced factors that have important roles in controlling IFV replication (2) including the IFN-inducible transmembrane proteins 1, 2, and 3 (4), MX1 proteins (5), and 2′,5′-oligoadenylate synthetase (OAS)-RNAaseL system (6).

Proinflammatory cytokines and chemokines produced as a result of TLR3 and RIG-I activation during IFV infection are also important for the generation of the respiratory antiviral innate immune response. Infection of epithelial cells by IFV increases the expression of TNF-α, IL-6, IL-8, CCL2 (MIP-1), CCL5 (RANTES), CCL3 (MIP-1α), and CXCL10 (IP-10) (7). The production of these cytokines is complemented by activity of inflammasomes that induce the activation of caspase-1 and promote the generation of the active forms of IL-1β and IL-18 (**Figure 1**). IFV has been shown to activate mainly the NLRP3 inflammasome which is essential for the protection against the virus since several studies demonstrated that mice lacking NLRP3 or caspase-1 have decreased IL-1β and IL-18 secretion and increased mortality after IFV challenge (8–10).

The proinflammatory cytokines and chemokines are responsible for the activation of resident immune cells such as innate lymphoid cells, alveolar macrophages, and dendritic cells (DCs) as well as for the recruitment of neutrophils, macrophages, and lymphocytes into the respiratory tract (2, 7) (**Figure 2**). Respiratory cells infected with IFV express HA on their surface that is important for its recognition by NK cells (11). It was established that HA expressed by the infected cells is recognized by NKp44 and PKp46 receptors of NK cells that then mediated the lysis of IFV-infected cells (12). Macrophages activated during IFV infection produce IFNs, IL-6, TNF-α, and nitric oxide synthase that amplify the inflammatory response. In addition, macrophages limit the viral spread by the elimination of apoptotic-infected cells and through phagocyte-mediated opsonophagocytosis of IFV (7). The production of proinflammatory cytokines during the generation of the respiratory innate immune response against IFV also conditions the adaptive immune response, which includes the production of virus-specific systemic and mucosal antibodies as well as the induction of specific T cell responses (13).

After exposure to IFV there is an activation of antibody responses in the respiratory tract. Upper airway exposure results primarily in an IgA response while the contact of IFV with the deep lung induces an increased production of pathogen-specific IgG (14). Following exposure to IFV in the airways there is an antigen uptake and processing by DCs, activation of $CD4^+$ Th cells, and generation of IgA-producing plasma cells that populate airway lamina propria. Secretory IgA has a non-inflammatory protective function since these antibodies can bind to virus without activating complement or stimulating the release of inflammatory mediators by innate immune cells (14, 15). IgA prevents IFV from adhering to the epithelial surface by inducing viral agglutination, and masking adhesion epitopes. In the deep lung, when IFV reach the alveolar space, there is a differentiation and expansion of antibody-secreting plasma cells that are committed to the production of IgG. Induction of

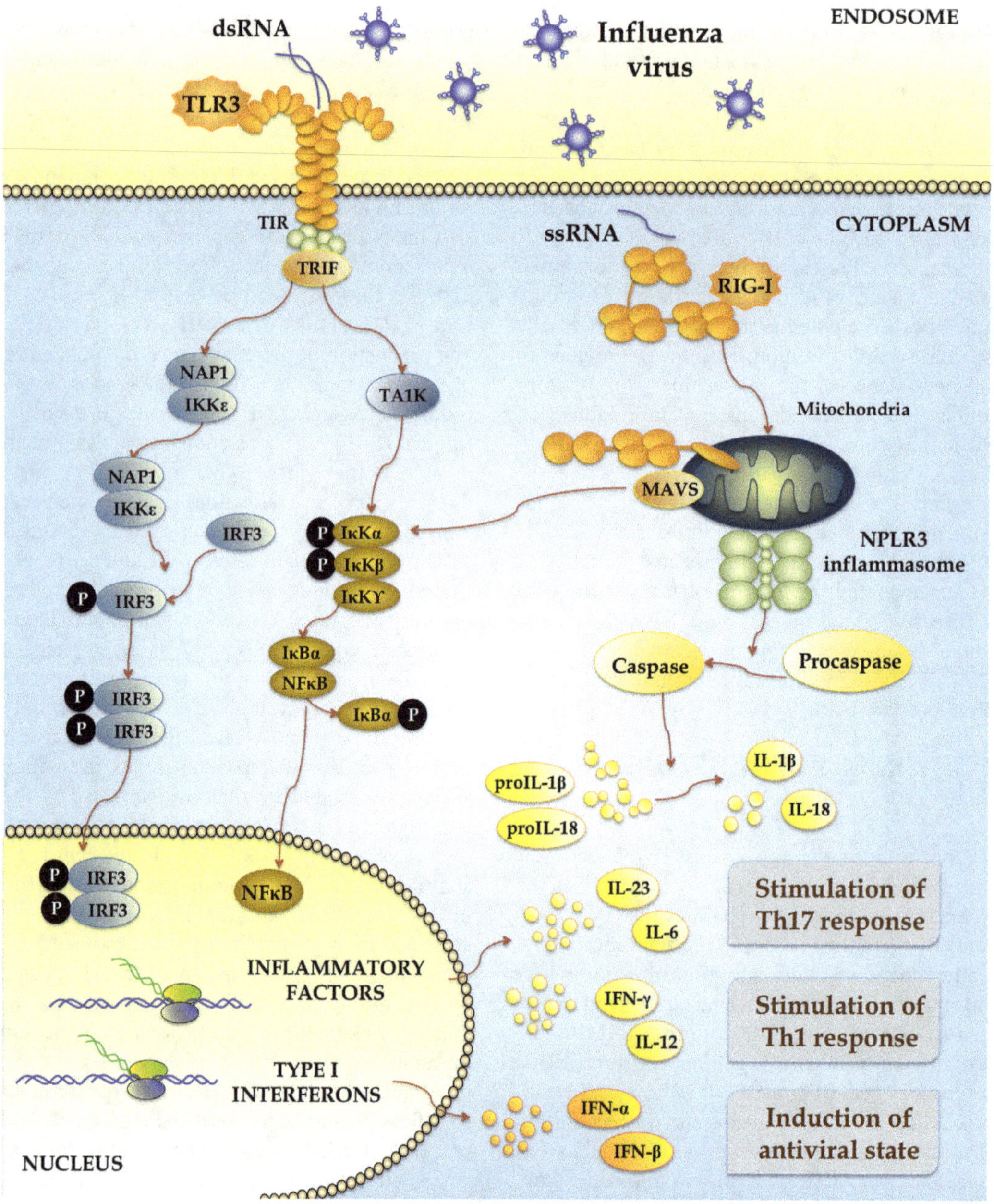

FIGURE 1 | **Signaling pathways activated by the recognition of influenza virus-associated molecular patterns by pattern-recognition receptors expressed in respiratory epithelial cells and immune cells.**

neutralizing respiratory and serum IgG antibodies is a key event in the defense against influenza infection since IgG prevents systemic spread (16). Influenza infection in the lungs also activates the cellular adaptive immune response by stimulating the production of IFN-γ by Th1 cells that effectively activate CD8+ T cells and macrophages, which clear virus and infected cells from the lungs (17). Therefore, during uncomplicated influenza, adaptive immune response ultimately results in clearance of IFV from the lungs through the activity of virus-specific antibodies and CD4+ and CD8+ T cells.

ROLE OF MICROBIOTA ON IFV INFECTION

The gut microbiome, which is defined as the collective group of microorganisms and their associated genes within the intestinal tract, is considered as a key player in the modulation of host intestinal immune responses (18, 19). In fact, the impact of gut commensal bacteria on the innate and adaptive immune responses to enteric pathogens has been recognized conclusively (20–22). However, the effect of gut microbiome on the immune

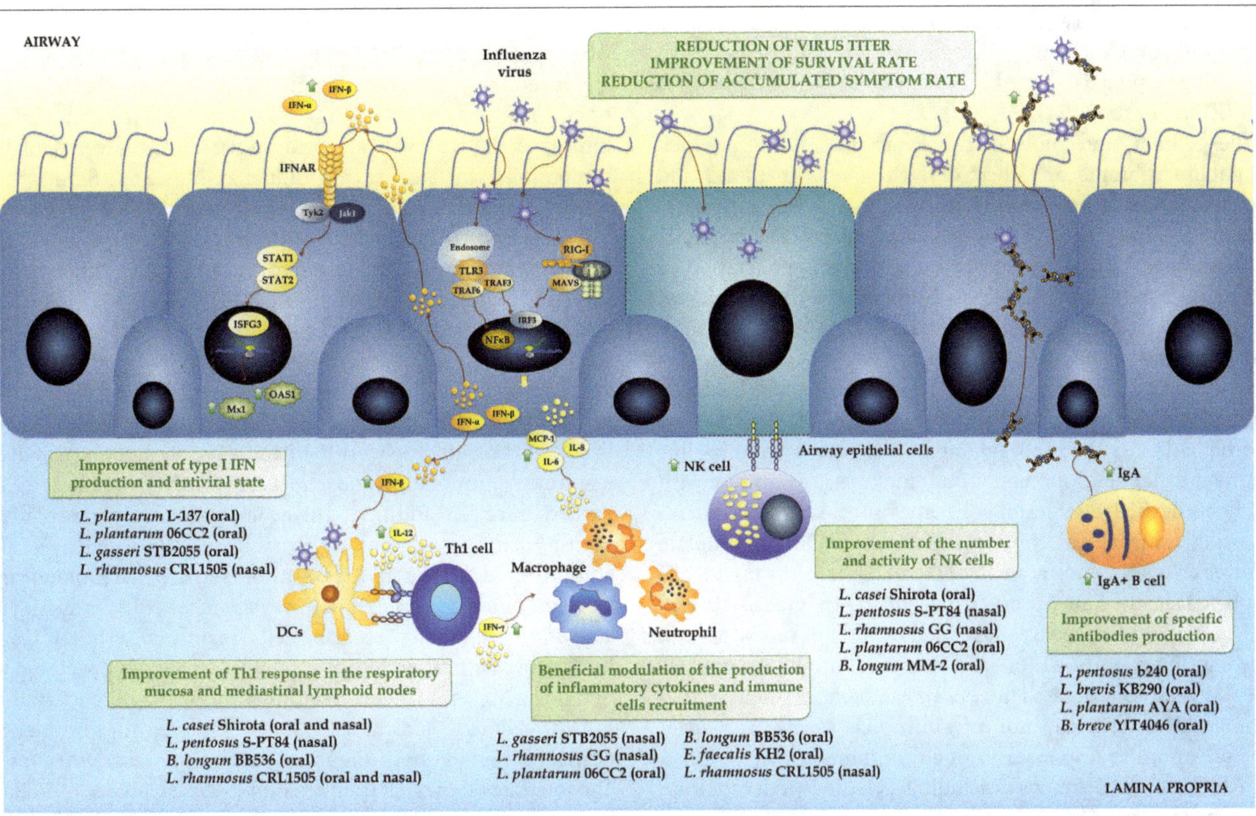

FIGURE 2 | Innate immune response against influenza virus in the respiratory mucosa mediated by the recognition of viral-associated molecular patterns by pattern-recognition receptors expressed in respiratory epithelial cells. Beneficial effects of immunobiotics administration on the resistance and immune response against Influenza Virus in the respiratory mucosa.

responses in distal mucosal sites and its impact in the outcome of respiratory infections has recently been exposed. In this regard, some studies have demonstrated an important role for intestinal microbiota in maintaining respiratory antiviral immunity against IFV (23, 24).

Iwasaki and colleagues observed that commensal bacteria within the gut, especially gram-positive bacterial populations, had an important role in supporting an appropriate immune response to IFV infection in the respiratory tract (23). The work demonstrated that oral antibiotic treatments impaired the resistance of mice to the intranasal infection with IFV as noted by the elevated lung viral titers when compared to non-antibiotic-treated animals. Results indicated that gut gram-positive bacteria provided protection by triggering an adequate inflammatory response through inflammasomes activation. In antibiotic-treated mice, synthesis of pro-IL-1β, pro-IL-18, and NLRP3 was impaired even at the steady state. In addition, depletion of gram-positive bacterial populations in the gut resulted in an alteration of the distribution and activation of respiratory DCs at steady state as well as in a diminished DCs migration from the lung to the draining lymph nodes, resulting in reduced activation of $CD8^+$ and $CD4^+$ T cells after influenza challenge (23). Alteration of respiratory DCs activities also correlated with impaired expansion of influenza-specific B cells and reduced influenza-specific antibodies.

By using germ-free and antibiotic-treated mice challenged with IFV, Abt et al. (24) showed that the absence or the alteration of intestinal microbiota induced an exacerbated weight loss, a greater drop in blood oxygen saturation, increased mortality, and elevated lung viral titers indicating a weaker ability to resist influenza. Even more, germ-free and antibiotic-treated mice infected with IFV experienced higher epithelial cell necrosis, peribronchiolar inflammation, severe bronchiole epithelial degeneration, and epithelial hyperplasia when compared to conventional animals (24). Interestingly, those effects were observed when both the PR8 strain and the X31-GP33 virus, a less pathogenic strain of IFV that causes minimal mortality and morbidity in conventional mice, were used. Consistent with the work by Ichinohe et al. (23), germ-free and antibiotic-treated mice challenged with IFV had an impaired adaptive immune response as shown by the lower influenza-specific antibodies (serum IgM and IgG), fewer number of IFV-specific T cells present in lungs, as well as a reduced capacity of specific T cells to produce effector cytokines such as TNF-α, MIP-1α, IL-2, and IFN-γ (24). Moreover, authors demonstrated that the alterations of adaptive immune responses were related to defects in the early innate immune response mediated by macrophages. In fact, transcriptional profiling and computational analyses of macrophages from antibiotic-treated mice indicated a reduced expression of antiviral genes including *Ifnb*, *Tnfa*, *Il1b*, *Irf7*, *Mx1*, and *Oas1a* when compared to conventional mice. In addition, functional assays of macrophages from antibiotic-treated mice demonstrated that those cells had a defective response to type I IFNs and an impaired capacity to limit IFV replication (24).

The cellular and molecular mechanisms through which the gut microbiome and their derived signals maintain and modulate immune responses in distal mucosal sites are poorly understood. Two possible mechanisms that are not mutually exclusive have been proposed to explain this beneficial effect of the gut microbiome. One possibility is that distal mucosal and peripheral immune cells are directly exposed to bacterial products that activate PRRs in the steady state and help to maintain the normal immune tone. There is evidence that bacterial products from gut commensals such as peptidoglycan can be absorbed and circulate throughout the host and help to modulate the normal development of immune cells (25). In line with this hypothesis, Iwasaki and colleagues speculated that bacterial products from gut commensals trigger PRRs to stimulate immune cells systemically and that factors released by those cells supported steady-state production of pro-IL-1β, pro-IL-18, and NLR proteins. This idea was sustained by their observation that intestinal injection of TLR ligands restored immune responses to IFV in antibiotic-treated mice (23). Another possibility is that commensal bacteria may indirectly influence systemic and distal mucosal immune responses through immune factors released from the intestinal mucosa including cytokines, chemokines, and grow factors.

These research works demonstrated that the gut microbiome provides signals to sustain antiviral innate immune defense mechanisms in the respiratory tract allowing robust and efficient effector responses upon challenge by viral pathogens such as IFV. Therefore, the role of the gut microbiome in regulating respiratory antiviral immunity represents an exciting area of research that could help to provide the scientific basis for the development of novel prevention strategies for lung infectious diseases. However, several questions need to be answered to identify new alternatives to improve antiviral respiratory defenses by modulating the microbiota. How the different microbial species from the gut microbiota influence the common mucosal immune system? Which PRRs are activated by the gut microbiota to functionally modulate antiviral immunity locally and in distal mucosal sites? Which cellular functions are modulated by the microbiota after PRR activation? Has the microbiota the ability to influence immune responses to other respiratory viruses? Are similar immune mechanisms activated by the microbiota in high-risk populations (infants, elderly, immunocompromised hosts) in which respiratory viral infections are more frequent and severe? Is it possible to beneficially modulate antiviral respiratory defenses by orally administering selected microorganisms with immunomodulatory capacities? Research from the last years has provided some answers for the last question.

BENEFICIAL EFFECTS OF IMMUNOBIOTICS ON IFV INFECTION

The first studies that assessed the capacity of immunobiotics to favorably modulate the immune response against IFV focused on the humoral immunity (**Table 1**). Yasui et al. (26) reported that the oral administration of *Bifidobacterium breve* YIT4064 improved the production of anti-IFV IgG antibodies in serum of IFV-infected mice. The YIT4064 strain reduced viral titers, improved the survival rate, and decreased the severity of the symptoms associated to the influenza infection. Similarly, it was shown that orally administered non-viable *Lactobacillus pentosus* b240 (27) or viable *Lactobacillus brevis* KB290 (28) were able to improve the levels of respiratory specific IgA and IgG antibodies of mice challenged with IFV. Moreover, the improved humoral response induced by these strains correlated with significant reduction of viral titers, body weight loss, and a decrease of the alterations of physical conditions induced by IFV. More recently, Kikuchi et al. (29) demonstrated a beneficial effect on the outcome to IFV infection related to an improved respiratory humoral response in *Lactobacillus plantarum* AYA-treated mice. In addition, the work proposed a mechanism for the distal immunomodulatory activity induced by orally administered immunobiotics. Authors showed that *L. plantarum* AYA fed to mice impacted in Peyer's patches (PPs) inducing an activation of antigen presenting cells (mainly $CD11b^+$ DCs) and increasing the production of IL-6. Those changes promoted an IgM-to-IgA class switch recombination, the differentiation of IgA^+ B cells into plasma cells, and improved the production of mucosal IgA in both the intestine and the respiratory tract. Those studies show that immunobiotics are capable to modulate the production of systemic and mucosal antibodies against influenza and therefore, to enhance the humoral immune response (**Figure 2**). However, the precise mechanism by which orally administered immunobiotics induce IgA production in distant mucosal sites remains unclear.

It was also demonstrated that immunobiotics are able to improve cellular immune response against IFV (**Figure 2**). In this regard, it was reported that orally administered *Lactobacillus casei* Shirota improved the outcomes of IFV infection of aged (30) and infant mice (31) by increasing systemic and respiratory NK cell activity and improving the production of IFN-γ and TNF-α by respiratory lymphocytes. Both studies also demonstrated that IFV titers were significantly reduced in aged and infant mice treated with the Shirota strain (30, 31). Similar to the mechanism proposed to explain the improvement of humoral response, it was postulated that immunobiotic *L. casei* Shirota stimulated Th1 cells and NK cells in PPs and induced a mobilization of those cells to lungs and respiratory-associated lymphoid tissues where they produced IFN-γ and enhanced the antiviral defenses. Several other studies corroborated these findings by showing similar effects for orally administered lactobacilli (32, 33). Immunobiotic *Lactobacillus* strains (*L. gasseri* TMC0356, *L. rhamnosus* GG, or *L. plantarum* 06CC2) beneficially modulated NK cells activity and Th1 response against IFV, diminished virus titers and reduced lung pathological changes (32, 33) (**Table 1**). More recently, Kawahara et al. (34) described the improvement of respiratory antiviral response by an orally administered bifidobacteria strain. It was shown that *Bifidobacterium longum* MM-2 increased respiratory NK cell activity and IFN-γ production resulting in improved clinical symptoms, reduced mortality, and decreased virus titers after IFV challenge.

TABLE 1 | Effect of immunobiotics on influenza virus (IFV) infection in mice models.

Immunobiotic strain	Viability	Administration protocol	Challenge	Mice	Immunobiotic effects	Effect on IFV infection	Reference
Effects on humoral immune response							
Bifidobacterium breve YIT4064	Non-viable	Oral *ad libitum* administration of food with 0.05% *B. breve* YIT4064 during 15 weeks before IFV challenge. Treatment was continued for 2 weeks after infection	IFV (H1N1) strain A/PR/8/34	Six-week-old male BALB/c	Improved the production of anti-IFV IgG antibodies in serum	Reduced viral titers, improved survival rate, and decreased severity of symptoms	(26)
Lactobacillus pentosus b240	Non-viable	*L. pentosus* was administered by gavage at doses of 0.4, 2, or 10 mg per mouse per day during 21 days before IFV challenge. Treatment was continued for 2 weeks after infection	IFV (H1N1) strain A/PR/8/34	Six-week-old female BALB/c	Improved levels of respiratory IgA and IgG specific antibodies	Reduced IFV titers	(27)
Lactobacillus brevis KB290	Viable	*L. brevis* was administered by gavage at a dose of 10^9 cells per mouse per day during 14 days before IFV challenge	IFV (H1N1) strain A/PR/8/34	Six to eight-week-old female BALB/c	Improved levels of IFV-specific IgA in the respiratory tract	Reduced body weight loss and decreased alterations of physical conditions	(28)
Lactobacillus plantarum AYA	Non-viable	Oral *ad libitum* administration of food with 5% of *L. plantarum* AYA (120 mg per mouse per day) during 28 days before IFV challenge	IFV (H3N2) strain X-31	Seven-week-old female BALB/c	Improved the production of IgA in the respiratory tract	Reduced body weight loss and decreased mortality	(29)
Effects on cellular immune response							
Lactobacillus casei Shirota	Non-viable	Oral *ad libitum* administration of food with 0.05% of *L. casei* Shirota during 4 weeks before IFV challenge	IFV (H1N1) strain A/PR/8/34	Fifteen-week-old female BALB/c	Improved systemic and respiratory NK cell activity and production of interferon (IFN)-γ and TNF-α by respiratory lymphocytes	Reduced IFV titers	(30)
L. casei Shirota	Viable	*L. casei* Shirota was administered by gavage at a dose of 10^9 cells per mouse 5 times/week for about 3 weeks (total, 17 times) before IFV challenge	IFV (H1N1) strain A/PR/8/34	Neonatal and infant mice	Improved systemic and respiratory NK cell activity and production of IFN-γ and TNF-α by respiratory lymphocytes	Reduced IFV titers, decreased accumulated symptom rate, and decreased mortality	(31)
Lactobacillus gasseri TMC0356	Viable	Ten milligrams of lyophilized bacteria in 200 µl of saline was administered orally per day during 14 days before IFV challenge. Treatment was continued for 5 days after infection	IFV (H1N1) strain A/PR/8/34	Five-week-old female BALB/c	Improved NK cell activity and production of IFN-γ	Reduced virus titers and diminished lung pathological changes	(32)
Lactobacillus rhamnosus GG	Viable	Ten milligrams of lyophilized bacteria in 200 µl of saline was administered orally per day during 14 days before IFV challenge. Treatment was continued for 5 days after infection	IFV (H1N1) strain A/PR/8/34	Five-week-old female BALB/c	Improved NK cell activity and production of IFN-γ	Reduced virus titers and diminished lung pathological changes	(32)
L. plantarum 06CC2	Non-viable	*L. plantarum* was administered by gavage twice daily during 2 days before IFV challenge (20 mg/mouse). Treatment was continued for 7 days after infection	IFV (H1N1) strain A/PR/8/34	Six-week-old female BALB/c	Beneficially modulated NK cells activity and improved Th1 response	Reduced virus titers and diminished lung pathological changes	(33)

(*Continued*)

TABLE 1 | **Continued**

Immunobiotic strain	Viability	Administration protocol	Challenge	Mice	Immunobiotic effects	Effect on IFV infection	Reference
Bifidobacterium longum MM-2	Viable	Oral administration of 2 × 10^9 cells per mouse per day during 14 days before IFV challenge. Treatment was continued for 2 days after infection	IFV (H1N1) strain A/PR/8/34	Six-week-old female BALB/c	Increased respiratory NK cell activity and IFN-γ production	Improved clinical symptoms, reduced mortality, and decreased virus titers	(34)
L. casei Shirota	Non-viable	Nasal administration of 20 or 200 μg per mouse per day during 3 days before IFV challenge	IFV (H1N1) strain A/PR/8/34	Ten to eleven-week-old female BALB/c	Increased levels of IL-12, IFN-γ, and TNF-α in mediastinal lymphoid nodes and lungs	Decreased virus titers and increased survival rates	(35)
L. pentosus S-PT84	Non-viable	Nasal administration of 20 or 200 μg per mouse per day during 3 days before IFV challenge	IFV (H1N1) strain A/PR/8/34	Eight to twelve-week-old female BALB/c	Increased IL-12, IFN-α, and NK cell activity in the respiratory tract. Increased levels of IL-12 and IFN-γ in mediastinal lymphoid nodes	Decreased virus titers and increased survival rates	(36)
L. rhamnosus GG	Viable	Nasal administration of 200 μg per mouse per day during 3 days before IFV challenge	IFV (H1N1) strain A/PR/8/34	Seven-week-old female BALB/c	Increased respiratory NK cell activity	Reduced IFV titers, decreased accumulated symptom rate, and increased survival rates	(37)
L. rhamnosus	Viable	Sublingual administration of 10^8 cells per mouse per day during 7 days before IFV challenge	IFV (H1N1) strain A/FMI/33	Adult female BALB/c	Improved levels of IgA specific antibodies, IL-12, and decreased levels of TNF-α and IL-6 in lungs. Increased NK cell activity in spleen. Increased CD25 expression by $CD4^+$ and $CD8^+$ in lung and mediastinal lymphoid nodes	Increase of the survival rates and decrease in the lung lesion scores	(38)
Effects on innate immune response							
L. plantarum L-137	Non-viable	Intragastric administration of 5–100 mg/kg of mouse per day during 7 days before IFV challenge. Treatment was continued for 7 days after infection	IFV (H1N1) strain A/NWS/47	Seven-week-old female C57BL/6	Improved production of type I IFNs	Reduced viral loads in lungs and improved survival	(39)
L. gasseri SBT2055	Viable	Oral administration of 10^8 or 10^9 cells per mouse per day during 7–21 days before IFV challenge	IFV (H1N1) strain A/PR/8/34	Five to seven-week-old male C57BL/6	Enhanced lung expression of the antiviral genes *Mx1* and *Oas1a* and differentially regulated inflammatory response	Enhanced survival rates, reduced lung viral titers and diminished lung inflammatory damage	(40)
L. rhamnosus CRL1505	Viable	Oral administration of 10^8 cells per mouse per day during 5 days before IFV challenge	IFV (H1N1) strain A/PR/8/34	Six-week-old male BALB/c	Differentially regulated levels and kinetics of inflammatory cells (neutrophils and macrophages) and cytokines (TNF-α, IL-6, IL-10, and type I IFNs) Diminished coagulation activation in blood and respiratory tract	Decreased IFV titers in lungs, lessened pulmonary damage, and increased survival	(41)
L. rhamnosus CRL1505	Viable and non-viable	Nasal administration of 10^8 cells per mouse per day during 2 days before IFV challenge	IFV (H1N1) strain A/PR/8/34	Six-week-old male BALB/c	Differentially regulated levels and kinetics of inflammatory cells (neutrophils and macrophages) and cytokines (TNF-α, IL-6, IL-10, and type I IFNs) Diminished coagulation activation in blood and respiratory tract	Decreased IFV titers in lungs, lessened pulmonary damage, and increased survival	(42)

(*Continued*)

TABLE 1 | Continued

Immunobiotic strain	Viability	Administration protocol	Challenge	Mice	Immunobiotic effects	Effect on IFV infection	Reference
Enterococcus faecalis KH2	Viable and non-viable	Intragastric administration of 8.5 × 10^{10} cell per kg of mouse per day during 7 or 12 days before IFV challenge	IFV (H1N1) strain A/WSN/33	Adult male C57BL/6	Diminished concentrations of proinflammatory factors especially MCP-1	Reduced mortality, weight loss, and lung viral titers	(43)
L. pentosus b240	Non-viable	Oral administration of 10^{10} cells per mouse per day during 21 days before IFV challenge. Oral treatment was continued for 14 days after infection	IFV (H1N1) pdm strain A/California/04/09	Six-week-old female BALB/c	Downregulated expression of the immune related genes *Cyr61*, *Egr1*, and *Fos*, and genes related to Acyl-CoA-mediated metabolism. Upregulated expression of the antiviral gene Rsad2 in the lungs	Prolonged mouse survival. No effect on virus titers and no apparent differences in the extent of lung damage	(44)

Research work has also demonstrated that nasal administration of immunobiotics is an interesting alternative to improve cellular response against influenza infection (35–37) (**Table 1**). Hori et al. (35) observed that BALB/c mice nasally treated with non-viable *L. casei* Shirota had increased levels of IL-12, IFN-γ, and TNF-α in mediastinal lymphoid nodes and lungs. This improved cellular respiratory immunity correlated with a beneficial clinical outcome to IFV challenge. Similar observations were performed with nasally administered *L. pentosus* S-PT84 (36) and *L. rhamnosus* GG (37).

Other recent studies have also demonstrated the ability of immunobiotics to improve respiratory innate antiviral defenses in the respiratory tract (**Table 1**; **Figure 2**). It was reported that orally administered non-viable *L. plantarum* L-137 improved protection against IFV by increasing type I IFN production (39). The work clearly demonstrated that the increased production of IFN-β induced by the immunobiotic strain correlated with the reduction of viral loads in lungs as well as the improved survival of infected mice. More recently, it was shown that *L. gasseri* SBT2055 enhanced survival rates and reduced lung viral titers in mice infected with IFV (40). Interestingly, authors observed that the lung expression of the antiviral genes *Mx1* and *Oas1a* was enhanced in *L. gasseri* SBT2055-treated mice and that the inflammatory response triggered by IFV was differentially regulated inducing a lower inflammatory damage (40).

Our group has also reported a beneficial regulation of the IFV-triggered inflammatory response by immunobiotics. Lung damage induced by IFV is known to be produced by virus replication as well as the uncontrolled inflammatory response that is characterized by a hypersecretion of proinflammatory cytokines, especially TNF-α, IL-1β, and IL-6 (45). The adequate production of inflammatory factors is necessary to protect against IFV infection together with an appropriate regulation with anti-inflammatory cytokines to prevent the damage of lung tissue. Thus, the proper balance of cytokines is a key factor in determining the outcome of IFV infection. In this regard, we observed that orally (41) or nasally (42) administered immunobiotic *L. rhamnosus* CRL1505 differentially regulated the levels and kinetics of inflammatory cells and cytokines in mice after IFV challenge. In our experimental model, we observed increased levels of respiratory TNF-α, IL-6, neutrophils, and macrophages in CRL1505-treated mice early after the challenge with IFV. Later, proinflammatory cytokines and infiltrated cells started to decrease in immunobiotic-treated animals in contrast to control mice, in which those parameters continued increasing. The trend toward lower inflammatory factors and cells registered later during IFV infection in *L. rhamnosus* CRL1505-treated mice correlated with a reduced severity of pulmonary damage when compared to control mice (41, 42).

Chen et al. (43) also investigated the ability of orally administered *Enterococcus faecalis* KH2 to beneficially modulate the innate immune response to influenza infection. Authors observed that KH2 strain protected C57BL/6 mice against IFV as observed by the reduced mortality, weight loss, and lung viral titers. As expected, IFV enhanced the levels of proinflammatory mediators in the respiratory tract including IL-6, TNF-α, IFN-γ, IL-1β, IL-17, and MCP-1 while the treatment with *E. faecalis* significantly diminished the concentrations of proinflammatory factors, especially MCP-1. Considering that monocyte migration mediated by MCP-1 has been linked to several respiratory inflammatory disorders including IFV infection, authors investigated the role of MCP-1/CCR2 pathway in the immunobiotic effect of *E. faecalis* KH2. The work reported that the protective activity of the KH2 strain was abrogated when recombinant MCP-1 was administered concomitantly (43).

It is not clear how immunobiotics initiates the cross-talk with the immune system in order to modulate the respiratory antiviral immunity. It is not known exactly which PRRs are activated by immunobiotics in the intestinal or respiratory mucosa to functionally modulate antiviral immunity locally and in distal mucosal sites, respectively. Neither it has been determined with exactitude which cellular functions are modulated by immunobiotics immediately after PRR activation. Research from the last decade has demonstrated that the immunomodulatory effects of probiotic bacteria are the consequence of complex interactions between several bacterial molecules and host receptors located in different immune and non-immune cells (46, 47). It has also been shown that the immunomodulatory properties of immunobiotics are dependent on the strains. Therefore, studies carried out with certain strains cannot be easily extrapolated to other bacteria, even those of the same genus and species (48, 49). Consequently, it is still necessary to carry out deeper studies to find out the molecular mechanisms by which immunobiotics beneficially influence the respiratory antiviral immunity.

The studies mentioned before showed the potential of immunobiotics to be used for the reduction of the incidence and severity of IFV infections. However, in addition to deepening the knowledge of their mechanisms of action, several other points should be considered for the efficient application of immunobiotics in humans.

For example, it is necessary to determine the best time as well as the most appropriate route for their administration. Immunobiotics used as components of functional foods can be included in diets on a regular basis and thus help to improve respiratory defenses, especially in high-risk populations and during the seasons with the highest incidence of respiratory infections occurs. In this sense, in a randomized controlled trial we demonstrated that *L. rhamnosus* CRL1505 (administered in a yogurt formulation) improved mucosal immunity and reduced the incidence and severity of intestinal and respiratory infection in children (50). Hence, the incidence of infectious events was reduced from 66% in the placebo group to 34% in the group that received the probiotic yogurt. Furthermore, there was also a significant reduction in the occurrence of indicators of disease severity such as fever and the need for antibiotic treatment in children receiving the probiotic yogurt. This immunobiotic yogurt (YOGURITO®) has been included into official National Nutritional Programs in Argentina and is given daily to children at schools in several provinces thanks to the Government actions. Epidemiological studies in the schools receiving the immunobiotic product have shown a reduction in the incidence of infections and in the associated school absenteeism (Alvarez et al., unpublished results).

On the other hand, as mentioned earlier the nasal administration of immunobiotics is more efficient than the oral administration to enhance respiratory immunity. This route of administration poses a practical disadvantage considering that the treatments with immunobiotics showed favorable results when they were used before the infectious challenges. In this way, it would be necessary to predict the exact moment in which the viral pathogen will be in contact with the host in order to carry out the prophylactic immunobiotic treatment. This option could be used for example during a school or work outbreak in which cases of respiratory infections occur and it is desired to prevent or reduce the severity of infections in asymptomatic individuals. For an intervention of these characteristics, it would be also important to determine the exact time after the contact with the virus in which it is possible to administer immunobiotics to achieve the beneficial effect. In a recent study, Percopo et al. (51) have defined this as "the window of opportunity." The work evaluated the effect of the nasal administration of live or inactivated *L. plantarum* NCIMB 8826 in a mice model of severe respiratory infection with the pneumonia virus of mice (PVM) and found that immunobiotic treatment promoted full survival from acute PVM infection when administered within 1 day after virus challenge (51). Similar studies would be of value in IFV infection models.

Another point of interest is related to the duration of the improvement of respiratory defenses after the last immunobiotic administration. Our studies have showed that the immunomodulatory effect of some nasally administered immunobiotics persisted for at least 15 days (Villena et al., unpublished results). Other studies have also reported short-term protection after nasal treatment with different immunobiotic strains (43). Interestingly, Garcia-Crespo et al. (52) found that adult mice primed nasally with *L. plantarum* NCIMB 8826 or *Lactobacillus reuteri* F275 were completely protected against lethal PVM infection and that protection persisted for at least 5 months after the initial priming. These findings open an interesting challenge in the study of immunobiotics to improve the defenses against IFV, since it would be very useful to establish the duration of the protective effect for each strain and treatment, since in the majority of cases these long-term studies were not taken into account.

IFV infections often result in mild to moderate lung infection; however, life-threatening disease can occur. It has been demonstrated that the most severe disease outcomes are associated with secondary bacterial pneumonia caused primarily by *Staphylococcus aureus* or *Streptococcus pneumoniae* (53). Taking into account the high incidence of viral infections and the frequency of associated secondary bacterial infections which contribute to aggravate the health status of the host and reduce its chance of recovery, various approaches for preventing and treating influenza and secondary bacterial pneumonia are been investigated. A wide range of antibiotics and anti-inflammatory drugs has been tested in mice [reviewed in Ref. (54)]. It would be of interest to evaluate the potential beneficial effect of immunobiotics on these circumstances. In this regard, preliminary studies from our laboratory showed that nasally administered *L. rhamnosus* CRL1505 is able to improve survival, reduce bacterial cell counts in lung and blood, and limit lung inflammatory damage caused by *S. pneumoniae* infection in mice produced after the infection with IFV or respiratory syncytial virus (RSV) (Villena et al., unpublished results). These results opened an interesting topic for future investigations.

Finally, it would be also of interest to investigate whether immunobiotic treatments may influence other physiological systems involved in the defenses against viral respiratory infections such as the coagulation system. Our group has made some progress in this regard, as mentioned below.

RESPIRATORY IMMUNE-COAGULATIVE RESPONSE AND IFV

Coagulation is an extremely ordered process that involves the interaction of three key components: endothelial cells (ECs), platelets, and coagulation factors. Tissue injury that activates ECs typically initiates coagulation that is characterized by the binding of platelets to activated ECs and the formation of the platelet plug. Almost simultaneously, tissue factor (TF) released by ECs result in factor X activation, which induces thrombin and the generation of fibrin strands to strengthen the platelet plug leading to a stable platelet–fibrin clot. All these processes are tightly regulated by anticoagulant and fibrinolytic mechanisms to avoid thrombotic and/or haemorrhagic complications. A key role has been attributed to ECs in the temporal and special regulation of coagulation activation. Resting ECs avoid the inappropriate plug formation by controlling platelet adhesion and activation and generating several anticoagulant factors providing a non-thrombogenic barrier (55, 56). Once activated or injured, ECs expose collagen to blood, increase platelet binding and aggregation, reduce the expression physiological anticoagulant factors, increase the expression of TF and von willebrand factor, and suppress the fibrinolytic activity (57, 58). All these changes in the hemostatic system facilitate thrombosis in the infected or inflammated tissue.

Both hemorrhagic and thrombotic complications have been described during IFV infection. Influenza is able to cause pulmonary hemorrhage and edema related to coagulopathy or induce uncontrolled thrombosis through an over-activated coagulation (**Figure 3**) (55, 58). Animal models have helped to explain the mechanisms by which IFV infection activates coagulation and key role has been attributed to TF. It was described that IFV activates coagulation by enhancing TF production, thrombin generation and fibrin deposition in C57BL/6 mice (59). In a mice model of IFV infection, it was recently shown that wild-type animals increased lung TF expression and activation of coagulation but presented alveolar hemorrhage (60). Moreover, selective deletion of TF in epithelial cells from lung significantly reduced TF expression after IFV infection and had higher alveolar hemorrhage and

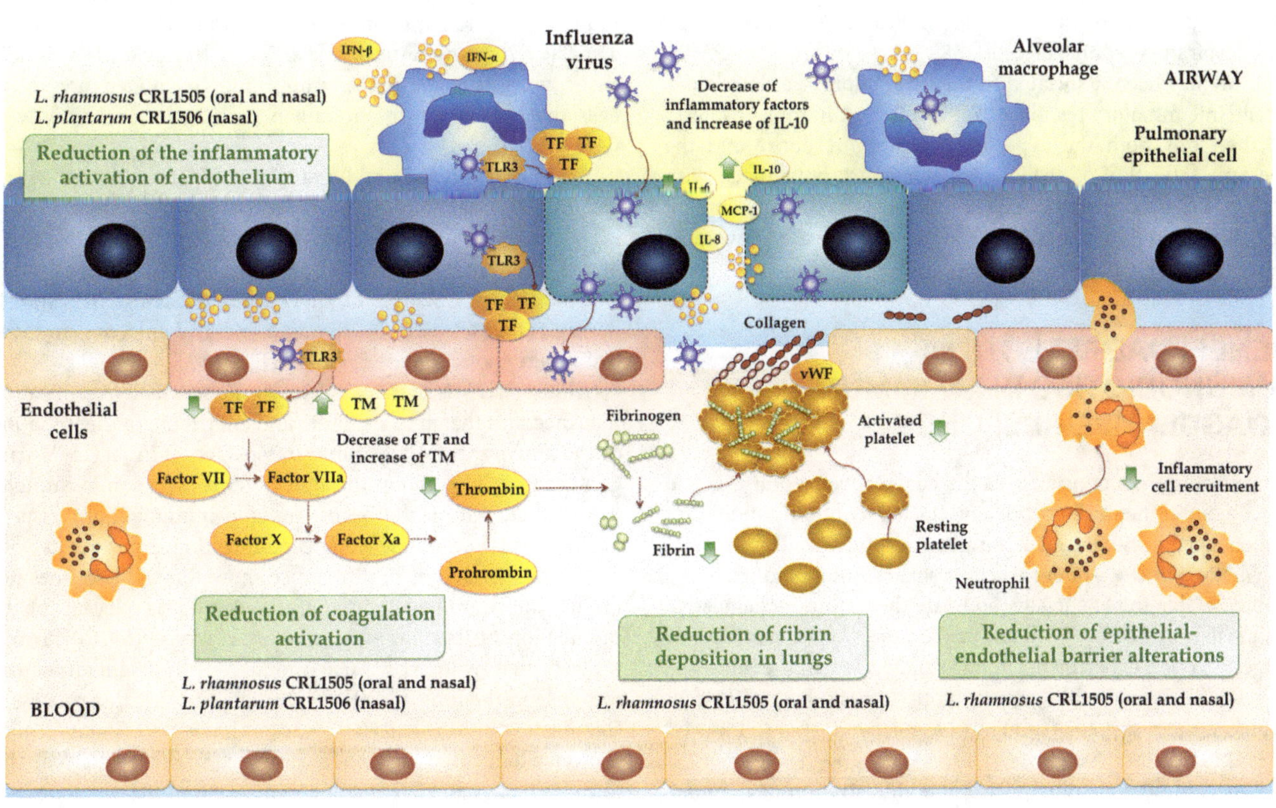

FIGURE 3 | Activation of the immuno-coagulative response by influenza virus in the respiratory mucosa. Beneficial effects of immunobiotics administration on the immuno-coagulative response triggered by toll-like receptor 3 or Influenza Virus in the respiratory mucosa.

reduced survival than controls. On the contrary, deficiency of TF in either respiratory myeloid cells or ECs did not enhanced alveolar hemorrhage or modified survival of IFV-infected mice (60). These results indicate that an appropriate modulation in the production of TF in the lung during IFV infection is necessary to maintain tissue hemostasis avoiding hemorrhage and excessive fibrin deposition. Production of TF by lung epithelial cells will be required to maintain alveolar hemostasis during IFV infection, while excessive release of TF by macrophages and ECs would contribute to pathology and lung tissue injury (59, 60).

It is considered that ECs may play an important role in the pathogenesis of IFV. Influenza infection is able to induce alveolar edema and pulmonary hemorrhage through the alteration of ECs via several mechanisms, including direct damage and loss of tight junctions and apoptosis (61). In addition, recognition of damage-associated molecular patterns such as HMGB1 or oxidized phospholipids through TLR4 activates ECs to drive lung injury (62). Direct stimulation of TLR3 by viral RNA also results in the upregulation of TF and the downregulation of thrombomodulin (TM) in ECs (63). At the same time, the inflammatory activation of ECs leads to the activation of the coagulation cascade. Inflammation caused by IFV infection increases various proinflammatory cytokines such as TNF-α, IL-1β, and IL-6 that induce the secretion of TF by ECs and monocytes (58). In addition to their roles in coagulation, activated proteins such as thrombin, FXa, and FVIIa also enhance the inflammatory response. The inflammatory potentiating abilities of coagulation factors are mediated through their activation of protease-activated receptors (PARs) that are expressed in platelets, ECs, macrophages, and respiratory epithelial cells (58). The TF/thrombin/PAR-1 pathway has been associated to the promotion of a deleterious innate inflammatory response to IFV infection in mice (64, 65).

Therefore, both the hyper-inflammatory response and the aberrant activation of coagulation, which are potentiated with each other, are involved in severe influenza pneumonia and are key events that have to be controlled in order to reach a favorable resolution of the infectious process.

BENEFICIAL EFFECTS OF IMMUNOBIOTICS IN IFV IMMUNE-COAGULATIVE RESPONSE

Considering the importance of the coagulative response in the outcome of influenza infection and the ability of immunobiotics to beneficially influence the immune response to this respiratory pathogen, we wonder whether some immunobiotic strains would be able to beneficially modulate the immuno-coagulative response triggered by IFV. For this purpose, we performed challenge-infection experiments in mice and evaluated the influence of viable and non-viable immunobiotic *L. rhamnosus* CRL1505 strain on the respiratory immuno-coagulative response induced by IFV (41, 42).

Our data demonstrated that oral administration of *L. rhamnosus* CRL1505 to mice significantly reduced lung viral titers and tissue damage after the challenge with IFV (41). We later explored the capacity of nasally administered *L. rhamnosus* CRL1505, alive or heat killed, to reduce the influenza burden of disease (42). Those treatments induced a significant decrease in IFV titers in lungs, lessened pulmonary damage, and increased survival. Interestingly, a similar effect was achieved with the nasal administration of viable and non-viable CRL1505 strain. Moreover, the nasal route was more efficient than the oral administration to protect mice against IFV infection (41, 42). The protective effect achieved by the immunobiotic strain was related to its ability to modulate the respiratory antiviral immune response, particularly to its capacity to improve the levels of IFN-γ and IFN-β in the respiratory tract (**Figure 2**). Type I IFNs trigger the activation of the JAK-STAT pathway and increase the expression of antiviral genes. In addition, IFN-γ is produced by immune cells, especially Th1 cells, and it further improves antiviral immune response by inducing activation of NK cells and macrophages. Therefore, the modulation of type I IFNs and IFN-γ would be responsible of the reduction of viral loads in IFV-infected mice previously treated with the CRL1505 strain, similarly to other immunobiotic strains as mentioned before (**Table 1**). We demonstrated that the CRL1505 strain increased the levels of gut $CD3^+CD4^+IFN\text{-}\gamma^+$ T cells, induce a mobilization of these lymphocytes into the lung and enhanced the respiratory production of IFN-γ and the activity of local antigen presenting cells (41, 66, 67). It was also noted that nasal administration was more effective than the oral route to increase pulmonary $CD3^+CD4^+IFN\text{-}\gamma^+$ T cells (41, 42). The mechanism by which nasally administered viable or heat-killed *L. rhamnosus* CRL1505 improves $IFN\text{-}\gamma^+$ T cells population is not clear. However, our studies support the possibility that the immunobiotic strain *L. rhamnosus* CRL1505 impact in the nasal-associated lymphoid tissue or bronchial-associated lymphoid tissue producing an innate imprinting in antigen presenting cells that contribute to the enhanced number and activity of $CD3^+CD4^+IFN\text{-}\gamma^+$ T cells.

Our studies also showed that immunobiotic treatments were able to beneficially modulate the activation of coagulation during respiratory viral infection, an effect that was not reported before (41, 42). Then, our studies were the first in demonstrating a beneficial modulation of the immune-coagulative response during respiratory TRL3 activation and IFV infection induced by immunobiotic microorganisms (**Figure 3**).

Although IFV is an ssRNA virus, it generates dsRNA replication intermediates that activate TLR3 and contribute to the initiation of the antiviral respiratory immune response. In fact, IFV triggers type I IFN secretion through TLR3 recognition in immune (myeloid DCs or macrophages) and non-immune (fibroblasts or pneumocytes) cells (68). Challenge-infection experiments with respiratory viruses in $TLR3^{-/-}$ mice showed that TLR3 does not modify the clearance of viral pathogens but it is relevant for the modulation of the lung inflammatory response (69, 70). It was showed that wild-type mice mount a robust inflammatory response in the lung after IFV infection and that this process is significantly diminished in $TLR3^{-/-}$ animals (70). $TLR3^{-/-}$ mice showed a longer survival when compared wild type animals and this effect was associated with a reduction of inflammatory cells recruitment and lower levels of inflammatory factors in the respiratory tract. Other *in vivo* studies also demonstrated that TLR3 activation by poly(I:C) enhanced proinflammatory cytokines and

TABLE 2 | Effect of probiotics on influenza virus (IFV) infection in humans.

Strain	Viability	Route	Population studied	Effects	Reference
Lactobacillus fermentum CECT5716	Viable	Oral (capsule)	Randomized, double-blinded, and placebo-controlled human clinical trial in adults	Coadjuvant capability for anti-IFV vaccine. Lower incidence of influenza-like illness during 5 months after vaccination Increased proportion of NK cells, higher induction of Th1 cytokines and augmented specific T-helper and T-cytotoxic lymphocytes. Increased antigen specific IgA	(83)
Lactobacillus casei DN-114 001	Viable	Oral (fermented dairy drink Actimel®)	Randomized, multicentre, double-blind, and controlled studies in elderly population over 70 years of age	Coadjuvant capability for anti-influenza vaccine. Improved IFV-specific antibody titers after vaccination	(84)
Lactobacillus GG		Oral (capsule)	Randomized, double-blind, and placebo-controlled pilot study in adults	Coadjuvant capability for anti-IFV vaccine. Increased protective titer 28 days after vaccination for the H3N2 strain	(85)
Lactobacillus plantarum L-137	Non-viable (heat killed)	Oral (capsule)	Randomized, double-blind, and placebo-controlled pilot study in adults	Improved levels of interferon (IFN)-β before vaccination	(86)
Bifidobacterium animalis ssp. *lactis* BB-12w and *Lactobacillus paracasei* ssp. *paracasei* 431w	Viable	Oral (capsule and acidified dairy drink)	Randomized, double-blind, placebo-controlled, and parallel-group study in adults	Coadjuvant capability for anti-IFV vaccine. Improved vaccine-specific secretory IgA in saliva. Significant higher levels of vaccine-specific plasma IgG, IgG1, and IgG3	(87)
Lactobacillus rhamnosus strains GG and LC705	Viable	Macrophage stimulation	Human primary macrophages	Quantitative different IL-1β and type I IFN gene expression levels in macrophages. Diminished IFV replication and production of viral proteins in macrophages	(88)
Lactobacillus pentosus b240	Non-viable (heat killed)	Oral (tablet)	Randomized, double-blind, and placebo-controlled trial in elderly population over 65 years of age	Significant reduction of the incidence rate of the common cold	(89)
L. paracasei MoLac-1	Non-viable (heat killed)	Oral (jelly)	Randomized, double-blind, and placebo-controlled trial in elderly nursing home resident volunteers	Coadjuvant capability for anti-IFV vaccine. Improvement of hemagglutination inhibition titers against all different types of influenza antigens analyzed. Improvement in antibody titers against A/H3N2	(90)
L. rhamnosus GG	Viable	Oral (supplemented milk)	Randomized, double-blinded, and placebo-controlled in children of 2–6 years of age	Probiotic intervention did not reduce significantly the occurrence of the examined respiratory viruses, but the children that received the *GG* strain had fewer days with respiratory symptoms	(91)
Lactobacillus brevis KB290	Viable	Oral (fermented drink)	Open-label, parallel-group trial in children of 6–12 years of age	Reduced incidence of IFV infection in schoolchildren	(92)
L. rhamnosus GG	Viable	Oral (added to breast milk or formula)	Randomized, double-blind, and placebo-controlled trial in infants between the first and third days of life	Significant reduction in the incidence of viral respiratory tract infections	(93)
Lactococcus lactis ssp. *lactis* JCM5805	Viable	Oral (fermented dairy drink)	Randomized, placebo-controlled, and double-blind trial in adults	Significant decrease in major symptoms of influenza-like illness. IFN-α elicited by A/H1N1 on peripheral blood mononuclear cells prepared from volunteers tended to be higher, and IFN-stimulated gene 15 was significantly higher	(94)

antiviral factors expression (71), altered vascular permeability (72), and incremented the levels of D-dimers indicating that coagulation and fibrinolysis were triggered. In line with these findings, it was observed that the levels of D-dimers in TLR3$^{-/-}$ mice were significantly lower than in wild-type animals after poly(I:C) administration (63). In addition, by using siRNA technology it was demonstrated that TLR3 is a key receptor in the induction of the procoagulant state in ECs (63). Challenge of those cells with the TLR3 agonist poly(I:C) induced a decrease of TM and an enhancement of TF expression in a time- and dose-dependent manner. The results obtained in our own *in vivo* experiments were in line with these preceding reports (41, 42). We observed that three daily doses of nasally administered poly(I:C) to BALB/c mice induced a marked enhancement of inflammatory cells (neutrophils and macrophages) and proinflammatory mediators (IL-1β, TNF-α, IL-8, and IL-6) in the respiratory tract. Moreover, TLR3 activation also induced an increase in TF expression and thrombin–antithrombin complex (TATc) levels in the lung while it reduced TM expression. These inflammatory–coagulative modifications were accompanied by respiratory tissue alterations and impairment of lung function (41, 42).

Of interest, we demonstrated that orally (41) or nasally (42) administered immunobiotics before the challenge with poly(I:C) differentially modulated the inflammatory-coagulative response. *L. rhamnosus* CRL1505 was able to reduce and increase the expression of TF and TM, respectively, after the respiratory activation of TLR3. Thus, the CRL1505 strain significantly diminished coagulation activation in blood and in the respiratory tract after the nasal stimulation with poly(I:C).

We also evaluated pulmonary coagulation during IFV infection (41, 42). The respiratory virus induced activation of coagulation in the lungs of infected mice as demonstrated by the increased levels of respiratory TATc. These procoagulant changes were related to alterations in the expression of TM and TF in lungs. Our findings are in line with previous studies in humans and animal models of influenza infection demonstrating increased lung fibrin deposition and enhanced numbers of intravascular thrombi in the respiratory tract (59, 73, 74). We demonstrated that immunobiotic treatment is able to significantly diminish the activation of coagulation in IFV-challenged mice. In fact, lower levels of respiratory TATc and a reduced expression of TF was observed in *L. rhamnosus* CRL1505-treated mice infected with IFV when compared to controls (41, 42).

As mentioned before, IFV promote a procoagulant state directly through its capacity to infect ECs and monocytes stimulating the expression of TF (75, 76). In addition, IFV induce activation of coagulation indirectly by the enhancement of proinflammatory factors such as IL-6 (75, 76). Therefore, the ability of immunobiotics to modulate the IFV-triggered immune-coagulative response could be explained by their direct influence on viral replication related to the enhancement of the antiviral state in the respiratory mucosa, and indirectly through the modulation of the inflammatory response. Considering this last point, we performed experiments using anti-IL-10R blocking antibodies in order to evaluate the role of the regulation of the inflammatory response in the reduction of coagulation activation. Results showed that IL-10 is important for the regulation of coagulation induced by the immunobiotic *L. rhamnosus* CRL1505 (41). Blocking of IL-10R abolished the capacity of the CRL1505 strain to change the expression of TM and TF in the lungs. This was in line with our previous studies evaluating the ability of *L. rhamnosus* CRL1505 to confer protection against inflammatory damage induced by TLR3 activation or RSV infection, which showed that IL-10 is a key factor for the reduction of lung injury (67). Additionally, it was demonstrated that lethal disease caused by IFV infection is prevented by IL-10 administration through the reduction of lung immunopathology (77). Moreover, TF expression and procoagulant activity of macrophages and ECs are reduced by IL-10 (78, 79).

Therefore, we demonstrated that immunobiotic administration induce an early increase in the levels of TNF and IL-6 in the respiratory tract after poly(I:C), RSV, or IFV challenge, while the levels of those proinflammatory factors are significantly reduced later during infection (41, 42, 67). The early increase of proinflammatory mediators and the augmented levels of IFN-γ explain the ability of *L. rhamnosus* CRL1505 to diminish viral replication while the improved production of IL-10 would lead to a beneficial modulation of the immune-coagulative response which results in a reduced severity of lung damage. It has been suggested that respiratory viral infections increase the risk of venous thromboembolism and ischemic heart disease through ECs perturbation, coagulation activation, reduction of anticoagulant factors, and inhibition of fibrinolysis (80–82). Then, our studies suggest that immunobiotics could be an interesting alternative not only to reduce the incidence and/or severity of respiratory viral infections, but in addition to reduce the risk of atherothrombotic alterations associated to respiratory viral infections.

CONCLUSION

Research from the last decade has clearly demonstrated that beneficial microorganisms are able to modulate respiratory tract immunity and promote the resolution and lessen the severity of respiratory infections caused by pathogens such as IFV. Studies in animal models have demonstrated that orally or nasally administered immunobiotics are able to improve protection against IFV by three main mechanisms. First, immunobiotics increase the respiratory antiviral state by their capacity to improve levels of type I IFNs, the number and activity of antigen presenting cells, NK cells, $CD4^+IFN\text{-}\gamma^+$ T, and IgA^+ B lymphocytes, as well as the levels of systemic and mucosal specific antibodies. Second, immunobiotics beneficially modulate the IFV-triggered respiratory inflammatory response by inducing changes in the levels and kinetics of proinflammatory factors and immunoregulatory cytokines such as IL-10 that allow the clearance of virus with a minimal inflammatory lung tissue damage. Finally, as demonstrated by our recent research works, immunobiotics modulate lung immune-coagulative response triggered by TLR3 activation or IFV infection, mainly by down-regulating lung TF and restoring TM levels. Studies in animal models suggest that immunobiotics would influence principally the innate immune response, modulating in that way the early antiviral inflammatory response and the subsequent cellular and humoral immune responses. Therefore, immunobiotics would have mainly an adjuvant effect. However, the exact molecular mechanisms by which immunobiotics differentially modulate the innate antiviral immune response against IFV remain to be elucidated.

Additionally, a growing number of studies in humans have examined the effect of immunobiotics on the incidence and severity of IFV infection. Considering the impact of immunobiotics in the innate immune response clinical studies have evaluated principally their potential adjuvant effects on IFV vaccination (**Table 2**). Although mechanistic studies have not been addressed in depth, there is promising evidence for beneficial effects of immunobiotics on human respiratory health and resistance against IFV. These observations might be helpful to propose new preventive approaches to improve IFV control using immunobiotics by developing functional foods, pharmabiotics, or vaccine adjuvants.

AUTHOR CONTRIBUTIONS

HZ, SA, HK, and JV have designed, written, and revised the review article.

REFERENCES

1. Cohen M, Zhang XQ, Senaati HP, Chen HW, Varki NM, Schooley RT, et al. Influenza A penetrates host mucus by cleaving sialic acids with neuraminidase. *Virol J* (2013) 10:321. doi:10.1186/1743-422X-10-321
2. Tripathi S, White MR, Hartshorn KL. The amazing innate immune response to influenza A virus infection. *Innate Immun* (2015) 21(1):73–98. doi:10.1177/1753425913508992
3. Hsu AC, Parsons K, Barr I, Lowther S, Middleton D, Hansbro PM, et al. Critical role of constitutive type I interferon response in bronchial epithelial cell to influenza infection. *PLoS One* (2012) 7(3):e32947. doi:10.1371/journal.pone.0032947
4. Everitt AR, Clare S, Pertel T, John SP, Wash RS, Smith SE, et al. IFITM3 restricts the morbidity and mortality associated with influenza. *Nature* (2012) 484(7395):519–23. doi:10.1038/nature10921
5. Cilloniz C, Pantin-Jackwood MJ, Ni C, Carter VS, Korth MJ, Swayne DE, et al. Molecular signatures associated with Mx1-mediated resistance to highly pathogenic influenza virus infection: mechanisms of survival. *J Virol* (2012) 86(5):2437–46. doi:10.1128/JVI.06156-11
6. Ronni T, Matikainen S, Sareneva T, Melen K, Pirhonen J, Keskinen P, et al. Regulation of IFN-alpha/beta, MxA, 2′,5′-oligoadenylate synthetase, and HLA gene expression in influenza A-infected human lung epithelial cells. *J Immunol* (1997) 158(5):2363–74.
7. Goraya MU, Wang S, Munir M, Chen JL. Induction of innate immunity and its perturbation by influenza viruses. *Protein Cell* (2015) 6(10):712–21. doi:10.1007/s13238-015-0191-z
8. Thomas PG, Dash P, Aldridge JR Jr, Ellebedy AH, Reynolds C, Funk AJ, et al. The intracellular sensor NLRP3 mediates key innate and healing responses to influenza A virus via the regulation of caspase-1. *Immunity* (2009) 30(4):566–75. doi:10.1016/j.immuni.2009.02.006
9. Allen IC, Scull MA, Moore CB, Holl EK, McElvania-TeKippe E, Taxman DJ, et al. The NLRP3 inflammasome mediates in vivo innate immunity to influenza A virus through recognition of viral RNA. *Immunity* (2009) 30(4):556–65. doi:10.1016/j.immuni.2009.02.005
10. Ichinohe T, Lee HK, Ogura Y, Flavell R, Iwasaki A. Inflammasome recognition of influenza virus is essential for adaptive immune responses. *J Exp Med* (2009) 206(1):79–87. doi:10.1084/jem.20081667
11. Mendelson M, Tekoah Y, Zilka A, Gershoni-Yahalom O, Gazit R, Achdout H, et al. NKp46 O-glycan sequences that are involved in the interaction with hemagglutinin type 1 of influenza virus. *J Virol* (2010) 84(8):3789–97. doi:10.1128/JVI.01815-09
12. Arnon TI, Lev M, Katz G, Chernobrov Y, Porgador A, Mandelboim O. Recognition of viral hemagglutinins by NKp44 but not by NKp30. *Eur J Immunol* (2001)31(9):2680–9.doi:10.1002/1521-4141(200109)31:9<2680::AID-IMMU 2680>3.0.CO;2-A
13. Kreijtz JH, Fouchier RA, Rimmelzwaan GF. Immune responses to influenza virus infection. *Virus Res* (2011) 162(1–2):19–30. doi:10.1016/j.virusres.2011.09.022
14. Iwasaki A. Exploiting mucosal immunity for antiviral vaccines. *Annu Rev Immunol* (2016) 34:575–608. doi:10.1146/annurev-immunol-032414-112315
15. Favre L, Spertini F, Corthesy B. Secretory IgA possesses intrinsic modulatory properties stimulating mucosal and systemic immune responses. *J Immunol* (2005) 175(5):2793–800. doi:10.4049/jimmunol.175.5.2793
16. Chiu C, Ellebedy AH, Wrammert J, Ahmed R. B cell responses to influenza infection and vaccination. *Curr Top Microbiol Immunol* (2015) 386:381–98. doi:10.1007/82_2014_425
17. Braciale TJ, Sun J, Kim TS. Regulating the adaptive immune response to respiratory virus infection. *Nat Rev Immunol* (2012) 12(4):295–305. doi:10.1038/nri3166
18. Ignacio A, Morales CI, Camara NO, Almeida RR. Innate sensing of the gut microbiota: modulation of inflammatory and autoimmune diseases. *Front Immunol* (2016) 7:54. doi:10.3389/fimmu.2016.00054
19. Arrieta MC, Finlay BB. The commensal microbiota drives immune homeostasis. *Front Immunol* (2012) 3:33. doi:10.3389/fimmu.2012.00033
20. Baumler AJ, Sperandio V. Interactions between the microbiota and pathogenic bacteria in the gut. *Nature* (2016) 535(7610):85–93. doi:10.1038/nature18849
21. Pamer EG. Resurrecting the intestinal microbiota to combat antibiotic-resistant pathogens. *Science* (2016) 352(6285):535–8. doi:10.1126/science.aad9382
22. Thiemann S, Smit N, Strowig T. Antibiotics and the intestinal microbiome: individual responses, resilience of the ecosystem, and the susceptibility to infections. *Curr Top Microbiol Immunol* (2016). doi:10.1007/82_2016_504
23. Ichinohe T, Pang IK, Kumamoto Y, Peaper DR, Ho JH, Murray TS, et al. Microbiota regulates immune defense against respiratory tract influenza A virus infection. *Proc Natl Acad Sci U S A* (2011) 108(13):5354–9. doi:10.1073/pnas.1019378108
24. Abt MC, Osborne LC, Monticelli LA, Doering TA, Alenghat T, Sonnenberg GF, et al. Commensal bacteria calibrate the activation threshold of innate antiviral immunity. *Immunity* (2012) 37(1):158–70. doi:10.1016/j.immuni.2012.04.011
25. Clarke TB, Davis KM, Lysenko ES, Zhou AY, Yu Y, Weiser JN. Recognition of peptidoglycan from the microbiota by Nod1 enhances systemic innate immunity. *Nat Med* (2010) 16(2):228–31. doi:10.1038/nm.2087
26. Yasui H, Kiyoshima J, Hori T, Shida K. Protection against influenza virus infection of mice fed *Bifidobacterium* breve YIT4064. *Clin Diagn Lab Immunol* (1999) 6(2):186–92.
27. Kobayashi N, Saito T, Uematsu T, Kishi K, Toba M, Kohda N, et al. Oral administration of heat-killed *Lactobacillus pentosus* strain b240 augments protection against influenza virus infection in mice. *Int Immunopharmacol* (2011) 11(2):199–203. doi:10.1016/j.intimp.2010.11.019
28. Waki N, Yajima N, Suganuma H, Buddle BM, Luo D, Heiser A, et al. Oral administration of *Lactobacillus brevis* KB290 to mice alleviates clinical symptoms following influenza virus infection. *Lett Appl Microbiol* (2014) 58(1):87–93. doi:10.1111/lam.12160
29. Kikuchi Y, Kunitoh-Asari A, Hayakawa K, Imai S, Kasuya K, Abe K, et al. Oral administration of *Lactobacillus plantarum* strain AYA enhances IgA secretion and provides survival protection against influenza virus infection in mice. *PLoS One* (2014) 9(1):e86416. doi:10.1371/journal.pone.0086416
30. Hori T, Kiyoshima J, Shida K, Yasui H. Augmentation of cellular immunity and reduction of influenza virus titer in aged mice fed *Lactobacillus casei* strain Shirota. *Clin Diagn Lab Immunol* (2002) 9(1):105–8. doi:10.1128/CDLI.9.1.105-108.2002
31. Yasui H, Kiyoshima J, Hori T. Reduction of influenza virus titer and protection against influenza virus infection in infant mice fed *Lactobacillus casei* Shirota. *Clin Diagn Lab Immunol* (2004) 11(4):675–9. doi:10.1128/CDLI.11.4.675-679.2004
32. Kawase M, He F, Kubota A, Harata G, Hiramatsu M. Oral administration of lactobacilli from human intestinal tract protects mice against influenza virus infection. *Lett Appl Microbiol* (2010) 51(1):6–10. doi:10.1111/j.1472-765X.2010.02849.x
33. Takeda S, Takeshita M, Kikuchi Y, Dashnyam B, Kawahara S, Yoshida H, et al. Efficacy of oral administration of heat-killed probiotics from Mongolian dairy products against influenza infection in mice: alleviation of influenza infection by its immunomodulatory activity through intestinal immunity. *Int Immunopharmacol* (2011) 11(12):1976–83. doi:10.1016/j.intimp.2011.08.007
34. Kawahara T, Takahashi T, Oishi K, Tanaka H, Masuda M, Takahashi S, et al. Consecutive oral administration of *Bifidobacterium longum* MM-2 improves the defense system against influenza virus infection by enhancing natural killer cell activity in a murine model. *Microbiol Immunol* (2015) 59(1):1–12. doi:10.1111/1348-0421.12210
35. Hori T, Kiyoshima J, Shida K, Yasui H. Effect of intranasal administration of *Lactobacillus casei* Shirota on influenza virus infection of upper respiratory tract in mice. *Clin Diagn Lab Immunol* (2001) 8(3):593–7. doi:10.1128/CDLI.8.3.593-597.2001

36. Izumo T, Maekawa T, Ida M, Noguchi A, Kitagawa Y, Shibata H, et al. Effect of intranasal administration of *Lactobacillus pentosus* S-PT84 on influenza virus infection in mice. *Int Immunopharmacol* (2010) 10(9):1101–6. doi:10.1016/j.intimp.2010.06.012
37. Harata G, He F, Hiruta N, Kawase M, Kubota A, Hiramatsu M, et al. Intranasal administration of *Lactobacillus rhamnosus* GG protects mice from H1N1 influenza virus infection by regulating respiratory immune responses. *Lett Appl Microbiol* (2010) 50(6):597–602. doi:10.1111/j.1472-765X.2010.02844.x
38. Lee YN, Youn HN, Kwon JH, Lee DH, Park JK, Yuk SS, et al. Sublingual administration of *Lactobacillus rhamnosus* affects respiratory immune responses and facilitates protection against influenza virus infection in mice. *Antiviral Res* (2013) 98(2):284–90. doi:10.1016/j.antiviral.2013.03.013
39. Maeda N, Nakamura R, Hirose Y, Murosaki S, Yamamoto Y, Kase T, et al. Oral administration of heat-killed *Lactobacillus plantarum* L-137 enhances protection against influenza virus infection by stimulation of type I interferon production in mice. *Int Immunopharmacol* (2009) 9(9):1122–5. doi:10.1016/j.intimp.2009.04.015
40. Nakayama Y, Moriya T, Sakai F, Ikeda N, Shiozaki T, Hosoya T, et al. Oral administration of *Lactobacillus gasseri* SBT2055 is effective for preventing influenza in mice. *Sci Rep* (2014) 4:4638. doi:10.1038/srep04638
41. Zelaya H, Tsukida K, Chiba E, Marranzino G, Alvarez S, Kitazawa H, et al. Immunobiotic lactobacilli reduce viral-associated pulmonary damage through the modulation of inflammation-coagulation interactions. *Int Immunopharmacol* (2014) 19(1):161–73. doi:10.1016/j.intimp.2013.12.020
42. Zelaya H, Tada A, Vizoso-Pinto MG, Salva S, Kanmani P, Aguero G, et al. Nasal priming with immunobiotic *Lactobacillus rhamnosus* modulates inflammation-coagulation interactions and reduces influenza virus-associated pulmonary damage. *Inflamm Res* (2015) 64(8):589–602. doi:10.1007/s00011-015-0837-6
43. Chen MF, Weng KF, Huang SY, Liu YC, Tseng SN, Ojcius DM, et al. Pretreatment with a heat-killed probiotic modulates monocyte chemoattractant protein-1 and reduces the pathogenicity of influenza and enterovirus 71 infections. *Mucosal Immunol* (2016). doi:10.1038/mi.2016.31
44. Kiso M, Takano R, Sakabe S, Katsura H, Shinya K, Uraki R, et al. Protective efficacy of orally administered, heat-killed *Lactobacillus pentosus* b240 against influenza A virus. *Sci Rep* (2013) 3:1563. doi:10.1038/srep01563
45. Armstrong SM, Wang C, Tigdi J, Si X, Dumpit C, Charles S, et al. Influenza infects lung microvascular endothelium leading to microvascular leak: role of apoptosis and claudin-5. *PLoS One* (2012) 7(10):e47323. doi:10.1371/journal.pone.0047323
46. Lebeer S, Vanderleyden J, De Keersmaecker SC. Host interactions of probiotic bacterial surface molecules: comparison with commensals and pathogens. *Nat Rev Microbiol* (2010) 8(3):171–84. doi:10.1038/nrmicro2297
47. Bermudez-Brito M, Plaza-Diaz J, Munoz-Quezada S, Gomez-Llorente C, Gil A. Probiotic mechanisms of action. *Ann Nutr Metab* (2012) 61(2):160–74. doi:10.1159/000342079
48. Kitazawa H, Villena J. Modulation of respiratory TLR3-anti-viral response by probiotic microorganisms: lessons learned from *Lactobacillus rhamnosus* CRL1505. *Front Immunol* (2014) 5:201. doi:10.3389/fimmu.2014.00201
49. Villena J, Kitazawa H. Modulation of intestinal TLR4-inflammatory signaling pathways by probiotic microorganisms: lessons learned from *Lactobacillus jensenii* TL2937. *Front Immunol* (2014) 4:512. doi:10.3389/fimmu.2013.00512
50. Villena J, Salva S, Núñez M, Corzo J, Tolaba R, Faedda J, et al. Probiotics for everyone! The novel immunobiotic *Lactobacillus rhamnosus* CRL1505 and the beginning of Social Probiotic Programs in Argentina. *Int J Biotechnol Wellness Ind* (2012) 1:189–98.
51. Percopo CM, Rice TA, Brenner TA, Dyer KD, Luo JL, Kanakabandi K, et al. Immunobiotic *Lactobacillus* administered post-exposure averts the lethal sequelae of respiratory virus infection. *Antiviral Res* (2015) 121:109–19. doi:10.1016/j.antiviral.2015.07.001
52. Garcia-Crespo KE, Chan CC, Gabryszewski SJ, Percopo CM, Rigaux P, Dyer KD, et al. *Lactobacillus* priming of the respiratory tract: heterologous immunity and protection against lethal pneumovirus infection. *Antiviral Res* (2013) 97(3):270–9. doi:10.1016/j.antiviral.2012.12.022
53. Rynda-Apple A, Robinson KM, Alcorn JF. Influenza and bacterial superinfection: illuminating the immunologic mechanisms of disease. *Infect Immun* (2015) 83(10):3764–70. doi:10.1128/IAI.00298-15
54. Robinson KM, Kolls JK, Alcorn JF. The immunology of influenza virus-associated bacterial pneumonia. *Curr Opin Immunol* (2015) 34:59–67. doi:10.1016/j.coi.2015.02.002
55. Short KR, Veldhuis Kroeze EJ, Reperant LA, Richard M, Kuiken T. Influenza virus and endothelial cells: a species specific relationship. *Front Microbiol* (2014) 5:653. doi:10.3389/fmicb.2014.00653
56. van Hinsbergh VW. Endothelium – role in regulation of coagulation and inflammation. *Semin Immunopathol* (2012) 34(1):93–106. doi:10.1007/s00281-011-0285-5
57. Armstrong SM, Darwish I, Lee WL. Endothelial activation and dysfunction in the pathogenesis of influenza A virus infection. *Virulence* (2013) 4(6):537–42. doi:10.4161/viru.25779
58. Yang Y, Tang H. Aberrant coagulation causes a hyper-inflammatory response in severe influenza pneumonia. *Cell Mol Immunol* (2016) 13(4):432–42. doi:10.1038/cmi.2016.1
59. Keller TT, van der Sluijs KF, de Kruif MD, Gerdes VE, Meijers JC, Florquin S, et al. Effects on coagulation and fibrinolysis induced by influenza in mice with a reduced capacity to generate activated protein C and a deficiency in plasminogen activator inhibitor type 1. *Circ Res* (2006) 99(11):1261–9. doi:10.1161/01.RES.0000250834.29108.1a
60. Antoniak S, Tatsumi K, Hisada Y, Milner JJ, Neidich SD, Shaver CM, et al. Tissue factor deficiency increases alveolar hemorrhage and death in influenza A virus-infected mice. *J Thromb Haemost* (2016) 14(6):1238–48. doi:10.1111/jth.13307
61. Teijaro JR, Walsh KB, Cahalan S, Fremgen DM, Roberts E, Scott F, et al. Endothelial cells are central orchestrators of cytokine amplification during influenza virus infection. *Cell* (2011) 146(6):980–91. doi:10.1016/j.cell.2011.08.015
62. Tsai SY, Segovia JA, Chang TH, Morris IR, Berton MT, Tessier PA, et al. DAMP molecule S100A9 acts as a molecular pattern to enhance inflammation during influenza A virus infection: role of DDX21-TRIF-TLR4-MyD88 pathway. *PLoS Pathog* (2014) 10(1):e1003848. doi:10.1371/journal.ppat.1003848
63. Shibamiya A, Hersemeyer K, Schmidt Woll T, Sedding D, Daniel JM, Bauer S, et al. A key role for Toll-like receptor-3 in disrupting the hemostasis balance on endothelial cells. *Blood* (2009) 113(3):714–22. doi:10.1182/blood-2008-02-137901
64. Khoufache K, Berri F, Nacken W, Vogel AB, Delenne M, Camerer E, et al. PAR1 contributes to influenza A virus pathogenicity in mice. *J Clin Invest* (2013) 123(1):206–14. doi:10.1172/JCI61667
65. Antoniak S, Owens AP III, Baunacke M, Williams JC, Lee RD, Weithauser A, et al. PAR-1 contributes to the innate immune response during viral infection. *J Clin Invest* (2013) 123(3):1310–22. doi:10.1172/JCI66125
66. Villena J, Chiba E, Tomosada Y, Salva S, Marranzino G, Kitazawa H, et al. Orally administered *Lactobacillus rhamnosus* modulates the respiratory immune response triggered by the viral pathogen-associated molecular pattern poly(I:C). *BMC Immunol* (2012) 13:53. doi:10.1186/1471-2172-13-53
67. Chiba E, Tomosada Y, Vizoso-Pinto MG, Salva S, Takahashi T, Tsukida K, et al. Immunobiotic *Lactobacillus rhamnosus* improves resistance of infant mice against respiratory syncytial virus infection. *Int Immunopharmacol* (2013) 17(2):373–82. doi:10.1016/j.intimp.2013.06.024
68. Kawai T, Akira S. Toll-like receptor and RIG-I-like receptor signaling. *Ann N Y Acad Sci* (2008) 1143:1–20. doi:10.1196/annals.1443.020
69. Rudd BD, Smit JJ, Flavell RA, Alexopoulou L, Schaller MA, Gruber A, et al. Deletion of TLR3 alters the pulmonary immune environment and mucus production during respiratory syncytial virus infection. *J Immunol* (2006) 176(3):1937–42. doi:10.4049/jimmunol.176.3.1937
70. Le Goffic R, Balloy V, Lagranderie M, Alexopoulou L, Escriou N, Flavell R, et al. Detrimental contribution of the toll-like receptor (TLR)3 to influenza A virus-induced acute pneumonia. *PLoS Pathog* (2006) 2(6):e53. doi:10.1371/journal.ppat.0020053
71. Gitlin L, Barchet W, Gilfillan S, Cella M, Beutler B, Flavell RA, et al. Essential role of mda-5 in type I IFN responses to polyriboinosinic:polyribocytidylic acid and encephalomyocarditis picornavirus. *Proc Natl Acad Sci U S A* (2006) 103(22):8459–64. doi:10.1073/pnas.0603082103
72. Wang T, Town T, Alexopoulou L, Anderson JF, Fikrig E, Flavell RA. Toll-like receptor 3 mediates West Nile virus entry into the brain causing lethal encephalitis. *Nat Med* (2004) 10(12):1366–73. doi:10.1038/nm1140

73. Hwang DM, Chamberlain DW, Poutanen SM, Low DE, Asa SL, Butany J. Pulmonary pathology of severe acute respiratory syndrome in Toronto. *Mod Pathol* (2005) 18(1):1–10. doi:10.1038/modpathol.3800247
74. Muramoto Y, Ozaki H, Takada A, Park CH, Sunden Y, Umemura T, et al. Highly pathogenic H5N1 influenza virus causes coagulopathy in chickens. *Microbiol Immunol* (2006) 50(1):73–81. doi:10.1111/j.1348-0421.2006.tb03764.x
75. Visseren FL, Bouwman JJ, Bouter KP, Diepersloot RJ, de Groot PH, Erkelens DW. Procoagulant activity of endothelial cells after infection with respiratory viruses. *Thromb Haemost* (2000) 84(2):319–24.
76. Bouwman JJ, Visseren FL, Bosch MC, Bouter KP, Diepersloot RJ. Procoagulant and inflammatory response of virus-infected monocytes. *Eur J Clin Invest* (2002) 32(10):759–66. doi:10.1046/j.1365-2362.2002.01041.x
77. Sun J, Cardani A, Sharma AK, Laubach VE, Jack RS, Muller W, et al. Autocrine regulation of pulmonary inflammation by effector T-cell derived IL-10 during infection with respiratory syncytial virus. *PLoS Pathog* (2011) 7(8):e1002173. doi:10.1371/journal.ppat.1002173
78. Poitevin S, Cochery-Nouvellon E, Dupont A, Nguyen P. Monocyte IL-10 produced in response to lipopolysaccharide modulates thrombin generation by inhibiting tissue factor expression and release of active tissue factor-bound microparticles. *Thromb Haemost* (2007) 97(4):598–607.
79. Ben-Hadj-Khalifa S, Nguyen P, Mahjoub T, Hezard N. Anticoagulant properties of the anti-inflammatory cytokine IL-10 in a factor Xa-activated human monocyte model. *Eur Cytokine Netw* (2012) 23(3):87–92.
80. Smeeth L, Thomas SL, Hall AJ, Hubbard R, Farrington P, Vallance P. Risk of myocardial infarction and stroke after acute infection or vaccination. *N Engl J Med* (2004) 351(25):2611–8. doi:10.1056/NEJMoa041747
81. Smeeth L, Cook C, Thomas S, Hall AJ, Hubbard R, Vallance P. Risk of deep vein thrombosis and pulmonary embolism after acute infection in a community setting. *Lancet* (2006) 367(9516):1075–9. doi:10.1016/S0140-6736(06)68474-2
82. Esmon CT. Crosstalk between inflammation and thrombosis. *Maturitas* (2004) 47(4):305–14. doi:10.1016/j.maturitas.2003.10.015
83. Olivares M, Diaz-Ropero MP, Sierra S, Lara-Villoslada F, Fonolla J, Navas M, et al. Oral intake of *Lactobacillus fermentum* CECT5716 enhances the effects of influenza vaccination. *Nutrition* (2007) 23(3):254–60. doi:10.1016/j.nut.2007.01.004
84. Boge T, Remigy M, Vaudaine S, Tanguy J, Bourdet-Sicard R, van der Werf S. A probiotic fermented dairy drink improves antibody response to influenza vaccination in the elderly in two randomised controlled trials. *Vaccine* (2009) 27(41):5677–84. doi:10.1016/j.vaccine.2009.06.094
85. Davidson LE, Fiorino AM, Snydman DR, Hibberd PL. *Lactobacillus* GG as an immune adjuvant for live-attenuated influenza vaccine in healthy adults: a randomized double-blind placebo-controlled trial. *Eur J Clin Nutr* (2011) 65(4):501–7. doi:10.1038/ejcn.2010.289
86. Arimori Y, Nakamura R, Hirose Y, Murosaki S, Yamamoto Y, Shidara O, et al. Daily intake of heat-killed *Lactobacillus plantarum* L-137 enhances type I interferon production in healthy humans and pigs. *Immunopharmacol Immunotoxicol* (2012) 34(6):937–43. doi:10.3109/08923973.2012.672425
87. Rizzardini G, Eskesen D, Calder PC, Capetti A, Jespersen L, Clerici M. Evaluation of the immune benefits of two probiotic strains *Bifidobacterium animalis* ssp. *lactis*, BB-12(R) and *Lactobacillus paracasei* ssp. *paracasei*, *L. casei* 431(R) in an influenza vaccination model: a randomised, double-blind, placebo-controlled study. *Br J Nutr* (2012) 107(6):876–84. doi:10.1017/S000711451100420X
88. Miettinen M, Pietila TE, Kekkonen RA, Kankainen M, Latvala S, Pirhonen J, et al. Nonpathogenic *Lactobacillus rhamnosus* activates the inflammasome and antiviral responses in human macrophages. *Gut Microbes* (2012) 3(6):510–22. doi:10.4161/gmic.21736
89. Shinkai S, Toba M, Saito T, Sato I, Tsubouchi M, Taira K, et al. Immunoprotective effects of oral intake of heat-killed *Lactobacillus pentosus* strain b240 in elderly adults: a randomised, double-blind, placebo-controlled trial. *Br J Nutr* (2013) 109(10):1856–65. doi:10.1017/S0007114512003753
90. Akatsu H, Arakawa K, Yamamoto T, Kanematsu T, Matsukawa N, Ohara H, et al. *Lactobacillus* in jelly enhances the effect of influenza vaccination in elderly individuals. *J Am Geriatr Soc* (2013) 61(10):1828–30. doi:10.1111/jgs.12474
91. Kumpu M, Lehtoranta L, Roivainen M, Ronkko E, Ziegler T, Soderlund-Venermo M, et al. The use of the probiotic *Lactobacillus rhamnosus* GG and viral findings in the nasopharynx of children attending day care. *J Med Virol* (2013) 85(9):1632–8. doi:10.1002/jmv.23623
92. Waki N, Matsumoto M, Fukui Y, Suganuma H. Effects of probiotic *Lactobacillus brevis* KB290 on incidence of influenza infection among schoolchildren: an open-label pilot study. *Lett Appl Microbiol* (2014) 59(6):565–71. doi:10.1111/lam.12340
93. Luoto R, Ruuskanen O, Waris M, Kalliomaki M, Salminen S, Isolauri E. Prebiotic and probiotic supplementation prevents rhinovirus infections in preterm infants: a randomized, placebo-controlled trial. *J Allergy Clin Immunol* (2014) 133(2):405–13. doi:10.1016/j.jaci.2013.08.020
94. Sugimura T, Takahashi H, Jounai K, Ohshio K, Kanayama M, Tazumi K, et al. Effects of oral intake of plasmacytoid dendritic cells-stimulative lactic acid bacterial strain on pathogenesis of influenza-like illness and immunological response to influenza virus. *Br J Nutr* (2015) 114(5):727–33. doi:10.1017/S0007114515002408

16

Intestinal Dysbiosis is Associated with Altered Short-Chain Fatty Acids and Serum-Free Fatty Acids in Systemic Lupus Erythematosus

Javier Rodríguez-Carrio[1], Patricia López[2], Borja Sánchez[1], Sonia González[3], Miguel Gueimonde[1], Abelardo Margolles[1], Clara G. de los Reyes-Gavilán[1]* and Ana Suárez[2]*

[1] Department of Microbiology and Biochemistry of Dairy Products, Instituto de Productos Lácteos de Asturias (IPLA-CSIC), Villaviciosa, Asturias, Spain, [2] Area of Immunology, Department of Functional Biology, University of Oviedo, Oviedo, Asturias, Spain, [3] Area of Physiology, Department of Functional Biology, University of Oviedo, Oviedo, Asturias, Spain

Edited by:
Ian Marriott,
University of North Carolina at Charlotte, USA

Reviewed by:
Martin Rumbo,
National University of La Plata (CONICET)
Paola Gauggin Cano,
Centro de Referencia Para Lactobacilos (CONICET)

***Correspondence:**
Abelardo Margolles
amargolles@ipla.csic.es;
Clara G. de los Reyes-Gavilán
greyes_gavilan@ipla.csic.es

Metabolic impairments are a frequent hallmark of systemic lupus erythematosus (SLE). Increased serum levels of free fatty acids (FFA) are commonly found in these patients, although the underlying causes remain elusive. Recently, it has been suggested that factors other than inflammation or clinical features may be involved. The gut microbiota is known to influence the host metabolism, the production of short-chain fatty acids (SCFA) playing a potential role. Taking into account that lupus patients exhibit an intestinal dysbiosis, we wondered whether altered FFA levels may be associated with the intestinal microbial composition in lupus patients. To this aim, total and specific serum FFA levels, fecal SCFA levels, and gut microbiota composition were determined in 21 SLE patients and 25 healthy individuals. The *Firmicutes* to *Bacteroidetes* (F/B) ratio was strongly associated with serum FFA levels in healthy controls (HC), even after controlling for confounders. However, this association was not found in lupus patients, where a decreased F/B ratio and increased FFA serum levels were noted. An altered production of SCFA was related to the intestinal dysbiosis in lupus, while SCFA levels paralleled those of serum FFA in HC. Although a different serum FFA profile was not found in SLE, specific FFA showed distinct patterns on a principal component analysis. Immunomodulatory omega-3 FFA were positively correlated to the F/B ratio in HC, but not in SLE. Furthermore, divergent associations were observed for pro- and anti-inflammatory FFA with endothelial activation biomarkers in lupus patients. Overall, these findings support a link between the gut microbial ecology and the host metabolism in the pathological framework of SLE. A potential link between intestinal dysbiosis and surrogate markers of endothelial activation in lupus patients is supported, FFA species having a pivotal role.

Keywords: free fatty acids, systemic lupus erythematosus, dysbiosis, microbiota, short-chain fatty acids

INTRODUCTION

Epidemiological studies have consistently shown an increase in the prevalence and severity of a number of metabolic disorders in patients with systemic lupus erythematosus (SLE) compared to the general population (1–3). Among them, metabolic syndrome, disturbed glucose metabolism, or altered lipid metabolism are the most relevant. These disorders are related to an increased risk of cardiovascular disease (CVD) development, the most important cause of mortality in SLE (4, 5), thus highlighting the clinical relevance of the metabolic alterations in SLE.

Immune dysregulation and chronic inflammation are known to promote endothelial dysfunction in SLE (6, 7). Increased levels of pro-inflammatory cytokines [such as tumor necrosis factor alpha (TNFα), interleukin-8 (IL-8), and monocyte chemoattractant protein-1 (MCP-1)], adipokines, and autoantibodies are associated with the progression of endothelial dysfunction toward atherosclerosis development (6). At the local level, these mediators can impair the balance between endothelial repair and damage, whereas a number of systemic effects can be also triggered, including a shift to a pro-oxidant status (8) and altered lipid metabolism. In this scenario, although the underlying mechanisms are not totally understood, the relationship between systemic inflammation, metabolic disorders, and CVD may be explained, at least in part, by the free fatty acids (FFA) (9). FFA are fatty acid molecules released from adipocytes and several cell types upon lipolysis (10). Increased FFA levels in serum have been described in several metabolic disorders. Moreover, elevated serum FFA have also been found in immune-mediated diseases, such as SLE or rheumatoid arthritis, although striking differences were noted between both conditions (11). Rather than inflammatory or clinical parameters, the body mass index (BMI) was found to be the main predictor of FFA serum levels in lupus (11). However, these clinical studies did not allow the elucidation of the exact mediators and mechanisms involved.

Obesity is the result of an imbalance between energy intake and expenditure, which results in an excess of fat accumulation. However, several epidemiological studies have identified people with low BMI exhibiting markers of metabolic dysfunction (12, 13). Similarly, healthy metabolic profiles are found in a subset of obese subjects (14, 15), hence suggesting that metabolic dysfunction (that is, impaired fatty acid mobilization) rather than adiposity should be considered as the underlying cause. Therefore, it is feasible that factors related to energy intake and expenditure may underlie altered FFA levels and thus, metabolic disorders.

A mounting body of evidence shows that the gut microbiota can influence the host metabolism as well as the energy harvest and storage (16–18). Actually, the gut microbiota is seen by some authors as a separate endocrine organ involved, through a molecular cross talk with the host, in the maintenance of energy homeostasis and fat deposition (19). Currently, extensive research efforts have been focused on deciphering the basis of the cross talk between the microbiota and the host metabolism in the development and progression of host diseases and have revealed the relevance of the intestinal microbiota–host metabolism axis mediated by different bacterial and host metabolites (20, 21). Thus, it may be speculated that changes in the intestinal microbial ecology could disrupt this homeostatic cross talk and precipitate the development of pathological outcomes in the host.

Recently, we have reported that SLE patients exhibit an altered intestinal composition compared to healthy subjects, mainly characterized by a decreased abundance of members of the *Firmicutes* phylum and an overrepresentation of those of *Bacteroidetes* (22). However, the clinical impact of this SLE-associated intestinal dysbiosis remains to be elucidated. Taking into account the former assumptions, we hypothesized that altered gut microbiota composition in SLE may underlie increased FFA serum levels. Accordingly, the main aims of the present report were (i) to analyze the potential association between the microbiota composition and FFA serum levels, (ii) to elucidate whether microbial metabolites can have a role in this interaction, (iii) to evaluate whether a different profile of FFA can be found in lupus patients, and (iv) to study the associations of these parameters with clinically relevant serum biomarkers.

MATERIALS AND METHODS

Ethical Approval

Ethical approval for this study was obtained from the Institutional Review Board (Comité de Ética de Investigación Clínica del Principado de Asturias) in compliance with the Declaration of Helsinki. All participants were informed and gave a signed informed consent prior their inclusion in the study.

Patients and Controls

Our study involved 21 SLE patients, all fulfilling classification criteria for SLE. According to the 1982 revised criteria from the American College of Rheumatology, a definitive SLE diagnosis can be established when a patient exhibit at least 4 out of the 11 SLE criteria (malar rash, discoid lesions, photosensitivity, oral ulcers, arthritis, serositis, renal disorders, neurological disorder, cytopenia, raised anti-DNA titers, and positivity to antinuclear antibodies) (23). A complete clinical examination, including Systemic Lupus Erythematosus Disease Activity Index (SLEDAI) calculation and anti-dsDNA autoantibodies assessment, was performed at the time of sampling. All patients were in remission (SLEDAI <8) at the sampling time. Information on clinical features along the disease course as well as the therapies received during the last 6 months was obtained from their clinical records. A group of 25 age- [median 43.50 (range 23.00–63.00) years] and gender-matched (23 females) healthy individuals recruited from the general population was included as the healthy controls (HC). Patients and controls did not differ in age ($p = 0.293$) and gender distribution ($p = 0.495$). Exclusion criteria were the history of recent infections, diagnosis of metabolic diseases, or the use of antibiotics, glucocorticoids, or monoclonal antibodies in the previous 6 months.

Upon acceptance of the individuals to participate in the study, a strict overnight fast (more than 8 h) blood sample was obtained in tubes without anticoagulant. Serum was collected, divided into aliquots, and samples were stored at −80°C until experimental procedures were performed. Additionally, basic serum blood lipid analyses were carried out on fresh samples at the time of sampling, by standardized procedures.

Quantification of Total FFA Serum Levels

Total FFA serum levels were analyzed by a colorimetric enzymatic assay using a commercial kit (NEFA kit half-microtest, Roche Life

Sciences, Penzberg, Germany) following the instructions from the manufacturer. Final absorbance was measured at 546 nm, and the detection limit was 0.2 mM.

Assessment of Serum FFA Profiles

Individual FFA were analyzed in serum samples following a methyl-*tert*-butylether-based extraction protocol (MTBE) as previously described (24), with minor modifications. Briefly, serum samples (100 µl) were spiked with 5 µl of internal standard (600 ppm heptadecanoic acid). Proteins were precipitated by the addition of 200 µl methanol chromasolv grade (Sigma Aldrich, MO, USA). Organic phases were obtained by the addition of 1,200 µl MTBE chromasolv grade (Sigma) followed by an incubation in an ultrasound water bath at 15°C for 30 min. Finally, organic phases were isolated by centrifugation at 5,000 rpm (7 min, 15°C) after the addition of 200 µl milliQ water. The extraction protocol was repeated once with 100 µl MetOH, 500 µl MTBE, and 100 µl milliQ H_2O. Lipid extracts were dried in a miVac centrifugal evaporator (Genevac Ltd., UK) and redissolved in 100 µl of water:acetonitrile (38:62).

The analyses of fatty acids in the samples were performed in a Dionex Ultimate 3000 HPLC system (Thermo Scientific, Bremen, Germany) equipped with a column Zorbax Eclipse Plus C18 (50 mm × 2.1 mm, 1.8 µm). Mobile phases A and B were water and acetonitrile, respectively, both containing 0.1% of formic acid. Fatty acids were separated in an injection volume of 2 µl by a gradient program as follows: 62% B (held for 4.5 min) followed by a linear increase up to 100% B in 10 min (held for 1 min). The column temperature was set at 45°C. Mass detection was carried out in a Bruker Impact II q-ToF mass spectrometer with electrospray ionization, operating in the negative mode. The settings of the mass spectrometer were as follows: spray voltage 4.5 kV; drying gas flow 12 l/min; drying gas temperature 250°C; and nebulizer pressure 44 psi.

For quantification, calibration curves for each compound were prepared by dissolution of the pure standards in methanol to adequately encompass the expected concentration of the analytes in the samples. The calibration ranges were as follows: 0.4–12.5 µg/ml for EPA and γ-linolenic; 1.2–37.5 µg/ml for DHA and linolenic; 2.3–75 µg/ml for AA and palmitoleic; 3.9–125 µg/ml for linoleic; and 7.8–250 µg/ml for oleic, palmitic, and stearic acids. A good linearity was observed in all cases ($r^2 > 0.994$). Heptadecanoic acid was used as internal standard to account for potential biases during the extraction protocol.

Analysis of Fecal Microbiota

Fecal sample collection and metagenomic analyses of fecal microbiota were performed as previously reported (22). Briefly, fresh fecal material was processed within 3 h from collection and immediately homogenized and stored at −80°C. Fecal DNA was extracted with a QIAampDNA stool minikit (Qiagen, Strasse, Germany). Then, 16S rRNA gene sequences were amplified, and 16S rRNA and gene-based amplicons were sequenced by an Ion Torrent PGM sequencing platform as described elsewhere (22).

Analysis of Short-Chain Fatty Acids (SCFA) in Fecal Samples

Analysis of SCFA (acetate, propionate, and butyrate) was performed by gas chromatography. Briefly, 1 g of fecal samples was diluted 1:10 in sterile PBS and homogenized in a LabBlender 400 stomacher (Seward Medical, London, UK) at full speed for 4 min. Then, supernatants were obtained by centrifugation (10.000 × *g*, 30 min, 4°C), filtered through 0.2-µm filters, mixed with 1:10 of ethyl butyric acid (2 mg/ml) as an internal standard, and stored at −80°C until analysis.

A gas chromatograph 6890N (Agilent Technologies Inc., Palo Alto, CA, USA) connected to a mass spectrometry (MS) 5973N detector (Agilent Technologies) and to a flame ionization detector was used for identification and quantification of SCFA. Data were collected using the Enhanced ChemStation G1701DA software (Agilent). Samples (1 µl) were injected into the gas chromatograph equipped with an HP-Innowax capillary column (60-m length by 0.25-mm internal diameter, with a 0.25-µm film thickness; Agilent) using He as a gas carrier (flow rate of 1.5 ml/min). The temperature of the injector was kept at 220°C, and the split ratio was 50:1. Chromatographic conditions were as follows: initial oven temperature of 120°C, 5°C/min up to 180°C, 1 min at 180°C, and a ramp of 20°C/min up to 220°C to clean the column. In the MS detector, the electron impact energy was set at 70 eV. The data collected were in the range of 25 to 250 atomic mass units (at 3.25 scans/s).

SCFA were identified by comparison of their mass spectra with those held in the HP-Wiley 138 library (Agilent) and by comparison of their retention times with those of the corresponding standards (Sigma Aldrich, St. Louis, MO, USA). The peaks were quantified as relative abundances with respect to the internal standard. The concentration (in millimolar) of each SCFA was calculated using the linear regression equations ($R^2 \geq 0.99$) from the corresponding standard curves.

Analysis of Serum Biomarkers

Soluble Biomarkers

Serum levels of vascular endothelial growth factor (VEGF), granulocyte monocyte colony-stimulating factor (GM-CSF), and IL-8 were analyzed by Cytometric Bead Arrays (BD Biosciences, NJ, USA) using a BD FACS Canto II and FACS Diva software. Detection limits were 4.5, 0.2, and 1.2 pg/ml, respectively.

Epidermal growth factor (EGF), TNFα, MCP-1, interferon gamma-inducible protein-10 (IP-10), and leptin serum levels were assessed by plate immunoassays using commercial kits by Peprotech (NJ, USA), following manufacturer's instructions. Detection limits were 3.9, 3.9, 8, 3.9, and 24 pg/ml, respectively.

Malondialdehyde (MDA)

Malondialdehyde serum levels were determined by means of a colorimetric method using a commercial kit (LPO-596, Byoxytech, Oxis International, France). Final absorbance was read at 586 nm.

Anthropometric Measures

Height was measured using a stadiometer with an accuracy of ±1 mm (Año-Sayol, Barcelona, Spain). The subjects stood barefoot, in an upright position and with the head positioned in the Frankfort horizontal plane. Weight was measured on a scale with an accuracy of ±100 g (Seca, Hamburg, Germany).

Nutritional Assessments

Dietary intakes were assessed by means of an annual semiquantitative validated food frequency questionnaire including 160 items (25). During an interview by trained dietitians, subjects were asked, item by item, whether they usually ate each food and, if so, how much they usually ate. For this purpose, three different serving sizes of each cooked food were presented in pictures to the participants so that they could choose from up to seven serving sizes (from "less than the small one" to "more than the large one"). For some of the foods consumed, amounts were recorded in household units, by volume, or by measuring with a ruler. Information on the cooking practices, number and amount of ingredients used in each recipe, and other relevant information for the study was collected. Methodological issues concerning dietary assessment have been detailed elsewhere (25). The consumption of foods was converted into energy intake (kilocalories per day), macronutrients (carbohydrates, lipids, and proteins, grams per day), and total fiber (grams per day) using the nutrient food composition tables developed by the Centro de Enseñanza Superior de Nutrición Humana y Dietética (CESNID) (26). CESNID, a foundation, involves different institutions, universities, and companies related to the food and nutrition area, and its food composition databases are supported by the Spanish Association of Nutrition and Dietetics.

Statistical Analyses

Continuous variables were expressed as median (interquartile range) or mean ± SD. Mann–Whitney *U*, Student's *t* or Kruskal–Wallis tests were performed to assess statistical differences. Correlations were analyzed by Spearman's rank or Pearson tests, depending on the distribution of the data. Categorical variables were summarized as *n* (%), and differences were analyzed by χ^2 tests. A principal component analysis (PCA) was performed to avoid potential bias due to collinearity. The adequacy of the data was studied by Kaiser–Meyer–Olkin test and Bartlett test of sphericity. The number of components retained was based on eigenvalues (>1), and loadings greater than 0.5 were used to identify the variables comprising each component. Unsupervised cluster analysis was performed based on squared Euclidean distances, and Ward's Minimum Variance method was used to identify the clusters. Heatmaps were generated under R package *heatmap.2*. SPSS 21.0, R 3.0.3, and GraphPad Prism 5.0 for Windows were used.

RESULTS

Total FFA Serum Levels in SLE Patients: Association with Intestinal Dysbiosis

The concentration of total FFA was measured in serum samples from 21 SLE patients and 25 matched HC (**Table 1**). SLE patients exhibited higher FFA serum levels (**Table 1**). Differences between groups in the levels of FFA remained significant after adjusting for age and gender ($p = 0.024$). Moreover, no associations were found with demographical parameters, cholesterol and triglycerides levels, and dietary intakes (**Table 2**). Furthermore, FFA were neither related to clinical manifestations (**Table 3**) (all $p > 0.050$) nor disease activity ($r = -0.349, p = 0.169$), duration ($r = -0.005$,

TABLE 1 | Serum-free fatty acids (FFA) levels, nutritional parameters and blood lipid profiles of the healthy controls (HC) and systemic lupus erythematosus (SLE) patients recruited in this study.

	HC (n = 25)	SLE (n = 21)	p
FFA assessment			
Total FFA (mM)	0.27 (0.17)	0.41 (0.26)	0.045
Blood lipid analyses			
Total cholesterol (mg/dl)	191.50 (49.00)	200.00 (61.25)	0.732
HDL-cholesterol (mg/dl)	62.00 (14.75)	62.00 (24.00)	0.740
LDL-cholesterol (mg/dl)	114.50 (50.00)	111.50 (57.50)	0.530
Triglycerides (mg/dl)	68.50 (54.25)	71.55 (45.25)	0.715
Nutritional parameters			
Total energy (kcal/day)	1,888.88 (226.53)	2,186.11 (208.16)	0.069
Carbohydrates (g/day)	202.50 (51.60)	205.46 (102.95)	0.944
Lipids (g/day)	78.13 (29.32)	79.42 (63.57)	0.789
Proteins (g/day)	96.98 (15.81)	102.60 (34.30)	0.782
Fiber (g/day)	24.68 (6.17)	26.47 (6.57)	0.609
Body mass index (kg/m^2)	24.96 (4.47)	24.58 (7.78)	0.715

Variables are represented as median (interquartile range) or n (%) unless otherwise stated. Differences in demographical and blood lipid variables were assessed by Mann–Withney U tests, whereas differences in daily intakes were analyzed by multivariate analyses adjusted for confounders. Energy was adjusted by gender and age, whereas the rest of the nutrients were adjusted by gender, age, and energy.

TABLE 2 | Analysis of the correlation between serum FFA levels and demographical and nutritional features in healthy controls (HC) and systemic lupus erythematosus (SLE) patients.

	HC	SLE
Age	$r = -0.260$ $p = 0.231$	$r = -0.179$ $p = 0.451$
Total cholesterol	$r = -0.108$ $p = 0.625$	$r = -0.203$ $p = 0.390$
HDL-cholesterol	$r = 0.220$ $p = 0.313$	$r = 0.114$ $p = 0.633$
LDL-cholesterol	$r = -0.028$ $p = 0.898$	$r = -0.248$ $p = 0.291$
Triglycerides	$r = -0.224$ $p = 0.305$	$r = -0.078$ $p = 0.743$
BMI	$r = 0.247$ $p = 0.268$	$r = 0.214$ $p = 0.366$
Total energy	$r = 0.082$ $p = 0.710$	$r = -0.212$ $p = 0.369$
Carbohydrates	$r = -0.107$ $p = 0.628$	$r = -0.311$ $p = 0.182$
Lipids	$r = -0.048$ $p = 0.826$	$r = -0.220$ $p = 0.352$
Proteins	$r = 0.010$ $p = 0.964$	$r = -0.005$ $p = 0.985$
Fiber	$r = 0.125$ $p = 0.568$	$r = -0.394$ $p = 0.086$

Correlations were assessed by Spearman ranks tests (r coefficient and p-value is indicated for each parameter).

TABLE 3 | Demographical and clinical parameters of the systemic lupus erythematosus (SLE) patients.

	SLE (n = 21)
Age, (years), mean (range)	48.35 (27.00–70.00)
Gender, (f/m)	21/0
Age at diagnosis, (years)	33.00 (14.50)
Disease duration, (years), median (range)	7.00 (2.00–24.00)
SLEDAI score	4.00 (3.25)
Clinical manifestations, *n*(%)	
Malar rash	12 (57.1)
Photosensitivity	16 (76.2)
Discoid lesions	6 (28.6)
Arthritis	10 (47.6)
Oral ulcers	10 (47.6)
Serositis	4 (19.0)
Renal disorder	3 (14.3)
Neurological disorder	0 (0.0)
Cytopenia	11 (52.4)
Autoantibodies, *n*(%)	
ANAs	21 (100)
Anti-dsDNA titer, (U/ml), mean ± SD	25.30 ± 33.89
Anti-SSa	11 (52.4)
Anti-SSb	2 (9.5)
Anti-Sm	2 (9.5)
Anti-RNP	1 (4.8)
Treatments, *n* (%)	
None or NSAIDs	3 (14.2)
Antimalarials	18 (85.7)

Variables are represented as median (interquartile range) or n(%), unless otherwise stated.

TABLE 4 | Association between serum-free fatty acids (FFA) levels and gut microbiota composition in healthy controls (HC) and systemic lupus erythematosus patients (SLE).

	HC	SLE)
Actinobacteria	r = 0.075 p = 0.733	r = −0.415 p = 0.069
Bacteroidetes	**r = 0.721** **p < 0.0001**	r = 0.311 p = 0.182
Firmicutes	**r = −0.574** **p = 0.007**	r = −0.117 p = 0.622
Cyanobacteria	r = −0.120 p = 0.539	r = −0.401 p = 0.080
Euryarchaeota	r = −0.213 p = 0.328	r = −0.063 p = −0.792
Fusobacteria	r = −0.052 p = 0.812	r = 0.139 p = 0.560
Lentisphaerae	r = 0.272 p = 0.210	r = 0.019 p = 0.937
Proteobacteria	r = −0.158 p = 0.471	r = 0.230 p = 0.329
Tenericutes	r = −0.105 p = 0.634	r = −0.220 p = 0.227
TM7	r = 0.015 p = 0.945	r = 0.018 p = 0.939
Verrucomicrobia	r = −0.325 p = 0.130	r = 0.209 p = 0.376
Synergistetes	r = −0.211 p = 0.334	r = −0.104 p = 0.661

The associations between serum FFA levels and the abundance of microbial groups at the level of phyla in HC and SLE patients were analyzed by Spearman ranks tests (r coefficient and p-value is indicated for each parameter). Statistical analyses with a p-value below 0.050 are highlighted in bold.

$p = 0.982$), or anti-dsDNA levels ($r = -0.350, p = 0.130$) in SLE. Therefore, parameters other than those indicated may explain the altered serum FFA levels registered in SLE.

Then, we wondered whether gut microbial composition may account for the increased FFA serum levels in SLE. To this aim, the associations between FFA levels and the main intestinal microbial groups analyzed by a metagenomic approach as already described (22) were assessed. As previously reported, diminished *Firmicutes* to *Bacteroidetes* (F/B) ratio characterized the intestinal dysbiosis found in SLE compared to healthy subjects [1.94 (1.51) vs 4.27 (5.93), $p < 0.001$] (22). Among the phyla analyzed (*Actinobacteria, Bacteroidetes, Firmicutes, Cyanobacteria, Euryarchaeota, Fusobacteria, Lentisphaerae, Proteobacteria, Tenericutes,* TM7, *Verrucomicrobia,* and *Synergistetes*), FFA levels displayed opposite correlations with the *Firmicutes* and *Bacteroidetes* groups in HC, but not in lupus patients (**Table 4**). Consequently, a negative association with the F/B ratio was observed in HC, but not in SLE (**Figure 1**). Moreover, this association remained significant after adjusting for potential confounders (**Table 5**). Therefore, F/B ratio was found to be the main predictor of FFA serum levels in HC, whereas this effect was not seen in lupus patients, hallmarked by a decreased F/B ratio and elevated FFA levels.

Since some heterogeneity within groups in the FFA levels was observed and in order to gain more insight into the connections between gut microbiota and serum FFA, further analyses were performed. Focusing on the main microbial groups at the level of phyla, individuals were classified into groups by means of a cluster analysis. Interestingly, two main clusters were identified (thereafter referred to as clusters I and II) (**Figure 2A**), mainly differing in the F/B ratio (8.84 ± 5.53 vs 1.70 ± 0.76, respectively; $p < 0.0001$). Notably, a distinct distribution of individuals was observed, as HC were mainly found within the cluster I (14/25), whereas SLE patients were marginally present in this group (3/21, $p = 0.004$). On the one hand, this result highlights a shift in the microbiota composition in SLE patients compared to HC, hence supporting an association between a biased distribution of the intestinal microbial groups and elevated FFA serum levels. More importantly, when FFA levels were compared among HC and SLE subjects stratified by microbial clusters, it was noted that HC grouping within the cluster II exhibited similar FFA serum levels as SLE patients (**Figure 2B**), thus reinforcing the relevance of the microbiota composition on the FFA serum levels.

Overall, our findings disclose a strong association between FFA levels in serum and specific groups of the gut microbiota in healthy individuals, but not in lupus patients where a profound intestinal dysbiosis was registered.

SCFA and FFA Levels

Our results point to a relationship between the gut microbiota and the host metabolism at the systemic level, but the actual mediators are unclear. Since SCFA may affect the human metabolism

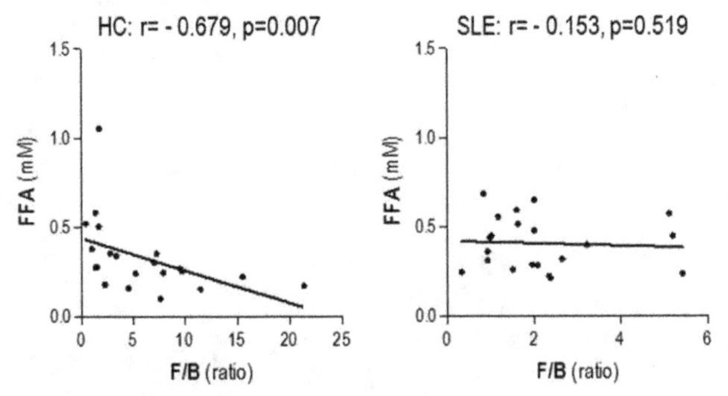

FIGURE 1 | Serum-free fatty acids (FFA) levels and *Firmicutes* to *Bacteroidetes* (F/B) ratio. The association between serum FFA levels and the F/B ratio was analyzed by Spearman's ranks correlation tests.

TABLE 5 | *Firmicutes/Bacteroidetes* (F/B) ratio is the main predictor of FFA levels in healthy controls (HC) but not in systemic lupus erythematosus (SLE) patients.

		β	*B* [95% CI]	*p*
HC	F/B ratio	−0.636	−0.334 [−0.557, −0.111]	**0.007**
	Age	−0.354	−0.652 [−1.436, 0.132]	0.093
	Gender	0.150	0.114 [−0.179, 0.407]	0.405
	BMI	−0.039	−0.002 [−0.022, 0.018]	0.832
	CRP	0.191	0.133 [−0.170, 0.436]	0.352
	Total energy	−0.010	0.001 [−0.044, 0.042]	0.961
	Lipids	0.276	0.003 [−0.004, 0.010]	0.315
	Carbohydrates	−0.372	−0.002 [−0.004, 0.001]	0.073
	Proteins	0.092	0.001 [−0.005, 0.007]	0.690
	Fiber	−0.223	−0.007 [−0.020, 0.005]	0.239
SLE	F/B ratio	−0.025	−0.014 [−0.332, 0.303]	0.923
	Age	−0.229	−0.336 [−1.315, 0.643]	0.466
	BMI	0.415	0.012 [−0.008, 0.032]	0.205
	CRP	0.186	0.072 [−0.191, 0.335]	0.558
	Total energy	−0.072	−0.007 [−0.045, 0.031]	0.687
	Lipids	−0.193	−0.001 [−0.005, 0.003]	0.698
	Carbohydrates	−0.265	−0.001 [−0.003, 0.002]	0.649
	Proteins	0.369	0.002 [−0.002, 0.006]	0.308
	Fiber	−0.351	−0.006 [−0.019, 0.008]	0.365

The association between F/B ratio and FFA serum levels in HC was studied by multiple lineal regression analysis including demographical parameters and nutritional intakes as potential confounders. HC: R^2 (model) = 0.762; SLE: R^2 (model) = 0.426. Statistical analyses with a p-value below 0.050 are highlighted in bold.

and an altered gut microbiota composition leads to a dysregulated SCFA production, the associations between fecal SCFA levels and those of serum FFA were analyzed.

On the one hand, higher levels of all SCFA studied were observed in lupus patients compared to HC (**Table 6**). However, no differences were found between SLE and HC when relative proportions were compared (all $p > 0.050$). On the other hand, all SCFA exhibited a positive correlation with FFA serum levels in HC (**Table 6**).

Importantly, the F/B ratio was negatively correlated to the fecal levels of propionate and butyrate in HC but not in SLE patients (**Figure 3**). Notably, stronger associations were found in HC when only *Bacteroidetes* abundance was considered: propionate ($r = 0.653, p < 0.001$) and butyrate ($r = 0.623, p = 0.002$).

In order to gain further insight into the relevance of the intestinal microbiota and the SCFA production and serum FFA levels, we performed additional analyses by stratifying subjects according to the clusters obtained from the microbiota analysis (**Figure 2**) instead of their clinical condition. Interestingly, a negative association between F/B ratio and fecal SCFA was found in cluster I (propionate: $r = -0.621$, $p = 0.024$ and butyrate: $r = -0.654$, $p = 0.015$), but not in those grouped in cluster II (propionate: $r = -0.015, p = 0.940$ and butyrate: $r = 0.220, p = 0.271$). Overall, this picture mirrors that of found for the HC vs SLE populations according to our previous findings and confirms a pivotal role of the intestinal microbiota in this scenario. However, SCFA and FFA levels did not remain associated after stratifying the whole population by the clusters, hence suggesting the involvement of additional factors, such as the clinical condition, to explain the connection between gut microbiota composition, SCFA, and serum FFA levels.

All these results highlight a role for the gut microbiota in the maintenance of serum FFA levels, SCFA having a potential role orchestrating this interaction. Additional factors, such as disease status, may also influence the outcome of the associations between gut microbiota composition and the interaction SCFA–FFA. Indeed, altered gut microbiota composition found in SLE patients was linked to an altered SCFA production and increased FFA levels in serum, thus supporting this hypothesis.

FFA Profiling in SLE Patients

Although elevated FFA levels were found in SLE, whether a global increase in all FFA species underlies this finding, or if some specific FFA were altered was not clear. To address this issue, a number of FFA species were measured, and the differences between SLE and HC were studied.

Overall, no striking differences were observed between patients and controls (**Table 7**). However, since some collinearity among FFA species existed, a PCA was carried out on the FFA species analyzed to avoid potential biases. PCA demonstrated a good adequacy of the data (KMO statistic = 0.781, Barlett sphericity test $p = 10^{-44}$), and three components were identified (eigenvalues >1) explaining 77.53% of the total variance. Based on their loadings, PC1 (53.32% variance explained) retained γ-linolenic, palmitoleic, palmitic, oleic, linolenic, linoleic, and arachidonic acids, and PC2 (13.95% variance explained) mainly retained EPA and DHA. Finally, PC3 (10.26% variance explained) only retained stearic acid (**Figure 4**).

On the one hand, these results underlie the outstanding heterogeneity of FFA species, a clearly distinct pattern of grouping depending on their chemical structure (chain length or double-bond position) not being found. Globally, saturated, monounsaturated, and w6 fatty acids were grouped together within the PC1, whereas the most important anti-inflammatory w3 FFA did in the PC2. Stearic acid, of controversial immunological and metabolic role, was grouped in the third component. Hence, these findings support a functional, rather than structural, relationship of FFA.

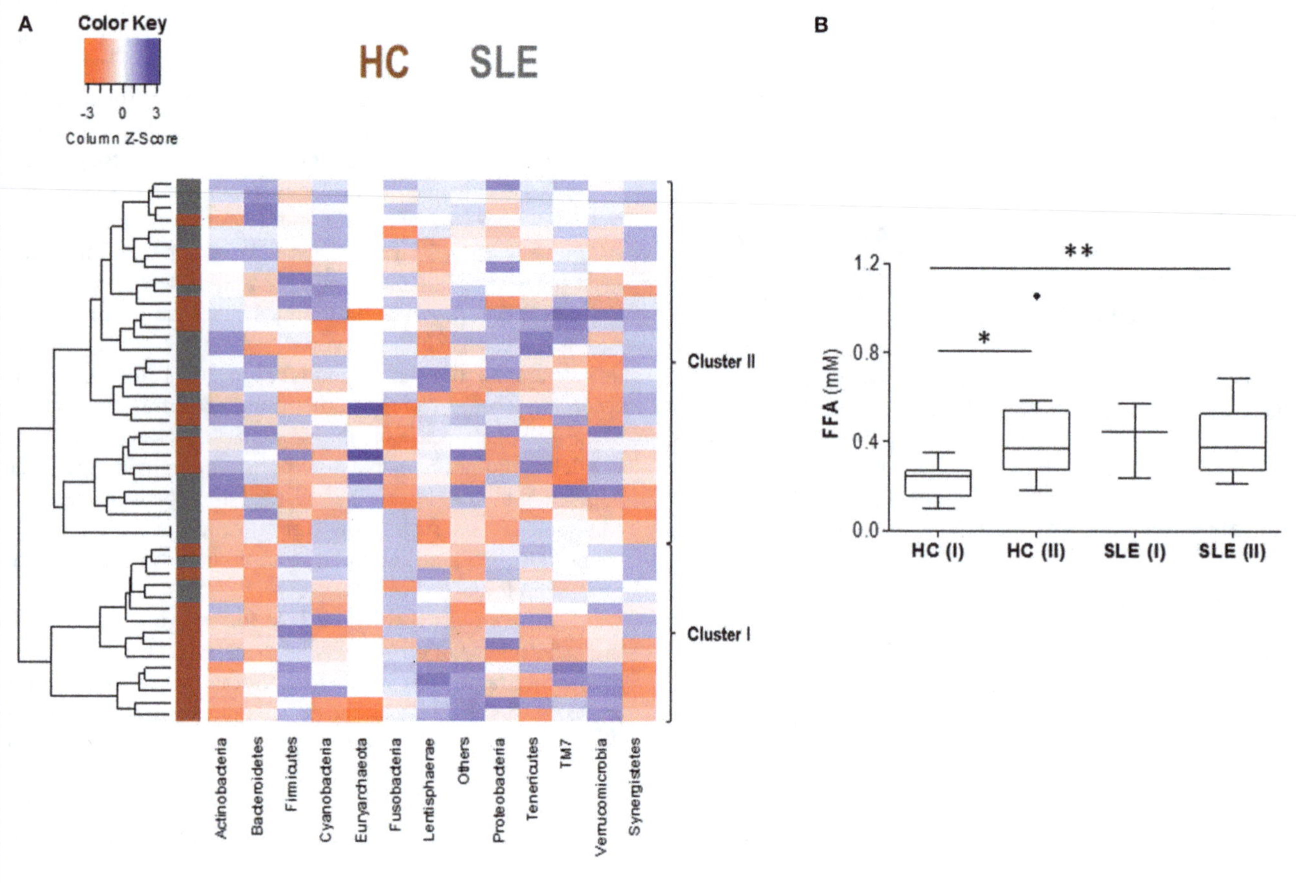

FIGURE 2 | Cluster analysis revealed a link between gut microbiota composition and total free fatty acids (FFA) serum levels. (A) Heatmap plotting gut microbiota composition, based on the main phyla, in healthy controls (HC) and systemic lupus erythematosus (SLE) patients. Tiles are colored based on the abundance of each group, red and blue colors indicating low or high levels, respectively. Each row represents an individual, and the vertical colored bar at the left represents HC (dark red) or SLE patient (gray). Two clusters were identified and are highlighted at the right (clusters I and II). **(B)** Comparison of total FFA serum levels among groups after stratifying by disease status (HC or SLE) and microbiota clusters (I or II). Boxes represent median and interquartile range, whereas whiskers represent minimum and maximum values. Differences were assessed by Kruskal–Wallis test and Dunn–Bonferroni *post hoc* correction for multiple comparisons tests. $^{*}p < 0.050$, $^{**}p < 0.010$.

TABLE 6 | Analysis of fecal short-chain fatty acids (SCFA) levels and their correlation with serum-free fatty acids (FFA) levels in healthy controls (HC) and systemic lupus erythematosus (SLE) patients.

	HC	SLE	*p*
SCFA levels (mM)			
Acetate	41.14 (12.30)	57.63 (19.63)	**0.005**
Propionate	11.96 (8.72)	20.61 (9.80)	**0.003**
Butyrate	7.78 (3.97)	10.50 (7.14)	0.075
SCFA–FFA correlations			
Acetate	$\mathbf{r = 0.770}$ $\mathbf{p < 0.001}$	$r = 0.067$ $p = 0.793$	
Propionate	$\mathbf{r = 0.790}$ $\mathbf{p < 0.001}$	$r = 0.230$ $p = 0.359$	
Butyrate	$\mathbf{r = 0.764}$ $\mathbf{p < 0.001}$	$r = -0.066$ $p = 0.795$	

The differences between fecal SCFA levels found in lupus patients and those in HC were analyzed by Mann–Withney U tests; whereas the correlation analyses were performed by Spearman rank's tests. Variables are summarized as median (interquartile range). Statistical analyses with a p-value below 0.050 are highlighted in bold.

On the other hand, no differences in the PCA scores were registered between SLE and HC groups (PC1: $p = 0.169$, PC2: $p = 0.378$, and PC3: $p = 0.916$), thus suggesting that SLE patients did not exhibit a different FFA profile compared to HC.

Finally, whether PCA scores could be related to gut microbiota composition was analyzed. Notably, F/B ratio was positively correlated with the PC2 score (**Table 8**) in HC but not in SLE, thereby suggesting a beneficial effect of gut microbiota composition on the serum FFA pool in healthy individuals. Again, when the phyla were independently studied, *Bacteroidetes* exhibited a stronger correlation with PC2 score ($r = -0.433$, $p = 0.039$) than that of *Firmicutes* ($r = 0.411$, $p = 0.052$) in HC individuals. Thus, gut microbiota seems to quantitatively and qualitatively impact the FFA serum pool.

FFA and Serum Biomarkers in SLE Patients

Since some associations between gut microbiota and specific FFA PCA scores were observed, we aimed to evaluate whether these

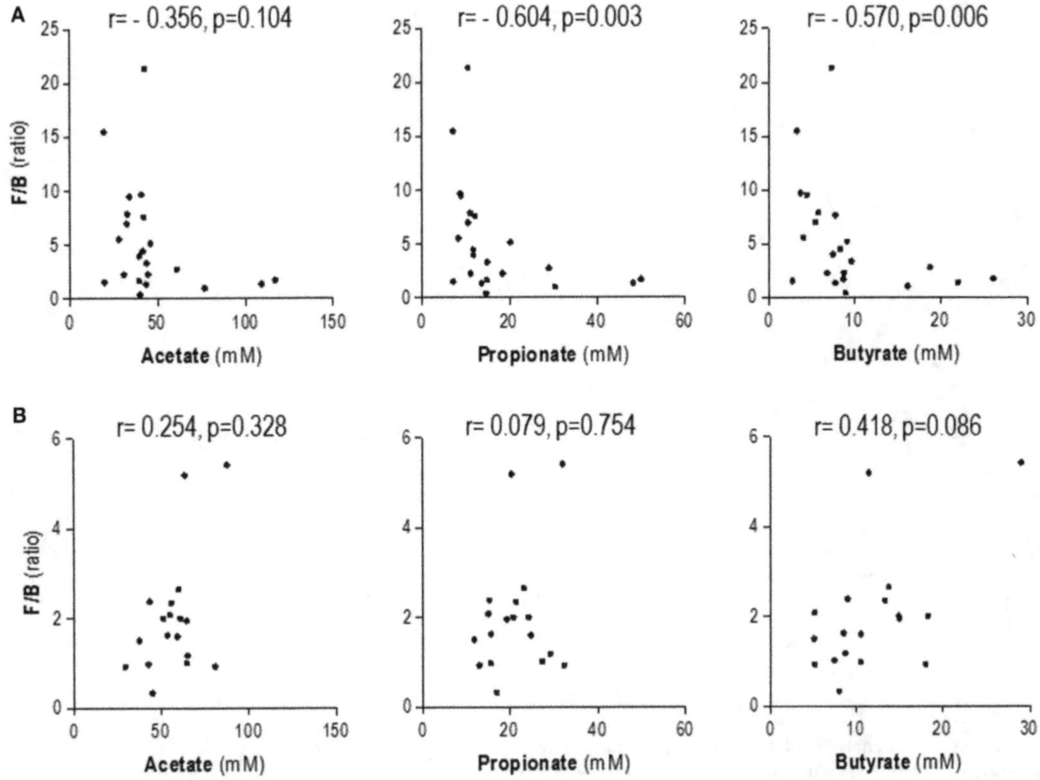

FIGURE 3 | Association between fecal short-chain fatty acids (SCFA) levels and *Firmicutes* to *Bacteroidetes* ratio. Correlation analyses by Spearman's ranks tests were performed in order to analyze the association between fecal SCFA levels and those of serum-free fatty acids in healthy controls **(A)** and systemic lupus erythematosus patients **(B)**.

TABLE 7 | Specific free fatty acids (FFA) in healthy controls (HC) and systemic lupus erythematosus (SLE) patients.

FFA (μg/ml)	HC	SLE	p
Palmitic (16:0)	32.76 (15.59)	30.35 (8.37)	0.982
Stearic (18:0)	28.51 (12.95)	29.12 (6.19)	0.873
Palmitoleic (16:1ω7)	1.93 (1.62)	2.67 (0.99)	0.351
Oleic (18:1ω9)	27.76 (20.61)	34.39 (17.77)	0.467
Linoleic (18:2ω6)	6.99 (6.47)	10.26 (7.35)	0.246
γ-Linoleic (18:3ω6)	0.08 (0.08)	0.10 (0.06)	0.785
AA (20:4ω6)	1.96 (1.68)	2.74 (1.74)	**0.045**
Linolenic (18:3ω3)	0.18 (0.17)	0.20 (0.16)	0.539
EPA (20:5ω3)	0.07 (0.15)	0.15 (0.17)	0.363
DHA (22:6ω3)	1.47 (1.46)	1.65 (1.76)	0.209

The differences in specific FFA serum levels between control and patients were assessed by Mann–Withney U tests. Variables are summarized as median (interquartile range). Statistical analyses with a p-value below 0.050 are highlighted in bold.

parameters could be related to some relevant serum biomarkers in lupus. To this end, a panel of serum biomarkers of endothelial activation (VEGF, GM-CSF, EGF, IL-8, TNFα, MCP-1, IP-10, and leptin) and oxidative stress (MDA) were measured (**Table 9**).

First, the associations between these biomarkers and the gut microbiota composition were analyzed. Interestingly, the F/B ratio was negatively associated to leptin ($r = -0.369$, $p = 0.006$) and MCP-1 serum levels ($r = -0.304$, $p = 0.025$) in the whole group.

On the other hand, divergent associations were noted among FFA PCA scores and these biomarkers in SLE patients. Whereas PC1 was positively correlated with biomarkers of endothelial activation [VEGF ($r = 0.444$, $p = 0.044$), IL-8 ($r = 0.522$, 0.015), and EGF ($r = 0.400$, $p = 0.070$)], negative associations were observed for PC2 [EGF ($r = -0.425$, $p = 0.055$), MCP-1 ($r = -0.640$, $p = 0.002$), IP-10 ($r = -0.397$, $p = 0.075$), TNFα ($r = -0.410$, $p = 0.065$), and MDA ($r = -0.375$, $p = 0.057$)]. Interestingly, negative associations were also found for PC3 [VEGF ($r = -0.534$, $p = 0.013$) and IL-8 ($r = -0.459$, $p = 0.036$)]. No associations were observed in the HC.

All these findings seem to point to a link between gut microbiota, FFA serum pool, and biomarkers of endothelial activation in lupus, thus emphasizing the systemic effect of the gut microbiota in this condition. Additionally, differences among FFA PCA are in line with their proposed functional diversity.

DISCUSSION

Over the last decade, several studies have revealed a number of interactions between the gut microbiota and the host in homeostatic conditions. Accordingly, dysbiosis has been consistently related to different pathological situations, from immune-mediated to metabolic diseases (27–29). In this sense, we have recently reported the existence of an intestinal dysbiosis in SLE

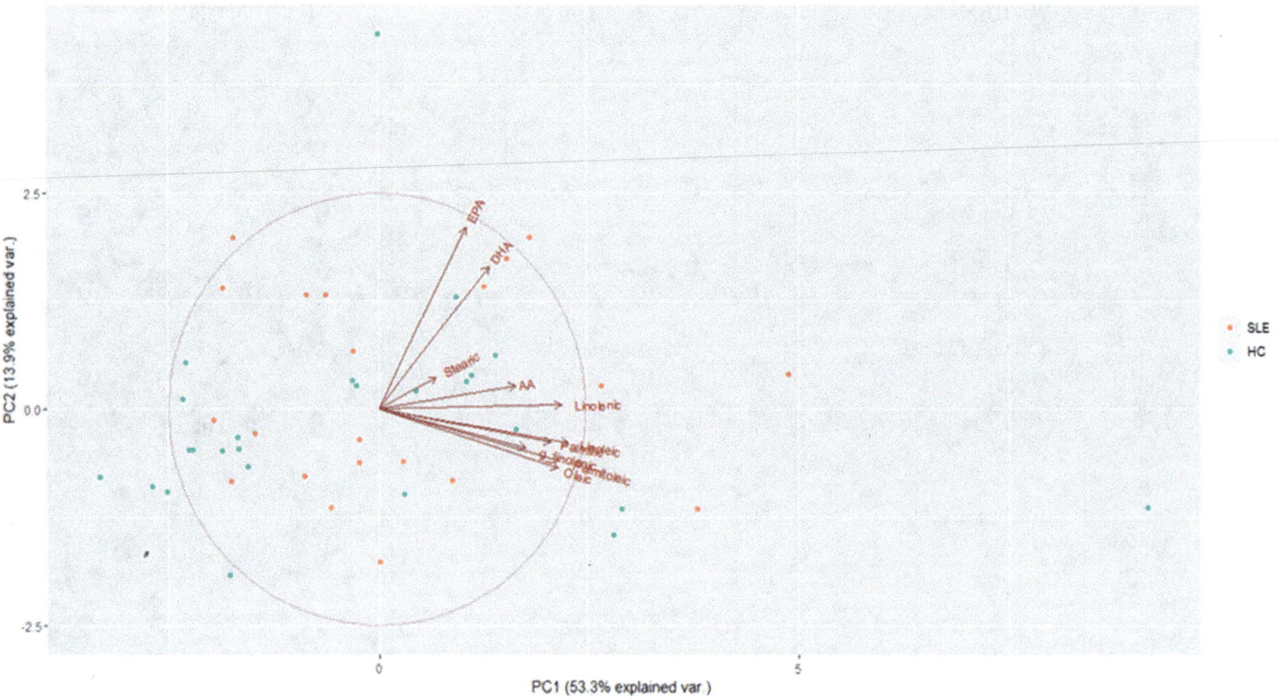

FIGURE 4 | Principal component analysis (PCA) of specific free fatty acids (FFA) profiling. Biplot obtained in the PCA of specific FFA serum levels. PC1 and PC2 are represented in the horizontal and vertical axes, respectively. Arrows represent the vectors showing the associations among the raw variables entered in the analysis. Individuals are represented in colored dots: healthy controls (HC) (turquoise) and systemic lupus erythematosus (SLE) (red).

TABLE 8 | Associations between *Firmicutes* to *Bacteroidetes* ratio and free fatty acids-principal component analysis scores in healthy controls (HC) and systemic lupus erythematosus (SLE) patients.

	HC	SLE
PC1	$r = -0.246$ $p = 0.257$	$r = 0.078$ $p = 0.736$
PC2	**$r = 0.437$** **$p = 0.037$**	$r = 0.110$ $p = 0.635$
PC3	$r = -0.075$ $p = 0.734$	$r = 0.089$ $p = 0.700$

Correlations between these parameters were assessed by Pearson correlation tests. Statistical analyses with a p-value below 0.050 are highlighted in bold.

TABLE 9 | Levels of serum biomarkers analyzed in healthy controls (HC) and systemic lupus erythematosus (SLE) patients.

	HC	SLE	p
Vascular endothelial growth factor [VEGF] (pg/ml)	83.38 (49.49)	70.73 (98.87)	0.326
Granulocyte monocyte colonystimulating factor [GM-CSF] (pg/ml)	0.35 (0.92)	0.35 (2.77)	0.424
Epidermal growth factor [EGF] (pg/ml)	114.29 (81.35)	65.57 (78.61)	**0.019**
Interleukin-8 [IL-8] (pg/ml)	14.69 (22.51)	27.85 (21.92)	**0.016**
Tumor necrosis factor alpha [TNFα] (pg/ml)	174.40 (309.4)	188.14 (292.92)	0.789
Monocyte chemoattractant protein-1 [MCP-1] (pg/ml)	444.55 (481.45)	616.13 (402.07)	**0.011**
Interferon gamma-inducible protein-10 [IP-10] (pg/ml)	98.82 (148.81)	167.67 (152.76)	**0.019**
Leptin (ng/ml)	7.73 (7.14)	14.16 (20.20)	**<0.001**
Malondialdehyde [MDA] (μM)	2.78 (0.71)	2.90 (0.44)	0.658

The differences in serum levels between control and patients were assessed by Mann–Withney U tests. Variables are summarized as median (interquartile range). Statistical analyses with a p-value below 0.050 are highlighted in bold.

(22). Additional studies from our group allowed us to associate the dysbiotic state with the dysregulated Treg/Th17 responses found in lupus patients (30). In the present report, we go a step further by addressing the study of the potential connections between the intestinal dysbiosis and the metabolic impairment in SLE, focusing on the role of FFA. Thus, gut microbiota may not only be related to disease pathogenesis itself but also to some comorbidities frequently present in lupus patients. Since the origin of such alterations is ill-defined, these new findings allow us to gain some insight into this complex situation and may help to delineate new therapeutic targets. Actually, the experimental modulation of the gut microbiota has yielded promising results in other scenarios (17). In fact, the lupus-like immune over-activation was partially reestablished *in vitro* by the supplementation with specific bacterial strains (30). Thus, our study warrants future research to assess whether this therapy may be also advisable to counteract the metabolic alterations in SLE patients.

Metabolic disorders, including metabolic syndrome, are common hallmarks of SLE and other related diseases (31–33).

However, the underlying causes of these traits are not well defined. The findings herein presented suggest that gut microbiota may play a role in this condition. This notion can explain why a wide range of diseases, with striking differences in their clinical presentations, are associated with similar comorbidities (such as metabolic alterations). Thus, it is feasible to think that similar patterns of intestinal dysbiosis may underlie this situation. This idea is supported by the altered F/B ratios that were reported in other diseases exhibiting increased serum FFA levels (34–36). The fact that this ratio is a continuum may explain the differences in prevalence and severity of metabolic complications among different conditions. However, it must be remarked that studies on the alterations in the F/B ratio have yielded contradictory results in different contexts, such as obesity (37–39). Schwiertz and colleagues have recently published a reduced F/B ratio in obese and overweighed individuals in a large study population (40). Similarly, the enrichment of *Firmicutes* in the intestinal ecosystem has been related to improved lipid absorption and homeostasis in animal models (41). It must be taken into account that differences in sequencing techniques, data analysis, and characteristics of the recruited populations may be an important source of discrepancy in this field. Thus, the associations of the microbiota with metabolic traits in different scenarios must be interpreted with caution, since direct comparison is not always possible. Additional studies focusing on the F/B ratio in non-obese healthy population are warranted.

The association between the F/B ratio and the serum levels of FFA emphasizes the ability of the gut microbiota to promote systemic responses in the host. Moreover, it supports that gut microbiota can modulate the energy metabolism of the host (42). However, the identification of the actual mediators involved and the potential impact of this interaction in pathological conditions is currently lacking in the literature. Our findings in the present work point to the SCFA as potential orchestrators of the cross talk between gut microbiota and the host metabolism. Although these compounds are thought to be of key relevance in the interactions between intestinal microbial populations and the host (16), their link with the lipid metabolism remains controversial. Our results suggest that the SCFA production paralleled the FFA serum levels in healthy individuals. However, this association was absent in the pathological framework of lupus, where an increased SCFA production, together with elevated FFA serum levels, was noted. These results are in line with those from other metabolic conditions [reviewed in Ref. (43)]. Additionally, our analyses revealed that this aberrant SCFA production can be linked to an altered microbial gut composition, as a reduced F/B ratio was related to increased SCFA fecal levels. In this scenario, the potential involvement of the propionate deserves a special mention. Propionate is mainly produced by *Bacteroidetes* species (44), thereby supporting its negative association with the F/B ratio observed. It is important to note that increased propionate fecal levels have been reported in obese individuals exhibiting a decreased F/B ratio (40). Furthermore, exposure of human intestinal organoids to propionate led to an upregulation of genes belonging to lipolytic pathways (45). Moreover, experimental evidence from animal models and *ex vivo* experiments with human material have identified a mechanistic link between exposure to propionate and increased lipolysis mediated by the increased expression of the enzyme lipoprotein lipase (46–48). Moreover, a homeostatic role for propionate on glucose metabolism and regulation of energy intake has also been proposed. However, which is the actual role for propionate in human diseases required further elucidation. Taken together, our finding may provide a possible explanation for the elevated FFA serum levels in SLE, altered SCFA production, and overrepresentation of *Bacteroidetes* in the intestinal microbiota playing a pivotal role. The stronger associations of *Bacteroidetes* alone compared with those of the F/B ratio are in line with this point.

Another important result of our study was the association between FFA and some biomarkers of endothelial activation. Because of their nature, FFA are considered as common mediators between immunity, inflammation, and metabolism. Although some authors have previously proposed a role for the gut microbiota in the etiology of metabolic alterations and CVD (49), the actual players are far from being clear. Interestingly, experimental studies revealed a mechanistic link between propionate and leptin expression by human adipose and omental tissues (50), which is in line with our results. Nevertheless, the exact significance of this finding *in vivo* is not known. Taking into account the effects of FFA on inflammation, oxidative stress, and expression of adhesion molecules (51–53), our results may support a role for FFA as a link between the (altered) gut microbiota, host metabolism, and disease status. It is interesting to note that differences among FFA in their ability to promote endothelial activation *in vivo* or *in vitro* have been demonstrated (54–56), which is in line with the associations found in our study. Importantly, these biomarkers are considered as early preclinical indicators of CVD development in the long term (57–60). Taking this into account, these associations may point to a very early role of the altered gut microbiota in the etiology of these complications. This is reinforced by the negative association between the intestinal dysbiosis in lupus and the levels of the protective IgM antibodies against phosphorylcholine (30). These antibodies are known to enhance apoptotic-cell clearance and induce anti-inflammatory pathways, explaining its negative association with markers of subclinical atherosclerosis (61) and CVD development (62) in lupus.

Finally, our approach did not identify a different FFA serum profile in SLE patients in comparison to HC. Although a similar pattern of grouping of FFA species in the PCA was observed in rheumatoid arthritis patients by our group (24), differences among FFA species between patients and controls were not observed in the case of lupus. Interestingly, no differences in plasma FFA profiling were observed in a previous study with lupus patients (63), although slight alterations in the polyunsaturated fatty acids were reported in those with a previous history of CVD. Our results are, at least in part, in line with these findings, although differences in the experimental procedures between both studies are important. It is worthy to note that our group of patients was characterized by a low disease activity, even in the absence of glucocorticoid and immunosuppressive drugs. Thus, a larger study involving SLE patients with a higher degree of disease activity is warranted. However, despite no differences being found in the specific FFA levels, the results from the PCA emphasize the heterogeneity among FFA classes and suggest that FFA, despite being mostly unaltered, can develop different roles under different milieu. This hypothesis is in line with current evidence in this field (64, 65) and stresses the underestimated significance of FFA as key mediators for the human health.

Due to the lack of direct mechanistic data in our approach, these results pose the question on whether the microbiota composition is responsible of the altered FFA levels or if, alternatively, increased FFA levels may lead to changes in the gut ecology. Based on the literature currently available, several research studies seem to align with the former idea. The fact that no changes in the gut microbiota were related to disease duration (in spite of the wide range of disease duration studied in the present report) is also in line with this idea, probably suggesting that intestinal dysbiosis could be present at the preclinical stages of the disease. Similarly, experiments of fecal transplantation in obese and lean mice also support the causative role of the microbiota in shaping the host metabolism (66). However, due to the role of FFA on inflammation, it is tempting to speculate that these molecules can prompt a shift toward a systemic pro-inflammatory state, which can, in turn, disrupt the intestinal microbiota. Experimental studies with mice have revealed that diet-induced obesity is accompanied by changes in the gut microbiota and damaged intestinal barrier (67, 68). Interestingly, a diet with high ω6 content resulted in intestinal dysbiosis in mice, the inflammatory pathways playing a crucial role (69). Moreover, ω3 fatty acids seem to counteract the effects of diet- or antibiotics-induced dysbiosis through different mechanisms (70, 71). Additionally, an antibacterial effect was observed for some FFA (72). Therefore, it is feasible that a bidirectional cross talk between the gut microbiota and host metabolism is established, with immune circuits participating in this interaction.

In summary, our data indicate that increased serum FFA levels in SLE patients may be associated with changes in the gut ecosystem in the framework of lupus dysbiosis. The association between serum FFA and SCFA supports this notion. Additionally, different associations between FFA species and serum biomarkers of endothelial activation were found, hence not only underscoring the heterogeneity among FFA compounds but also shedding new light on the gut–metabolism–CVD axis. Although the reduced sample size and the lack of a mechanistic data are the limitations of our study, to the best of our knowledge this is the first report supporting a connection between gut microbiota, FFA, and biomarkers of endothelial activation. Moreover, we have provided a proof of concept evidence on the involvement of the intestinal dysbiosis in the metabolic alterations in lupus.

AUTHOR CONTRIBUTIONS

All the authors listed made substantial contributions to the design of the work, analysis, or interpretation of the results obtained; involved in drafting the manuscript, revising it critically for intellectual content, and approving the final version; and agreed to be accountable for all aspects of the work in ensuring that questions related to the accuracy or integrity of any part of the work are appropriately investigated and resolved.

ACKNOWLEDGMENTS

The authors acknowledge the excellent technical assistance of Ana M. Hernández-Barranco (IPLA) with the analysis of SCFA in fecal samples as well as of the staff of the scientific core facilities from the University of Oviedo (Unidad de Espectrometría y Espectrofotometría, Servicios Científico-Técnicos, Universidad de Oviedo) with the FFA analysis. The authors also show our deepest gratitude to all the study volunteers.

REFERENCES

1. Saegusa J, Irino Y, Yoshida M, Tanaka S, Kogata Y, Kageyama G, et al. GC/MS-based metabolomics detects metabolic alterations in serum from SLE patients. *Clin Exp Rheumatol* (2014) 32(1):148.
2. Demir S, Artim-Esen B, Şahinkaya Y, Pehlivan Ö, Alpay-Kanıtez N, Omma A, et al. Metabolic syndrome is not only a risk factor for cardiovascular diseases in systemic lupus erythematosus but is also associated with cumulative organ damage: a cross-sectional analysis of 311 patients. *Lupus* (2016) 25:177–84. doi:10.1177/0961203315603140
3. Parker B, Bruce IN. The metabolic syndrome in systemic lupus erythematosus. *Rheum Dis Clin North Am* (2010) 36:81–97, viii. doi:10.1016/j.rdc.2009.12.004
4. Bartels CM, Buhr KA, Goldberg JW, Bell CL, Visekruna M, Nekkanti S, et al. Mortality and cardiovascular burden of systemic lupus erythematosus in a US population-based cohort. *J Rheumatol* (2014) 41:680–7. doi:10.3899/jrheum.130874
5. Esdaile JM, Abrahamowicz M, Grodzicky T, Li Y, Panaritis C, Berger R, et al. Traditional Framingham risk factors fail to fully account for accelerated atherosclerosis in systemic lupus erythematosus. *Arthritis Rheum* (2001) 44:2331–7. doi:10.1002/1529-0131(200110)44:10<2331::AID-ART395>3.0.CO;2-I
6. Bartoloni E, Shoenfeld Y, Gerli R. Inflammatory and autoimmune mechanisms in the induction of atherosclerotic damage in systemic rheumatic diseases: two faces of the same coin. *Arthritis Care Res* (2011) 63:178–83. doi:10.1002/acr.20322
7. Symmons DP, Gabriel SE. Epidemiology of CVD in rheumatic disease, with a focus on RA and SLE. *Nat Rev Rheumatol* (2011) 7:399–408. doi:10.1038/nrrheum.2011.75
8. López-Pedrera C, Barbarroja N, Jimenez-Gomez Y, Collantes-Estevez E, Aguirre MA, Cuadrado MJ. Oxidative stress in the pathogenesis of atherothrombosis associated with anti-phospholipid syndrome and systemic lupus erythematosus: new therapeutic approaches. *Rheumatology (Oxford)* (2016) 55(12):2096–108. doi:10.1093/rheumatology/kew054
9. Boden G. Obesity and free fatty acids. *Endocrinol Metab Clin North Am* (2008) 37:635–46, viii–ix. doi:10.1016/j.ecl.2008.06.007
10. de Jong AJ, Kloppenburg M, Toes RE, Ioan-Facsinay A. Fatty acids, lipid mediators, and T-cell function. *Front Immunol* (2014) 5:483. doi:10.3389/fimmu.2014.00483
11. Ormseth MJ, Swift LL, Fazio S, Linton MF, Raggi P, Solus JF, et al. Free fatty acids are associated with metabolic syndrome and insulin resistance but not inflammation in systemic lupus erythematosus. *Lupus* (2013) 22:26–33. doi:10.1177/0961203312462756
12. Saito I. Epidemiological evidence of type 2 diabetes mellitus, metabolic syndrome, and cardiovascular disease in Japan. *Circ J* (2012) 76:1066–73. doi:10.1253/circj.CJ-11-1519
13. Shaw JE, Zimmet PZ, George K, Alberti MM. Metabolic syndrome-do we really need a new definition? *Metab Syndr Relat Disord* (2005) 3:191–3. doi:10.1089/met.2005.3.191
14. Chang Y, Jung H-S, Yun KE, Cho J, Ahn J, Chung EC, et al. Metabolically healthy obesity is associated with an increased risk of diabetes independently of nonalcoholic fatty liver disease. *Obesity (Silver Spring)* (2016) 24:1996–2003. doi:10.1002/oby.21580
15. Cheng FW, Gao X, Mitchell DC, Wood C, Rolston DD, Still CD, et al. Metabolic health status and the obesity paradox in older adults. *J Nutr Gerontol Geriatr* (2016) 35:161–76. doi:10.1080/21551197.2016.1199004

16. Canfora EE, Jocken JW, Blaak EE. Short-chain fatty acids in control of body weight and insulin sensitivity. *Nat Rev Endocrinol* (2015) 11:577–91. doi:10.1038/nrendo.2015.128
17. Boulangé CL, Neves AL, Chilloux J, Nicholson JK, Dumas ME. Impact of the gut microbiota on inflammation, obesity, and metabolic disease. *Genome Med* (2016) 8:42. doi:10.1186/s13073-016-0303-2
18. Brestoff JR, Artis D. Commensal bacteria at the interface of host metabolism and the immune system. *Nat Immunol* (2013) 14:676–84. doi:10.1038/ni.2640
19. Clarke G, Stilling RM, Kennedy PJ, Stanton C, Cryan JF, Dinan TG. Minireview: gut microbiota: the neglected endocrine organ. *Mol Endocrinol* (2014) 28:1221–38. doi:10.1210/me.2014-1108
20. Sharon G, Garg N, Debelius J, Knight R, Dorrestein PC, Mazmanian SK. Specialized metabolites from the microbiome in health and disease. *Cell Metab* (2014) 20:719–30. doi:10.1016/j.cmet.2014.10.016
21. Marchesi JR, Adams DH, Fava F, Hermes GD, Hirschfield GM, Hold G, et al. The gut microbiota and host health: a new clinical frontier. *Gut* (2016) 65:330–9. doi:10.1136/gutjnl-2015-309990
22. Hevia A, Milani C, López P, Cuervo A, Arboleya S, Duranti S, et al. Intestinal dysbiosis associated with systemic lupus erythematosus. *mBio* (2014) 5:e1548–1514. doi:10.1128/mBio.01548-14.Invited
23. Tan EM, Cohen AS, Fries JF, Masi AT, McShane DJ, Rothfield NF, et al. The 1982 revised criteria for the classification of systemic lupus erythematosus. *Arthritis Rheum* (1982) 25:1271–7. doi:10.1002/art.1780251101
24. Rodríguez-Carrio J, Alperi-López M, López P, Ballina-García FJ, Suárez A. Non-esterified fatty acids profiling in rheumatoid arthritis: associations with clinical features and Th1 response. *PLoS One* (2016) 11:e0159573. doi:10.1371/journal.pone.0159573
25. Cuervo A, Hevia A, López P, Suárez A, Sánchez B, Margolles A, et al. Association of polyphenols from oranges and apples with specific intestinal microorganisms in systemic lupus erythematosus patients. *Nutrients* (2015) 7:1301–17. doi:10.3390/nu7021301
26. Centro de Enseñanza Superior de Nutrición Humana y Dietética (CESNID). *Tablas de composición de alimentos por medidas caseras de consumo habitual en España*. Barcelona: McGraw-Hill Publicaciones y Ediciones de la Universidad de Barcelona (2008).
27. Tilg H, Adolph TE. Influence of the human intestinal microbiome on obesity and metabolic dysfunction. *Curr Opin Pediatr* (2015) 27:496–501. doi:10.1097/MOP.0000000000000234
28. Peterson CT, Sharma V, Elmén L, Peterson SN. Immune homeostasis, dysbiosis and therapeutic modulation of the gut microbiota. *Clin Exp Immunol* (2015) 179:363–77. doi:10.1111/cei.12474
29. Honda K, Littman DR. The microbiota in adaptive immune homeostasis and disease. *Nature* (2016) 535:75–84. doi:10.1038/nature18848
30. López P, de Paz B, Rodríguez-Carrio J, Hevia A, Sánchez B, Margolles A, et al. Th17 responses and natural IgM antibodies are related to gut microbiota composition in systemic lupus erythematosus patients. *Sci Rep* (2016) 6:24072. doi:10.1038/srep24072
31. Parker B, Ahmad Y, Shelmerdine J, Edlin H, Yates AP, Teh LS, et al. An analysis of the metabolic syndrome phenotype in systemic lupus erythematosus. *Lupus* (2011) 20:1459–65. doi:10.1177/0961203311416695
32. Sidiropoulos PI, Karvounaris SA, Boumpas DT. Metabolic syndrome in rheumatic diseases: epidemiology, pathophysiology, and clinical implications. *Arthritis Res Ther* (2008) 10:207. doi:10.1186/ar2397
33. Parker B, Urowitz MB, Gladman DD, Lunt M, Donn R, Bae SC, et al. Impact of early disease factors on metabolic syndrome in systemic lupus erythematosus: data from an international inception cohort. *Ann Rheum Dis* (2015) 74:1530–6. doi:10.1136/annrheumdis-2013-203933
34. Wong VW-S, Tse C-H, Lam TT-Y, Wong GL-H, Chim AM-L, Chu WC-W, et al. Molecular characterization of the fecal microbiota in patients with nonalcoholic steatohepatitis – a longitudinal study. *PLoS One* (2013) 8:e62885. doi:10.1371/journal.pone.0062885
35. Zhu L, Baker SS, Gill C, Liu W, Alkhouri R, Baker RD, et al. Characterization of gut microbiomes in nonalcoholic steatohepatitis (NASH) patients: a connection between endogenous alcohol and NASH. *Hepatology* (2013) 57:601–9. doi:10.1002/hep.26093
36. Larsen N, Vogensen FK, van den Berg FWJ, Nielsen DS, Andreasen AS, Pedersen BK, et al. Gut microbiota in human adults with type 2 diabetes differs from non-diabetic adults. *PLoS One* (2010) 5:e9085. doi:10.1371/journal.pone.0009085
37. Ley RE, Turnbaugh PJ, Klein S, Gordon JI. Microbial ecology: human gut microbes associated with obesity. *Nature* (2006) 444:1022–3. doi:10.1038/4441022a
38. Ley RE, Bäckhed F, Turnbaugh P, Lozupone CA, Knight RD, Gordon JI. Obesity alters gut microbial ecology. *Proc Natl Acad Sci U S A* (2005) 102:11070–5. doi:10.1073/pnas.0504978102
39. Raman M, Ahmed I, Gillevet PM, Probert CS, Ratcliffe NM, Smith S, et al. Fecal microbiome and volatile organic compound metabolome in obese humans with nonalcoholic fatty liver disease. *Clin Gastroenterol Hepatol* (2013) 11: 868-75.e1–3. doi:10.1016/j.cgh.2013.02.015
40. Schwiertz A, Taras D, Schäfer K, Beijer S, Bos NA, Donus C, et al. Microbiota and SCFA in lean and overweight healthy subjects. *Obesity (Silver Spring)* (2010) 18:190–5. doi:10.1038/oby.2009.167
41. Semova I, Carten JD, Stombaugh J, Mackey LC, Knight R, Farber SA, et al. Microbiota regulate intestinal absorption and metabolism of fatty acids in the zebrafish. *Cell Host Microbe* (2012) 12:277–88. doi:10.1016/j.chom.2012.08.003
42. Bäckhed F, Ding H, Wang T, Hooper LV, Koh GY, Nagy A, et al. The gut microbiota as an environmental factor that regulates fat storage. *Proc Natl Acad Sci U S A* (2004) 101:15718–23. doi:10.1073/pnas.0407076101
43. Ríos-Covián D, Ruas-Madiedo P, Margolles A, Gueimonde M, de Los Reyes-Gavilán CG, Salazar N. Intestinal short chain fatty acids and their link with diet and human health. *Front Microbiol* (2016) 7:185. doi:10.3389/fmicb.2016.00185
44. Salonen A, Lahti L, Salojärvi J, Holtrop G, Korpela K, Duncan SH, et al. Impact of diet and individual variation on intestinal microbiota composition and fermentation products in obese men. *ISME J* (2014) 8:2218–30. doi:10.1038/ismej.2014.63
45. Lukovac S, Belzer C, Pellis L, Keijser BJ, de Vos WM, Montijn RC, et al. Differential modulation by *Akkermansia muciniphila* and *Faecalibacterium prausnitzii* of host peripheral lipid metabolism and histone acetylation in mouse gut organoids. *MBio* (2014) 5:e01438–14. doi:10.1128/mBio.01438-14
46. Lee SH, Hossner KL. Coordinate regulation of ovine adipose tissue gene expression by propionate. *J Anim Sci* (2002) 80:2840–9. doi:10.2527/2002.80112840x
47. Merkel M, Eckel RH, Goldberg IJ. Lipoprotein lipase: genetics, lipid uptake, and regulation. *J Lipid Res* (2002) 43:1997–2006. doi:10.1194/jlr.R200015-JLR200
48. Al-Lahham S, Roelofsen H, Rezaee F, Weening D, Hoek A, Vonk R, et al. Propionic acid affects immune status and metabolism in adipose tissue from overweight subjects. *Eur J Clin Invest* (2012) 42:357–64. doi:10.1111/j.1365-2362.2011.02590.x
49. Harris K, Kassis A, Major G, Chou CJ. Is the gut microbiota a new factor contributing to obesity and its metabolic disorders? *J Obes* (2012) 2012:879151. doi:10.1155/2012/879151
50. Al-Lahham SH, Roelofsen H, Priebe M, Weening D, Dijkstra M, Hoek A, et al. Regulation of adipokine production in human adipose tissue by propionic acid. *Eur J Clin Invest* (2010) 40:401–7. doi:10.1111/j.1365-2362.2010.02278.x
51. Mathew M, Tay E, Cusi K. Elevated plasma free fatty acids increase cardiovascular risk by inducing plasma biomarkers of endothelial activation, myeloperoxidase and PAI-1 in healthy subjects. *Cardiovasc Diabetol* (2010) 9:9. doi:10.1186/1475-2840-9-9
52. Tripathy D, Aljada A, Dandona P. Free fatty acids (FFA) and endothelial dysfunction; role of increased oxidative stress and inflammation. – to: Steinberg et al. (2002) Vascular function, insulin resistance and fatty acids. *Diabetologia* (2003) 46:300–1. doi:10.1007/s00125-002-1027-y
53. Steinberg HO, Baron AD. Vascular function, insulin resistance and fatty acids. *Diabetologia* (2002) 45:623–34. doi:10.1007/s00125-002-0800-2
54. Ishida T, Naoe S, Nakakuki M, Kawano H, Imada K. Eicosapentaenoic acid prevents saturated fatty acid-induced vascular endothelial dysfunction: involvement of long-chain Acyl-CoA synthetase. *J Atheroscler Thromb* (2015) 22:1172–85. doi:10.5551/jat.28167
55. Newens KJ, Thompson AK, Jackson KG, Williams CM. Endothelial function and insulin sensitivity during acute non-esterified fatty acid elevation: effects of fat composition and gender. *Nutr Metab Cardiovasc Dis* (2015) 25:575–81. doi:10.1016/j.numecd.2015.03.004
56. Loaiza A, Carretta MD, Taubert A, Hermosilla C, Hidalgo MA, Burgos RA. Differential intracellular calcium influx, nitric oxide production, ICAM-1 and IL8 expression in primary bovine endothelial cells exposed to nonesterified fatty acids. *BMC Vet Res* (2016) 12:38. doi:10.1186/s12917-016-0654-3

57. Weber C, Schober A, Zernecke A. Chemokines: key regulators of mononuclear cell recruitment in atherosclerotic vascular disease. *Arterioscler Thromb Vasc Biol* (2004) 24:1997–2008. doi:10.1161/01.ATV.0000142812.03840.6f
58. Zuojun H, Lingyu H, Wei H, Henghui Y, Chonggang Z, Jingsong W, et al. Interference of IP-10 expression inhibits vascular smooth muscle cell proliferation and intimal hyperplasia in carotid artery: a new insight in the prevention of restenosis. *Cell Biochem Biophys* (2012) 62:125–35. doi:10.1007/s12013-011-9270-9
59. Boring L, Gosling J, Cleary M, Charo IF. Decreased lesion formation in CCR2-/- mice reveals a role for chemokines in the initiation of atherosclerosis. *Nature* (1998) 394:894–7. doi:10.1038/29788
60. Apostolakis S, Vogiatzi K, Amanatidou V, Spandidos DA. Interleukin 8 and cardiovascular disease. *Cardiovasc Res* (2009) 84:353–60. doi:10.1093/cvr/cvp241
61. Grönwall C, Reynolds H, Kim JK, Buyon J, Goldberg JD, Clancy RM, et al. Relation of carotid plaque with natural IgM antibodies in patients with systemic lupus erythematosus. *Clin Immunol* (2014) 153:1–7. doi:10.1016/j.clim.2014.03.017
62. Su J, Hua X, Concha H, Svenungsson E, Cederholm A, Frostegård J. Natural antibodies against phosphorylcholine as potential protective factors in SLE. *Rheumatology (Oxford)* (2008) 47:1144–50. doi:10.1093/rheumatology/ken120
63. Aghdassi E, Ma DW, Morrison S, Hillyer LM, Clarke S, Gladman DD, et al. Alterations in circulating fatty acid composition in patients with systemic lupus erythematosus: a pilot study. *JPEN J Parenter Enteral Nutr* (2011) 35:198–208. doi:10.1177/0148607110386378
64. Perreault M, Roke K, Badawi A, Nielsen DE, Abdelmagid SA, El-Sohemy A, et al. Plasma levels of 14:0, 16:0, 16:1n-7, and 20:3n-6 are positively associated, but 18:0 and 18:2n-6 are inversely associated with markers of inflammation in young healthy adults. *Lipids* (2014) 49:255–63. doi:10.1007/s11745-013-3874-3
65. Alcock J, Lin HC. Fatty acids from diet and microbiota regulate energy metabolism. *F1000Research* (2015) 4:738. doi:10.12688/f1000research.6078.1
66. Ridaura VK, Faith JJ, Rey FE, Cheng J, Duncan AE, Kau AL, et al. Gut microbiota from twins discordant for obesity modulate metabolism in mice. *Science* (2013) 341:1241214. doi:10.1126/science.1241214
67. Kless C, Müller VM, Schüppel VL, Lichtenegger M, Rychlik M, Daniel H, et al. Diet-induced obesity causes metabolic impairment independent of alterations in gut barrier integrity. *Mol Nutr Food Res* (2015) 59:968–78. doi:10.1002/mnfr.201400840
68. Cani PD, Bibiloni R, Knauf C, Waget A, Neyrinck AM, Delzenne NM, et al. Changes in gut microbiota control metabolic endotoxemia-induced inflammation in high-fat diet-induced obesity and diabetes in mice. *Diabetes* (2008) 57:1470–81. doi:10.2337/db07-1403
69. Ghosh S, Molcan E, DeCoffe D, Dai C, Gibson DL. Diets rich in n-6 PUFA induce intestinal microbial dysbiosis in aged mice. *Br J Nutr* (2013) 110:515–23. doi:10.1017/S0007114512005326
70. Kaliannan K, Wang B, Li XY, Bhan AK, Kang JX. Omega-3 fatty acids prevent early-life antibiotic exposure-induced gut microbiota dysbiosis and later-life obesity. *Int J Obes (Lond)* (2016) 40:1039–42. doi:10.1038/ijo.2016.27
71. Ghosh S, DeCoffe D, Brown K, Rajendiran E, Estaki M, Dai C, et al. Fish oil attenuates omega-6 polyunsaturated fatty acid-induced dysbiosis and infectious colitis but impairs LPS dephosphorylation activity causing sepsis. *PLoS One* (2013) 8:e55468. doi:10.1371/journal.pone.0055468
72. Shin SY, Bajpai VK, Kim HR, Kang SC. Antibacterial activity of bioconverted eicosapentaenoic (EPA) and docosahexaenoic acid (DHA) against foodborne pathogenic bacteria. *Int J Food Microbiol* (2007) 113:233–6. doi:10.1016/j.ijfoodmicro.2006.05.020

17

Specific Strains of Lactic Acid Bacteria Differentially Modulate the Profile of Adipokines *In Vitro*

Emanuel Fabersani[1], María Claudia Abeijon-Mukdsi[1,2], Romina Ross[2,3], Roxana Medina[1,3], Silvia González[3] and Paola Gauffin-Cano[1,2]*

[1] Centro de Referencia para Lactobacilos (CERELA) – CONICET, Tucumán, Argentina, [2] Facultad Ciencias de la Salud, Universidad del Norte Santo Tomás de Aquino (UNSTA), Tucumán, Argentina, [3] Universidad Nacional de Tucumán (UNT), Tucumán, Argentina

Edited by:
Haruki Kitazawa,
Tohoku University, Japan

Reviewed by:
Arlette Santacruz,
Tecnológico de Monterrey, Mexico
Maria Carmen Cenit,
Hospital Doctor Peset, Spain

***Correspondence:**
Paola Gauffin-Cano
pgauffin@cerela.org.ar

Obesity induces local/systemic inflammation accompanied by increases in macrophage infiltration into adipose tissue and production of inflammatory cytokines, chemokines, and hormones. Previous studies have shown that probiotics could improve the intestinal dysbiosis induced by metabolic diseases such as obesity, diabetes, and metabolic syndrome. Microorganisms could (directly or indirectly) affect adipokine levels due to their capacity to induce translocation of several intestinal microbial antigens into systemic circulation, which could lead to metabolic endotoxemia or produce immunomodulation in different organs. The aim of the present study was to select non-inflammatory lactic acid bacteria (LAB) strains with the capacity to modulate adipokine secretion by the adipose tissue. We wish to elucidate the role of potential probiotic strains in the regulation of the cross talking between immune cells such as macrophages and adipose cells. Mouse macrophage cell line RAW 264.7 was used for evaluating the ability of 14 LAB strains to induce cytokine production. The LAB strains were chosen based on their previously studied beneficial properties in health. Then, in murine adipocyte culture and macrophage–adipocyte coculture, we determined the ability of these strains to induce cytokines and leptin secretion. Tumor necrosis factor alpha, interleukin 6 (IL-6), IL-10, monocyte chemoattractant protein-1, and leptin levels were measured in cell supernatants. We also performed the detection and quantification of leptin receptor (Ob-Rb) expression in macrophage cell lines stimulated by these LAB strains. Differential secretion profile of cytokines in macrophage cells induced by LAB strains was observed. Also, the levels of Ob-Rb expression diverged among different LAB strains. In LAB-stimulated coculture cells (adipocytes and macrophages), we observed differential production of leptin and cytokines. Furthermore, we detected lower production levels in single culture than cocultured cells. The principal component analysis showed an association between the four clusters of strains established according to their inflammatory profiles and leptin adipocyte production and leptin receptor expression in macrophages. We conclude that coculture is the most appropriate system for selecting strains with the ability to modulate adipokine secretion. The use of microorganisms with low and medium inflammatory properties and ability to modulate leptin levels could be a strategy for the treatment of some metabolic diseases associated with dysregulation of immune response.

Keywords: adipokine, leptin, lactic acid bacteria, probiotics, macrophage, adipocyte

INTRODUCTION

Since the discovery of leptin, 21 years ago (1), the adipose tissue was the focus of several functional studies, in such a way that nowadays it could be considered as a potent endocrine and immune organ (2–5). This feature is due to the peculiarity of the different cells that form this tissue: adipocytes, preadipocytes, endothelial cells, fibroblasts, and numerous immune cells including macrophages, B cells, T cells, and neutrophils mainly. The cross talk between these cells affects the composition of the adipose tissue-produced molecules (6, 7). By means of these molecules, called adipokines, the adipose tissue influences the regulation of several important physiological functions such as appetite, satiety, energy expenditure, insulin sensitivity and secretion, glucose and lipid metabolism, fat distribution, endothelial function, blood pressure, neuroendocrine regulation, and immune function. Under conditions of adipose tissue dysfunction, frequently associated with obesity or undernourishment, the secretion of adipokines is dysregulated, affecting physiological functions and the host's health (8–13). Currently, more than 600 adipokines are known. The most studied ones include leptin, adiponectin, resistin, visfatin, plasminogen activator inhibitor-1, tissue factor, tumor necrosis factor alpha (TNF-α), transforming growth factor beta, monocyte chemoattractant protein-1 (MCP-1), interleukin 6 (IL-6), and IL-8 (9). Leptin and adiponectin are adipose-derived factors with particular interest due to their potential as therapeutics in obesity treatment (14). Syndromes of malnutrition associated with excess/lack or dysfunction of adipose tissue certainly belong to these kinds of diseases (10).

Previous studies showed that adipokine levels could be affected by changes in the gut structure or in the composition of microbiota (13). Scientific evidence from both animal and human studies supports the relationship between the composition and function of intestinal microbiota and the alterations observed in metabolic and inflammatory syndromes. Consequently, the design of more effective dietary strategies for improving the treatment and prevention of metabolic diseases *via* modification of the gut microbiota composition or function is of increasing interest (15). In this context, Cani et al. (16) reported that changes in gut microbiota (following a high-fat diet or genetically induced obesity) contribute to increased gut permeability, metabolic endotoxemia [higher serum lipopolysaccharide (LPS) levels], and low-grade inflammation-induced metabolic disorders (insulin resistance and diabetes), while its restoration by prebiotic and probiotic strategies ameliorate those adverse effects. Potential probiotic strains have been shown to play a role in nutritional disorders, including both under and overnutrition in human and animal studies (17–25).

In this context, we demonstrated that oral administration of potential probiotic bacteria to a high-fat diet-induced obesity mice model ameliorates the alterations of leptin and cytokine levels along with partial restoration of the obesity-induced dysbiosis (21, 22). Recently, *in vitro* and *in vivo* studies demonstrated the influence of lactobacilli and bifidobacteria on adipokine levels (18, 21, 26). Considering the pleiotropic role of leptin in energy balance, the administration of commensal bacteria able to regulate its secretion and function could be an attractive strategy for the management of malnutrition (undernutrition and obesity), but appropriate strains need to be selected (27).

Circulating levels of leptin, an adipocyte-secreted hormone, are decreased or increased in undernutrition or obesity, respectively, and have thus been proposed to be a link between nutritional status and immune function (28–30). Papathanassoglou et al. (31) suggested the notion that nutritional status, acting via leptin-dependent mechanisms, may alter the nature and vigor of the immune response. Moreover, these authors showed that Ob-Rb, the leptin receptor, is expressed in normal mouse lymphocyte subsets and that leptin plays a role in lymphocyte survival, which alters the Ob-Rb/STAT-3-mediated signaling in T cells (31). In addition, it has been suggested that microbial products associated with immunobiotics (immunoregulatory probiotics) can also cross the intestinal barrier, being able to modulate distant tissues (such as adipose tissue) through the induction of changes in cytokine profiles (32). Miyazawa et al. in an *in vitro* study using conditioned medium showed that different lactobacilli may suppress differentiation of preadipocytes through macrophage activation and alter the immune responses of macrophages to adipose cells (33).

Therefore, we consider significant to establish a suitable criterion for the selection of immunobiotic strains with anti-inflammatory properties and ability to modulate leptin production. These bacterial capacities in this "next-generation of probiotics" would be useful to be applied in alternative treatments for diseases in which the profile of adipokines is deregulated (obesity, metabolic syndrome) (27).

The aim of the present study was to select non-inflammatory lactic acid bacteria (LAB) strains with capacity to modulate adipokine secretion in the adipose tissue. The LAB strains were selected for this study by their probiotic properties previously determined (17, 23, 34–38). To achieve this purpose, first we evaluated in murine macrophages the ability of different strains to induce the secretion of cytokines and chemokines (pro-inflammatory and anti-inflammatory responses) involved in metabolic inflammation (TNF-α, IL-6, IL-10, and MCP-1). The infiltration of adipose tissue by macrophages is an important event causing increased inflammatory process in obesity (39–41). In addition, leptin and cytokines and one chemokine secretion in murine adipocytes (mono- and coculture with macrophages) were investigated in order to understand the role of potential probiotic strains in the adipokine modulation. We also evaluated the leptin receptor (Ob-Rb) expression in macrophages, a molecule constitutively expressed in immune cells such as macrophages, B cells, and T cells (31).

MATERIALS AND METHODS

Bacterial Strains and Culture Conditions

Lactic acid bacteria strains were obtained from the Centro de Referencia para Lactobacilos (CERELA, Tucumán, Argentina) culture collection. They were isolated in our laboratory from regional products and stools of healthy infants. All the employed bacteria used in this work could potentially be considered as probiotic strains or as starter cultures for meat or milk fermentation.

Probiotic properties previously determined were immunomodulation, production of conjugated linoleic acid, feruloyl esterase activity, protection against intestinal infections, etc (17, 23, 34–38).

Strains used in this study were *Lactobacillus casei* CRL431, *L. acidophilus* CRL258, *L. acidophilus* CRL1063, *L. casei* CRL66, *L. casei* CRL72, *L. casei* CRL117, *L. fermentum* CRL1446, *Lactococcus lactis* CRL1434, *L. plantarum* CRL350, *L. plantarum* CRL352, *L. plantarum* CRL353, *L. plantarum* CRL355, *L. paracasei* CRL575, and *L. rhamnosus* CRL576.

Bacteria were cultured in Man–Rogosa–Sharpe (MRS) broth (Britania, Buenos Aires, Argentina) at 37°C for 22 h (stationary growth phase). Cells were harvested by centrifugation (10,000 rpm for 10 min), washed twice with phosphate-buffered saline (PBS, 130 mM sodium chloride, 10 mM sodium phosphate, pH 7.4), and re-suspended in PBS containing 20% (v/v) glycerol. Aliquots of these suspensions were frozen and stored at −80°C until used for *in vitro* stimulation of macrophage and adipocyte cells. The number of viable cells after freezing and thawing was determined by colony-forming unit counting on MRS agar after 48 h incubation in microaerophilia. For each strain tested, more than 90% cells remained alive upon thawing, and no significant differences were found during storage time (2 months). One fresh aliquot was thawed for every new experiment to avoid variability in the viability of cultures in the experiments.

Ability of LAB Strains to Induce Cytokine Secretion by Macrophages

Mouse macrophage cell line RAW 264.7 was used for evaluating the ability of different LAB strains to induce cytokine production as previously determined (21). Cells were cultured overnight into 24-well flat-bottom polystyrene microtiter plates (Costar® 24 Well Clear TC-Treated Multiple Well Plates, Individually Wrapped, Sterile #3524) at a concentration of 1×10^5 cells per milliliter in Dulbecco's Modified Eagle's Medium (DMEM—Gibco #41965-039). Medium was changed before stimulation, and then cells were incubated in the presence of 100 µl of a cell suspension (1×10^7 CFU/ml) of each strain for 24 h. Purified LPS from *Escherichia coli* serotype O26: B6 (Sigma Chemical Co, USA, #L2654) was used as a positive control, at a final concentration of 1 µg/ml. Cell viability was assessed by the Trypan blue assay. Non-stimulated Raw 264.7 cells were also evaluated as controls of basal cytokine production (control negative). The cell culture supernatants were collected, centrifuged (10,000 rpm for 10 min), and stored at −20°C until cytokine determination.

Detection and Quantification of Obesity Receptor (Ob-Rb) Expression

Macrophages were collected by vigorous pipetting after stimulation with different bacterial strains and immediately washed twice with PBS. Cells (10^6) were incubated with primary polyclonal antibody rabbit antimouse leptin receptor (Ob-R H300: sc8325, Santa Cruz Biotechnology, Inc.) in PBS-bovine serum albumin (1% w/v), dilution 1/250 (v/v) for 1 h at room temperature, washed twice with PBS-BSA (5%, w/v), and incubated with FITC-conjugated secondary antibodies goat antirabbit IgG-FITC (IgG-FITC: sc-2012 Santa Cruz Biotechnology, Inc.) for an additional 1 h at room temperature in darkness. Cells were washed twice and resuspended in 500 µl PBS (1%, w/v). LPS-stimulated and non-stimulated macrophages were used as positive and negative controls of the leptin receptor expression. Macrophage Ob-Rb (+) was quantified using flow cytometry (BD/FACSCalibur). Gates were set to exclude cell debris and non-specific Ab binding, and results were analyzed using the FACS analysis software (CellQuest; BD Biosciences). Unstained controls were used for setting compensation and gates.

Immunofluorescence microscopy was used to detect the Ob-Rb leptin receptor in the macrophages. The cells were cultured overnight into 24-well flat-bottom polystyrene microtiter plates [Costar® 24 Well Clear TC-Treated Multiple Well Plates, Individually Wrapped, Sterile (Product #3524)] containing glass coverslips 12 mm in diameter, at a concentration of 10^5 cells per milliliter in DMEM, then, the cells were washed twice with PBS 1× and fixed with paraformaldehyde 1% (SIGMA P6148-500G) in PBS, and incubated with primary and secondary antibodies as previously described for flow cytometry. Finally, a drop of mounting medium (SIGMA F4680, USA) was placed on the labeled cells and then the coverslip, following visualization in a fluorescence microscope (Carl Zeiss—Axio Scope.A1).

Isolation of Murine Adipocytes

Adipocytes from epididymal adipose tissue were isolated from 6-week old Balb/c male mice by collagenase digestion (collagenase from *Clostridium histolyticum* Type II #C6885 SIGMA, USA) as previously described (42, 43). Briefly, adipose tissues from four to six mice were pooled for adipocyte isolation. Tissue was digested during an hour incubation period at 37°C in DMEM high glucose supplemented with 10% (v/v) fetal bovine serum (FBS), penicillin/streptomycin, and containing 1.5 mg/ml collagenase II under constant agitation. The suspension was subsequently centrifuged at 500 rpm for 5 min at room temperature. The mature adipocyte floated to the surface, and the stromal vascular cells (capillary, endothelial, mast, macrophage, and epithelial cells) were deposited at the bottom. The stromal vascular cells were removed by aspiration, and the fat cells were washed with 10 ml of DMEM high glucose supplemented with 10% FBS and penicillin/streptomycin and centrifuged at 400 rpm for 2 min. This procedure was repeated twice. Two aliquots (10 µl) of cell suspension were stained with Trypan blue and counted on a hemocytometer to estimate the concentration of adipocyte cells. The experimental protocol was approved by the Animal Protection Committee of CERELA (CRL-BIOT-EF-2012/2A) and complied with current Argentinean laws.

Ability of LAB Strains to Induce Cytokine and Leptin Secretion by Murine Adipocytes Culture and Macrophage-Adipocyte Coculture

Adipocyte Culture

Adipocyte cells in 0.5 mL of plating medium were inoculated into 24-well plates at a concentration of 5×10^5 cells/wells, to study the ability of different strains to induce leptin and cytokine production. The cells were maintained in a humidified 5% CO_2 atmosphere for 24 h at 37°C. Medium was changed before the LAB stimulation, and then adipocytes were incubated in the presence of 100 μl of a cell suspension 1×10^7 CFU/ml of each strain for 24 h. Purified LPS from *E. coli* serotype O26:B6 was used at a concentration of 1 μg/ml as a positive control. Non-stimulated adipocytes cells were also evaluated as controls of basal leptin and cytokine production (control negative). Cell viability was assessed by the Trypan blue assay.

Macrophage–Adipocyte Coculture

Experiments of murine adipocytes and macrophages (cell line RAW 264.7) were performed by triplicate in two independent experiments with each strain. Adipocytes were seeded at a concentration of 10^4 cells/ml into 24-well plates, and macrophage cells were previously cultured at a concentration of 10^4 cells/ml. The cells were cocultured in a humidified 5% CO_2 atmosphere for 24 h at 37°C. Media were changed before stimulation, and then cells were incubated in the presence of 100 μl of each strain suspension (1×10^7 CFU/ml) during 24 h at 37°C in a humidified 5% CO_2 atmosphere. Purified LPS from *E. coli* serotype O26:B6 was used at a concentration of 1 μg/ml as a positive control. Non-stimulated coculture cells were also evaluated as controls of basal leptin and cytokine production (control negative). The coculture supernatants were collected and stored at −20°C until cytokines, chemokine, and leptin were quantified.

Detection of Cytokines and Adipokines

Tumor necrosis factor alpha, IL-6, MCP-1, and IL-10 were quantified in cell supernatants using the BD™ Cytometric Bead Array Mouse Inflammation Kit (BD Bioscience, 560485, San Diego, CA, USA). Leptin concentrations were measured in cell supernatants with a DuoSet kit (R&D Systems, Minneapolis). The assays were performed according to the manufacturer's instructions.

Statistical Analyses

Statistical analyses were performed using SPSS version 17.0 software (SPSS Inc., Chicago, IL, USA). The data were normally distributed and significant differences were determined by applying one-way ANOVA with *post hoc* Tukey's test or Fisher's least significant difference test. In every case, P-values < 0.05 were considered statistically significant. Principal component analysis (PCA), as a descriptive/exploratory technique, was used in order to reveal relationships between the variables. Further interpretations of any relationships among strains, cytokine and leptin levels, and Ob-Rb expression were obtained using PCA and Pearson correlation coefficients. PCA analysis was performed using the software XLSTAT (18.06).

RESULTS

Differential Secretion Pattern of Cytokines/Chemokine Induced by Different LAB in Macrophages

Results in **Figure 1** show the ability of viable LAB to induce cytokines/chemokine production in macrophages. Production of TNF-α and IL-6 (pro-inflammatory cytokines), IL-10 (regulatory cytokine), and MCP-1 (pro-inflammatory chemokine) by macrophages stimulated with several strains was determined. Large differences in the inflammatory profile among surveyed strains were observed. These results showed that the inflammatory property is strain-dependent. All strains induced lower secretion of pro-inflammatory and regulatory cytokines and chemokine than positive control.

Tumor necrosis factor alpha showed values lower than LPS stimulus (positive control), with exception of CRL1063 strains. CRL66 and CRL575 produced the lowest TNF-α secretions (**Figure 1A**). The highest secretion of IL-6 was observed when the cells were stimulated with strain CRL1434. Intermediate values of IL-6 were observed with CRL66, CRL431, CRL1063, CRL576, CRL575, and CRL372 strains, while with CRL1446, CRL117, CRL72, CRL350, CRL353, CRL355, and CRL143 strains, the lowest values of IL-6 were obtained (**Figure 1B**). In addition, CRL 1063 induced the highest production of MCP-1 followed by CRL431, CRL72, CRL352, and CRL143 (**Figure 1C**). Regarding anti-inflammatory cytokine IL-10, the highest levels were obtained in cells stimulated by strains CRL1434 and CRL575, followed by strains CRL1063, CRL72, CRL350, and CRL143 (**Figure 1D**).

The PCA (**Figure 1E**) revealed an association between strains into four different groups, according to the inflammatory mediators induced. The cluster I included the CRL355, CRL353, CRL350, CRL576, CRL66, and CRL575 strains. This cluster also comprises the negative control that represents the baseline cytokine secretion, which is positioned far from other strains with a lower inflammatory profile. The cluster II included the CRL117, CRL1446, CRL72, CRL431, and CRL352 strains and in the cluster III, CRL1063 was very closely located in the limit between quadrants II and III. The cluster IV only included the strain CRL1434 with a high inflammatory profile next to LPS stimulus (positive control), since this stimulus produced the highest inflammatory cytokine secretion compared to all studied strains.

Expression of the Ob-Rb on Macrophage RAW 264.7

The influence of different LAB strains on Ob-Rb (leptin receptor) expression in macrophages is shown in **Figure 2**. Basal Ob-Rb expression was detected in approximately 7.5% of control macrophages (10^6 cells; negative control or non-stimulated cells; **Figures 2A,B**). Cells were subsequently stimulated during 24 h by either different LAB or LPS (control positive). Ob-Rb-positive cells increased to a maximum value of about 38% after LPS stimulation, while the percentages of LAB-stimulated macrophages positive for Ob-Rb were lower, except for CRL1434. Levels of Ob-Rb expression diverged among different LAB stimuli. The most significant increase in the percentage of Ob-Rb (+) cells was observed when strain CRL1434 was used as stimulus. The strains CRL66 and CRL1063 induced similar Ob-Rb expression to positive control. CRL1446, CRL431, CRL576, CRL575, and CRL143 strains increased the positive macrophages compared to the basal control. For the other studied LAB strains, no significant changes in Ob-Rb expression were observed compared to negative control. The qualitative immunohistochemistry analyses were also performed in macrophages (**Figure 2C**).

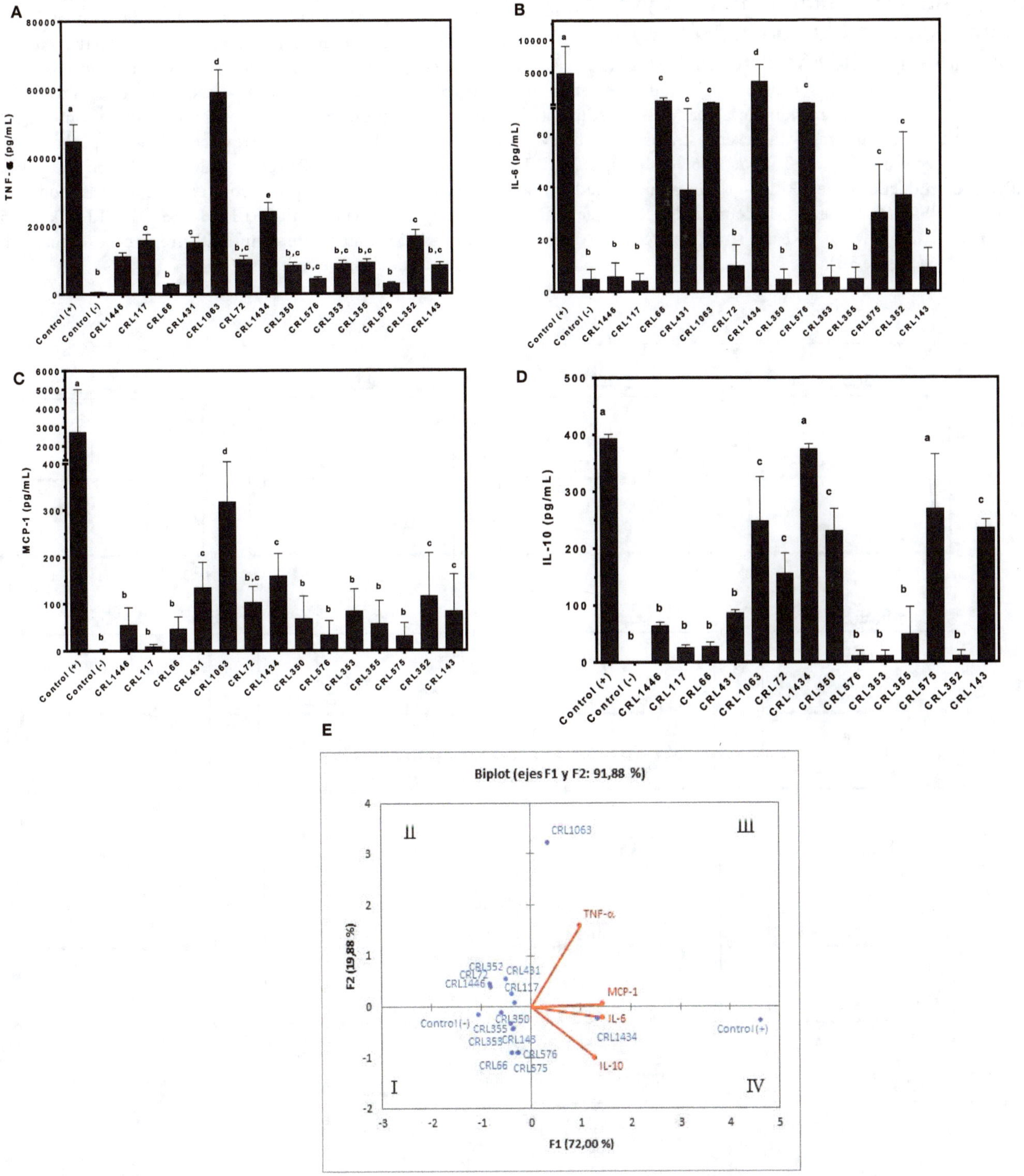

FIGURE 1 | Production of tumor necrosis factor alpha (TNF-α), interleukin 6 (IL-6), monocyte chemoattractant protein-1 (MCP-1), and IL-10 by RAW 264.7 cells stimulated with different lactic acid bacteria (LAB) strains. Cytokines/chemokine and leptin concentrations were assayed in supernatants from LAB-stimulated RAW 264.7 cells. Macrophages were treated for 24 h with bacterial cell suspensions, and TNF-α **(A)**, IL-6 **(B)**, MCP-1 **(C)**, and IL-10 **(D)** levels were quantified using cytometric bead array kit and leptin levels, using enzyme-linked immunosorbent assay test. Purified lipopolysaccharide from *Escherichia coli* was used as a positive control. Non-stimulated cells were evaluated as controls of basal cytokine levels (negative control). The stimulating strains were CRL431, CRL258, CRL1063, CRL66, CRL72, CRL117, CRL1446 CRL1434, CRL350, CRL352, CRL353, CRL355, CRL575, and *L.* CRL576 strains. Results are expressed as mean ± SD of triplicate measures determined in two independent experiments. Mean values in the same graphic with different letters (a–d) were significantly different ($P < 0.05$). The relationships among strains, cytokines/chemokine wer obtained using (PCA) and Pearson correlation coefficients. In the biplot obtained by PCA **(E)**, points are coded by stimulating strains and controls. The position of some points was slightly modified to avoid overlapping of the labels.

Differential Production of and Cytokines/Chemokine and Leptin in Adipocytes Stimulated with Different LAB Strains

To evaluate whether LAB may directly induce secretion of leptin, cytokines, and chemokine in adipocytes, we stimulated murine adipocyte cultures with several strains. We observed different effects of LAB on TNF-α, IL-6, IL-10, and MCP-1 adipocyte production. The CRL1434 strain induced the highest values of TNF-α; MCP-1 and IL-10 compared to the other strains (**Figures 3A,C,D**), while CRL350 strain induced the highest levels of IL-6 (**Figure 3B**).

As shown in **Figure 3E**, leptin production is modulated by LAB in a strain-dependent manner. We showed that LPS was able to induce a significantly higher leptin production compared to negative control. Similar effect was observed for CRL66 and CRL575 strains. The CRL1434 and CRL143 strains induced more leptin production than positive control. In contrast, lower levels of leptin secretion were secreted by adipocytes treated with the CRL431, CRL1063, CRL72, CRL355, and CRL352 strains compared to negative control. Leptin levels produced by adipocyte stimulated with CRL1446, CRL117, CRL350, CRL576, and CRL353 strains were significantly from those detected in the negative and positive controls.

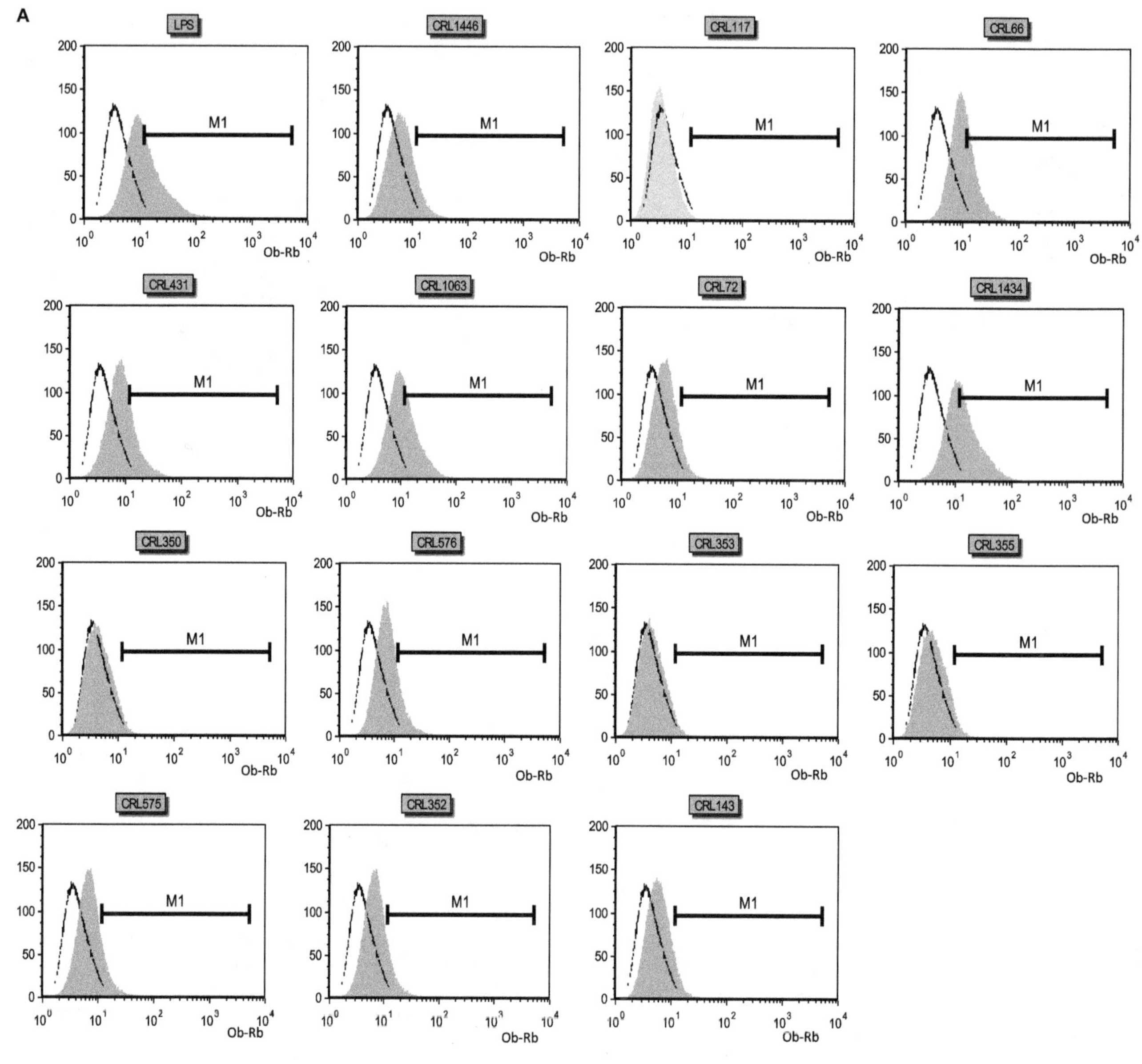

FIGURE 2 | Continued

B

C

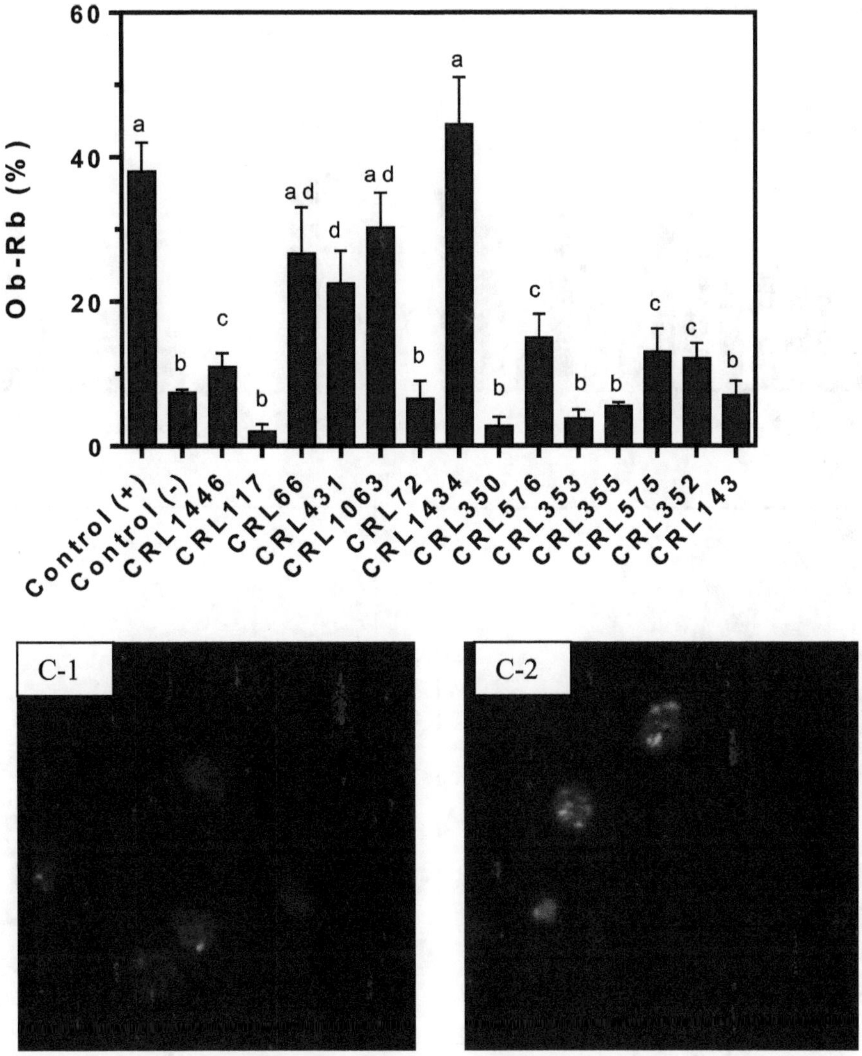

FIGURE 2 | Leptin receptor (Ob-Rb) expression in RAW 264.7 cells. RAW 264.7 cells after lactic acid bacteria (LAB) stimulation were incubated with a polyclonal rabbit antimouse Ob-Rb Ab and a secondary FITC-conjugated Ab (antirabbit IgG). Ten thousand cells were analyzed per sample at an argon laser flow cytometry scanner. **(A)** Histograms correspond to the analysis of Ob-Rb expression by non-stimulated (negative control) and LAB-stimulated RAW 264.7 cells. The stimulating strains were CRL431, CRL258, CRL1063, CRL66, CRL72, CRL117, CRL1446 CRL1434, CRL350, CRL352, CRL353, CRL355, CRL575, and CRL576. Lipopolysaccharide (LPS) was used as a positive control. Open black line represents fluorescent labeling of Ob-Rb positive cells of negative control, and gray areas represent other strains stimulus. **(B)** Percentage of Ob-Rb expression in RAW 264.7 cells. The bars represent the different LAB strains. The results are expressed as media of percentages of cells Ob-Rb (+) ± SD of two experiments. Mean values in the same graphic with different letters (a–d) were significantly different ($P < 0.05$). **(C)** Microphotograph representative of the Ob-Rb expression in non-stimulated macrophages (negative control, C-1) and LPS-stimulated macrophages culture (positive control, C-2).

Differential Production of Cytokines/Chemokine and Leptin by Cocultured Cells (Adipocytes and Macrophages) Stimulated with Different LAB Strains

To assess whether LAB may directly induce production of TNF-α, IL-6, MCP-1, IL-10, and leptin by the macrophage–adipocyte coculture, we stimulated these cells with the bacterial strains (**Figure 4**). Different effects of LAB on cytokine production in the cell coculture were observed (**Figures 4A–D**). All strains induced lower cytokines production than positive control. The CRL1434 strain was the most effective stimulating both inflammatory (TNF-α, IL-6, and MCP-1) and anti-inflammatory (IL-10) cytokines secretion. The CRL431, CRL1063, CRL72, CRL355, and CRL352 strains induced significantly higher TNF-α values than CRL1446, CRL66, CRL350, CRL576, CRL353, CRL575, and CRL143 (**Figure 4A**). Regarding IL-6 production, almost all strains induced intermediated levels between positive and negative controls (**Figure 4B**). The CRL431 strain was the most potent inductor of MCP-1 secretion (**Figure 4C**), meanwhile CRL1434 strain was the best inductor of IL-10 secretion (**Figure 4D**).

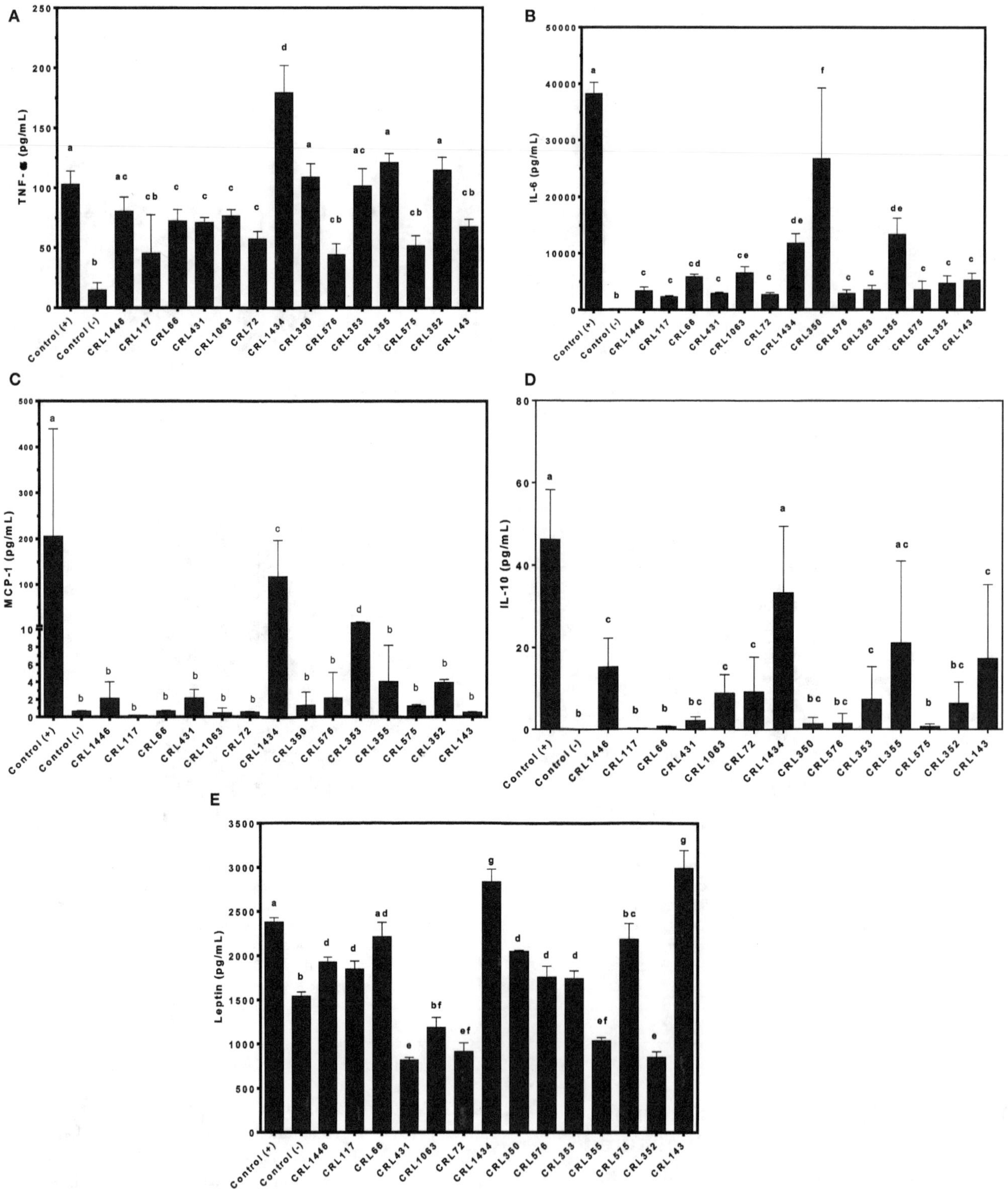

FIGURE 3 | Production of TNF-α (A), interleukin 6 (IL-6) (B), monocyte chemoattractant protein-1 (MCP-1) (C), IL-10 (D), and leptin (E) by lactic acid bacteria (LAB)-stimulated mice adipocytes. Cytokines/chemokine and leptin concentrations were assayed in supernatants from LAB-stimulated mice adipocytes. Adipocytes were treated for 24 h with bacterial cell suspensions, and TNF-α, IL-6, MCP-1, and IL-10 levels were quantified using Cytometric Bead Array Kit and leptin levels, using enzyme-linked immunosorbent assay test. LPS was used as a positive control. Non-stimulated cells were evaluated as controls of basal cytokine levels (negative control). The stimulating strains were CRL431, CRL258, CRL1063, CRL66, CRL72, CRL117, CRL1446 CRL1434, CRL350, CRL352, CRL353, CRL355, CRL575, and *L.* CRL576 strains. Results are expressed as mean ± SD of triplicate measures determined in two independent experiments. Mean values in the same graphic with different letters (a–g) were significantly different ($P < 0.05$).

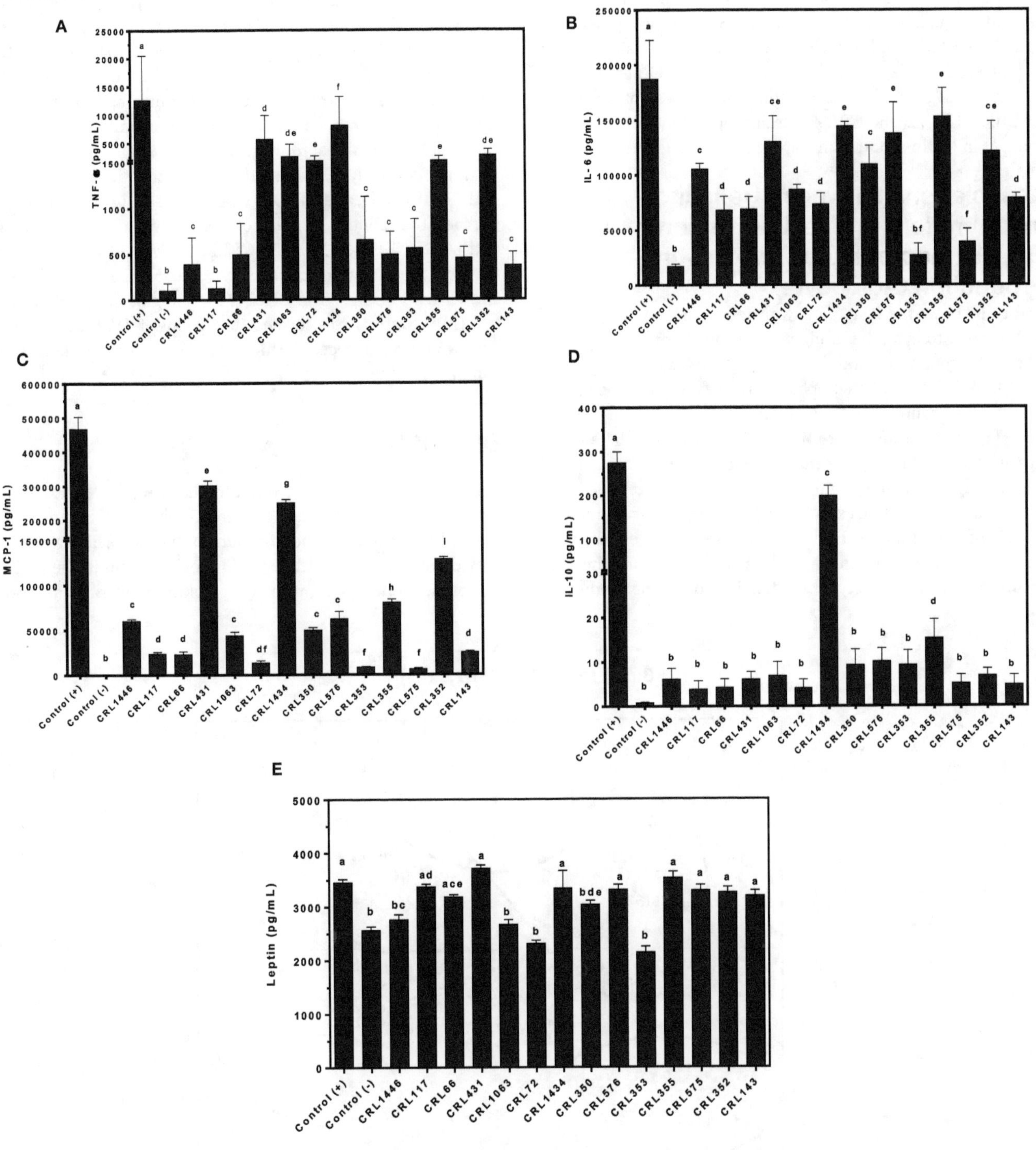

FIGURE 4 | Production of tumor necrosis factor alpha (TNF-α), interleukin 6 (IL-6), monocyte chemoattractant protein-1 (MCP-1), IL-10, and leptin by macrophage/adipocyte coculture stimulated with lactic acid bacteria (LAB) strains. Cytokines/chemokine and leptin concentrations were assayed in supernatants from LAB-stimulated macrophage/adipocyte coculture. Cells were treated for 24 h with bacterial cell suspensions and TNF-α, IL-6, MCP-1, and IL-10 levels were quantified using Cytometric Bead Array Kit and leptin levels, using enzyme-linked immunosorbent assay test. LPS was used as a positive control. Non-stimulated cells were evaluated as controls of basal cytokine levels (negative control). The stimulating strains were CRL431, CRL258, CRL1063, CRL66, CRL72, CRL117, CRL1446 CRL1434, CRL350, CRL352, CRL353, CRL355, CRL575, and *L.* CRL576 strains. Results are expressed as mean ± SD of triplicate measures determined in two independent experiments. Mean values in the same graphic with different letters (a–i) were significantly different ($P < 0.05$). Production levels of **(A)** TNF-α, **(B)** IL-6, **(C)** MCP-1, **(D)** IL-10, and **(E)** leptin.

Leptin production was also modulated by LAB in a strain-dependent manner. The CRL17, CRL66, CRL431, CRL1434, CRL576, CRL355, CRL575, CRL352, and CRL143 strains induced similar levels of leptin than positive control. Other group of strains (CRL1446 and CRL350) induced mid-levels of leptin. The CRL1063, CRL72, and CRL353 strains did not induce significant changes in leptin production compared with negative control.

Associations between Strain and Inflammatory Profile, Expression of the Ob-Rb (Macrophage), and Leptin Production (Adipocyte)

Figure 5 shows the PCA plots with focus on grouping of LAB with respect to cytokines and leptin produced by macrophage–adipocyte coculture, both associated with expression of the Ob-Rb in RAW 264.7 macrophages. PCA revealed the presence of different groups of LAB with significant biological correlation (**Figure 5**) according to the studied variables. The analysis clearly discriminated between LAB with different capacity for modulating adipokine production. The analysis revealed that two components can be extracted, which together accounted for 87.31% of the variability. However, the first component accounts for 71.33% of the variance and discriminated better the LAB according to their capacity for modulating adipokine production and was more influenced by TNF-α and MCP-1; however, all variables were positively correlated. Second component separates better the strains with regard to their influence on leptin and IL-6 levels. So, the first and second factors discriminate LAB strains in four clusters according to their inflammatory profiles, leptin (from adipocyte to macrophage) production and leptin receptor expression (only in macrophages).

In the cluster I, we observed strong correlations between the CRL72, CRL1063, and CRL353 strains. This group also comprises the negative control (basal control). The cluster II includes CRL1446, CRL66, CRL575, CRL143, CRL350, and CRL117 strains. The cluster III includes the CRL352, CRL576, CRL355, and CRL431 strains. The CRL1434 strain close to positive control (LPS control) was located in the cluster IV. Stimulus with CRL1434 strain induced the highest inflammatory cytokine levels compared to the other strains studied.

DISCUSSION

This study supports the hypothesis that LAB have capacity to induce adipokine secretion in strain-dependent manner, and this ability is related to their immune properties. This report also provides additional evidence for the role of leptin in the regulation of the immune system and the cytokine network. In addition,

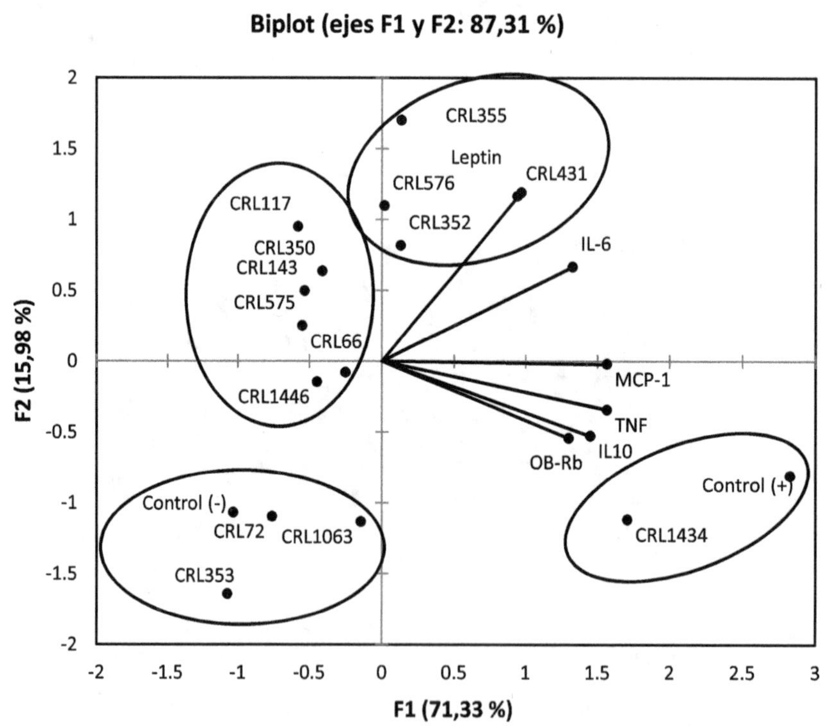

FIGURE 5 | Biplots obtained by principal component analysis (PCA) of cytokines/chemokine and leptin production by macrophage/adipocyte coculture associated with expression of the Ob-Rb receptor in macrophages. Levels of TNF-α, IL-6, MCP-1, IL-10, and leptin produced by macrophage/adipocyte cocultures were associated with the expression of Ob-Rb in macrophages in biplots obtained by PCA. Non-stimulated cells were evaluated as controls basal (negative control) of cytokines/chemokine and leptin levels and Ob-Rb expression. LPS was used as a positive control. In the biplots, points are coded by stimulating strains (CRL431, CRL258, CRL1063, CRL66, CRL72, CRL117, CRL1446 CRL1434, CRL350, CRL352, CRL353, CRL355, CRL575, and *L.* CRL576) and controls. The position of some points was slightly modified to avoid overlapping of the labels.

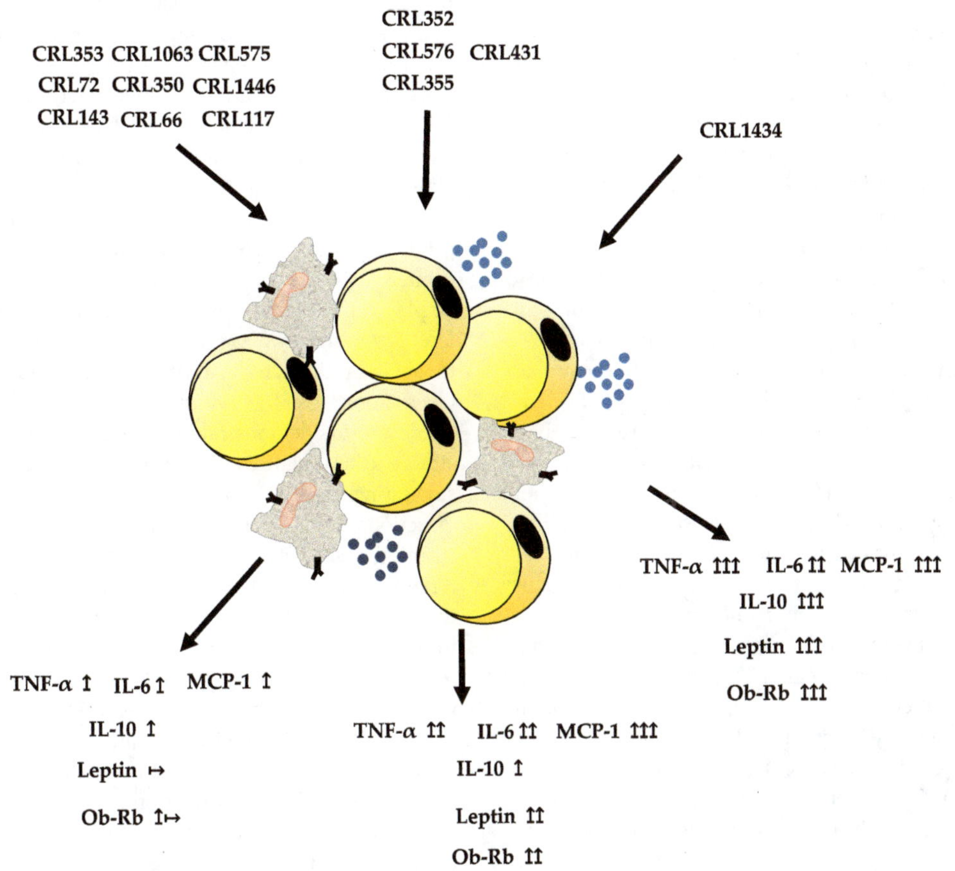

FIGURE 6 | **Possible inmuno- and adipokine modulation of lactic acid bacteria in an *in vitro* macrophage/adipocyte system.**

we showed a strategy of *in vitro* selection of immunobiotic strains (immunoregulatory probiotics) to prevent or improve immuno-metabolic alterations associated with malnutrition.

The mechanisms by which commensal bacterial strains (particularly lactobacilli and bifidobacteria) may confer health benefits on the host's health have been extensively studied (15). LAB are known to exert a wide range of effects on the immune and endocrine systems and, therefore, potentially in the whole body metabolism. However, these effects may be strain-specific and properties of one strain cannot be extrapolated to another even if belonging to the same species (44). Several beneficial microorganisms, generally known as immunobiotics (38), have been investigated for their potential use to treat or prevent nutritional disorders (undernutrition and obesity), which are further associated with immune deregulation (17, 21, 38, 45, 46).

Obesity induces low-grade inflammation characterized by chronic elevations in circulating inflammatory cytokines and adipokines (47, 48). Adipose tissue is constituted by active endocrine cells that secret a number of adipokines, which play pivotal roles in the regulation of various physiological and pathological processes in which adipose tissue is involved (49). At the adipose tissue level, inflammatory pathways are induced due in part to dynamic quantitative and phenotypic changes in adipose tissue leukocytes, principally macrophages (48, 50). According to Weisberg et al. (39), in mouse models, macrophage content could increase to about 50% of total non-adipocyte cells in obese mice. Macrophages infiltrated in white adipose tissue are the principal source of IL-6 and TNF-α (51). TNF-α is a pro-inflammatory cytokine, which has also been implicated as a mediator in induction of insulin resistance and adipose tissue inflammation (52). IL-6 has long been regarded as a pro-inflammatory molecule, but recent findings suggest that it also has many anti-inflammatory effects (53). IL-10 is a strong anti-inflammatory cytokine due to its ability to suppress the release of TNF-α and IL-1b from macrophages. In addition, IL-10 would affect Th1-lymphocyte actions (54). Regarding this, it was suggested that the C-C chemokine receptor 2 and its ligand CCL2 or MCP-1 are necessary for accumulation of inflammatory macrophages (39).

The results showed in this work indicate that adipocyte–macrophage coculture could be used for the screening and the selection of new immunobiotic strains, with the potential to functionally modulate adipose inflammation when orally administered. On the other hand, several authors have demonstrated that the gut microbiota could be modified by oral administration of LAB, and it has been identified as an important modifier of systemic inflammatory reactions influencing remote tissues (21). In addition, it is important to mention that there is no direct contact between intestinal bacteria and adipose tissue, but this contact could be indirectly mediated through translocation of bacterial products (e.g., LPS, DNA, etc.), which reach peripheral tissues and can stimulate innate immune receptors such as the mammalian toll-like receptors (TLRs) (55, 56). TLRs are germ line-encoded receptors expressed by cells of the innate immune system, adipocytes or intestinal epithelia, which are stimulated by structural motifs characteristically expressed by bacteria, viruses, and fungi known as pathogen-associated molecular patterns (57). Food-derived fatty acids, as well as intestinal bacteria-derived fatty acids could be sensed by TLRs, resulting in activation of the immune system (55). Taking this into account, we and other authors suggested that disruption of the mucosal barrier, as occurs in obesity and or undernutrition, leads to the exposure of a multitude of commensal-derived TLR ligands that could interact with TLR-expressing immune cells and adipocytes (55, 56). Batra et al. (58) demonstrated that expression and responsiveness of TLRs (TLR 1–9) in murine preadipocytes and adipocytes are both strongly regulated by leptin. This, coupled with the demonstrated pro-inflammatory actions of leptin in a variety of immune cells and other cell types (59), led us to propose that inflammatory responses could be regulated by leptin-modulating strains.

Adipose tissue consists of active endocrine cells that secrete a large number of adipokines, mainly leptin, adiponectin, and inflammatory cytokines such as TNF-α, IL-6, IL-1, IL-10, and MCP-1. These factors play a key role in the regulation of various physiological and pathological processes in which adipose tissue is involved (49, 60). For this purpose, we evaluated the ability of LAB to induce changes in the secretion of adipokines, cytokines, and chemokines involved in metabolic inflammation (IL-6, IL-10, TNF-α, MCP-1, and leptin), macrophages and adipocytes. Main cells that compose the adipose tissue (6, 61).

In order to establish the influence of cross talk between the main cells of adipose tissue, a coculture technique using macrophages and adipocytes was developed. According to Aravindhan and Madhumitha, metainflammation is due to the dysfunction of the immune system: at optimal level it confers protection against pathogens; at the suboptimal level it leads to immunodeficiency; and at supraoptimal level it leads to inflammation (62). Taking this into account, it is necessary to know the inflammatory profile of potential probiotic LAB. In this study, we first examined the ability of LAB to induce the production of different pro-inflammatory and anti-inflammatory responses in murine macrophage cell line, since the high infiltration of adipose tissue by macrophages occurs in obesity (39–41). Macrophages are phagocytic cells that participate in the innate and adaptive immune system. They are also one of the major cells that are in contact with the microorganisms in the intestine (63). This contact can be performed by phagocytosis or by recognition through different receptors, such as those PMAMs, including TLRs. In addition to the intestine, macrophages are found in various tissues, being one of the main immune cells of the visceral adipose tissue, in both lean and obese subjects, where they can represent between 5 and 60% of the immune cells of the adipose tissue (64, 65).

In the metabolic disorders, the number and level of activation of macrophages are altered (66), so that metabolic parameters, such as insulin resistance associated, may be affected (67) or the response to infections associated with malnutrition (68, 69). The main reason is due to the level of dynamic polarization between classically activated macrophages M1 (producers of pro-inflammatory cytokines) and alternatively activated macrophages M2 (anti-inflammatory cytokine producers) present in the adipose tissue (6). The level of activation is associated with a particular cytokine profile, and this is dysregulated in metabolic disorders (70). We demonstrated large differences in the inflammatory profile among evaluated strains, suggesting that the inflammatory property is strain-dependent, and different functional roles could be played by studied strains. We showed, in and other work, different cytokine profiles produced by macrophages induced by lactobacilli, bifidobacteria, and bacteroides strains (21, 71). Similar observations were previously reported by Medina et al. (72). These authors demonstrated different abilities of *Bifidobacterium* strains to modulate *in vitro* production of cytokines by PBMCs, suggesting that they could drive immune responses in different directions. Maassen et al. (73) showed that different *Lactobacillus* strains induce distinct mucosal cytokine profiles and possess differential intrinsic adjuvant properties. These authors suggested that rational *Lactobacillus* strain selection provides a strategy to influence cytokines expression and thereby influence immune responses. Considering only our results of inflammatory profile in macrophages, strains such as CRL72, CRL1446, CRL352, CRL431, and CRL117 with a medium inflammatory profile could provide protection against the early stage of infection *via* Th1 with TNF-α and IL-6 production (74).

According to Jaedicke et al. (59), increased leptin concentrations in obesity may drive monocytes into a more activated, macrophage-like, pro-inflammatory state, possibly by affecting expression of TLRs and CD14, thereby enhancing LPS responsiveness and contributing to increased inflammation. Furthermore, knowing that leptin enhances T cell proliferation and Th1 pro-inflammatory cytokine production *in vitro* (31), we proceed to evaluate leptin and cytokines production by adipocytes in mono and coculture and the presence of a functional Ob-Rb (leptin receptor) in macrophages. Other authors showed that bacterial strains have different ability to modulate leptin secretion by adipocytes (26, 75, 76).

We evaluated whether Ob-Rb expression is regulated during macrophage activation by different LAB strains. Ob-Rb positive cells increased after LPS stimulation (positive control) and its expression diverged among different LAB stimuli. A previous study demonstrated that macrophages and B and T lymphocytes constitutively express low levels of Ob-Rb, and that this expression is upregulated, in terms of both percentage of positive cells and receptor density, in response to activation of these immune cells (31). We observed that "more inflammatory" strains produced more leptin as well as increased Ob-Rb receptor expression on macrophages, which is according to the notion of pro-inflammatory property of leptin and its adverse role in obesity (28).

Stimulating adipocytes/RAW264.7 cells with LAB results in marked upregulation of cytokine and leptin production in comparison with an adipocyte culture. Other authors, using the coculture system, showed inhibition of the cycle of stimulation of adipocytes and macrophages through the inhibition of macrophage-mediated pro-inflammatory cytokines and upregulation of adiponectin in adipocytes (77). These favorable effects may suppress chronic inflammation in adipose tissue. De Palma et al. also demonstrated, in another coculture system (PBMC and Caco cells), that some microorganisms had different behavior (cytokine production) using individual cell cultures (78). Furthermore, we observed significant production of IL-6 and MCP-1 in a coculture compared to the effect in macrophage cells; these two molecules are related to macrophage infiltration and insulin resistance in adipose tissue (40, 79). In addition, it is estimated that between 15 and 35% of the systemic IL-6 levels come from adipose tissue in obese individuals (79).

In our study, we used viable LAB strains and observed a modulation, strain dependent, on the production of leptin in adipocytes in mono- and coculture with macrophages. However, like other authors, we suggest that mediators produced by other cells in adipose tissue, such as macrophages, influence the secretory capacity of adipocytes and vice versa, because of the difference in the secretion of leptin, cytokines, and chemokine, comparing mono- and coculture (80, 81).

We observed that CRL431 strain showed a significant reduction in leptin levels compared to control (—), when adipocytes were stimulated, but significantly higher levels than LPS in macrophage–adipocyte–LAB coculture. A similar pattern occurred with strain CRL1434, which showed significantly higher leptin levels of LPS by stimulating adipocytes, but in the coculture system it presented values similar to LPS. This clearly reflects the intercommunication between these two cells (macrophages and adipocytes) and that LAB can affect the production of adipokines in this system.

In order to determine an association between the different strains, regarding their inflammatory profile, Ob-Rb receptor induction and their effect on leptin production, the PCA was carried out. In this study, CRL355, CRL431, CRL576, and CRL352 strains that induced high levels of leptin could be exploited in diseases with low concentrations of leptin. On the contrary, downregulation of circulating leptin levels may be considered as possible strategy to intervene on some inflammatory and autoimmune conditions (28). In the latter situation, strains such as CRL117, CRL350, CRL143 CRL575, CRL1446, and CRL66 could be useful. Miyazawa et al. demonstrated that increased pro-inflammatory cytokines (IL-6, IL-12, and TNF-α) inhibited the differentiation of a fibroblast cell line (3T3L1) in adipocytes, suggesting that acute inflammation stimulated by lactobacilli could be the mechanism by which adipogenic differentiation is suppressed, leading to adipocyte hypertrophy (33).

We suggest that the CRL575, CRL143, CRL117, CRL352, CRL576, CRL355, CRL431, and CRL1434 strains that induce high levels of leptin (either in adipocytes or in the Mac-Adi-BL system) could be oriented to the use in nutritional therapies for diseases that occur with reduced levels of leptin. In an opposite case, decreased levels of this adipokine would be necessary for the intervention of inflammatory or autoimmune pathologies (28), where CRL72, CRL66, and CRL1446 strains could be used.

It is noteworthy that CRL1446 strain induced a decline in leptin production. This strain has antioxidant, hypoglycemic, and hypocholesterolemic properties in animal studies (23, 82), thereby could be an interesting alternative for treating obesity, which is characterized by high leptin levels. CRL431 strain, which is a probiotic microorganism that demonstrated positive immunological effects in undernourished hosts (17, 38), was located, in the PCA analysis, next to strains that induced middle leptin production. Other authors showed the specific effect of LAB on the response of porcine adipocytes to TNF-α stimulation using conditioned media from LAB-stimulated intestinal immune cells (32). They suggested that lactobacilli may suppress differentiation of preadipocytes through macrophage activation and production of Th1 cytokines and could be effective in improving Th1 response not only in the gut but also in the systemic compartment as well. Then, our data show that different LAB strains could be capable of regulating adipokine expression in adipose tissue and suggest that they could have the potential to functionally modulate adipose inflammation when orally administered.

We conclude that macrophage/adipocyte coculture is the most appropriate system for the selection of strains with the ability to modulate cytokine and leptin secretion. Our results showed that a stimulation of adipocyte monoculture with LAB strains exerts different effects than those observed in macrophage/adipocyte cocultures. This could be explained by the strong relationship between macrophages content and adipocytes in the adipose tissue, which boosts production of pro-inflammatory molecules and acute-phase proteins associated with obesity. Therefore, the regulation of TNF-α, IL-6, MCP-1, IL-10, and leptin and Ob-Rb receptor could be considered as biomarkers for immunobiotic strains. The use of microorganisms with low and middle inflammatory properties and ability to modulate leptin levels could be a strategy for the treatment of some metabolic diseases associated with immune abnormalities. In **Figure 6**, we show the possible inmuno- and adipokine modulation of LAB in an *in vitro* adipocyte system. This approach could be easily applicable in obesity and immune-deficient conditions like undernutrition. So, preclinical studies are currently being developed with the oral administration of CRL1446, CRL1434, and CRL431 (selected LAB in this work) in different experimental models of malnutrition (data no showed). The elucidation of the mechanisms involved in the modulation of adipose inflammation by LAB strains requires further studies associated with Ob-Rb and TLR expression.

AUTHOR CONTRIBUTIONS

Conceived and designed the experiments: EF and PG-C. Performed the experiments: EF, RR, and MCAM. Analyzed the data: EF, RR, MCAM, RM, and PG-C. Wrote draft and the final version of the manuscript: SG and PG-C.

ACKNOWLEDGMENTS

We sincerely thank Dr. Yolanda Sanz [Microbial Ecology, Nutrition and Health Research Unit, Institute of Agrochemistry and Food Technology (IATA), National Research Council (CSIC), Valencia, Spain], for her helpful advice about this study and during preparation of this manuscript. This work was supported by BID PICT-2011 no. 0804, CONICET-PIP215, and UNSTA grants.

REFERENCES

1. Zhang Y, Proenca R, Maffei M, Barone M, Leopold L, Friedman JM. Positional cloning of the mouse obese gene and its human homologue. *Nature* (1994) 372:425–32. doi:10.1038/372425a0
2. Gimeno RE, Klaman LD. Adipose tissue as an active endocrine organ: recent advances. *Curr Opin Pharmacol* (2005) 5:122–8. doi:10.1016/j.coph.2005.01.006
3. Grant RW, Dixit VD. Adipose tissue as an immunological organ. *Obesity (Silver Spring)* (2015) 23:512–8. doi:10.1002/oby.21003
4. Havel PJ. Update on adipocyte hormones: regulation of energy balance and carbohydrate/lipid metabolism. *Diabetes* (2004) 53(Suppl 1):S143–51. doi:10.2337/diabetes.53.2007.S143
5. Rezaee F, Dashty M. Role of adipose tissue in metabolic system disorders. *J Diabetes Metab* (2013) S13:2–8. doi:10.4172/2155-6156.S13-008
6. Mraz M, Haluzik M. The role of adipose tissue immune cells in obesity and low-grade inflammation. *J Endocrinol* (2014) 222:R113–27. doi:10.1530/JOE-14-0283
7. Rajala MW, Scherer PE. Minireview: the adipocyte – at the crossroads of energy homeostasis, inflammation, and atherosclerosis. *Endocrinology* (2003) 144:3765–73. doi:10.1210/en.2003-0580
8. Blüher M. Adipose tissue dysfunction in obesity. *Exp Clin Endocrinol Diabetes* (2009) 117:241–50. doi:10.1055/s-0029-1192044
9. Blüher M. Clinical relevance of adipokines. *Diabetes Metab J* (2012) 36:317–27. doi:10.4093/dmj.2012.36.5.317
10. Blüher M. Adipokines – removing road blocks to obesity and diabetes therapy. *Mol Metab* (2014) 3:230–40. doi:10.1016/j.molmet.2014.01.005
11. Blüher M, Mantzoros CS. From leptin to other adipokines in health and disease: facts and expectations at the beginning of the 21st century. *Metabolism* (2015) 64:131–45. doi:10.1016/j.metabol.2014.10.016
12. Catalán V, Gómez-Ambrosi J, Rodríguez A, Salvador J, Frühbeck G. Adipokines in the treatment of diabetes mellitus and obesity. *Expert Opin Pharmacother* (2009) 10:239–54. doi:10.1517/14656560802618811
13. Sahin-Efe A, Katsikeris F, Mantzoros CS. Advances in adipokines. *Metabolism* (2012) 61:1659–65. doi:10.1016/j.metabol.2012.09.001
14. Houde A-A, Légaré C, Biron S, Lescelleur O, Biertho L, Marceau S, et al. Leptin and adiponectin DNA methylation levels in adipose tissues and blood cells are associated with BMI, waist girth and LDL-cholesterol levels in severely obese men and women. *BMC Med Genet* (2015) 16:29. doi:10.1186/s12881-015-0174-1
15. Sanz Y, Rastmanesh R, Agostonic C. Understanding the role of gut microbes and probiotics in obesity: how far are we? *Pharmacol Res* (2013) 69:144–55. doi:10.1016/j.phrs.2012.10.021
16. Cani PD, Possemiers S, Van de Wiele T, Guiot Y, Everard A, Rottier O, et al. Changes in gut microbiota control inflammation in obese mice through a mechanism involving GLP-2-driven improvement of gut permeability. *Gut* (2009) 58:1091–103. doi:10.1136/gut.2008.165886
17. Gauffin-Cano P, Aguero G, Perdigon G. Adjuvant effects of *Lactobacillus casei* added to a renutrition diet in a malnourished mouse model. *Biocell* (2002) 26:35–48.
18. Sato M, Uzu K, Yoshida T, Hamad EM, Kawakami H, Matsuyama H, et al. Effects of milk fermented by *Lactobacillus gasseri* SBT2055 on adipocyte size in rats. *Br J Nutr* (2008) 99:1013–7. doi:10.1017/S0007114507839006
19. Kondo S, Xiao J-Z, Satoh T, Odamaki T, Takahashi S, Sugahara H, et al. Antiobesity effects of *Bifidobacterium breve* strain B-3 supplementation in a mouse model with high-fat diet-induced obesity. *Biosci Biotechnol Biochem* (2010) 74:1656–61. doi:10.1271/bbb.100267
20. Chang BJ, Park SU, Jang YS, Ko SH, Joo NM, Kim SI, et al. Effect of functional yogurt NY-YP901 in improving the trait of metabolic syndrome. *Eur J Clin Nutr* (2011) 65:1250–5. doi:10.1038/ejcn.2011.115
21. Gauffin Cano P, Santacruz A, Trejo FM, Sanz Y. *Bifidobacterium* CECT 7765 improves metabolic and immunological alterations associated with obesity in high-fat diet fed mice. *Obesity* (2013) 21:2310–21. doi:10.1002/oby.20330
22. Moya-Pérez A, Neef A, Sanz Y. *Bifidobacterium pseudocatenulatum* CECT 7765 reduces obesity-associated inflammation by restoring the lymphocyte-macrophage balance and gut microbiota structure in high-fat diet-fed mice. *PLoS One* (2015) 10:e0126976. doi:10.1371/journal.pone.0126976
23. Mukdsi A, Gauffin Cano M, González S, Medina R. Administration of *Lactobacillus fermentum* CRL1446 increases intestinal feruloyl esterase activity in mice. *Lett Appl Microbiol* (2012) 54(1):18–25. doi:10.1111/j.1472-765X.2011.03166.x
24. Nabavi S, Rafraf M, Somi MH, Homayouni-Rad A, Asghari-Jafarabadi M. Effects of probiotic yogurt consumption on metabolic factors in individuals with nonalcoholic fatty liver disease. *J Dairy Sci* (2014) 97:7386–93. doi:10.3168/jds.2014-8500
25. Nunez IN, Galdeano CM, Carmuega E, Weill R, de Moreno de Leblanc A, Perdigon G. Effect of a probiotic fermented milk on the thymus in Balb/c mice under non-severe protein-energy malnutrition. *Br J Nutr* (2013) 110(3):500–8. doi:10.1017/S0007114512005302
26. Bleau C, Lamontagne L, Savard R. New *Lactobacillus acidophilus* isolates reduce the release of leptin by murine adipocytes leading to lower interferon-gamma production. *Clin Exp Immunol* (2005) 140:427–35. doi:10.1111/j.1365-2249.2005.02785.x
27. Cani PD, Van Hul M. Novel opportunities for next-generation probiotics targeting metabolic syndrome. *Curr Opin Biotechnol* (2015) 32:21–7. doi:10.1016/j.copbio.2014.10.006
28. La Cava A, Alviggi C, Matarese G. Unraveling the multiple roles of leptin in inflammation and autoimmunity. *J Mol Med (Berl)* (2004) 82:4–11. doi:10.1007/s00109-003-0492-1
29. Matarese G, Moschos S, Mantzoros CS. Leptin in immunology. *J Immunol* (2005) 174:3137–42. doi:10.4049/jimmunol.174.6.3137
30. Cai C, Shi FD, Matarese G, La Cava A. Leptin as clinical target. *Recent Pat Inflamm Allergy Drug Discov* (2009) 3:160–6. doi:10.2174/187221309789257379
31. Papathanassoglou E, El-Haschimi K, Li XC, Matarese G, Strom T, Mantzoros C. Leptin receptor expression and signaling in lymphocytes: kinetics during lymphocyte activation, role in lymphocyte survival, and response to high fat diet in mice. *J Immunol* (2006) 176:7745–52. doi:10.4049/jimmunol.176.12.7745
32. Suzuki M, Tada A, Kanmani P, Watanabe H, Aso H, Suda Y, et al. Advanced application of porcine intramuscular adipocytes for evaluating anti-adipogenic and anti-inflammatory activities of immunobiotics. *PLoS One* (2015) 10:e0119644. doi:10.1371/journal.pone.0119644
33. Miyazawa K, He F, Yoda K, Hiramatsu M. Potent effects of, and mechanisms for, modification of crosstalk between macrophages and adipocytes by lactobacilli. *Microbiol Immunol* (2012) 56:847–54. doi:10.1111/j.1348-0421.2012.00512.x
34. de LeBlanc Ade M, Castillo NA, Perdigon G. Anti-infective mechanisms induced by a probiotic *Lactobacillus* strain against *Salmonella enterica* serovar Typhimurium infection. *Int J Food Microbiol* (2010) 138:223–31. doi:10.1016/j.ijfoodmicro.2010.01.020
35. Gerez CL, Torres MJ, de Valdez GF, Rollán G. Control of spoilage fungi by lactic acid bacteria. *Biol Control* (2013) 64:231–7. doi:10.1016/j.biocontrol.2012.10.009
36. Novotny Núñez I, Maldonado Galdeano C, de Moreno de LeBlanc A, Perdigón G. *Lactobacillus casei* CRL 431 administration decreases inflammatory cytokines in a diet-induced obese mouse model. *Nutrition* (2015) 31:1000–7. doi:10.1016/j.nut.2015.02.006
37. Terán V, Pizarro PL, Zacarías MF, Vinderola G, Medina R, Van Nieuwenhove C. Production of conjugated dienoic and trienoic fatty acids by lactic acid bacteria and bifidobacteria. *J Funct Foods* (2015) 19:417–25. doi:10.1016/j.jff.2015.09.046
38. Villena J, Salva S, Aguero G, Alvarez S. Immunomodulatory and protective effect of probiotic *Lactobacillus casei* against *Candida albicans* infection in malnourished mice. *Microbiol Immunol* (2011) 55:434–45. doi:10.1111/j.1348-0421.2011.00334.x
39. Weisberg SP, McCann D, Desai M, Rosenbaum M, Leibel RL, Ferrante AW. Obesity is associated with macrophage accumulation in adipose tissue. *J Clin Invest* (2003) 112:1796–808. doi:10.1172/JCI200319246
40. Kanda H, Tateya S, Tamori Y, Kotani K, Hiasa K, Kitazawa R, et al. MCP-1 contributes to macrophage infiltration into adipose tissue, insulin resistance, and hepatic steatosis in obesity. *J Clin Invest* (2006) 116:1494–505. doi:10.1172/JCI26498
41. Fujisaka S, Usui I, Bukhari A, Ikutani M, Oya T, Kanatani Y, et al. Regulatory mechanisms for adipose tissue M1 and M2 macrophages in diet-induced obese mice. *Diabetes* (2009) 58:2574–82. doi:10.2337/db08-1475
42. Rodbell M. The metabolism of isolated fat cells. IV. Regulation of release of protein by lipolytic hormones and insulin. *J Biol Chem* (1966) 241:3909–17.

43. Bernstein RL, Hyun WC, Davis JH, Fulwyler MJ, Pershadsingh HA. Flow cytometric analysis of mature adipocytes. *Cytometry* (1989) 10:469–74. doi:10.1002/cyto.990100416
44. Dogi CA, Galdeano CM, Perdigón G. Gut immune stimulation by non pathogenic Gram (+) and Gram (-) bacteria. Comparison with a probiotic strain. *Cytokine* (2008) 41:223–31. doi:10.1016/j.cyto.2007.11.014
45. Agüero G, Villena J, Racedo S, Haro C, Alvarez S. Beneficial immunomodulatory activity of *Lactobacillus casei* in malnourished mice pneumonia: effect on inflammation and coagulation. *Nutrition* (2006) 22:810–9. doi:10.1016/j.nut.2006.03.013
46. Yin Y-N. Effects of four bifidobacteria on obesity in high-fat diet induced rats. *World J Gastroenterol* (2010) 16:3394. doi:10.3748/wjg.v16.i27.3394
47. Sanz Y, Santacruz A, Gauffin P. Gut microbiota in obesity and metabolic disorders. *Proc Nutr Soc* (2010) 69:434–41. doi:10.1017/S0029665110001813
48. Glass CK, Olefsky JM. Inflammation and lipid signaling in the etiology of insulin resistance. *Cell Metab* (2012) 15:635–45. doi:10.1016/j.cmet.2012.04.001
49. Desruisseaux MS, Nagajyothi F, Trujillo ME, Tanowitz HB, Scherer PE. Adipocyte, adipose tissue, and infectious disease. *Infect Immun* (2007) 75:1066–78. doi:10.1128/IAI.01455-06
50. Cho KW, Morris DL, Lumeng CN. Flow cytometry analyses of adipose tissue macrophages. *Methods in Enzymology* Elsevier (2014). p. 297–314. Available from: http://linkinghub.elsevier.com/retrieve/pii/B9780124116191000161
51. Antuna-Puente B, Feve B, Fellahi S, Bastard J-P. Adipokines: the missing link between insulin resistance and obesity. *Diabetes Metab* (2008) 34:2–11. doi:10.1016/j.diabet.2007.09.004
52. Moller DE. Potential role of TNF-alpha in the pathogenesis of insulin resistance and type 2 diabetes. *Trends Endocrinol Metab* (2000) 11:212–7. doi:10.1016/S1043-2760(00)00272-1
53. Wolf J, Rose-John S, Garbers C. Interleukin-6 and its receptors: a highly regulated and dynamic system. *Cytokine* (2014) 70:11–20. doi:10.1016/j.cyto.2014.05.024
54. Opal SM, Depalo VA. Anti-inflammatory cytokines. *Chest J* (2000) 117:1162–72. doi:10.1378/chest.117.4.1162
55. Wolowczuk I, Verwaerde C, Viltart O, Delanoye A, Delacre M, Pot B, et al. Feeding our immune system: impact on metabolism. *Clin Dev Immunol* (2008) 2008:639803. doi:10.1155/2008/639803
56. Raybould HE. Gut microbiota, epithelial function and derangements in obesity: gut microbiota, epithelial function and derangements in obesity. *J Physiol* (2012) 590:441–6. doi:10.1113/jphysiol.2011.222133
57. Akira S, Uematsu S, Takeuchi O. Pathogen recognition and innate immunity. *Cell* (2006) 124:783–801. doi:10.1016/j.cell.2006.02.015
58. Batra A, Pietsch J, Fedke I, Glauben R, Okur B, Stroh T, et al. Leptin-dependent toll-like receptor expression and responsiveness in preadipocytes and adipocytes. *Am J Pathol* (2007) 170:1931–41. doi:10.2353/ajpath.2007.060699
59. Jaedicke KM, Roythorne A, Padget K, Todryk S, Preshaw PM, Taylor JJ. Leptin up-regulates TLR2 in human monocytes. *J Leukoc Biol* (2013) 93:561–71. doi:10.1189/jlb.1211606
60. Wu C-C, Weng W-L, Lai W-L, Tsai H-P, Liu W-H, Lee M-H, et al. Effect of *Lactobacillus plantarum* strain K21 on high-fat diet-fed obese mice. *Evid Based Complement Alternat Med* (2015) 2015:e391767. doi:10.1155/2015/391767
61. Ferrante AW. The immune cells in adipose tissue. *Diabetes Obes Metab* (2013) 15(Suppl 3):34–8. doi:10.1111/dom.12154
62. Aravindhan V, Madhumitha H. Metainflammation in diabetic coronary artery disease: emerging role of innate and adaptive immune responses. *J Diabetes Res* (2016) 2016:6264149. doi:10.1155/2016/6264149
63. Cerovic V, Bain CC, Mowat AM, Milling SWF. Intestinal macrophages and dendritic cells: what's the difference? *Trends Immunol* (2014) 35:270–7. doi:10.1016/j.it.2014.04.003
64. Michaud A, Drolet R, Noël S, Paris G, Tchernof A. Visceral fat accumulation is an indicator of adipose tissue macrophage infiltration in women. *Metabolism* (2012) 61:689–98. doi:10.1016/j.metabol.2011.10.004
65. Morris DL, Singer K, Lumeng CN. Adipose tissue macrophages: phenotypic plasticity and diversity in lean and obese states. *Curr Opin Clin Nutr Metab Care* (2011) 14:341–6. doi:10.1097/MCO.0b013e328347970b
66. Lee B-C, Lee J. Cellular and molecular players in adipose tissue inflammation in the development of obesity-induced insulin resistance. *Biochim Biophys Acta* (2014) 1842:446–62. doi:10.1016/j.bbadis.2013.05.017
67. Martí A, Marcos A, Martínez JA. Obesity and immune function relationships. *Obes Rev* (2001) 2:131–40. doi:10.1046/j.1467-789x.2001.00025.x
68. Heilbronn LK, Campbell LV. Adipose tissue macrophages, low grade inflammation and insulin resistance in human obesity. *Curr Pharm Des* (2008) 14:1225–30. doi:10.2174/138161208784246153
69. Keusch GT. The history of nutrition: malnutrition, infection and immunity. *J Nutr* (2003) 133:36S–340S.
70. Cildir G, Akıncılar SC, Tergaonkar V. Chronic adipose tissue inflammation: all immune cells on the stage. *Trends Mol Med* (2013) 19:487–500. doi:10.1016/j.molmed.2013.05.001
71. Gauffin Cano P, Santacruz A, Moya Á, Sanz Y. Bacteroides uniformis CECT 7771 ameliorates metabolic and immunological dysfunction in mice. *PLoS One* (2012) 7(7):e41079. doi:10.1371/journal.pone.0041079
72. Medina M, Izquierdo E, Ennahar S, Sanz Y. Differential immunomodulatory properties of *Bifidobacterium logum* strains: relevance to probiotic selection and clinical applications: immunomodulatory properties of B. longum strains. *Clin Exp Immunol* (2007) 150:531–8. doi:10.1111/j.1365-2249.2007.03522.x
73. Maassen CB, van Holten-Neelen C, Balk F, den Bak-Glashouwer MJ, Leer RJ, Laman JD, et al. Strain-dependent induction of cytokine profiles in the gut by orally administered *Lactobacillus* strains. *Vaccine* (2000) 18:2613–23. doi:10.1016/S0264-410X(99)00378-3
74. Sanz Y, Nadal I, Sánchez E. Probiotics as drugs against human gastrointestinal infections. *Recent Pat Antiinfect Drug Discov* (2007) 2:148–56. doi:10.2174/157489107780832596
75. McMullen MH, Hamilton-Reeves JM, Bonorden MJ, Wangen KE, Phipps WR, Feirtag JM, et al. Consumption of *Lactobacillus acidophilus* and *Bifidobacterium longum* does not alter phytoestrogen metabolism and plasma hormones in men: a pilot study. *J Altern Complement Med* (2006) 12:887–94. doi:10.1089/acm.2006.12.887
76. Sousa R, Halper J, Zhang J, Lewis SJ, Li WI. Effect of *Lactobacillus acidophilus* supernatants on body weight and leptin expression in rats. *BMC Complement Altern Med* (2008) 8:5. doi:10.1186/1472-6882-8-5
77. Kusunoki H, Taniyama Y, Otsu R, Rakugi H, Morishita R. Anti-inflammatory effects of hepatocyte growth factor on the vicious cycle of macrophages and adipocytes. *Hypertens Res* (2014) 37:500–6. doi:10.1038/hr.2014.41
78. De Palma G, Cinova J, Stepankova R, Tuckova L, Sanz Y. Pivotal advance: bifidobacteria and Gram-negative bacteria differentially influence immune responses in the proinflammatory milieu of celiac disease. *J Leukoc Biol* (2010) 87:765–78. doi:10.1189/jlb.0709471
79. Bastard J-P, Lagathu C, Caron M, Capeau J. Point-counterpoint: interleukin-6 does/does not have a beneficial role in insulin sensitivity and glucose homeostasis. *J Appl Physiol* (2007) 102:821–2; author reply 825.
80. Ouchi N, Parker JL, Lugus JJ, Walsh K. Adipokines in inflammation and metabolic disease. *Nat Rev Immunol* (2011) 11(2):85–97. doi:10.1038/nri2921
81. Huh JY, Park YJ, Ham M, Kim JB. Crosstalk between adipocytes and immune cells in adipose tissue inflammation and metabolic dysregulation in obesity. *Mol Cells* (2014) 37(5):365–71. doi:10.14348/molcells.2014.0074
82. Russo M, Fabersani E, Abeijón-Mukdsi MC, Ross R, Fontana C, Benítez-Páez A, et al. *Lactobacillus fermentum* CRL1446 ameliorates oxidative and metabolic parameters by increasing intestinal feruloyl esterase activity and modulating microbiota in caloric-restricted mice. *Nutrients* (2016) 8:E415. doi:10.3390/nu8070415

18

The Role of Microbiota and Immunobiotics in Granulopoiesis of Immunocompromised Hosts

Susana Salva[1] and Susana Alvarez[1,2]**

[1] *Immunobiotechnology Laboratory, CERELA-CONICET, Tucuman, Argentina,* [2] *Applied Biochemistry Institute, Universidad Nacional de Tucumán, Tucuman, Argentina*

Edited by:
Juarez Antonio Simões Quaresma, Federal University of Pará, Brazil

Reviewed by:
Maryam Dadar, Razi Vaccine and Serum Research Institute, Iran
Paras K. Anand, Imperial College London, UK

***Correspondence:**
Susana Salva
ssalva@cerela.org.ar;
Susana Alvarez
salvarez@cerela.org.ar

The number of granulocytes is maintained by a regulated balance between granulopoiesis in the bone marrow and clearance and destruction in peripheral tissues. Granulopoiesis plays a fundamental role in the innate immune response. Therefore, factors affecting the normal granulopoiesis lead to alterations in innate defenses and reduce the resistance against infections. In this study, we give a description on recent advances regarding the molecular and cellular events that regulate steady-state and emergency granulopoiesis, which are crucial processes for the generation of protective innate immune responses. Particular attention will be given to emergency granulopoiesis alterations in immunosuppression states caused by malnutrition and chemotherapy. The role of microbiota in maintaining a steady-state granulopoiesis and the immunological mechanisms involved are also discussed. Moreover, we describe the findings of our laboratory demonstrating that the dietary supplementation with immunobiotics is an interesting alternative to improve steady-state and emergency granulopoiesis, the respiratory innate immune response, and the resistance against respiratory pathogens in immunocompromised hosts.

Keywords: immunobiotics, granulopoiesis, immunocompromised hosts, respiratory infections, *Lactobacillus rhamnosus* CRL1505

INTRODUCTION

The microbiota is a complex community of bacteria, fungi, archaea, and viruses that colonize the mucosal surfaces and skin of the human body (1). The gut microbiota is typically integrated by bacteria and specifically by members of the divisions *Bacteroidetes* and *Firmicutes* (2). However, each individual's microbiota is unique, and its composition depends on multiple factors, such as, diet, lifestyle, host genetic, use of antibiotics, and environment (3–5). The gut microbiota plays a fundamental role in the health maintenance of its host. In particular, we highlight that microbiota is able to control immunity in distant tissues through its capacity to regulate hematopoiesis at primary immune sites as the bone marrow (BM) (6). On the other hand, the immunomodulatory probiotic lactic acid bacteria (immunobiotics) are capable to improve the recovery of myeloid cells production affected by malnutrition or chemotherapy, and to increase the immune response against bacterial pathogens (7, 8). The mechanisms for systemic immunomodulation by the microbiota provide a probable mechanism for immunobiotics activity, demonstrating that translocated microbial products benefit the host by enhancing systemic innate immune function.

In this mini review, we examine the interaction between microbiota and immune system, and how this crosstalk affects the maintenance of a steady-state granulopoiesis that is crucial for the generation of protective innate immune responses. We also revise the alterations of emergency granulopoiesis in immunosuppression states caused by malnutrition and chemotherapy. In addition, we discuss

TABLE 1 | Regulation of granulopoiesis by microbiota and immunobiotics.

Experiemental models	Outcome
Microbiota-granulopoiesis crosstalk	
Polymyxin treated and germ-free (GF) mice (18)	Decreased levels of splenic and bone marrow (BM) progenitor cells forming GM-CFU colonies
Kanamycin-treated mice (17)	Decreased numbers of granulocytes in the BM and blood
GF mice Antibiotic-treated mice Nod1-deficient mice (23)	Translocation of peptidoglycan from the gut to neutrophils in the BM Peptidoglycan concentrations in sera correlate with neutrophil function Antimicrobial capacity of neutrophils depends on recognition of microbiota-derived peptidoglycan from Gram-negative bacteria *via* the pattern-recognition receptor Nod1 but not Nod2 orTLR4 Consistent with impaired innate priming Nod1-deficient mice were unable to control *Streptococcus pneumoniae* early sepsis
GF mice *TLR4*$^{-/-}$ mice *TRIF*$^{-/-}$ mice *MyD88*$^{-/-}$ mice (14)	Total lack of microbial colonization is associated with decreased neutrophil numbers and decreased G-CSF levels in the steady state *In vivo* feedback is impaired in *TLR4*$^{-/-}$ and *TRIF*$^{-/-}$, but not *MyD88*$^{-/-}$ animals Steady-state neutrophil homeostasis is G-CSF-dependent and regulated through pattern-recognition receptors, thereby directly linking toll-like receptor (TLR)-triggering to granulopoiesis
MyD88-deficient mice (20)	Loss of MyD88 reduce numbers and proliferation rate of hematopoietic stem cells in the BM
GF mice (27)	Reduction of neutrophil recruitment to the peritoneal cavity in response to diverse stimuli including microbial components and sterile ligands Microbiota-derived signals *via* a MyD88-dependent pathway are required to precondition the neutrophil inflammatory response
Antibiotic treated neonatal mice GF neonatal mice (16)	Decreased numbers of circulating and BM neutrophils and lower granulocyte-macrophages in the BM Decreased number of interleukin (IL)-17-producing cells in the intestine and production of G-CSF Increased susceptibility to *Escherichia coli* K1 and *Klebsiella pneumoniae* sepsis, which could be partially reversed by administration of G-CSF. Microbiota-derived components, such as LPS *via* TLR4/MyD88 signaling, induced IL-17 production mainly by group 3 innate lymphoid cells in the intestine and increased plasma levels of G-CSF leading to granulocytosis
GF mice (19)	Damage of differentiation of specific myeloid cell progenitors of both yolk sac and BM origin Innate immune defects lead to impaired early responses to pathogens
GF mice (21)	Complexity of the intestinal microbiota correlates with the number of BM myeloid cells Transfer of sterile filtered, boiled serum from colonized mice was sufficient to expand the BM myeloid cell pool of GF mice in a MyD88/Toll-IL-I receptor-containing adaptor molecule-dependent manner, indicating that heat-stable, circulating, commensal-derived products may be responsible for maintaining steady-state myelopoiesis levels
Antibiotic-treated mice (28)	Impairment of resistance to lung infection with *K. pneumoniae* and reduction of ROS-mediated bacterial killing by alveolar macrophages and required Nod1- and Nod2- but not TLR-dependent signaling
GF mice Antibiotic-treated mice (29)	Reduction steady-state numbers of tissue-resident and BM-derived phagocytes rendered GF and antibiotic-treated mice susceptible to acute systemic *Lysteria monocytogenes* infection
Neonatal non-obese diabetic mice (22)	The gut microbiota enriched in *Staphylococcus* in neonatal non-obese diabetic mice, correlated with increased immature granulocytes in the liver and spleen
Immunobiotics-granulopoiesis crosstalk	
Protein-malnourished mice (33)	Protein malnutrition altered B cell development in BM. The treatment of malnourished mice with *Lactobacillus rhamnosus* CRL1505 was able to induce a recovery of B cells that would explain its ability to increase immunity against infections
Protein-malnourished mice (35)	Repletion of malnourished mice with supplemental *Lactobacillus rhamnosus* improved neutrophils recruitment, phagocytic activity, and resistance against pneumococcal infection
Protein-malnourished mice (7)	Protein-malnutrition impaired the emergency myelopoiesis induced by the generation of the innate immune response against pneumococcal infection Repletion of malnourished mice with *Lactobacillus rhamnosus* CRL1505 was able to accelerate the recovery of granulopoiesis and improve innate immunity
Chemotherapy-treated mice (8)	*Lactobacillus casei* CRL431 and *Lactobacillus rhamnosus* CRL1506 accelerated the recovery of Cy-caused myelosuppression and the recovery of the immune response against the opportunistic pathogen *Candida albicans*
Chemotherapy-treated mice (53)	*Bifidobacterium longum* BB536 increased resistance to sepsis caused by an intestinal infection of *Pseudomonas aeruginosa* in mice treated with Cy
Chemotherapy-treated mice (42, 54)	*Lactobacillus plantarum* HY7712 as *Lactobacillus casei* HY7213 accelerated the recovery of Cy-induced immunosuppression by immunopotentiating NK cells and cytotoxic T lymphocytes derived from BM and spleen, in addition to restoring the phagocytic capacity of peritoneal macrophages
Chemotherapy-treated mice (55)	*Lactobacillus plantarum* stimulated the proliferation of splenocytes from mice immunocompromised by Cy treatment in response to LPS

the research of our laboratory demonstrating that dietary supplementation with immunobiotics is an interesting alternative to improve steady-state and emergency granulopoiesis, respiratory innate immune response, and resistance against respiratory pathogens in immunocompromised hosts.

GRANULOPOIESIS AND ITS REGULATION BY THE GUT MICROBIOTA

Granulocytes are key players of the innate immune response. They are short-lived cells, and their number is kept by a balance between BM granulopoiesis and peripheral tissues' clearance and destruction (9). These cells are continuously generated in steady-state conditions from long-lived self-renewing hematopoietic stem cells (HSCs) that give rise to short-lived HSCs and multipotent progenitors (MPPs) in BM. MPPs differentiate into common lymphoid and myeloid progenitors (CMP). CMPs give rise to granulocyte-macrophage (GMP), megakaryocyte-erythrocytes, and dendritic cell progenitors. Neutrophils, monocytes, as well as other granulocyte populations derive from GMPs (10). In front of an infectious challenge, neutrophils are recruited in large numbers to the infected tissues, the hematopoietic system must rapidly respond to the demand of these cells by turning from the steady-state to an emergency granulopoiesis (11).

The tissue macrophages activate the LRX family transcription factors during the ingestion of apoptotic neutrophils in steady-state granulopoiesis. This, in turn, suppresses the pro-inflammatory cytokines' production (12). Those macrophages decrease their production of interleukin (IL)-23 and thereby reduce the stimulus for IL-17 production by innate lymphoid cells, natural killer T cells, γδ-T cells, or Th17 cells. The reduced IL-17 levels account for low G-CSF expression (13). Involvement of IL-23/IL-17/G-CSF axis in regulation of granulopoiesis was confirmed in several independent murine models (14) and human studies (15). Moreover, steady-state neutrophil homeostasis is G-CSF-dependent and regulated through pattern-recognition receptors (PRRs), thereby directly linking Toll-like receptor (TLR)-triggering to granulopoiesis (14). Microbiota-derived components, such as LPS *via* TLR4/MyD88 signaling, induced intestinal IL-17 production and increased plasma levels of G-CSF leading to granulocytosis (16). Studies using antibiotics-treated and germ-free (GF) mice showed a decrease in GMPs in BM, and a lower number of neutrophils in the periphery (16–20). Furthermore, it was reported that a live complex flora is needed to restore granulopoiesis completely (21, 22). By using MyD88-deficient mice, it was shown that MyD88-dependent TLR signaling induced by microbiota can impact on the early hematopoietic development and terminal myeloid differentiation (20, 21) (**Table 1**).

During emergency granulopoiesis, pathogen-associated molecule patterns (PAMPs) are detected by PRRs of innate immune system. In addition, bacteria and bacteria-derived products (e.g., LPS) are sensed by TLR-expressing endothelial cells. Consequently, the granulopoiesis and the neutrophils' release into the circulation are produced by the increased amounts of G-CSF and GM-CSF (11). A large body of evidence suggests that circulating microbiota-derived products or pathogens may reach the BM or extramedullar sites, where they can be directly sensed by HSPCs and committed myeloid progenitors (23, 24). On the other hand, circulating HSCs can encounter bacteria or their products in the periphery before re-entering the BM (10). LPS-sensing by hematopoietic cells is dispensable for the induction of emergency granulopoiesis. TLR4 and MyD88 expression of non-hematopoietic cell type is absolutely required for this process (25, 26). Thus, levels of growth factors determine the rate at which neutrophils are induced the proliferation and differentiation of neutrophil precursors by JAK–STAT pathways. In this context, transcription factor C/EBP-α regulates steady-state granulopoiesis, whereas C/EBP-β is critical for triggering emergency granulopoiesis in response to GM-CSF (11). On the other hand, recent studies demonstrate that microbiota priming is required for neutrophil extravasation to injured tissues after inflammatory stimuli (27). In addition, antimicrobial capacity of neutrophils was shown to be dependent on the recognition of microbiota-derived peptidoglycan from Gram-negative bacteria *via* Nod1 but not Nod2 or TLR4 (23). An example of the systemic effect of gut microbiota on granulopoiesis during infection has been provided by a research work demonstrating that early innate resistance to *Klebsiella pneumoniae* lung infection was impaired in microbiota-depleted mice, and that the peptidoglycan translocated from the gut was able to modulate the systemic innate immunity (28). Therefore, factors affecting the normal granulopoiesis lead to alterations in innate defenses and reduce the resistance against pathogens (23, 28, 29) (**Table 1**).

GRANULOPOIESIS AND MALNOURISHED HOSTS

Granulopoietic homeostasis requires an important cellular renewal, because of the cells' generation and death. Approximately $0.5–1.0 \times 10^{11}$ granulocytes are generated each day during steady-state conditions in adults (11). In contrast to local infection that can be contained by the innate immune response, in severe infections, the emergency granulopoiesis is triggered and neutrophilia occurs. Therefore, the hematopoietic system is capable of rapid adaptation when augmenting cellular output several-fold levels to respond to the higher demand for neutrophils (10). Steady-state growth and development, physical activity, and response to serious illness are affected by nutritional status (30). In agreement to several research works, we have established that malnutrition affects the hematopoietic tissue that has a high turnover rate and cell proliferation, inducing a damage of blood cells production and causing hypoplasia and histological alterations of BM (31–33). This is characterized by a reduction of hematopoietic space, which is occupied by components of extracellular matrix (31, 33). These histological alterations may be responsible for the damage of the hematopoietic niches, which may influence the crosstalk between hematopoietic cells and the growth factors that regulate the granulopoiesis. In line with Borelli et al. (34), a reduction of GMPs was observed in BM of malnourished mice that could explain the reduction of myeloid cells of BM and blood (7, 35). Thus, nutritional deficiencies affect hematopoiesis, leading to an immunocompromised condition (35).

The relationship between malnutrition and infection can be viewed under two aspects: malnutrition compromising host defense, or infections either aggravating a previously existing deficient nutritional status or triggering malnutrition through disease pathogenesis. It was described that malnutrition alters both innate and adaptive immune responses as consequence of multiple abnormalities induced in the immune system (36). Herrera et al. (7) demonstrated that protein-malnutrition significantly reduces the capacity to recruit neutrophils into infected lungs and that this effect could be related to impairment in granulopoiesis. Several factors could be involved in the impairment of emergency granulopoiesis in malnourished mice, in addition to those mentioned above. CXCL12 expression in response to pneumococcal infection in BM requires special attention. The HSCs homing into BM is regulated by CXCL12 and their receptor CXCR4 (9). There is no change in the expression of CXCL12 during an infection in malnourished mice, which could be a mechanism for the preservation of HSCs in the BM. Malnutrition also impairs the expression of both GM-CSF and IL-1 in BM and contributes to the altered emergency granulopoietic response (7). It is known that the steady-state and emergency granulopoiesis are directed by GM-CSF while the BM stromal cells function is to support hematopoiesis mainly regulated by IL-1 (37). Hence, the neutrophilia induced by infection or inflammation is assisted by both GM-CSF and IL-1, which in turn accelerates granulopoiesis by expanding MPP and CMP compartments (38). Thus, the reduced capacity of malnourished hosts to develop adequate levels of GM-CSF may explain BM's defective response against an infectious challenge.

On the other hand, there is a great increase in the number of patients with secondary immunodeficiencies related to chemotherapeutic treatments. Cyclophosphamide (Cy) is a drug widely used as an antineoplastic alkylating agent because of its significant therapeutic range and broad spectrum of activity to treat different types of cancer (39). For the World Health Organization, Cy is one of the essential medicines needed in a health system (40). However, this drug induces serious side effects, such as apoptosis and necrosis in BM cells (41), alterations of basal and emergency hematopoiesis, immunosuppression (8, 42), increased susceptibility to infections (8, 43), and even change of intestinal microbiota composition (44). Because of the increased susceptibility to infections, chemotherapy is commonly used in combination with antibiotics in cancer therapy (45). Paradoxically, the consequent propagation of antibiotic resistance among pathogens and depletion of intestinal microbiota lead to increased vulnerability of these patients. For these reasons, it is vital to support treatments aimed at recovering the hematopoietic capacity to increase the efficiency of the immune response triggered in infectious hematopoietic alternative resources processes.

CAN ORAL ADMINISTRATION OF IMMUNOBIOTICS REGULATE GRANULOPOIESIS?

In the last years, a number of research project were meant to find alternative treatments to favor hematopoiesis, improve immunity, booster anticancer effects, and clear anticancer drugs (46). A long list of health benefits has been described for immunobiotics, are likely to modulate and enhance immunity functions in malnourished mice (8, 47–49) (**Table 1**).

Therefore, when the diet induced *Lactobacillus casei* CRL431 or *Lactobacillus rhamnosus* CRL1505, the recovery of the respiratory immunity in immunocompromised hosts was reduced from 21 to 7 days (32, 50, 51). Furthermore, the supplementation of repletion diet with immunobiotics induced recovery of mielopoyesis and normalization of emergency granulopoiesis in response to pneumococcal infection (7, 32). We demonstrated that the treatments with immunobiotics were efficient to recover the architecture of BM tissue, subendosteal epithelium, and BM cellularity altered by malnutrition (7). Moreover, the administration of *L. rhamnosus* CRL1505 induced the growth of mitotic pool cells, mature myeloid cells, and neutrophils in BM. Although the mechanisms involved are not completely elucidated, it is known that cell wall components reach the gut mucosa and from there to circulation during colonization of gut mucosa by commensal bacteria or probiotics. Indeed, the detection of peptidoglycan in the neutrophil fraction shows that it can accumulate in the BM (23). Considering these findings, a probable mechanism for the immunobiotic activity of the microbiota was observed, demonstrating that microbial products favor the systemic innate immune function of the host.

On the other hand, it was described that some immunobiotics can influence ILs levels in blood, which agree with our findings demonstrating the capacity of immunobiotics to normalize the levels of TNF-α, IL-1β, IL-4, IL-6, and IL-10 in malnourished mice (52). It is probably that the changes in ILs levels induced by immunobiotics could influence on the normalization of granulopoiesis. Moreover, we demonstrated for the first time that dietary supplementation with immunobiotics can modulate the production of GM-CSF in infected lungs and its expression in the BM. Moreover, immunobiotics modulate the CXCR4/CXCL12 signaling axis, which is associated with the recovery of hematopoiesis induced by *L. rhamnosus* CRL1505 (7). The detailed study of the mechanisms that explain the influence of immunobiotics on the regulation of granulopoiesis in BM is an interesting topic for future investigations.

Some works have described beneficial effects of immunobiotics on myelosuppression and immunosuppression in Cy-treated mice, although no deep mechanistic studies were performed (8, 42, 53–55) (**Table 1**). Taking into consideration the capacity of *L. casei* CRL431 and *L. rhamnosus* CRL1506 to modulate hematopoiesis in malnourished mice, we also aimed to evaluate the ability of these immunobiotic strains in Cy-treated mice. We showed that preventive treatment with immunobiotics is capable to increase GMPs in BM ($CD34^+$ and $CD34^+Gr\text{-}1^+$ cells), which enables a prompt recovery of peripheral blood neutrophils after Cy-administration (8). These immunobiotic treatments were also able to improve recruitment of phagocytic cells to the site of infection and increase resistance against *Candida albicans* (8). Further studies to evaluate the mechanisms involved in these activities are needed. However, these results support the idea that immunobiotic strains can improve the recovery from Cy-immunosuppression, enhancing myeloid population in BM. Therefore, immunobiotics can serve as alternatives to reduce the immunosuppression in patients treated with chemotherapy drugs.

CONCLUDING REMARKS

This review exposes wide evidence that the gut microbiota regulates granulocyte homeostasis, and therefore influences the host's innate immune response. Additionally, research from the last years demonstrated that the oral administration of immunobiotics improves the recovery of steady-state granulopoiesis and stimulate the emergency granulopoiesis in malnourished and Cy-immunocompromised host. Future research is needed in order to elucidate the mechanisms by which specific immunobiotic strains enhance the recovery of granulopoiesis in immunocompromised hosts. Although the use of colony-stimulating factors can reduce the increased risk of infections induced by chemotherapy treatments, they are also the cause of several important side effects including bone pain, low-grade fever, and fatigue. Interestingly, the results expressed provide the basis for new applications of immunobiotics in order to stimulate the production of neutrophils and other types of leukocytes in the BM which would strength the ability of the host to fight against infections, without the side effects observed for stimulating factors. Certainly, this immunobiotic effect would improve the quality of life of patients receiving chemotherapy.

AUTHOR CONTRIBUTIONS

SS and SA wrote and approved the manuscript.

REFERENCES

1. Clemente JC, Ursell LK, Parfrey LW, Knight R. The impact of the gut microbiota on human health: an integrative view. *Cell* (2012) 148:1258–70. doi:10.1016/j.cell.2012.01.035
2. Rabot S, Membrez M, Blancher F, Berger B, Moine D, Krause L, et al. High fat diet drives obesity regardless the composition of gut microbiota in mice. *Sci Rep* (2016) 6:32484. doi:10.1038/srep32484
3. Benson AK, Kelly SA, Legge R, Ma F, Low SJ, Kim J, et al. Individuality in gut microbiota composition is a complex polygenic trait shaped by multiple environmental and host genetic factors. *Proc Natl Acad Sci U S A* (2010) 107:18933–8. doi:10.1073/pnas.1007028107
4. Spor A, Koren O, Ley R. Unravelling the effects of the environment and host genotype on the gut microbiome. *Nat Rev Microbiol* (2011) 9:279–90. doi:10.1038/nrmicro2540
5. Becattini S, Taur Y, Pamer EG. Antibiotic-induced changes in the intestinal microbiota and disease. *Trends Mol Med* (2016) 22(6):458–78. doi:10.1016/j.molmed.2016.04.003
6. Gorjifard S, Goldszmid RS. Microbiota-myeloid cell crosstalk beyond the gut. *J Leukoc Biol* (2016) 100:865–79. doi:10.1189/jlb.3RI0516-222R
7. Herrera M, Salva S, Villena J, Barbieri N, Marranzino G, Alvarez S. Dietary supplementation with *Lactobacilli* improves emergency granulopoiesis in protein-malnourished mice and enhances respiratory innate immune response. *PLoS ONE* (2014) 9:e90227. doi:10.1371/journal.pone.0090227
8. Salva S, Marranzino G, Villena J, Agüero G, Alvarez S. Probiotic *Lactobacillus* strains protect against myelosuppression and immunosuppression in cyclophosphamide-treated mice. *Int Immunopharmacol* (2014) 22:209–21. doi:10.1016/j.intimp.2014.06.017
9. Naussef WM, Borregaard N. Neutrophils at work. *Nat Immunol* (2014) 15:602–11. doi:10.1038/ni.2921
10. Takizawa H, Boettcher S, Manz MG. Demand-adapted regulation of early hematopoiesis in infection and inflammation. *Blood* (2012) 119:2991–3002. doi:10.1182/blood-2011-12-380113
11. Manz MG, Boettcher S. Emergency granulopoiesis. *Nat Rev Immunol* (2014) 14:302–14. doi:10.1038/nri3660
12. A-Gonzalez N, Bensinger SJ, Hong C, Beceiro S, Bradley MN, Zelcer N, et al. Apoptotic cells promote their own clearance and immune tolerance through activation of the nuclear receptor LXR. *Immunity* (2009) 31:245–58. doi:10.1016/j.immuni.2009.06.018
13. Mei J, Liu Y, Dai N, Hoffmann C, Hudock KM, Zhang P, et al. Cxcr2 and Cxcl5 regulate the IL-17/G-CSF axis and neutrophil homeostasis in mice. *J Clin Invest* (2012) 122:974–86. doi:10.1172/JCI60588
14. Bugl S, Wirths S, Radsak MP, Schild H, Stein P, André MC, et al. Steady-state neutrophil homeostasis is dependent on TLR4/TRIF signaling. *Blood* (2013) 121:723–33. doi:10.1182/blood-2012-05-429589
15. Westerterp M, Gourion-Arsiquaud S, Murphy AJ, Shih A, Cremers S, Levine RL, et al. Regulation of hematopoietic stem and progenitor cell mobilization by cholesterol efflux pathways. *Cell Stem Cell* (2012) 11:195–206. doi:10.1016/j.stem.2012.04.024
16. Deshmukh HS, Liu Y, Menkiti OR, Mei J, Dai N, O'Leary CE, et al. The microbiota regulates neutrophil homeostasis and host resistance to *Escherichia coli* K1 sepsis in neonatal mice. *Nat Med* (2014) 20:524–30. doi:10.1038/nm.3542
17. Tada T, Yamamura S, Kuwano Y, Abo T. Level of myelopoiesis in the bone marrow is influenced by intestinal flora. *Cell Immunol* (1996) 173:155–111. doi:10.1006/cimm.1996.0261
18. Goris H, de Boer F, van der Waaij D. Myelopoiesis in experimentally contaminated specific-pathogen-free and germ free mice during oral administration of polymyxin. *Infect Immun* (1985) 50:437–41.
19. Khosravi A, Yáñez A, Price JG, Chow A, Merad M, Goodridge HS, et al. Gut microbiota promote hematopoiesis to control bacterial infection. *Cell Host Microbe* (2014) 15:374–81. doi:10.1016/j.chom.2014.02.006
20. Fiedler K, Kokai E, Bresch S, Brunner C. MyD88 is involved in myeloid as well as lymphoid hematopoiesis independent of the presence of a pathogen. *Am J Blood Res* (2013) 3:124–40.
21. Balmer ML, Schürch CM, Saito Y, Geuking MB, Li H, Cuenca M, et al. Microbiota-derived compounds drive steady-state granulopoiesis via MyD88/TICAM signaling. *J Immunol* (2014) 193:5273–83. doi:10.4049/jimmunol.1400762
22. Damlund DS, Metzdorff SB, Hasselby JP, Wiese M, Lundsager M, Nielsen DS, et al. Postnatal hematopoiesis and gut microbiota in NOD mice deviate fromC57BL/6 mice. *J Diabetes Res* (2016) 2016:6321980. doi:10.1155/2016/6321980
23. Clarke TB, Davis KM, Lysenko ES, Zhou AY, Yu Y, Weiser JN. Recognition of peptidoglycan from the microbiota by Nod1 enhances systemic innate immunity. *Nat Med* (2010) 16:228–31. doi:10.1038/nm.2087
24. Zeng MY, Cisalpino D, Varadarajan S, Hellman J, Warren HS, Cascalho M, et al. Gut microbiota-induced immunoglobulin G controls systemic infection by symbiotic bacteria and pathogens. *Immunity* (2016) 44:647–58. doi:10.1016/j.immuni.2016.02.006
25. Boettcher S, Ziegler P, Schmid MA, Takizawa H, van Rooijen N, Kopf M, et al. Cutting edge: LPS-induced emergency myelopoiesis depends on TLR4-expressing non-hematopoietic cells. *J Immunol* (2012) 188:5824–8. doi:10.4049/jimmunol.1103253
26. Boettcher S, Gerosa RC, Radpour R, Bauer J, Ampenberger F, Heikenwalder M, et al. Endothelial cells translate pathogen signals into G-CSF-driven emergency granulopoiesis. *Blood* (2014) 124:1393–403. doi:10.1182/blood-2014-04-570762
27. Karmarkar D, Rock KL. Microbiota signalling through MyD88 is necessary for a systemic neutrophilic inflammatory response. *Immunology* (2013) 140:483–92. doi:10.1111/imm.12159
28. Clarke TB. Early innate immunity to bacterial infection in the lung is regulated systemically by the commensal microbiota via nod-like receptor ligands. *Infect Immun* (2014) 82:4596–606. doi:10.1128/IAI.02212-14
29. Mittrücker HW, Seidel D, Bland PW, Zarzycka A, Kaufmann SH, Visekruna A, et al. Lack of microbiota reduces innate responses and enhances adaptive immunity against *Listeria monocytogenes* infection. *Eur J Immunol* (2014) 44:1710–5. doi:10.1002/eji.201343927
30. Rodriguez L, Cervantes E, Ortiz R. Malnutrition and gastrointestinal and respiratory infections in children: a public health problem. *Int J Environ Res Public Health* (2011) 8:1174–205. doi:10.3390/ijerph8041174
31. Vituri CL, Alvarez-Silva M, Tretin AZ, Borelli P. Alteration of the bone marrow in extracellular matrix in mice undernourished. *Braz J Med Biol Res* (2001) 33:889–95. doi:10.1590/S0100-879X2000000800004
32. Salva S, Villena J, Racedo S, Agüero G, Alvarez S. *Lactobacillus casei* addition to a repletion diet induced early normalization of cytokine profiles during

pneumococcal infection in malnourished mice. *Food Agric Immunol* (2008) 19:195–211. doi:10.1080/09540100802247243

33. Salva S, Merino MC, Agüero G, Gruppi A, Alvarez S. Dietary supplementation with probiotics improve hematopoiesis in malnourished mice. *PLoS One* (2012) 7:e31171. doi:10.1371/journal.pone.0031171
34. Herrera M, Salva S, Villena J, Barbieri N, Alvarez S. *Lactobacillus rhamnosus* CRL1505 enhances systemic and respiratory innate immune response in immunocompromised malnourished mice. *J Funct Foods* (2013) 5:1693–704. doi:10.1016/j.jff.2013.07.014
35. Borelli P, Blatt SL, Rogero MM, Fock RA. Haematological alterations in protein malnutrition. *Rev Bras Hematol Hemoter* (2004) 26:49–56. doi:10.1590/S1516-84842004000100010
36. Salva S, Villena J, Herrera M, Alvarez S. Immunobiotic and hematopoyesis: can immunobiotics beneficially modulate hemato-immune responses in immunocompromised hosts? In: Kitazawa H, Villena J, Alvarez S, editors. *Probiotics: Immunobiotics and immunogenics*. Science Publishers, CRC Press: United States (2013). p. 280–97.
37. Cain DW, Snowden PB, Sempowski GD, Kelsoe G. Inflammation triggers emergency granulopoiesis through a density-dependent feedback mechanism. *PLoS One* (2011) 6:e19957. doi:10.1371/journal.pone.0019957
38. Ueda Y, Cain DW, Kuraoka M, Kondo M, Kelsoe G. IL-1R type I-dependent hemopoietic stem cell proliferation is necessary for inflammatory granulopoiesis and reactive neutrophilia. *J Immunol* (2009) 182:6477–84. doi:10.4049/jimmunol.0803961
39. Emadi A, Jones RJ, Brodsky RA. Cyclophosphamide and cancer: golden anniversary. *Nat Rev Clin Oncol* (2009) 6:638–47. doi:10.1038/nrclinonc.2009.146
40. WHO. *Model List of Essential Medicines*. 19th ed. World Health Organization (2015). Available from: http://www.who.int/medicines/publications/essentialmedicines/en/
41. Zhang QH, Wu CF, Duan L, Yang JY. Protective effects of total saponins from stem and leaf of *Panax* ginseng against cyclophosphamide-induced genotoxicity and apoptosis in mouse bone marrow cells and peripheral lymphocyte cells. *Food Chem Toxicol* (2008) 46:93–302. doi:10.1016/j.fct.2007.08.025
42. Jang SE, Joh EH, Lee HY, Ahn YT, Lee JH, Huh CS, et al. *Lactobacillus plantarum* HY7712 ameliorates cyclophosphamide-induced immunosuppression in mice. *J Microbiol Biotechnol* (2013) 23:414–21. doi:10.4014/jmb.1210.10010
43. Chandramathi S, Suresh K, Anita ZB, Kuppusamy UR. Infections of *Blastocystishominis*and microsporidia in cancer patients: are they opportunistic? *Trans R Soc Trop Med Hyg* (2012) 106:267–9. doi:10.1016/j.trstmh.2011.12.008
44. Xu X, Zhang X. Effects of cyclophosphamide on immune system and gut microbiota in mice. *Microbiol Res* (2015) 171:97–106. doi:10.1016/j.micres.2014.11.002
45. van Vliet MJ, Harmsen HJ, de Bont ES, Tissing WJ. The role of intestinal microbiota in the development and severity of chemotherapy-induced mucositis. *PLoS Pathog* (2010) 6:e1000879. doi:10.1371/journal.ppat.1000879
46. Zhu XL, Liu JH, Li WD, Lin ZB. Promotion of myelopoiesis in myelosuppressed mice by *Ganodermalucidum* polysaccharides. *Frontiers Pharmacol* (2012) 3:20. doi:10.3389/fphar.2012.00020
47. Alvarez S, Villena J, Salva S. Humoral immunity against respiratory pathogens: can lactic acid bacteria improve it? In: Mohad RM, editor. *Research Advances in Infection and Immunity*. India:Global Research Network (2009). p. 1–19.
48. Villena J, Salva S, Núñez M, Corzo J, Tolaba R, Faedda J, et al. Probiotics for everyone! The novel immunobiotics *Lactobacillus rhamnosus* CRL1505 and the beginning of social probiotic programs in Argentina. *Int J Biotechnol Wellness Ind* (2012) 1:189.
49. Popova M, Molimard P, Courau S, Crociani J, Dufour C, Le Vacon F, et al. Beneficial effects of probiotics in upper respiratory tract infections and their mechanical actions to antagonize pathogens. *J Appl Microbiol* (2012) 113:1305–18. doi:10.1111/j.1365-2672.2012.05394.x
50. Villena J, Racedo S, Agüero G, Bru E, Medina M, Alvarez S. *Lactobacillus casei* improves resistance to pneumococcal respiratory infection in malnourished mice. *J Nutr* (2005) 135:1462–9.
51. Salva S, Nuñez M, Villena J, Ramón A, Font G, Alvarez S. Development of a fermented goats' milk containing *Lactobacillus rhamnosus*: *in vivo* study of health benefits. *J Sci Food Agric* (2011) 91:2355–62. doi:10.1002/jsfa.4467
52. Villena J, Oliveira ML, Ferreira PC, Salva S, Alvarez S. Lactic acid bacteria in the prevention of pneumococcal respiratory infection: future opportunities and challenges. *Int Immunopharmacol* (2011) 11:1633–45. doi:10.1016/j.intimp.2011.06.004
53. Matsumoto T, Ishikawa H, Tateda K, Yaeshima T, Ishibashi N, Yamaguchi K. Oral administration of *Bifidobacterium longum* prevents gut-derived *Pseudomona aeruginosa* sepsis in mice. *J Appl Microbiol* (2008) 104:672–80. doi:10.1111/j.1365-2672.2007.03593.x
54. Jang SE, Joh EH, Ahn YT, Han MJ, Kim DH. *Lactobacillus casei* HY7213 ameliorates cyclophosphamide-induced immunosuppression in mice by activating NK, cytotoxic T cells and macrophages. *Immunopharmacol Immunotoxicol* (2013) 35:396–402. doi:10.3109/08923973.2013.789055
55. Bujalance C, Moreno E, Jimenez-Valera M, Ruiz-Bravo A. A probiotic strain of *Lactobacillus plantarum* stimulates lymphocyte responses in immunologically intact and immunocompromised mice. *Int J Food Microbiol* (2007) 113:28–34. doi:10.1016/j.ijfoodmicro.2006.07.014

19

Detection of Increased Plasma Interleukin-6 Levels and Prevalence of *Prevotella copri* and *Bacteroides vulgatus* in the Feces of Type 2 Diabetes Patients

Aline Zazeri Leite[1], Nathália de Campos Rodrigues[2], Marina Ignácio Gonzaga[1], João Carlos Cicogna Paiolo[3], Carolina Arantes de Souza[3], Nadine Aparecida Vicentini Stefanutto[2], Wellington Pine Omori[4], Daniel Guariz Pinheiro[4], João Luiz Brisotti[1], Euclides Matheucci Junior[5,6], Vânia Sammartino Mariano[7] and Gislane Lelis Vilela de Oliveira[1]*

[1] Microbiome Study Group, School of Health Sciences Dr. Paulo Prata (FACISB), Barretos, Brazil, [2] QGene-Solutions and Logistics in Health, Sao Carlos, Brazil, [3] Board of Health from Barretos, Barretos, Brazil, [4] Department of Technology, School of Agricultural and Veterinarian Sciences, São Paulo State University (UNESP), Sao Paulo, Brazil, [5] DNA Consult Genetics and Biotechnology, Sao Carlos, Brazil, [6] Biotechnology Department, Sao Carlos Federal University, UFSCAR, Sao Carlos, Brazil, [7] Barretos Cancer Hospital (HCB), Barretos, Brazil

Edited by:
Julio Villena, Centro de Referencia para Lactobacilos, Argentina

Reviewed by:
Maryam Dadar, Razi Vaccine and Serum Research Institute, Iran
Susana Alvarez, Consejo Nacional de Investigaciones Científicas y Técnicas (CONICET), Argentina

***Correspondence:**
Gislane Lelis Vilela de Oliveira
glelisvilela@gmail.com

Intestinal dysbiosis and metabolic endotoxemia have been associated with metabolic disorders, such as obesity, insulin resistance, and type 2 diabetes (T2D). The main goal of the present study was to evaluate the intestinal dysbiosis in Brazilian T2D patients and correlate these data with inflammatory cytokines and lipopolysaccharides (LPS) plasma concentrations. This study was approved by the Ethics Committees from Barretos Cancer Hospital and all individuals signed the informed consent form. Stool samples were required for DNA extraction, and the V3/V4 regions of bacterial 16S were sequenced using an Illumina platform. Peripheral blood was used to quantify inflammatory cytokines and plasma LPS concentrations, by CBA flex and ELISA, respectively. Statistical analyses were performed using Mann–Whitney and Spearman's tests. Analysis of variance, diversity indexes, and analysis of alpha- and beta-diversity were conducted using an annotated Operational Taxonomic Unit table. This study included 20 patients and 22 controls. We observed significant differences ($P < 0.01$) in the microbiota composition (beta-diversity) between patients and controls, suggesting intestinal dysbiosis in Brazilian T2D patients. The prevalent species found in patients' feces were the Gram-negatives *Prevotella copri*, *Bacteroides vulgatus*, *Bacteroides rodentium*, and *Bacteroides xylanisolvens*. The proinflammatory interleukin-6 (IL-6) was significantly increased ($P < 0.05$) in patients' plasma and LPS levels were decreased. We find correlations between the proinflammatory interferon-gamma with Gram-negatives *Bacteroides* and *Prevotella* species, and a positive correlation between the LPS levels and *P. copri* reads. The *P. copri* and *B. vulgatus* species were associated with insulin resistance in previous studies. In this study, we suggested that the prevalence of Gram-negative species in the gut and the increased plasma IL-6 in patients could be linked to low-grade inflammation and insulin resistance. In conclusion, the *P. copri* and *B. vulgatus* species could represent an intestinal microbiota signature, associated with T2D development. Furthermore, the identification of these Gram-negative bacteria, and the detection of inflammatory markers, such as increased IL-6, could be used as diabetes predictive markers in overweight, obese and in genetically predisposed individuals to develop T2D.

Keywords: type 2 diabetes, dietary habits, intestinal microbiota, inflammatory cytokines, interleukin-6, metabolic endotoxemia

INTRODUCTION

Type 2 diabetes (T2D) is a chronic disease characterized by insulin resistance, glucose intolerance, fat deposition, dyslipidemia, and systemic inflammation (1). According to the International Diabetes Federation, diabetes will affect 642 million people worldwide until 2040 (2). T2D development involves genetic and environmental factors, and recent reports have implicated the gut microbiota in the regulation of glucose and lipid metabolism (3, 4). Consistently, some studies correlate important perturbations in the gut microbiota composition with systemic inflammation, which is observed in metabolic dysfunctions, such as insulin resistance, obesity, and T2D (3–5).

In humans, more than a trillion of microorganisms, primarily bacteria, colonize the oral-gastrointestinal tract and reside in the distal portion of the intestine (6, 7). The gut microbiota contributes to many of the host physiological processes, and in turn, the host offers niche and nutrients for the survival of these microbes (8–10). The main contributions of the gut microbiota include digestion and carbohydrate fermentation, vitamins synthesis, mucosal lymphoid tissue development, epithelial barrier maintenance, and the prevention of pathobionts colonization (11–13). Furthermore, the interaction between host immune system and gut microbiota is necessary for the maintenance of mucosal immune homeostasis and epithelial barrier integrity (14). However, the interruption of this healthy interaction, with an imbalance in the normal bacterial ecology in the gut, defined as intestinal dysbiosis, may contribute to the development of metabolic and chronic inflammatory diseases, such as T2D (14–16).

Some mechanisms have been proposed to explain the influence of the gut microbiota on insulin resistance and T2D, such as bacterial translocation, metabolic endotoxemia, defective secretion of incretins, and decreased butyrate concentrations (13, 17). We focused on metabolic endotoxemia, involving the release of proinflammatory cytokines, such as tumor necrosis factor (TNF), interleukin-1 (IL-1), and interleukin-6 (IL-6), in response to the activation of innate immune receptors by lipopolysaccharides (LPS). LPS are endotoxins present in the cell wall of Gram-negative bacteria, and these molecules are primarily responsible for the endotoxemia observed in metabolic disorders (18).

Changes in Gram-negative bacteria concentrations in the gut, combined with increased intestinal permeability, could promote LPS escape into the bloodstream and induce systemic inflammation (19). Inflammation is associated with insulin resistance because the proinflammatory cytokines block insulin signaling by inhibiting the phosphorylation of insulin receptors (20, 21). Furthermore, studies in animal models showed that high-fat diets promote an increase in Gram-negative bacteria in the gut and increased LPS absorption in the intestinal mucosa (21). In addition, induction of metabolic endotoxemia *via* intravenous administration of LPS in mice induces a fast increase in glycemia, insulinemia, and dyslipidemia (21, 22).

Recent reports have suggested that increased IL-6 plasma concentrations, C-reactive proteins, and intestinal dysbiosis are associated with obesity and T2D development (23–26). Some studies showed that proinflammatory bacteria, *Ruminococcus gnavus* and *Bacteroides* spp., are more prevalent in the feces of T2D patients (25, 26). However, butyrate-producing bacteria, such as *Roseburia intestinalis* and *Faecalibacterium prausnitzii*, with anti-inflammatory effects, were decreased in T2D patients (25).

Based on studies showing the importance of resilience of the intestinal microbiota in human health and studies showing that intestinal dysbiosis may be strongly associated with gut epithelial barrier disruption, bacterial translocation, and metabolic endotoxemia (3–5, 27), we hypothesized that the abundance of Gram-negative bacteria is greater in the feces of T2D patients and positively correlated with the plasma levels of proinflammatory cytokines and LPS. In the present study, we evaluated intestinal dysbiosis in Brazilian T2D patients and correlated these data with systemic inflammatory cytokines and plasma LPS concentrations.

MATERIALS AND METHODS

Patients and Controls Enrollment

Type 2 diabetes patients with fasting blood glucose levels greater than or equal to 126 mg/dL (2) were enrolled at the Board of Health from Barretos, Sao Paulo, Brazil, from June 1st, 2015 to July 30th, 2016. A physician from the endocrinology department selected a total of 20 patients, 11 females and 9 males, ranging from 36 to 75 years (mean age ± SD = 58.9 ± 8.4 years) for inclusion in the present study.

Healthy controls, without T2D familial history among grandparents, parents, and siblings, were enrolled. A total of 22 healthy controls, 12 males and 10 females, ranging from 36 to 69 years (mean age ± SD = 55.7 ± 8.3 years) were enrolled in the present study. The present study was performed in accordance with the recommendations of Ethics Committee from Barretos Cancer Hospital. All subjects provided written informed consent in accordance with the Declaration of Helsinki. The protocol was approved by the Barretos Cancer Hospital (Process number 903/2014). Subsequent to consent, the peripheral blood of patients and controls was collected and stool samples were requested, and its delivery occurred within 5 days.

All subjects who had used anti-inflammatories, antibiotics, and laxatives in the last 15 days prior to blood and feces collection were excluded in the present study. Similarly, all individuals who were vaccinated or administered corticosteroids in the last 30 days were not included. The presence of chronic diarrhea and surgeries, such as appendectomy, cholecystectomy, and bariatric surgery, were also considered as exclusion criteria for T2D patients and healthy controls.

Clinical data from T2D patients, such as body mass index (BMI), fasting blood glucose (close to blood collection), glycated hemoglobin ($HbA1_C$), and disease duration, were recorded. **Table 1** summarizes the demographic and clinical data from T2D patients.

Bacterial DNA Extraction, V3/V4 Amplification, and Sequencing

Bacterial DNA was extracted from 250 mg of stool using a PowerSoil DNA Isolation Kit (MO BIO Laboratories, QIAGEN, CA, USA), according to the manufacturer's instructions. The amount of DNA was determined using a Quantus fluorometer and adjusted to 5 ng/mL with Tris buffer (10 mM, pH 8.5). The V3 and V4 regions of the bacterial 16S were amplified by PCR using 2.5 mL of bacterial DNA, 5 mL of each primer and 12.5 mL of 2× KAPA HiFi HotStart Ready Mix (Kapa Biosystems, MA, USA). The PCR products were purified using an XP AMPure Beads Kit (BD Biosciences, CA, USA). DNA libraries were constructed according to the Illumina protocols, including steps of connecting adapters (Nextera XT Index Kit), purification steps (AMPure XP beads), quantification, and pre-denaturation (V3 MiSeq reagent kits). Sample sequencing was performed using an Illumina MiSeq platform system.

Cytokine Quantification Using a Cytometric Bead Array

Peripheral blood (10 mL) was collected from T2D patients and controls and plasma-EDTA was separated by centrifugation at 1,372 *g*, for 10 min, 4°C. Cytokine quantification was performed by cytometric bead array (Human Th1/Th2/Th17 Cytokine Kit, BD Biosciences, CA, USA). Plasma levels of IL-2, IL-4, IL-6, IL-10, IL-17A, TNF, and interferon-gamma (IFN-γ) were detected by flow cytometer FACSCanto™ II (BD Biosciences). The analyses were performed by using BDFCAP array™ software and results were expressed by conversion of the median fluorescence intensity in picograms per milliliter.

LPS Quantification by ELISA Assay

After centrifuging the blood samples, plasma-EDTA was stored at −80°C until the measurement of LPS. Plasma samples were used for LPS quantification, performed in duplicate, using a LPS ELISA Kit (LPS, Elabscience Biotechnology, MD, USA), according to the manufacturer's instructions. The absorbance was read at 450 nm, and the results are presented as nanograms per milliliter.

Statistical Analyses and Paired-End Data Processing

The comparisons between cytokines and LPS levels in patients and controls were performed using the Mann–Whitney test (28). The correlations among the relative abundance of microbiota with cytokines, LPS levels, and clinical data were performed

TABLE 1 | Demographic and clinical features obtained from 20 type 2 diabetes (T2D) patients.

Patients	Gender/age	Ethnicity	BMI (kg/m^2)	Fasting blood glucose (mg/dL)	$HbA1_C$ (%)	Disease duration (years)
T2D01	M/49	Caucasian	27.8	191.0	8.0	16
T2D02	M/58	Caucasian	40.1	255.1	8.6	10
T2D03	F/62	Caucasian	32.4	87.0	7.4	11
T2D04	M/63	Caucasian	27.8	100.0	9.8	20
T2D05	M/64	Asian	32.0	76.0	5.3	16
T2D06	F/61	Afrodescendent	37.8	175.3	8.2	10
T2D07	M/58	Afrodescendent	27.5	98.6	9.8	10
T2D08	M/68	Afrodescendent	30.1	ND	ND	1
T2D09	F/36	Caucasian	30.5	84.3	6.8	9
T2D10	F/61	Caucasian	29.1	271.0	8.0	5
T2D11	M/63	Caucasian	27.4	96.0	9.9	21
T2D12	F/66	Caucasian	37.8	258.0	9.2	9
T2D13	F/45	Caucasian	31.2	245.0	7.7	18
T2D14	F/54	Caucasian	26.0	174.0	8.0	8
T2D15	M/59	Afrodescendent	31.6	ND	ND	ND
T2D16	F/75	Caucasian	21.1	220.0	8.5	21
T2D17	M/60	Caucasian	21.8	ND	ND	6
T2D18	F/56	Caucasian	27.7	ND	ND	17
T2D19	F/63	Caucasian	28.0	ND	ND	1
T2D20	F/57	Caucasian	35.6	ND	ND	ND

M, male; F, female; BMI, body mass index (BMI > 25 = overweighted, BMI > 30 = obese); $HbA1_C$, glycated hemoglobin (reference: 4.0–6.0%); ND, not determined. Fasting blood glucose (reference < 126 mg/dL).

using the Spearman's test (29). *P* values less than 0.05 were considered statistically significant.

The paired-end reads from sequenced 16S amplified fragments were first assembled using PANDAseq v.2.10 (30) and subsequently processed using Cutadapt v.1.12 (31) to trim the Illumina adapter sequences, and PRINSEQ v.0.19.5 (32) to evaluate reads quality and to trim off low-quality bases from 3′ end from reads. Thus, we only retrieved high quality sequences between 350 and 500 bases in size to identify the Operational Taxonomic Units (OTUs) associated with each library. Chimeric sequence analyses, clustering, taxonomic assignment, and statistical analysis were performed using QIIME v.1.9.1 scripts (33), according to Souza and colleagues (34), with minor modifications, as described as follows. To obtain an OTU table, we first performed a multiple sequence alignment with MUSCLE v.3.8.31 (35), together with the pre-aligned 16S data from SILVA 119 database. Chimeric sequences were identified and removed and clustering was performed using the UPARSE protocol (36). The taxonomic assignment for each OTU was based on Ribosomal Database Project (RDP-II) (37) trainset 14 using MOTHUR v.1.25 (38). Analysis of variance, diversity index (Shannon and Observed species), and analysis of α- and β-diversity were conducted from the annotated OTU table.

TABLE 2 | Diversity and richness index results from alpha-diversity analyses.

Sample ID	Simpson	Shannon	Chao1	Observed Operational Taxonomic Units
T2D01	0.95	5.53	240.44	213
T2D04	0.95	5.26	194.55	167
T2D07	0.92	5.20	267.12	231
T2D08	0.91	4.46	107.00	99
T2D09	0.92	4.90	196.16	165
T2D11	0.92	5.00	219.05	182
T2D13	0.89	4.47	149.17	138
T2D14	0.93	4.98	215.15	180
T2D15	0.96	5.67	257.02	227
T2D17	0.92	5.17	272.06	209
CTL16	0.94	5.22	164.86	148
CTL22	0.94	4.90	172.76	127
CTL23	0.93	5.28	221.05	184
CTL29	0.95	5.36	205.35	178
CTL31	0.96	5.88	286.21	224
CTL32	0.93	4.56	108.50	83
CTL33	0.97	6.11	284.67	264
CTL34	0.91	4.78	200.62	159
CTL37	0.90	4.23	164.25	141
CTL41	0.89	4.47	197.60	148
CTL43	0.86	4.05	115.10	98
CTL44	0.94	5.02	138.50	110
CTL45	0.93	5.21	229.91	196
CTL46	0.90	4.22	132.00	94
CTL47	0.96	5.67	274.22	227
CTL49	0.97	5.94	262.88	231
CTL50	0.94	5.28	245.13	204
CTL51	0.91	4.64	161.00	143

RESULTS

Prevalence of Gram-Negative Species in the Feces of T2D Patients

To evaluate the intestinal dysbiosis in T2D patients, we analyzed the 16S ribosomal DNA sequences in stool samples obtained from patients and controls, targeting V3–V4 conserved regions. We calculated alpha and beta-diversity to evaluate differences in microbiota community in patients and healthy subjects. There were no significant differences ($P < 0.05$) in richness (Chao1 and observed OTUs) and evenness (Shannon and Simpson) measured according to the rarefaction curves between T2D patients and controls (**Table 2; Figures 1A,B**). However, using the weighted and unweighted UniFrac metric with Bonferroni's correction (beta-diversity), we observed that the microbial communities from T2D patients and healthy controls were not similar ($P = 0.01$) (**Figures 1C,D**).

To evaluate differences in phyla composition in the microbiota of feces samples obtained from patients and controls, we compare the relative abundances in both groups, represented by read percentages. The prevalent phyla in patients were Bacteroidetes [patient reads (*P*) = 47.97%; control reads (*C*) = 46.32%] and Firmicutes (*P* = 43.77%; *C* = 43.92%), the prevalent classes were Bacteroidia (*P* = 44.40%; *C* = 45.73%) and Clostridia (*P* = 35.31%; *C* = 34.39%), the prevalent orders were Bacteroidales (*P* = 44.41%; *C* = 45.73%) and Clostridiales (*P* = 35.31%; *C* = 34.39%), and the prevalent families were Bacteroidaceae (*P* = 21.09%; *C* = 27.19%), Ruminococcaceae (*P* = 19.05%; *C* = 17.99%), Prevotellaceae (*P* = 17.11%; *C* = 8.41%), and Lachnospiraceae (*P* = 11.00%; *C* = 12.43%) (**Figures 2A–D**). The prevalent genera in T2D patients were *Bacteroides* (*P* = 21.09%; *C* = 27.19%) and *Prevotella* (*P* = 14.07%; *C* = 7.03%). The prevalent species in the feces of T2D patients were *Prevotella copri* (*P* = 19%; *C* = 7%), *B. vulgatus* (*P* = 13%; *C* = 18%), *Bacteroides rodentium* (*P* = 9%; *C* = 13%), and *Bacteroides xylanisolvens* (*P* = 8%; *C* = 6%) (**Figures 2E,F**).

To identify correlations between intestinal microbiota composition and clinical data, we examined the correlations among IMC, fasting blood glucose and $HbA1_C$ with relative abundances of bacterial groups detected in the feces of T2D patients. There were no correlations among microbiota reads with IMC and fasting blood glucose. However, a negative correlation of the Ruminococcaceae reads with $HbA1_C$ percentages ($P = 0.021$, $\rho = -0.69$) was observed (**Figure 3**).

Proinflammatory IL-6 Is Increased in Plasma from T2D Patients

To evaluate the cytokine profile in plasma from T2D patients and controls, we quantified the plasma concentrations of IL-2, IL-4, IL-6, IL-10, IL-17A, IFN-γ, and TNF. IL-2 was undetectable in the vast majority of patient and control samples. IL-4 plasma concentrations, characteristic of Th2 responses, were similar in T2D (mean ± SEM: 0.181 ± 0.147 pg/mL) and controls (0.247 ± 0.203 pg/mL) (**Figure 4A**). The IL-6 concentration was significantly higher ($P = 0.001$) in patient plasma samples (3.081 ± 0.447 pg/mL) than in samples from the control group (1.547 ± 0.141 pg/mL) (**Figure 4B**). The concentration of IL-10, an anti-inflammatory cytokine, was increased ($P = 0.014$) in the plasma of patients (0.371 ± 0.231 pg/mL) compared with controls (0.197 ± 0.162 pg/mL) (**Figure 4C**). There were no

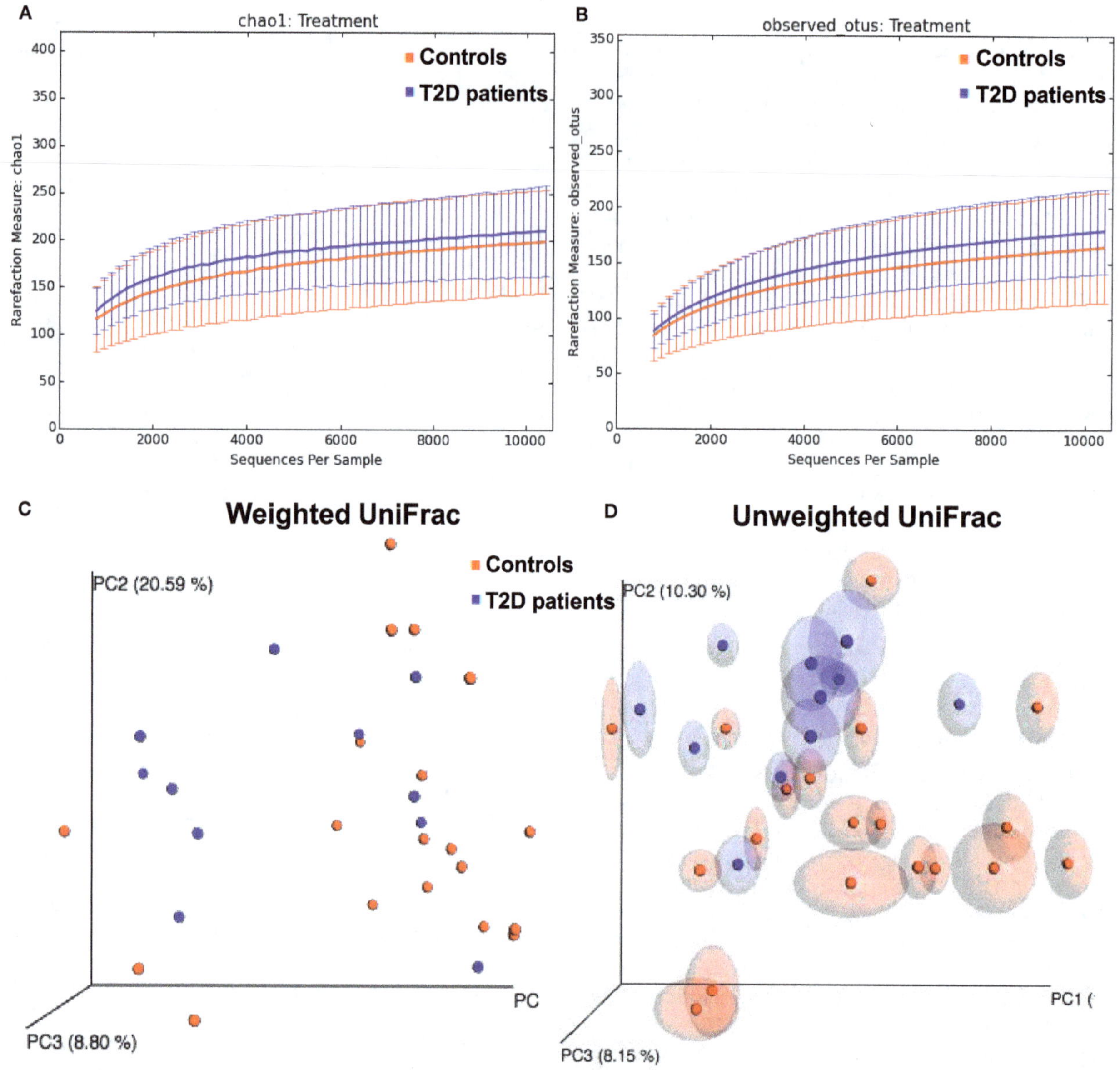

FIGURE 1 | Alpha and beta-diversity in gut microbiota from type 2 diabetes (T2D) patients. **(A,B)** Rarefaction curves comparing the species richness, Chao1, and observed Operational Taxonomic Unit (OTU) numbers. **(C,D)** PcoA plots with weighted and unweighted UniFrac metric with Bonferroni's correction.

significant differences ($P > 0.05$) in the plasma concentrations of proinflammatory cytokines IL-17A, IFN-γ, and TNF in patients (IL-17A: 6,089 ± 2,042 pg/mL; IFN-γ: 1.361 ± 0.921 pg/mL; TNF: 0.2714 ± 0,122 pg/mL) compared with controls (IL-17A: 5,491 ± 1,382 pg/mL; IFN-γ: 0.842 ± 0.149 pg/mL; TNF: 0.689 ± 0.391 pg/mL) (**Figures 4D–F**).

To identify correlations between intestinal microbiota composition and cytokines, we examined correlations between systemic levels of cytokines and relative abundances of bacterial groups in the feces of T2D patients. Significant correlations among the proinflammatory cytokine IFN-γ and relative abundances of Firmicutes ($P = 0.007$, $\rho = 0.75$), Clostridia ($P = 0.016$, $\rho = 0.69$), *Bacteroides* ($P = 0.014$, $\rho = -0.70$), and *Prevotella* ($P = 0.021$, $\rho = 0.66$) were observed (**Figures 5A–D**). Plasma levels of IL-17A were positively correlated with the relative abundances of Enterobacteriaceae ($P = 0.041$, $\rho = 0.58$) (**Figure 5E**). Furthermore, a positive correlation between Negativicutes reads with IL-6 ($P = 0.037$, $\rho = 0.59$) was observed (**Figure 5F**).

LPS Plasma Concentrations Were Different between Patients and Controls

To evaluate the metabolic endotoxemia in the plasma of T2D patients, we quantified LPS using an ELISA. We observed a

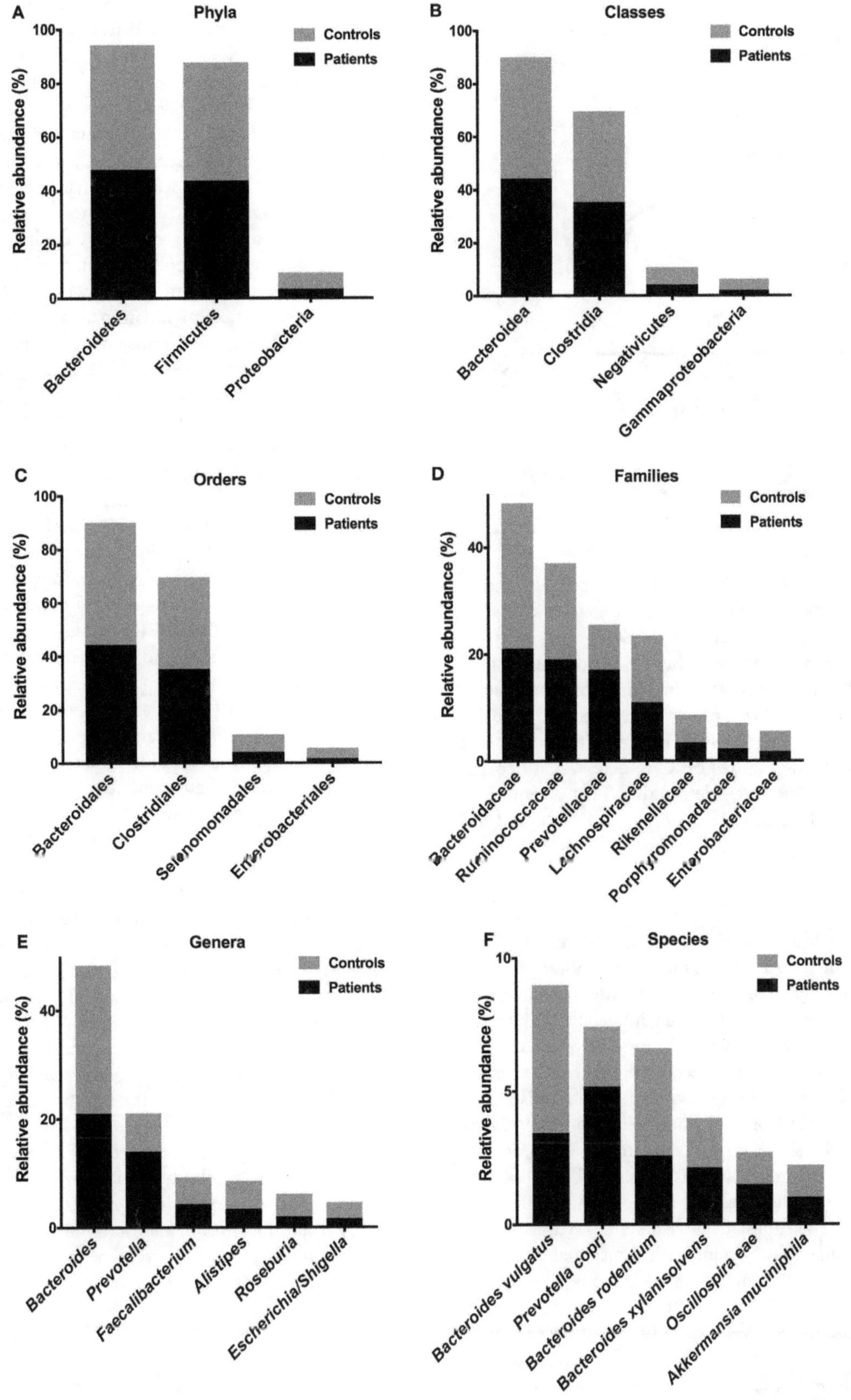

FIGURE 2 | Relative abundances of bacterial taxa in the feces of T2D patients. Prevalent phyla **(A)**, classes **(B)**, orders **(C)**, families **(D)**, genera **(E)**, and species **(F)**. Bars represent the reads percentages found in metagenomic analyses.

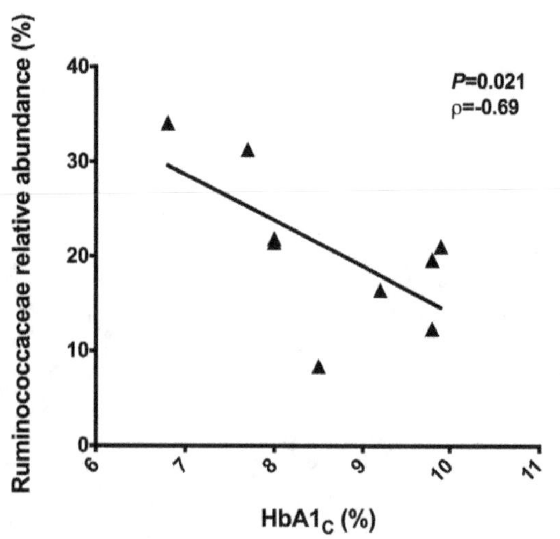

FIGURE 3 | Negative correlation between the Ruminococcaceae reads with the HbA1c percentages. Statistical analyses were performed using the Spearman's test. Significance was set at $P < 0.05$.

significant difference ($P = 0.009$) in the LPS concentration in plasma from T2D patients (mean ± SEM: 13.54 ± 0.86 ng/mL) and controls (16.98 ± 0.79 ng/mL) (**Figure 6A**).

An inverse correlation between the LPS concentration in the plasma of patients and the relative abundance of Proteobacteria ($P = 0.040$, $\rho = -0.58$) was observed. Moreover, a positive correlation was observed between LPS and *Prevotella* reads ($P = 0.041$, $\rho = 0.58$) (**Figures 6B,C**). There was no correlation among LPS plasma levels detected in T2D patients, with concentrations of IL-4, IL-6, IL-10, IL-17A, IFN-γ, and TNF cytokines.

DISCUSSION

The human body is inhabited by several different microbial ecosystems that colonize the body's mucous membranes (39, 40). Several studies have focused on the role of intestinal microbiota in health and disease, and factors that influence its dynamics, such as genetic and environmental factors (41, 42). A healthy intestinal microbiota is characterized by the presence of microorganisms that improve metabolism and confer resistance to infection and inflammation (43). Increasing evidence suggests that intestinal dysbiosis might be associated with the development of metabolic disorders, such as obesity and T2D (44–46). Here, we investigated the intestinal dysbiosis in Brazilian T2D patients and correlated these data with systemic inflammatory cytokines, LPS concentrations, and with clinical data.

The adult healthy gut microbiota is dominated by microorganisms belonging to the Firmicutes (Gram-positive) and Bacteroidetes (Gram-negative) phyla (39). Most bacteria in the adult human microbiota belong to the Firmicutes. and the prevalent species are *F. prausnitzii* and *Eubacterium rectale/Roseburia* spp. (47). These bacteria produce short-chain fatty acids, such as butyrate, which has anti-inflammatory effects (48). Butyrate inhibits NF-κB transcription factor signaling in intestinal epithelial cells and prevents the exposure of these cells to external factors, such as antigens derived from pathogenic microorganisms (47). The Bacteroidetes phylum is the second most populous in the human gut, with predominance of the *Bacteroides* and *Prevotella* genera (49). Studies have shown that *Prevotella* species predominantly activate TLR2 receptors and induce Th17 CD4 T cells polarization. The increased abundance of *Bacteroides* and *Prevotella* spp. is associated with gut inflammation, mainly mediated by proinflammatory Th17 cytokines. In addition, *Prevotella* spp. induce IL-8 and IL-6 secretion by epithelial cells, favoring Th17 responses and neutrophil recruitment (50). Thus, inflammation of the gut mucosa, mediated by *Prevotella* spp. promotes systemic dissemination of inflammatory mediators, increased intestinal permeability and translocation of bacterial products, which amplify and promote systemic inflammation (50).

In this study, we observed an intestinal dysbiosis in Brazilian T2D patients, with significant differences in the gut microbiota composition (beta-diversity) between patients and controls. Furthermore, we showed the prevalence of Gram-negative species in stool samples provided by patients, which is in agreement with previous studies (51, 52) and supports our hypothesis. The main Gram-negative species found in the present study were *P. copri*, *B. vulgatus*, *B. rodentium*, and *B. xylanisolvens*. The prevalence of Gram-negative bacteria suggests an increase in LPS levels, which can translocate through the intestinal barrier, and trigger systemic inflammation state and insulin resistance (51). Pedersen and colleagues showed that *P. copri* and *B. vulgatus* are associated with insulin resistance (52). In addition, studies in animal models have shown that *P. copri*, prevalent in our T2D patients, induce insulin resistance and glucose intolerance (52).

Alterations in the relative abundance of the Firmicutes and Bacteroidetes proportions have been reported in obesity and T2D (24, 53). Larsen and colleagues (2010) reported the diminished relative abundance of Firmicutes and Clostridia class in the diabetic group, while Bacteroidetes and Proteobacteria members were increased. These authors also observed a positive correlation between Bacteroidetes/Firmicutes and *Bacteroides-Prevotella/C. coccoides–E. rectale* ratios with plasma glucose concentrations (53). In the present study, we observed a negative correlation between Ruminococcaceae reads and HbA1c percentages. Ruminococcaceae are a family of common anaerobes, Gram-positive gut microbes that break down complex carbohydrates, and these bacteria are most common in the intestine of individuals with carbohydrate-enriched diets (54).

Studies in T2D patients have reported decreased *R. intestinalis* and *F. prausnitzii*, both butyrate-producing bacteria (25). The prevalence of *Lactobacillus gasseri*, *Streptococcus mutans*, and *Akkermansia muciniphila* have also been reported in T2D patients (25, 53). In the present study, *R. intestinalis* and *F. prausnitzii*, butyrate-producing bacteria, were not observed. *A. muciniphila* was detected at a lower relative abundance in T2D patients and controls. A previous study demonstrated that this Gram-negative specie mediates the negative effect of IFN-γ on glucose tolerance in mice (55). Moreover, IFN-γ-deficient mice showed improved glucose metabolism, likely reflecting diminished adipose inflammation, hepatic gluconeogenesis, and increased insulin sensitivity (56–58). In the present study, we

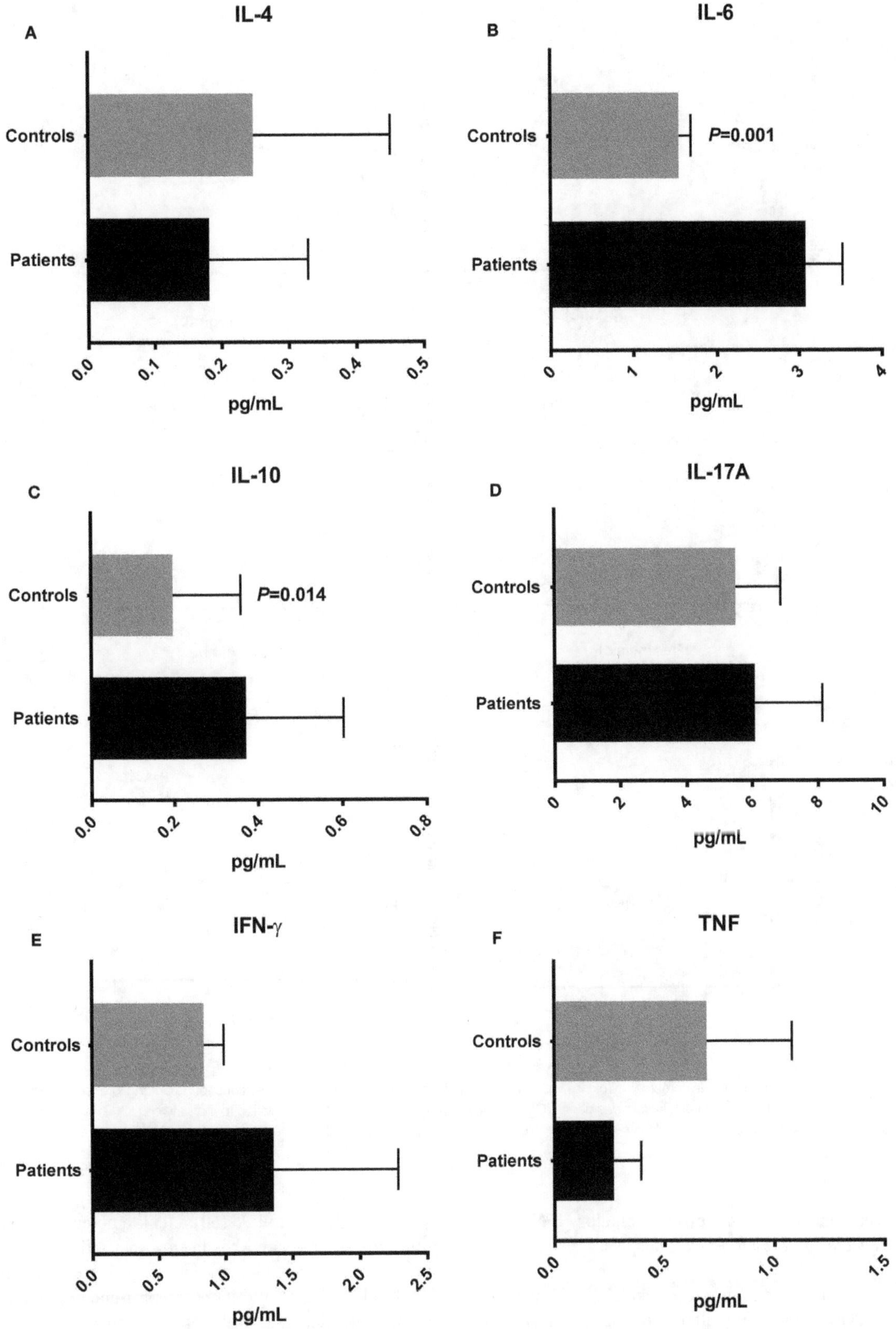

FIGURE 4 | Cytokine profile in type 2 diabetes patients and control subjects. Plasma concentrations of IL-4 **(A)**, interleukin-6 (IL-6) **(B)**, IL-10 **(C)**, IL-17A **(D)**, interferon-gamma (IFN-γ) **(E)**, and tumor necrosis factor (TNF) **(F)**. Statistical analyses were performed by Mann–Whitney test. Significance was set at $P < 0.05$.

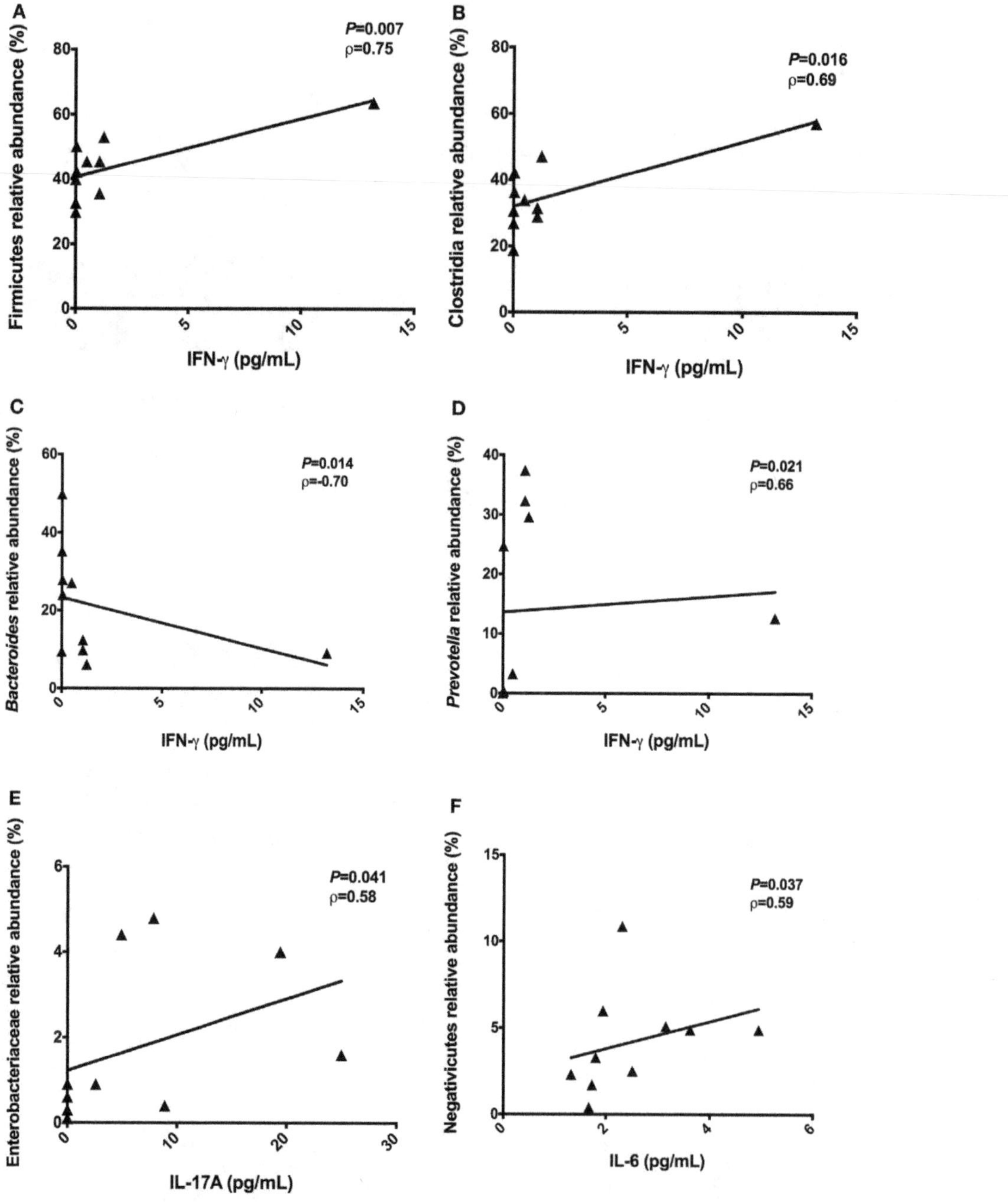

FIGURE 5 | Correlations between the proinflammatory cytokines with relative abundances of bacterial taxa. Correlations found among interferon-gamma (IFN-γ) and Firmicutes phylum **(A)**, Clostridia class **(B)**, *Bacteroides* genus **(C)**, and *Prevotella* genus **(D)**. Positive correlation found between IL-17A with Enterobacteriaceae family **(E)**. Positive correlation found between interleukin-6 (IL-6) with Negativicutes class **(F)**. Statistical analyses were performed by Spearman's test. Significance was set at $P < 0.05$.

observed correlations between the proinflammatory IFN-γ with Gram-negatives *Bacteroides* and *Prevotella* species, also supporting our hypothesis.

One of the mechanisms proposed to explain the imbalance in the intestinal microbiota, the altered regulation of fat storage, and the development of metabolic diseases is the metabolic endotoxemia (59). Intestinal dysbiosis may trigger a state of chronic low-grade inflammation, making the host susceptible to systemic exposure to LPS (60). LPS is a potent inducer of innate immune responses and has been associated with the adiposity, insulin resistance, and *de novo* triglycerides synthesis (60). LPS binds to TLR4 and its coreceptor and triggers the inflammatory cascade, resulting in NF-κB activation and secretion of proinflammatory cytokines, such as TNF, IL-1, and IL-6, which influence glucose metabolism and inhibit the phosphorylation of insulin receptors (20, 21, 60).

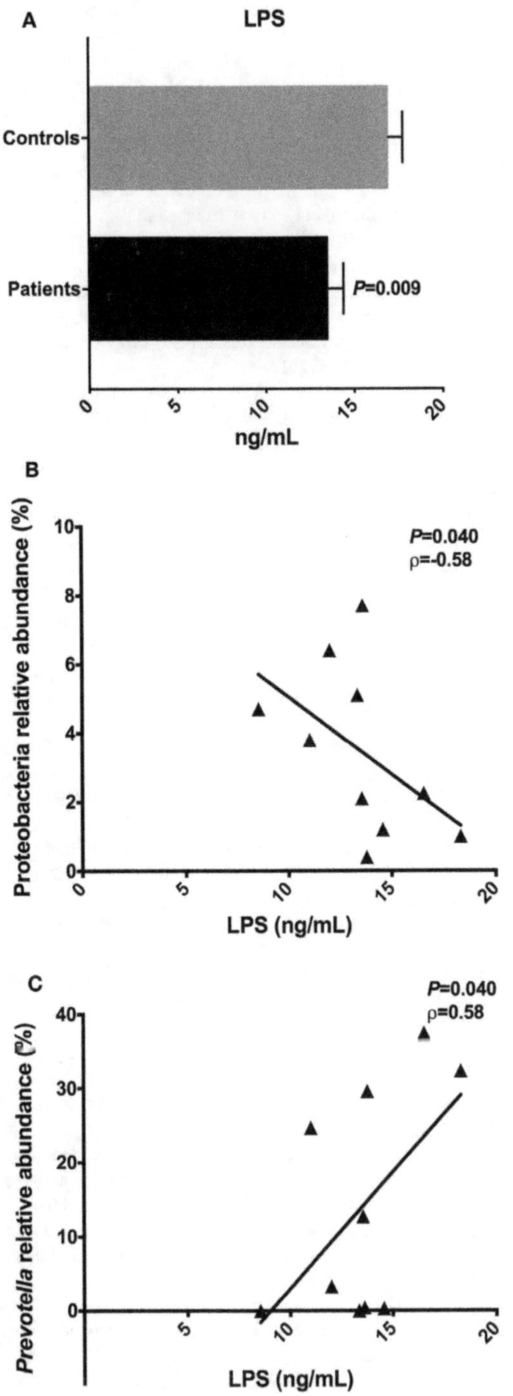

FIGURE 6 | Lipopolysaccharide (LPS) concentrations and the correlations with relative abundances of bacterial taxa. Plasma levels of the LPS in type 2 diabetes patients and controls **(A)**. Negative correlation found between the LPS with Proteobacteria phylum **(B)**. Positive correlation found between the LPS with *Prevotella* genus **(C)**. Statistical analyses were performed using the Mann–Whitney and the Spearman's test. Significance was set at $P < 0.05$.

In the present study, the proinflammatory IL-6 was increased in patients' plasma and positively correlate with Negativicutes abundance. IL-6 is secreted from several cell types, such as macrophages, monocytes, dendritic cells, and T-cells (20). The stimuli for IL-6 synthesis include IL-1, TNF, and LPS (20). IL-6 influences the antigen-specific responses and inflammatory reactions and is one of the main mediators of acute phase reactions (1, 23). Jayashree and colleagues showed increased serum levels of LPS, TNF, and IL-6 in T2D patients when compared with controls (24). The authors also reported correlations among LPS with glucose concentrations, $HbA1_C$ percentages, TNF, and IL-6 (24). In the present study, although there were no correlations between plasma inflammatory cytokines and LPS concentrations, the prevalence of Gram-negative species and the increased plasma IL-6 in patients could be associated with low-grade inflammation and insulin resistance.

Finally, we concluded that the *P. copri* and *B. vulgatus* species could represent an intestinal microbiota signature, associated with T2D development. Furthermore, the identification of these Gram-negative bacteria, and the detection of inflammatory markers, such as increased IL-6, could be used as diabetes predictive markers in overweight, obese, and genetically predisposed individuals to develop T2D.

ETHICS STATEMENT

This study was carried out in accordance with the recommendations of Ethics Committee from Barretos Cancer Hospital with written informed consent from all subjects. All subjects gave written informed consent in accordance with the Declaration of Helsinki. The protocol was approved by the Barretos Cancer Hospital (Process number 903/2014).

AUTHOR CONTRIBUTIONS

AL participated in patient enrollment, sample collection, DNA extraction, cytokine and LPS quantification, data acquisition, and manuscript writing; MG and CS participated in patient enrollment and sample collection; NR and NS participated in V3/V4 amplification, library construction, and sequencing; JB provided support for control sample collection; EJ provided support to Illumina platform sequencing; JP was responsible for all clinical aspects involving T2D patients. WO and DP performed bioinformatics analyses; VM participated in sample collection, DNA, cytokine and LPS quantification, and data acquisition; GO participated in experimental conception, patient enrollment, sample collection, cytokine and LPS quantification, data interpretation, and manuscript writing and revision.

ACKNOWLEDGMENTS

The authors would like to thank Johnny Rodrigues and Antoniel da Silva Fernandes for technical support at School of Healthy Sciences from Barretos Dr. Paulo Prata.

REFERENCES

1. Donath MY, Shoelson SE. Type 2 diabetes as an inflammatory disease. *Nat Rev Immunol* (2011) 11:98–107. doi:10.1038/nri2925
2. International Diabetes Federation. *International Diabetes Federation Atlas*. 7th ed. Brussels: Karakas Print (2015).
3. Tremaroli V, Bäckhed F. Functional interactions between the gut microbiota and host metabolism. *Nature* (2012) 489:242–9. doi:10.1038/nature11552
4. Van Olden C, Groen AK, Nieuwdorp M. Role of the intestinal microbiome in lipid and glucose metabolism in diabetes mellitus. *Clin Ther* (2015) 37:1172–7. doi:10.1016/j.clinthera.2015.03.008
5. Kau AL, Ahern PP, Griffin NW, Goodman AL, Goerdon JL. Human nutrition, the gut microbiome and the immune system. *Nature* (2011) 474:327–36. doi:10.1038/nature10213
6. Kamada N, Seo SU, Chen GY, Núñez G. Role of the gut microbiota in immunity and inflammatory disease. *Nat Rev Immunol* (2013) 13:321–35. doi:10.1038/nri3430
7. Karczewski J, Poniedzialek B, Adamski Z, Rzymski P. The effects of the microbiota on the host immune system. *Autoimmunity* (2014) 47:494–504. doi:10.3109/08916934.2014.938322
8. Hooper LV, Macpherson AJ. Immune adaptations that maintain homeostasis with the intestinal microbiota. *Nat Rev Immunol* (2010) 10:159–69. doi:10.1038/nri2710
9. Walsh CJ, Guinane CM, Hill C, Ross RP, O'Toole PW, Cotter PD. In silico identification of bacteriocin gene clusters in the gastrointestinal tract, based on the Human Microbiome Project's reference genome database. *BMC Microbiol* (2015) 15:183. doi:10.1186/s12866-015-0515-4
10. Doré J, Blottière H. The influence of diet on the gut microbiota and its consequences for health. *Curr Opin Biotechnol* (2015) 32:195–9. doi:10.1016/j.copbio.2015.01.002
11. Littman DR, Pamer EG. Role of the commensal microbiota in normal and pathogenic host immune responses. *Cell Host Microbe* (2011) 10:311–23. doi:10.1016/j.chom.2011.10.004
12. Renz H, Brandtzaeg P, Hornef M. The impact of perinatal immune development on mucosal homeostasis and chronic inflammation. *Nat Rev Immunol* (2012) 12(1):9–23. doi:10.1038/nri3112
13. Allin KH, Nielsen T, Pedersen O. Mechanisms in endocrinology: gut microbiota in patients with type 2 diabetes mellitus. *Eur J Endocrinol* (2015) 172:R167–77. doi:10.1530/EJE-14-0874
14. Honda K, Littman DR. The microbiota in adaptive immune homeostasis and disease. *Nature* (2016) 535:75–84. doi:10.1038/nature18848
15. Thaiss CA, Zmora N, Levy M, Elinav E. The microbiome and innate immunity. *Nature* (2016) 535:65–74. doi:10.1038/nature18847
16. Petersen C, Round JL. Defining dysbiosis and its influence on host immunity and disease. *Cell Microbiol* (2014) 16:1024–33. doi:10.1111/cmi.12308
17. Amar J, Chabo C, Waget A, Klopp P, Vachoux C, Bermúdez-Humarán LG, et al. Intestinal mucosal adherence and translocation of commensal bacteria at the early onset of type 2 diabetes: molecular mechanisms and probiotic treatment. *EMBO Mol Med* (2011) 3:559–72. doi:10.1002/emmm.201100159
18. Manco M, Putignani L, Bottazzo GF. Gut microbiota, lipopolysaccharides, and innate immunity in the pathogenesis of obesity and cardiovascular risk. *Endocr Rev* (2010) 31:817–44. doi:10.1210/er.2009-0030
19. Cani PD, Delzenne NM. The role of the gut microbiota in energy metabolism and metabolic disease. *Curr Pharm Des* (2009) 15:1546–58. doi:10.2174/138161209788168164
20. Chawla A, Nguyen KD, Goh YP. Macrophage-mediated inflammation in metabolic disease. *Nat Rev Immunol* (2011) 11:738–49. doi:10.1038/nri3071
21. Cani PD, Bibiloni R, Knauf C, Waget A, Neyrinck AM, Delzenne NM, et al. Changes in gut microbiota control metabolic endotoxemia-induced inflammation in high-fat diet-induced obesity and diabetes in mice. *Diabetes* (2008) 57:1470–81. doi:10.2337/db07-1403
22. Caricilli AM, Saad MJ. The role of gut microbiota on insulin resistance. *Nutrients* (2013) 5:829–51. doi:10.3390/nu5030829
23. Pickup JC, Mattock MB, Chusney GD, Burt D. NIDDM as a disease of the innate immune system: association of acute-phase reactants and interleukin-6 with metabolic syndrome X. *Diabetologia* (1997) 40:1286–92. doi:10.1007/s001250050822
24. Jayashree B, Bibin YS, Prabhu D, Shanthirani CS, Gokulakrishnan K, Lakshmi BS, et al. Increased circulatory levels of lipopolysaccharide (LPS) and zonulin signify novel biomarkers of proinflammation in patients with type 2 diabetes. *Mol Cell Biochem* (2014) 388:203–10. doi:10.1007/s11010-013-1911-4
25. Qin J, Li Y, Cai Z, Li S, Zhu J, Zhang F, et al. A metagenome-wide association study of gut microbiota in type 2 diabetes. *Nature* (2012) 490:55–60. doi:10.1038/nature11450
26. Everard A, Cani PD. Diabetes, obesity and gut microbiota. *Best Pract Res Clin Gastroenterol* (2013) 27:73–83. doi:10.1016/j.bpg.2013.03.007
27. Sommer F, Anderson JM, Bharti R, Raes J, Rosenstiel P. The resilience of the intestinal microbiota influences health and disease. *Nat Rev Microbiol* (2017). doi:10.1038/nrmicro.2017.58
28. Fay MP, Proschan MA. Wilcoxon-Mann-Whitney or t-test? On assumptions for hypothesis tests and multiple interpretations of decision rules. *Stat Surv* (2010) 4:1–39. doi:10.1214/09-SS051
29. Bonett DG, Wright TA. Sample size requirements for estimating Pearson, Kendall and Spearman correlations. *Psychometrika* (2000) 65:23–8. doi:10.1007/BF02294183
30. Masella AP, Bartram AK, Truszkowski JM, Brown DG, Neufeld JD. PANDAseq: paired-end assembler for Illumina sequences. *BMC Bioinformatics* (2012) 13:31. doi:10.1186/1471-2105-13-31
31. Martin M. Cutadapt removes adapter sequences from high-throughput sequencing reads. *EMBnet J* (2011) 17:10–2. doi:10.14806/ej.17.1.200
32. Schmieder R, Edwards R. Quality control and preprocessing of metagenomic datasets. *Bioinformatics* (2011) 27:863–4. doi:10.1093/bioinformatics/btr026
33. Caporaso JG, Kuczynski J, Stombaugh J, Bittinger K, Bushman FD, Costello EK, et al. QIIME allows analysis of high-throughput community sequencing data. *Nat Methods* (2010) 7:335–6. doi:10.1038/nmeth.f.303
34. De Souza RS, Okura VK, Armanhi JS, Jorrín B, Lozano N, da Silva MJ, et al. Unlocking the bacterial and fungal communities assemblages of sugarcane microbiome. *Sci Rep* (2016) 6:28774. doi:10.1038/srep28774
35. Edgar RC. MUSCLE: multiple sequence alignment with high accuracy and high throughput. *Nucleic Acids Res* (2004) 32:1792–7. doi:10.1093/nar/gkh340
36. Edgar RC. UPARSE: highly accurate OTU sequences from microbial amplicon reads. *Nat Methods* (2013) 10:996–8. doi:10.1038/nmeth.2604
37. Cole JR, Chai B, Farris RJ, Wang Q, Kulam SA, McGarrell DM, et al. The Ribosomal Database Project (RDP-II): sequences and tools for high-throughput rRNA analysis. *Nucleic Acids Res* (2005) 33:D294–6. doi:10.1093/nar/gki038
38. Schloss PD, Westcott SL, Rvabin T, Hall JR, Hartmann M, Hollister EB, et al. Introducing mothur: open-source, platform-independent, community-supported software for describing and comparing microbial communities. *Appl Environ Microbiol* (2009) 75:7537–41. doi:10.1128/AEM.01541-09
39. Eckburg PB, Bik EM, Bernstein CN, Purdom E, Dethlefsen L, Sargent M, et al. Diversity of the human intestinal microbial flora. *Science* (2005) 308:1635–8. doi:10.1126/science.1110591
40. Costello EK, Lauber CL, Hamady M, Fierer N, Gordon JI, Knight R. Bacterial community variation in human body habitats across space and time. *Science* (2009) 326:1694–7. doi:10.1126/science.1177486
41. Sommer F, Bäckhed F. The gut microbiota – masters of host development and physiology. *Nat Rev Microbiol* (2013) 11:227–38. doi:10.1038/nrmicro2974
42. Biedermann L, Rogler G. The intestinal microbiota: its role in health and disease. *Eur J Pediatr* (2015) 174:151–67. doi:10.1007/s00431-014-2476-2
43. Wu H, Tremaroli V, Bäckhed F. Linking microbiota to human diseases: a systems biology perspective. *Trends Endocrinol Metab* (2015) 26:758–70. doi:10.1016/j.tem.2015.09.011
44. Haro C, Montes-Borrego M, Rangel-Zúñiga OA, Alcalá-Díaz JF, Gómez-Delgado F, Pérez Martínez P, et al. Two healthy diets modulate gut microbial community improving insulin sensitivity in a human obese population. *J Clin Endocrinol Metab* (2016) 101:233–42. doi:10.1210/jc.2015-3351
45. Janssen AW, Kersten S. The role of gut microbiota in metabolic health. *FASEB J* (2015) 29:3111–23. doi:10.1096/fj.14-269514

46. Palau-Rodriguez M, Tulipani S, Queipo-Ortuño MI, Urpi-Sarda M, Tinahones FJ, Andres-Lacueva C. Metabolomic insights into the intricate gut microbial-host interaction in the development of obesity and type 2 diabetes. *Front Microbiol* (2016) 6:1151. doi:10.3389/fmicb.2015.01151
47. Kelly CJ, Zheng L, Campbell EL, Saeedi B, Scholz CC, Bavless AJ, et al. Crosstalk between microbiota-derived short-chain fatty acids and intestinal epithelial HIF augments tissue barrier function. *Cell Host Microbe* (2015) 17:662–71. doi:10.1016/j.chom.2015.03.005
48. Canabi RB, Costanzo MD, Leone L, Pedata M, Meli R, Calignano A. Potential beneficial effects of butyrate in intestinal and extraintestinal diseases. *World J Gastroenterol* (2011) 17:1519–28. doi:10.3748/wjg.v17.i12.1519
49. Wexler HM. Bacteroides: the good, the bad, and the nitty-gritty. *Clin Microbiol Rev* (2007) 20:593–621. doi:10.1128/CMR.00008-07
50. Larsen JM. The immune response to *Prevotella* bacteria in chronic inflammatory disease. *Immunology* (2017) 151:363–74. doi:10.1111/imm.12760
51. Crelly SJ, McTernan PG, Kusminski CM, Fisher FM, Da Silva NF, Khanolkar M, et al. Lipopolysaccharide activates an innate immune system response in human adipose tissue in obesity and type 2 diabetes. *Am J Physiol Endocrinol Metab* (2007) 292:E740–7. doi:10.1152/ajpendo.00302.2006
52. Pedersen HK, Gudmundsdottir V, Nielsen HB, Hyotylainen T, Nielsen T, Jensen BA, et al. Human gut microbes impact host serum metabolome and insulin sensitivity. *Nature* (2016) 535:376–81. doi:10.1038/nature18646
53. Larsen N, Vogensen FK, van den Berg FW, Nielsen DS, Andreasen AS, Pedersen BK, et al. Gut microbiota in human adults with type 2 differs from non-diabetic adults. *PLoS One* (2010) 5:e9085. doi:10.1371/journal.pone.0009085
54. La Reau AJ, Meier-Kolthoff JP, Suen G. Sequence-based analysis of the genus *Ruminococcus* resolves its phylogeny and reveals strong host association. *Microb Genom* (2016) 2:e000099. doi:10.1099/mgen.0.000099
55. Greer RL, Dong X, Moraes ACF, Zielke RA, Fernandes GR, Peremyslova E, et al. *Akkermansia muciniphila* mediates negative effects of IFN-γ on glucose metabolism. *Nat Commun* (2016) 7:13329. doi:10.1038/ncomms13329
56. Wong N, Fam BC, Cempako GR, Steinberg GR, Walder K, Kay TW, et al. Deficiency in interferon-gamma results in reduced body weight and better glucose tolerance in mice. *Endocrinology* (2011) 152:3690–9. doi:10.1210/en.2011-0288
57. Rocha VZ, Folco EJ, Sukhova G, Shimizu K, Gotsman I, Vernon AH, et al. Interferon-gamma, a Th1 cytokine, regulates fat inflammation: a role for adaptive immunity in obesity. *Circ Res* (2008) 103:467–76. doi:10.1161/CIRCRESAHA.108.177105
58. O'Rourke RW, White AE, Metcalf MD, Winters BR, Diggs BS, Zhu X, et al. Systemic inflammation and insulin sensitivity in obese IFN-γ knockout mice. *Metabolism* (2012) 61:1152–61. doi:10.1016/j.metabol.2012.01.018
59. Moya-Pérez A, Neef A, Sanz Y. *Bifidobacterium pseudocatenulatum* CECT 7765 reduces obesity-associated inflammation by restoring the lymphocyte-macrophage balance and gut microbiota structure in high-fat diet-fed mice. *PLoS One* (2015) 10:e0126976. doi:10.1371/journal.pone.0126976
60. Cani PD, Neyrinck AM, Fava F, Knauf C, Burcelin RG, Tuohy KM, et al. Selective increases of bifidobacteria in gut microflora improve high fat-diet-induced diabetes in mice through a mechanism associated with endotoxemia. *Diabetologia* (2007) 50:2374–83. doi:10.1007/s00125-007-0791-0

20

Transcriptomic Analysis of the Innate Antiviral Immune Response in Porcine Intestinal Epithelial Cells: Influence of Immunobiotic Lactobacilli

Leonardo Albarracin[1,2,3†], Hisakazu Kobayashi[3,4†], Hikaru Iida[3,4], Nana Sato[3,4], Tomonori Nochi[5,6], Hisashi Aso[5,6], Susana Salva[1,2], Susana Alvarez[1,2], Haruki Kitazawa[3,4] and Julio Villena[1,2,3]**

[1] Laboratory of Immunobiotechnology, Reference Centre for Lactobacilli (CERELA-CONICET), Tucuman, Argentina, [2] Immunobiotics Research Group, Tucuman, Argentina, [3] Food and Feed Immunology Group, Laboratory of Animal Products Chemistry, Graduate School of Agricultural Science, Tohoku University, Sendai, Japan, [4] Livestock Immunology Unit, International Education and Research Center for Food Agricultural Immunology (CFAI), Graduate School of Agricultural Science, Tohoku University, Sendai, Japan, [5] Cell Biology Laboratory, Graduate School of Agricultural Science, Tohoku University, Sendai, Japan, [6] Infection Immunology Unit, International Education and Research Center for Food Agricultural Immunology (CFAI), Graduate School of Agricultural Science, Tohoku University, Sendai, Japan

Edited by:
Juarez Antonio Simões Quaresma, Federal University of Pará, Brazil

Reviewed by:
Kieran G. Meade, Teagasc – The Irish Agriculture and Food Development Authority, Ireland
Haitao Guo, University of North Carolina at Chapel Hill, USA

***Correspondence:**
Haruki Kitazawa
haruki.kitazawa.c7@tohoku.ac.jp;
Julio Villena
jcvillena@cerela.org.ar

†These authors have contributed equally to this work.

Lactobacillus rhamnosus CRL1505 and *Lactobacillus plantarum* CRL1506 are immunobiotic strains able to increase protection against viral intestinal infections as demonstrated in animal models and humans. To gain insight into the host–immunobiotic interaction, the transcriptomic response of porcine intestinal epithelial (PIE) cells to the challenge with viral molecular associated pattern poly(I:C) and the changes in the transcriptomic profile induced by the immunobiotics strains CRL1505 and CRL1506 were investigated in this work. By using microarray technology and reverse transcription PCR, we obtained a global overview of the immune genes involved in the innate antiviral immune response in PIE cells. Stimulation of PIE cells with poly(I:C) significantly increased the expression of *IFN-α* and *IFN-β*, several interferon-stimulated genes, cytokines, chemokines, adhesion molecules, and genes involved in prostaglandin biosynthesis. It was also determined that lactobacilli differently modulated immune gene expression in poly(I:C)-challenged PIE cells. Most notable changes were found in antiviral factors (*IFN-α*, *IFN-β*, *NPLR3*, *OAS1*, *OASL*, *MX2*, and *RNASEL*) and cytokines/chemokines (*IL-1β*, *IL-6*, *CCL4*, *CCL5*, and *CXCL10*) that were significantly increased in lactobacilli-treated PIE cells. Immunobiotics reduced the expression of *IL-15* and *RAE1* genes that mediate poly(I:C) inflammatory damage. In addition, lactobacilli treatments increased the expression *PLA2G4A*, *PTGES*, and *PTGS2* that are involved in prostaglandin E2 biosynthesis. *L. rhamnosus* CRL1505 and *L. plantarum* CRL1506 showed quantitative and qualitative differences in their capacities to modulate the innate antiviral immune response in PIE cells, which would explain the higher capacity of the CRL1505 strain when compared to CRL1506 to protect against viral infection and inflammatory damage *in vivo*. These results provided valuable information for the deeper understanding of the host–immunobiotic interaction and their effect on antiviral immunity. The comprehensive transcriptomic analyses successfully identified a group of genes (*IFN-β*, *RIG1*, *RNASEL*, *MX2*, *A20*, *IL27*, *CXCL5*, *CCL4*, *PTGES*, and *PTGER4*), which can be used as prospective biomarkers for the screening of new antiviral immunobiotics in PIE cells and for the development of novel functional food and feeds, which may help to prevent viral infections.

Keywords: intestinal epithelial cells, immunotranscriptomic response, TLR3, *Lactobacillus rhamnosus* CRL1505, *Lactobacillus plantarum* CRL1506, antiviral response

INTRODUCTION

In the past decade, research has demonstrated that beneficial microbes with the capacity to modulate the mucosal immune system (immunobiotics) are a potential alternative to enhance resistance against viral infections. Immunobiotic lactic acid bacteria (LAB) are able to provide protection against viral infections by modulating innate and adaptive antiviral immunity. Several reports have shown that immunobiotic LAB improve protection against enteric viral infections and shorten the duration of diarrhea, reduce the number of episodes, diminish virus shedding, normalize gut permeability, and increase the production of virus-specific antibodies (1–3). Moreover, it was demonstrated that some immunobiotic strains, when orally administered, are able to increase respiratory defenses and reduce the susceptibility to respiratory viral infections improving virus clearance and diminishing inflammatory-mediated lung tissue damage (4–7).

In developing countries, viral mucosal infections such as bronchitis and diarrhea are the most common infectious diseases in children (8–10). The use of immunobiotics to improve the outcome of those viral infections has been proposed. In this regard, in a randomized controlled trial conducted by Villena et al. (4), the immunobiotic strain *Lactobacillus rhamnosus* CRL1505 (administered in a yogurt formulation) improved mucosal immunity and reduced the incidence and severity of intestinal and respiratory infection in children. The incidence of infectious events was reduced from 66% in the placebo group to 34% in the group that received the probiotic yogurt. Furthermore, there was also a significant reduction in the occurrence of indicators of disease severity such as fever and the need for antibiotic treatment in children receiving the probiotic yogurt (4). Studies in mice models have proved that orally administered *L. rhamnosus* CRL1505 improves antiviral immune responses in the intestinal mucosa (local effect) (5, 11) and the respiratory tract (distal effect) (6, 7). Of interest, it was demonstrated that these immunomodulatory capacities are strain specific since other immunobiotic strains such as *Lactobacillus plantarum* CRL1506 exert only local affects after oral administration (5–7, 11).

The interactions of intestinal epithelial cells (IECs) with luminal antigens and immune cells play a central role in determining the type of immune response triggered by microorganisms in the intestinal mucosa (12, 13). Therefore, by using a previously established porcine intestinal epithelial (PIE) cells that is able to respond to the dsRNA synthetic analog poly(I:C) and are permissive to rotavirus (14, 15), we aimed to evaluate the similarities and differences in the innate antiviral immune response induced by *L. rhamnosus* CRL1505 and *L. plantarum* CRL1506. We hypothesized that transcriptomic analyses using microarray technology in PIE cells could provide valuable information to gain insights in the mechanisms involved in the capacity of immunobiotics to modulate the innate antiviral immune response in the gastrointestinal tract and could provide some clues about their ability to stimulate immunity in distal mucosal sites such as the respiratory tract. Therefore, the aim of this study was to investigate the transcriptomic response of PIE cells to the challenge with viral molecular associated pattern poly(I:C) and the changes in that immunotranscriptomic profiles induced by the immunobiotics strains with antiviral capabilities *L. rhamnosus* CRL1505 and *L. plantarum* CRL1506. We obtained a global overview of the immune genes involved in the innate antiviral immune response in PIE cells that include type I interferons (IFNs), several IFN-stimulated genes (ISGs), cytokines, chemokines, adhesion molecules, and genes involved in prostaglandin biosynthesis. It was also determined that lactobacilli differently modulated immune gene expression in poly(I:C)-challenged PIE cells by increasing the expression of antiviral factors and cytokines/chemokines and reducing genes involved in poly(I:C)-mediated inflammatory damage. Moreover, the study allowed us to identify a group of genes that could be used as biomarkers for the screening of new antiviral immunobiotics in PIE cells.

MATERIALS AND METHODS

PIE Cells

PIE cells are intestinal non-transformed cultured cells originally derived from intestinal epithelia isolated from an unsuckled neonatal swine (16). When PIE cells are cultured, they assume a monolayer with a cobblestone and epithelial-like morphology and with close contact between cells (14, 16, 17). PIE cells were maintained in Dulbecco's modified Eagle's medium (DMEM) (Invitrogen Corporation, Carlsbad, CA, USA) supplemented with 10% fetal calf serum, 100 U/ml streptomycin, and 100 mg/ml penicillin at 37°C in an atmosphere of 5% CO_2. PIE cells grow rapidly and are well adapted to culture conditions even without transformation or immortalization (17–19).

Microorganisms

Lactobacillus rhamnosus CRL1505 and *L. plantarum* CRL1506 belong to CERELA Culture Collection and were originally isolated from goat milk (19). These strains were grown in Man-Rogosa-Sharpe broth at 37°C. For immunomodulatory assays, overnight cultures were harvested by centrifugation, washed three times with sterile PBS, counted in a Petroff-Hausser counting chamber, and resuspended in DMEM until use.

Immunomodulatory Effect of Lactobacilli in PIE Cells

Evaluation of the immunomodulatory activity of *L. rhamnosus* CRL1505 and *L. plantarum* CRL1506 was performed using PIE cells as described previously (19). PIE cells were seeded at 3×10^4 cells per well in 12-well type I collagen-coated plates (Sumitomo Bakelite Co., Tokyo, Japan) and cultured for 3 days. After changing medium, lactobacilli (5×10^8 cells/ml) were added, and 48 h later, each well was washed vigorously with medium at least three times to eliminate all stimulants. Then cells were stimulated with poly(I:C) (60 µg/ml) for 3, 6, 12, or 24 h for reverse transcription (RT)-PCR studies or for 12 h for microarray studies.

Microarray Analysis

Total RNA was isolated from lactobacilli-treated and control PIE cells using PureLink RNA Mini Kit (Life Technologies Inc., Gaithersburg, MD, USA) and treated with DNase. RNA integrity of all samples were evaluated by Agilent 2100 Bioanalyzer (Agilent Technologies, Santa Clara, CA, USA), using the RNA 6000 Nano Kit (20). Complementary DNA synthesis was performed using 200 ng of RNA. Hybridization with Porcine (V2) Gene Expression Microarray (Agilent Technologies) was performed at Hokkaido System Science Co. Scanning and digitization of Microarray were done by Agilent Technologies Microarray Scanner and Agilent Feature Extraction 10.7.3.1, respectively.

Data normalization and expression analysis were performed using GeneSpring software version 13.1 (Agilent Technologies). Significant genes up and downregulated in test samples [those stimulated with poly(I:C) or lactobacilli plus poly(I:C)] with respect to control samples [without poly(I:C) stimulation] were identified. Genes with significant changes in transcript abundance were selected on the basis of two criteria: a *t*-test *P* value of less than 0.05, which was considered statistically significant, and a cutoff in transcript abundance of at least twofold. Statistical analysis was conducted using the Limma package from BioConductor in R software (version 3.2.5). Results were expressed as log2 scale (log2 ratio). Genes whose expressions were log2 > 1 and $P < 0.05$ were annotated using PANTHER 11.1 (pantherdb.org). Genes were further analyzed according to Gene Ontology (GO) classification. Microarray data were submitted to NCBI-GEO under the accession number GSE93225.

Quantitative Expression Analysis by Two-Step Real-time Quantitative PCR (qPCR)

Two-step real-time qPCR was performed to characterize the expression of selected genes in PIE cells. Total RNA was isolated from each PIE cell sample using TRIzol reagent (Invitrogen). All cDNAs were synthesized using a Quantitect RT kit (Qiagen, Tokyo, Japan) according to the manufacturer's recommendations. Real-time qPCR was carried out using a 7300 real-time PCR system (Applied Biosystems, Warrington, UK) and the Platinum SYBR green qPCR SuperMix uracil-DNA glycosylase with 6-carboxyl-X-rhodamine (Invitrogen). The primers used in this study were described before (19, 20). The PCR cycling conditions were 2 min at 50°C, followed by 2 min at 95°C, and then 40 cycles of 15 s at 95°C, 30 s at 60°C, and 30 s at 72°C. The reaction mixtures contained 5 µl of sample cDNA and 15 µl of master mix, which included the sense and antisense primers. According to the minimum information for publication of quantitative real-time PCR experiments guidelines, β-actin was used as a housekeeping gene because of its high stability across porcine various tissues (14, 15, 20). Expression of β-actin was used to normalize cDNA levels for differences in total cDNA levels in the samples. The quality of the RNA in all experiments was checked by Agilent 2100 Bioanalyzer, and all samples were determined to be suitable for the qPCR assay considering values of A260/A280 and A260/A230 over 2.0 and the RIN value over 9.0.

Statistical Analysis

Statistical analyses were performed using GLM and REG procedures available in the SAS computer program (SAS, 1994). Comparisons between mean values were carried out using one-way ANOVA and Fisher's least significant difference test. For these analyses, *P* values <0.05 were considered significant.

RESULTS

Immunotranscriptomic Changes in PIE Cells after Poly(I:C) Challenge

The transcriptomic response of PIE cells to the challenge with poly(I:C) was first investigated. Microarray analysis was performed in PIE cells 12 h after the stimulation with poly(I:C). When these cells were compared with unchallenged PIE cells, it was found that there were 5,140 transcripts (representing 1,178 unique genes) and 3,359 transcripts (representing 788 unique genes) upregulated and downregulated, respectively (**Figures 1A,B**).

Of these differentially regulated genes, 165 were assigned to immune-related functions according to GO database (**Figures 1C,D**; Table S1 in Supplementary Material). Changes in the immunotranscriptome response in PIE cells after poly(I:C) stimulation included genes in the following GO Biological Process pathways: "immune system process," "regulation of defense response," "cell adhesion," "innate immune response," "regulation of viral process," "cellular response to interferon-gamma," and several pathways related to immune cells migration and chemotaxis (**Figure 1C**).

The most remarkable changes in PIE cells after stimulation with poly(I:C) were found in expression type I IFNs and antiviral factors, cytokines, chemokines, adhesion molecules, and prostaglandins.

A significant increase in the expression of *IFN-β* and *IFN-α* was observed in poly(I:C)-challenged PIE cells with fold changes (log_2 ratio) of 4.3 and 3.5, respectively (Table S1 in Supplementary Material). Increased expression of the IFN-induced antiviral factors *OAS1* (11.2), *OASL* (10.7), *IFIT1* (9.9), *IFIT3* (9.1), *IFIT2* (8.3), *MX1* (7.9), *MX2* (6.3), *OAS2* (6.3), *IFIT5* (3.0), *RNASEL* (2.2), and *RNASE4* (1.9) was also observed. In addition, a significant

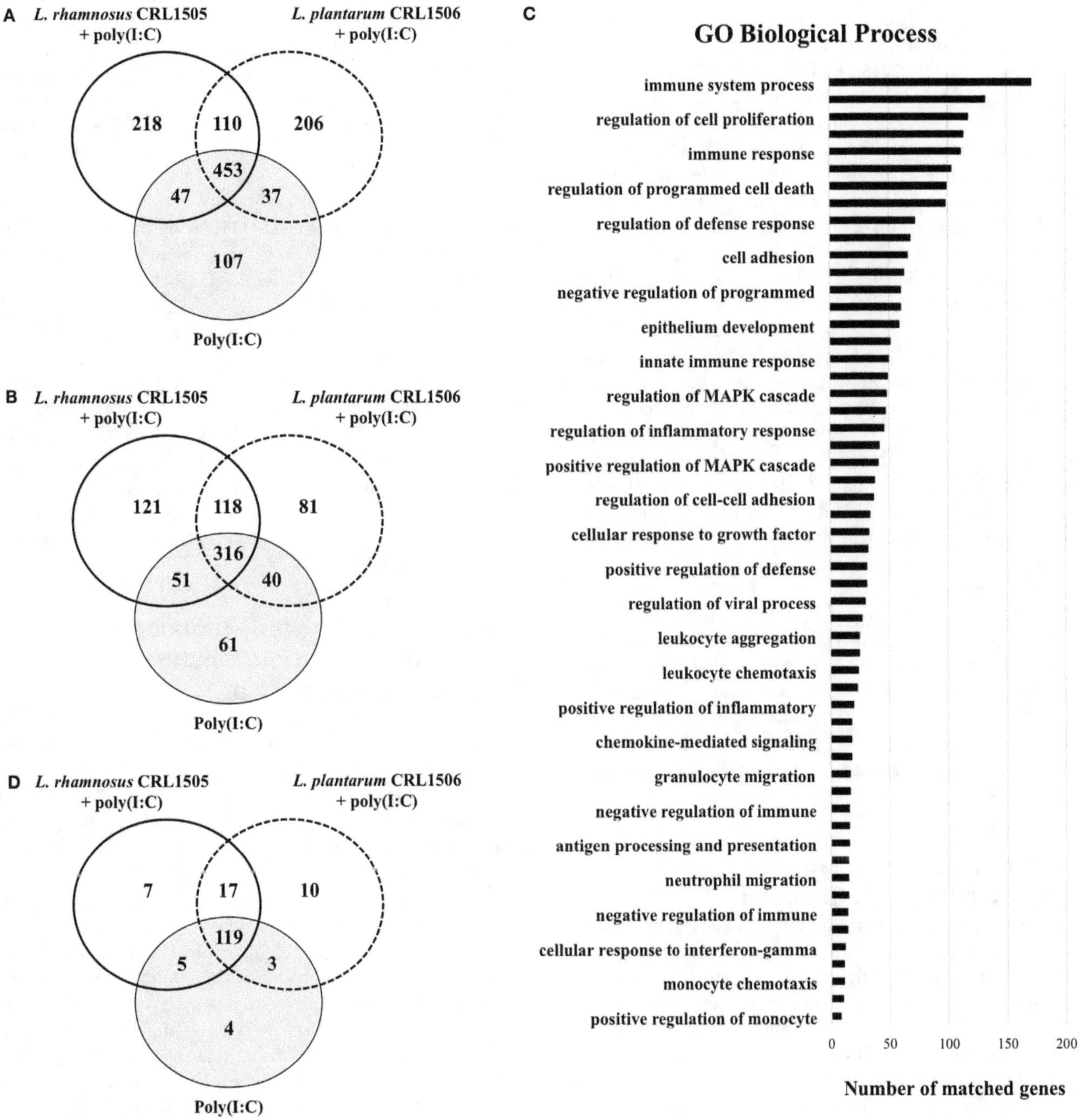

FIGURE 1 | Differentially regulated genes in porcine intestinal epithelial (PIE) cells treated with immunobiotic *Lactobacillus rhamnosus* CRL1505 or *Lactobacillus plantarum* CRL1506 and challenged with the viral molecular associated pattern poly(I:C). Non-lactobacilli-treated PIE cells challenged with poly(I:C) were used as controls. The changes in gene expression were evaluated by comparing the three mentioned groups with unchallenged PIE cells. Venn diagrams showing the number of differentially upregulated **(A)** and downregulated **(B)** genes for each experimental group. Number of matched genes categorized according to Gene Ontology (GO) database **(C)**. Venn diagram showing the number of differentially regulated genes that are known to have immune-related functions for each experimental group **(D)**.

upregulation of the transcriptional regulators *IRF7* (4.6), *STAT1* (4.3), *IRF1* (3.9), *IRF9* (2.5), and *STAT2* (2.2) were found in poly(I:C)-challenged PIE cells (Table S1 in Supplementary Material).

The stimulation of PIE cells with poly(I:C) significantly increased the expression of the inflammatory cytokines *IL-1α* (4.1), *IL-6* (4.0), and *IL-15* (1.8) (Table S1 in Supplementary Material). There was also a 3.9-fold increase in the expression of the sensor of the inflammasome polymeric complex *NPLR3*. Chemokines involved in monocyte and T lymphocyte recruitment and activation such as *CXCL10* (13.2), *CCL5* (8.4), *CXCL9* (8.1), *CCL4* (7.8), *CCL20* (5.9), *CCL23* (5.1), *CCL28* (2.9), *CCL8* (2.3), and *CCL2* (2.0) were increased after poly(I:C) stimulation. In addition, we observed a significant upregulation of the chemotactic factors for neutrophils *CXCL5* (2.5), *CXCL11* (10.3), and *CXCL8* (1.2) (Table S1 in Supplementary Material). Moreover, *CSF1* (2.9) and *CFS2* (2.9) that are factors able to stimulate the growth and differentiation of hematopoietic precursor cells from granulocytes and macrophages were also increased.

An upregulation of genes for adhesion molecules in PIE cells after stimulation with poly(I:C) was observed, including *SELE* (5.3), *VCAM-1* (4.0), *SELL* (2.6), *ICAM-1* (2.2), *EPCAM* (1.8), and *SELP* (1.8) (Table S1 in Supplementary Material). There was also a sevenfold increase in the expression of *LGALS9* (galectin 9), which is involved in epithelial–lymphocytes interaction.

The microarray analysis revealed increases in the expression of several genes related to prostaglandins biosynthesis in poly(I:C)-challenged PIE cells including *PTGS2* (5.0), *PTGIR* (3.6), *PTGIS* (1.6), *PTGER4* (1.6), and *PLA2G4A* (1.2). In addition, factors belonging to the complement system were upregulated including *C1R* (7.5), *C1S* (5.7), *C3* (2.9), and *CFB* (3.9) (Table S1 in Supplementary Material).

Changes in the expression of some pattern recognition receptors (PRRs) were detected including *TLR2* (1.6), and *PGLYRP2* (8.1). In addition, we detected changes in the viral innate immune receptors *TLR3* (2.8), *DDX58* (8.9) also known as retinoic acid inducible gene-I (*RIG-I*), *IFIH1* (5.4) also known as melanoma differentiation associated gene-5 (*MDA-5*), and *PKR* (3.2) (Table S1 in Supplementary Material). We also detected increases in the expression of serum amyloid A2 (*SAA2*) (8.6).

qPCR Analysis of Selected Genes in PIE Cells after Poly(I:C) Challenge

To further evaluate gene expression changes induced by poly(I:C) in PIE cells, qPCR was performed. From the 165 immune and immune-related genes differentially regulated by poly(I:C) (**Figure 1D**; Table S1 in Supplementary Material), we selected 39 belonging to IFN and IFN-induced antiviral factors, cytokines, chemokines, adhesion molecules, prostaglandins, *SAA2, A20, GZMA, LYZ,* and trefoil factor 1 (*TFF1*) to be studied by qPCR. We confirmed that the direction of the changes in gene expression was in agreement with results obtained in the microarray analysis in all the studied genes.

We detected a significant increase in the expression of *IFN*-β and *IFN*-α that reached a maximum value on hour 12 after poly(I:C) stimulation (**Figure 2**). *IRF3, RNASEL, MX1,* and *MX2* showed a peak on hour 12 after poly(I:C) challenge (**Figure 2**). Similarly, we observed increases in expression of *OAS1* and *OASL* with peaks at hour 24 and in *OAS2* with peaks between hours 6 and 12 after the poly(I:C) stimulation.

A significant increase in expression of *CCL4, CCL20, CXCL2,* and *CXCL5* with peaks on hour 3 after poly(I:C) challenge was also detected (**Figure 3**). Similarly, we observed increases in expression of *CCL8* and *CXCL10* with peaks at hour 6 and in *CCL11* and *CCL5* with peaks at hours 12 and 24, respectively. In addition, expression of *CCL23* increased from hour 3 and stayed in the same level between hours 6 and 24 after stimulation of PIE cells (**Figure 3**). *CXCL14* expression was significantly reduced after poly(I:C) challenge and returned to basal levels at hour 24. Poly(I:C) also increased the expression of the adhesion molecules *SELE, SELL, ICAM-1,* and *EPCAM* (Figure S1 in Supplementary Material).

Increased expression of *IL-1*β, *IL-5,* and *IL-15* was observed in poly(I:C)-challenged PIE cells (**Figure 4**) showing all of them their highest values after 6 h of stimulation. Amphiregulin (*AREG*) was also increased after poly(I:C) challenge with a peak at hour 24. On the contrary, *IL-9* expression was significantly reduced between hours 6 and 12 and returned to the basal levels at hour 24 (**Figure 4**).

We detected a significant increase in the expression of *PTGS2, PTGIR, PLA2G4A, PTGES,* and *PTGER4* (**Figure 4**). In addition, a slight increase in *PTGIS* was observed at hour 3, and a significant downregulation occurred at hour 24. A decrease in *PTGFRN* between hours 3 and 12 was also observed (**Figure 4**).

Finally, we observed upregulation of *GZMA, LYZ, TFF1,* and *SAA2* with peaks at hours 3, 6, 12, and 24, respectively (Figure S2 in Supplementary Material).

Modulation of Poly(I:C)-Induced Immunotranscriptome Changes in PIE Cells by Immunobiotics

Next, we analyzed microarray data to evaluate the effect of the immunobiotic strains *L. rhamnosus* CRL1505 and *L. plantarum* CRL1506 on the immunotranscriptomic response of PIE cells after the challenge with poly(I:C). For that purpose, PIE cells were stimulated with *L. rhamnosus* CRL1505 or *L. plantarum* CRL1506 and then challenged with poly(I:C). Comparative analysis of microarray profiles indicated that both CRL1505 and CRL1506 strains differentially modulated the expression of several genes related to the innate antiviral immune response in PIE cells after poly(I:C) stimulation (Table S2 in Supplementary Material).

The Venn diagram analysis was used to find genes that were uniquely and commonly modulated between lactobacilli-treated and control PIE cells (**Figure 1D**). Of the 165 differentially expressed genes in the Venn diagram analysis, 4 (*PPARA, TFF1, STAT3,* and *DUOX1*) were unique to the poly(I:C) challenge. Seven (*TNFRSF11B, C5, LOC100127164, PIK3R5, IL27, IL17RC,* and *IBSP*) and 10 (*NFIA, CADM4, CDH24, CCR7, IL1RAPL2, TNFAIP8L2, DPEP1, CDH19, BPIFA1,* and *TNFSF18*) unique genes were found in the CRL1505 stimulation plus poly(I:C) challenge and the CRL1506 stimulation plus poly(I:C) challenge groups, respectively. In addition, five genes (*RNASE6, PROC, VTN, CCL28,* and *PLG*) were common to CRL1505 treatment plus poly(I:C) and control, whereas three genes (*IL23RA, ITGA1,* and *IL20RB*) were common to CRL1506 treatment plus poly(I:C) and control. It was also observed that 119 genes were common to all the 3 treatments (**Figure 1D**). The cluster analysis in Figure S3 in Supplementary Material depicts the transcriptomic patterns of differentially modulated genes between lactobacilli-treated and control PIE cells. The treatment with CRL1505 plus poly(I:C)

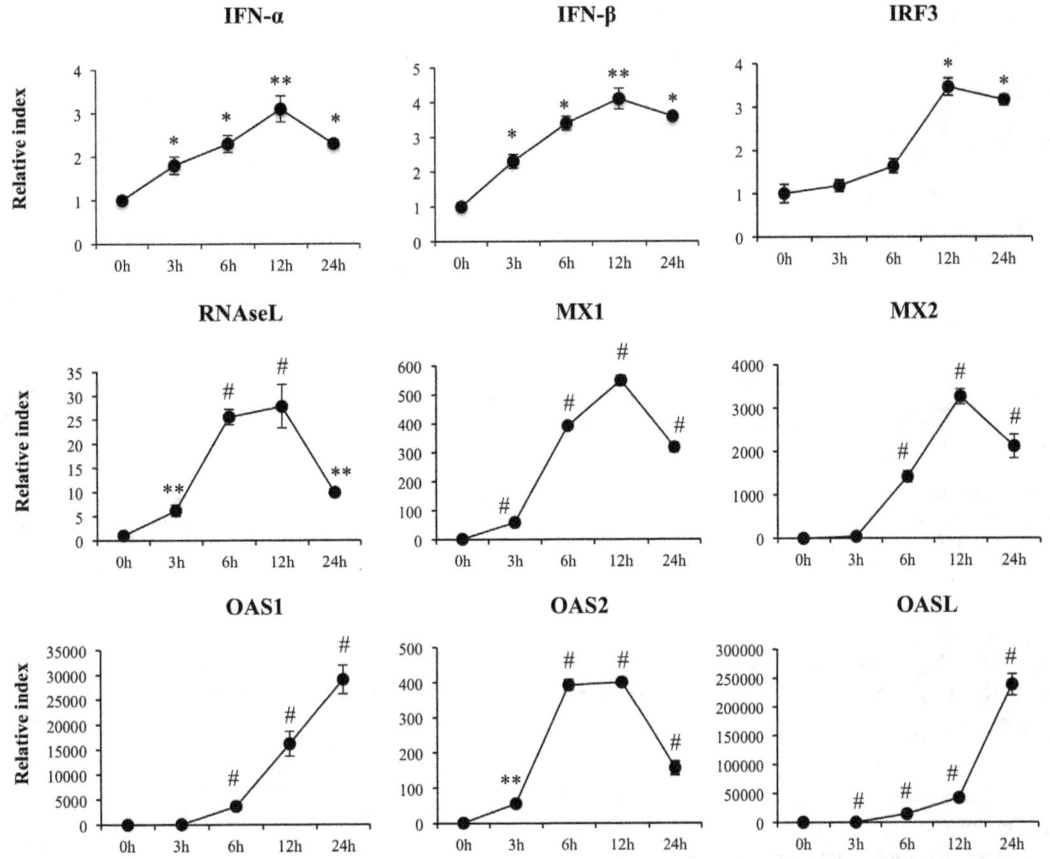

FIGURE 2 | Expression of type I interferons (*IFN*-β and *IFN*-α), IFN regulatory factor 3, and IFN-induced antiviral genes in porcine intestinal epithelial (PIE) cells after the challenge with the viral molecular associated pattern poly(I:C), analyzed by quantitative PCR. The results represent data from three independent experiments. Symbols indicate significant differences when compared to unchallenged control PIE cells (time 0 h) (*$P < 0.05$, **$P < 0.01$, #$P < 0.001$).

clustered closer to the treatment with CRL1506 plus poly(I:C) and both clustered separated from the control.

Closer examination of gene expression revealed differences in several genes sheared by immunobiotic-treated PIE cells and controls (Table S1 in Supplementary Material). Most remarkable differences were found in the genes belonging to IFN and IFN-induced antiviral factors, cytokines, chemokines, and adhesion molecules. Both lactobacilli treatment significantly increased *IFN-β*, *IFN-α*, *TLR3*, *OAS1*, *OASL*, *MX2*, *RNASEL*, *RNASE4*, and *STAT5A* when compared to controls. In addition, stimulation of PIE cells with *L. rhamnosus* CRL1505 plus poly(I:C) significantly increased the expression levels of *IFIT1*, *IFITM1*, *DDX58/RIG1*, *IFIH1/MDA5*, *IRF7*, *STAT1*, *NLRP3*, *IRF1*, *STAT2*, and *IRF2* when compared with PIE cells stimulated only with poly(I:C).

Although expression of *IL1A*, *IL6*, *IL8*, *AREG*, *CXCL10*, *CCL5*, *CCL4*, *CCL20*, *CCL23*, *CSF2*, *CCL3L1*, and *SELL* was upregulated in lactobacilli-treated PIE cells after the challenge with poly(I:C), the increases were significantly higher when compared to control PIE cells without lactobacilli treatment (Table S1 in Supplementary Material). *L. rhamnosus* CRL1505 plus poly(I:C) also increased the expression levels of *VEGFA*, *IL17RC*, *CXCL11*, *CCRL2*, *CXCL5*, *CXCL2*, *SELE*, *CDHR4*, and *EPCAM* when compared with PIE cells stimulated only with poly(I:C), an effect that was not observed with CRL1506 treatment. Interestingly, *IL27* was upregulated only in PIE cells receiving the CRL1505 strain plus poly(I:C). In addition, the expression levels of *IL15* and *RAE1* were reduced by lactobacilli treatments.

We also observed an increased expression of *PLA2G4A*, *PTGES*, and *PTGS2* genes in lactobacilli-treated PIE cells after the challenge with poly(I:C) when compared to the control cells, whereas *PTGER4* and *PTGER2* were diminished in lactobacillus-treated cells (Table S1 in Supplementary Material). *L. rhamnosus* CRL1505 plus poly(I:C) also increased the expression levels of *PTGIR*.

Expression of *TLR6*, *MYD88*, *NCOA1*, and *NFKB1* was significantly higher in lactobacilli-treated PIE cells after the challenge with poly(I:C) when compared to controls. In addition, the transcripts of other immune and immune-related genes including *GZMH*, *TFF1*, *LYZ*, *C1R*, *CFB*, *PLG*, *CFD*, *SAA2*, and *NOS2* were higher in lactobacilli-treated PIE cells than controls (Table S1 in Supplementary Material). Stimulation of PIE cells with *L. rhamnosus* CRL1505 plus poly(I:C) significantly increased the expression levels of *C1S*, *C3*, and *PLAU* when compared with PIE cells stimulated only with poly(I:C).

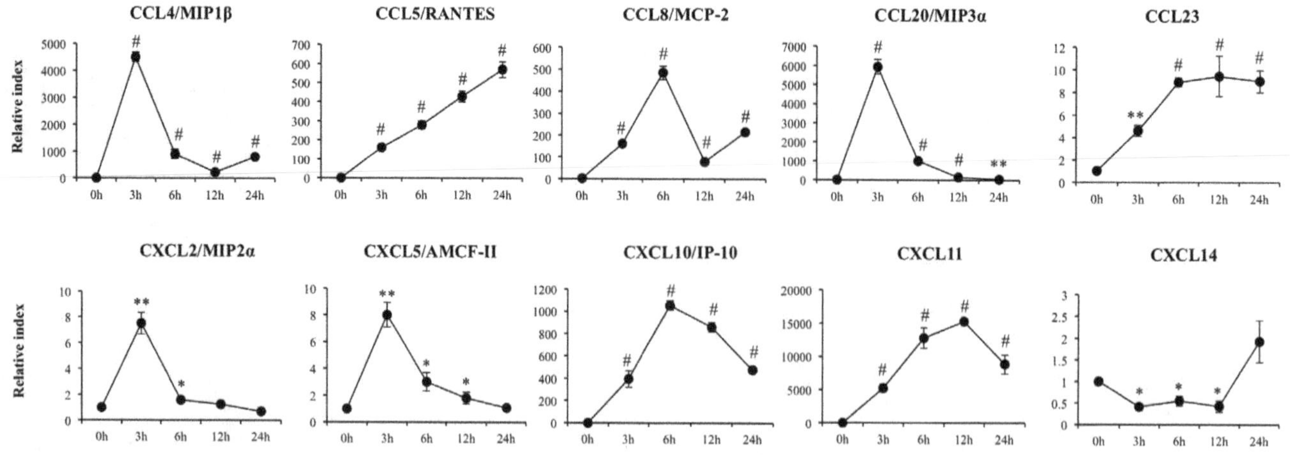

FIGURE 3 | **Expression of chemokines genes in porcine intestinal epithelial (PIE) cells after the challenge with the viral molecular associated pattern poly(I:C), analyzed by quantitative PCR.** The results represent data from three independent experiments. Symbols indicate significant differences when compared to unchallenged control PIE cells (time 0 h) (*$P < 0.05$, **$P < 0.01$, #$P < 0.001$).

qPCR Analysis of Selected Genes in PIE Cells after Stimulation with Immunobiotics and Poly(I:C) Challenge

To confirm the changes induced by *L. rhamnosus* CRL1505 and *L. plantarum* CRL1506 in the immunotranscriptome response of poly(I:C)-challenged PIE cells, qPCR was performed on selected genes. Genes with or without significant differences between lactobacilli-treated and non-treated PIE cells were chosen. The transcriptional changes evaluated by qPCR indicated a similar overall trend in the transcription.

Both *L. rhamnosus* CRL1505 and *L. plantarum* CRL1506 induced a significantly higher expression of *IFN-α* and *IFN-β* when compared with control poly(I:C)-challenged PIE cells (**Figure 5**). In addition, *IRF3* and the IFN-induced antiviral factors *RNASEL, MX2, OAS1,* and *OASL* were significantly higher in lactobacilli-treated PIE cells than in controls. Furthermore, *MX2* expression was higher in PIE cells treated with CRL1505 strain than those treated with CRL1506. Expression of *MX1* and *OAS2* in lactobacilli-treated PIE cells was not different from the control PIE cells after the challenge with poly(I:C) (**Figure 5**).

Expression of *CCL8* and *CXCL14* in lactobacilli-treated PIE cells was not different from the control PIE cells after the challenge with poly(I:C) (**Figure 6**). In contrast, the levels of *CCL23, CXCL8,* and *SELL* were significantly higher in lactobacilli-treated PIE cells when compared to the controls (**Figure 6**). In addition, both lactobacilli significantly increased the expression of *CCL4, CCL5, CCL20,* and *CXCL10*; however, values in *L. rhamnosus* CRL1505-treated PIE cells were higher than in cells treated with *L. plantarum* CRL1506. Only *L. rhamnosus* CRL1505 was able to increase the expression of *CXCL2, CXCL5, CXCL11, EPCAM, ICAM-1,* and *SELE* when compared to control PIE cells (**Figure 6**).

In agreement with the results from our microarray analysis, both lactobacilli strains were able to increase the expression of *IL-1β, IL-6,* and *AREG* and reduce the expression of *IL-15* and *PTGER4*, with no significant differences between them (**Figure 7**). Moreover, no differences in *TGF-β* or *PTGIS* were found between lactobacilli-treated and control PIE cells. Both lactobacilli significantly increased the expression of *PLA2G4A, PTGES,* and *PTGS2*; however, values in *L. rhamnosus* CRL1505-treated PIE cells were higher than in cells treated with *L. plantarum* CRL1506. In addition, only *L. rhamnosus* CRL1505 was able to significantly increase the expression of *IL-9* and *PTGIR* when compared to control PIE cells (**Figure 7**).

Expression of *TLR2* and *PGLYRP2* in CRL1505- or CRL1506-tretaed PIE cells was not different from the control PIE cells after the challenge with poly(I:C). In contrast, expression levels of *RIG1, TLR3,* and *TLR6* (**Figure 8**) were significantly higher in lactobacilli-treated PIE cells when compared to the controls. We also observed that *A20* (*TNFAIP3*) was reduced in lactobacilli-treated PIE cells when compared to the controls (**Figure 8**). *SAA2, GZMA, LYZ, TFF1,* and *C1R* were significantly upregulated in lactobacilli-treated PIE cells when compared to the controls (Figure S4 in Supplementary Material). Only *L. rhamnosus* CRL1505 was able to significantly increase the expression of *C3* when compared to control PIE cells, whereas both lactobacilli reduced the expression of *CFB* (Figure S4 in Supplementary Material).

DISCUSSION

It is known that IECs senses viral dsRNA through PRRs including TLR3, RIG-I, and MDA-5. After the recognition of dsRNA by those receptors, cellular signaling cascades are activated to react against viral infection. Antiviral PRRs activation leads to the production of cytokines, chemokines, IFNs, and IFN-regulated gene products that play a key role in establishing an antiviral state for virus clearance and restriction of spread (21).

High-throughput microarray technology has been employed for screening genes involved in the immune responses to enteric virus or poly(I:C) (22, 23). By using a human colon epithelial cell line (HT29 cells), Bagchi et al. (22) evaluated the

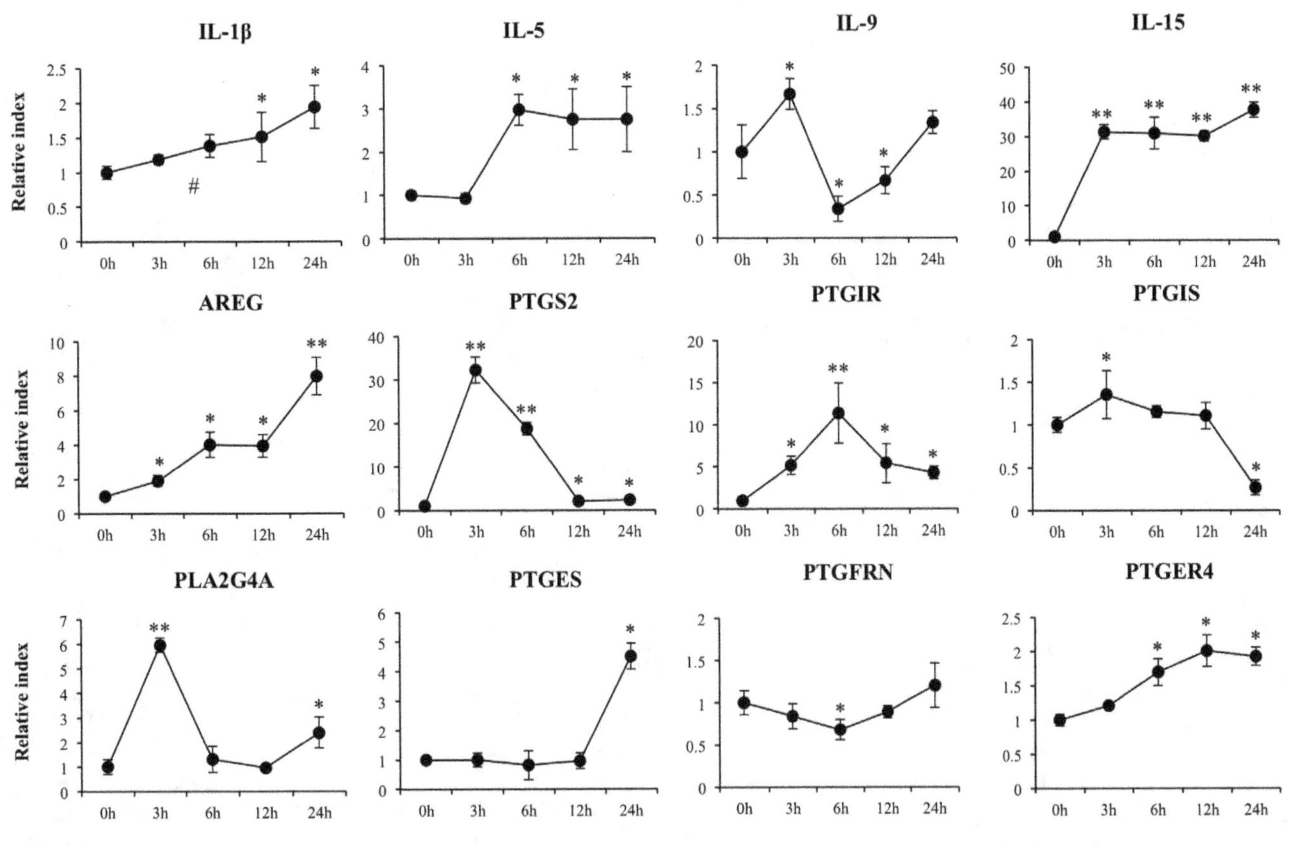

FIGURE 4 | Expression of cytokines and genes involved in prostaglandins biosynthesis in porcine intestinal epithelial (PIE) cells after the challenge with the viral molecular associated pattern poly(I:C), analyzed by quantitative PCR. The results represent data from three independent experiments. Symbols indicate significant differences when compared to unchallenged control PIE cells (time 0 h) (**P* < 0.05, ***P* < 0.01, #*P* < 0.001).

immunotranscriptomic response of IECs to the challenge with different rotavirus strains. Microarray data revealed a set of commonly differentially regulated genes for the three rotaviruses used in that work. Of interest, several IFN inducible genes (*OAS1*, *MX1*, *IL18*, *IITP3*, *TAP1*, and *RSAD2*) as well as several cytokines and chemokines (*CCL5*, *CXCL10*, *CXCL11*, *IL8*, and *CCL15*) were upregulated by rotavirus infection. Later, it was observed that the stimulation of HT29 cells with poly(I:C) enhanced the expression of several genes associated with the dsRNA recognition by PRRs including antiviral factors (*IRF1*, *ISG20*, *IFIT2*, *OASL*, and *STAT5*), and proinflammatory cytokines (*CSF1*, *CSF2*, *IL29*, *TNF-α*, *CXCL11*, and *CLCF1*) (23). Those transcriptomic studies indicated that poly(I:C) and rotavirus induce similar innate antiviral immunotranscriptomic responses in IECs.

Previously, the response of PIE cells to poly(I:C) challenge was evaluated, and it was found that MCP-1, IL-8, TNF-α, IL-6, and both IFN-α and IFN-β were upregulated in PIE cells after stimulation (14). The suitability of PIE cells as a model for studying immune signaling pathways after rotavirus infection was also evaluated. Our results showed that PIE cells have functional TLR3, RIG-I, and MDA-5 receptors, which are able to detect rotavirus infection and enhance the expression of IFN-β and the ISGs MxA and RNase L (15), which are important antiviral effectors of IFN pathway. In this study, we corroborated and deepen those findings by using microarray technology and qPCR. We demonstrated that stimulation with poly(I:C) significantly alters gene expression profiles of PIE cells. Of the transcripts differentially modulated by poly(I:C), several were assigned to immune-related functions. Our results showed that the activation of IRF3 and NF-kB pathways in PIE cells by poly(I:C) increased the expression of IFN-α and IFN-β, several ISGs (*OAS1*, *OASL*, *IFIT1*, *IFIT3*, *IFIT2*, *MX1*, *MX2*, *OAS2*, *IFIT5*, *RNASEL*, and *RNASE4*), cytokines (*IL-1β*, *IL-5*, and *IL-15*), and chemokines (*CCL4*, *CCL20*, *CXCL2*, *CXCL5*, *CCL8*, *CXCL10*, *CCL11*, *CCL5*, and *CCL23*). Moreover, some adhesion molecules were also significantly upregulated in PIE cells after poly(I:C) stimulation including *SELE*, *SELL*, *ICAM-1*, and *EPCAM*. In addition, we also observed a significant upregulation of the dsRNA detection sensors *TLR3*, *RIG1*, and *MDA5*. This is in agreement with studies in HT29 cells showing that RIG1 was upregulated by rotavirus infection (22).

These results are in line with the transcriptomics studies mentioned before and indicate that PIE cells are able to mount a complex innate antiviral immune response involving changes needed to induce a mucosal antiviral state and promote the recruitment of inflammatory cells to the intestinal tissue, which are intended to eliminate the viral pathogen (**Figure 9A**). These features also exhibit that PIE cells are an excellent laboratory tool

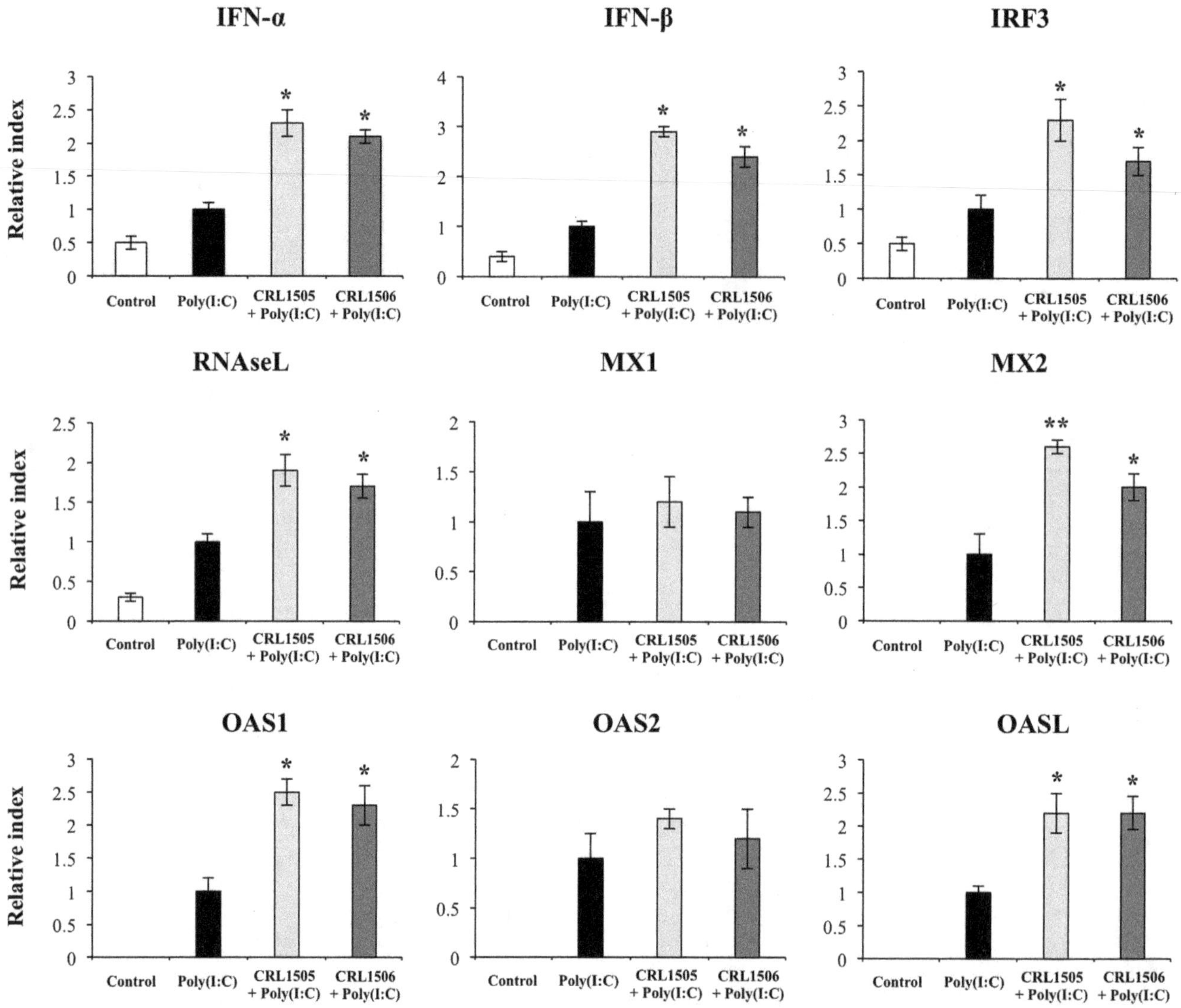

FIGURE 5 | Expression of type I interferons (*IFN*-β and *IFN*-α), IFN regulatory factor 3, and IFN-induced antiviral genes in porcine intestinal epithelial (PIE) cells treated with immunobiotic *Lactobacillus rhamnosus* CRL1505 or *Lactobacillus plantarum* CRL1506 and challenged with the viral molecular associated pattern poly(I:C), analyzed by quantitative PCR. Non-lactobacilli-treated PIE cells with or without poly(I:C) challenge were used as controls. The results represent data from three independent experiments. Asterisks indicate significant differences when compared to poly(I:C)-challenged control PIE cells (*$P < 0.05$, **$P < 0.01$).

to study treatments able to favorably modulate the innate antiviral response.

Several studies have shown that immunobiotics are able to beneficially modulate PRRs-mediated inflammatory response in the gut by regulating the functions of IECs (24). In this regard, our previous studies demonstrated that the immunobiotic strains *L. rhamnosus* CRL1505 and *L. plantarum* CRL1506 differentially regulated the expression of IFN-α, IFN-β, MCP-1, IL-8, and IL-6 in PIE cells after TLR3 activation (19). In line with those previous findings, we described here that the treatment of PIE cells with lactobacilli resulted in differential expression of several immune genes in response to the poly(I:C) challenge (**Figure 9B**), which include not only antiviral factors and cytokines as previously demonstrated but also adhesion molecules, complement factors, enzymes involved in prostaglandin biosynthesis, and PRRs. Most notable changes were found in *IFN*-α, *IFN*-β, *NPLR3*, *OAS1*, *OASL*, *MX2*, *RNASEL*, and *RNASE4* that were significantly increased in lactobacilli-treated PIE cells when compared to the controls. It is known that RNAse L, OAS, MX, and NPLR3 are important factors for the protection of the intestinal mucosa against rotavirus infection (25–27). This finding is of interest because it confirms our previous *in vitro* (19) and *in vivo* (11) studies demonstrating the antiviral capacity of *L. rhamnosus* CRL1505 and *L. plantarum* CRL1506.

In addition, it was observed that *L. rhamnosus* CRL1505 and *L. plantarum* CRL1506 differentially regulated the expression of

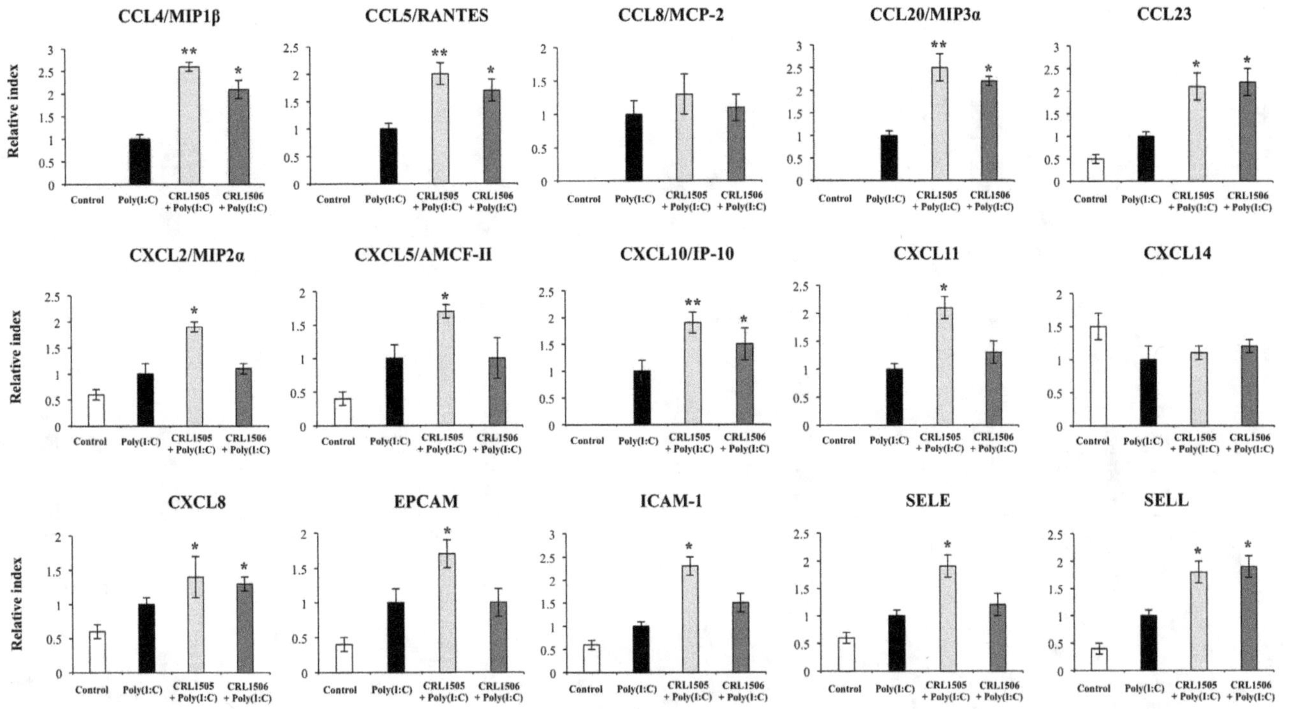

FIGURE 6 | Expression of chemokines and adhesion molecules genes in porcine intestinal epithelial (PIE) cells treated with immunobiotic *Lactobacillus rhamnosus* CRL1505 or *Lactobacillus plantarum* CRL1506 and challenged with the viral molecular associated pattern poly(I:C), analyzed by quantitative PCR. Non-lactobacilli-treated PIE cells with or without poly(I:C) challenge were used as controls. The results represent data from three independent experiments. Asterisks indicate significant differences when compared to poly(I:C)-challenged control PIE cells (*$P < 0.05$, **$P < 0.01$).

cytokines, chemokines, and adhesion molecules (**Figure 9B**). Expression levels of *IL-1β*, *IL-6*, *SELL*, *CCL4*, *CCL5*, *CCL20*, *CCL23*, *CXCL8*, and *CXCL10* were higher in lactobacilli-treated PIE cells than controls. In addition, *ICAM1*, *EPCAM*, *CXCL2*, *CXCL5*, and *CXCL11* were increased in CRL1505-tretated PIE cells. This pattern of cytokines/chemokines and adhesion molecules gene expression induced by lactobacilli would allow us to predict an improved recruitment and activation of immune cells to the gut mucosa, which could beneficially influence the elimination of the virus. It is also necessary to consider that in several viral infections, the excessive recruitment of inflammatory cells and/or their deregulated activation may contribute to the damage of the infected tissue rather than the resolution of the infection. It was reported that poly(I:C), when administered intraperitoneally to mice, mimics the local intestinal immune response elicited by an enteric viral infection (28, 29). Both purified dsRNA from rotavirus and poly(I:C) are able to induce severe mucosal damage in the gut *via* TLR3 activation including villous atrophy, mucosal erosion, and gut wall attenuation (28). It was demonstrated that TLR3 activation in IECs by poly(I:C) or rotavirus genomic dsRNA induce the expression of IL-15 and retinoic acid early inducible-1 (RAE1), which mediate epithelial destruction and mucosal injury by interacting with the NKG2D receptor expressed on CD3$^+$NK1.1$^+$CD8αα$^+$ intraepithelial lymphocytes (IELs) (30). Here, we found a significant reduction in the expression of *IL-15* and *RAE1* in PIE cells treated with lactobacilli. This is in line with our previous work that showed that mice pretreated with immunobiotic lactobacilli responded with reduced levels of TNF-α, IL-15, RAE1, and CD3$^+$NK1.1$^+$ CD8αα$^+$ IELs after TLR3 activation with poly(I:C) (11). Those changes significantly diminished the inflammatory damage of the intestinal mucosa.

Our transcriptomic study indicates that other regulatory mechanisms would be improved by lactobacilli to limit the inflammatory damage during intestinal viral infection. A significant upregulation of *AREG* and *TFF1* expression was observed in lactobacilli-treated PIE cells when compared to controls. Recently, it was demonstrated that the mucosal surfaces of lung and intestine are protected from detrimental inflammation by group 2 innate lymphoid cells (ILC2s). Monticelli et al. (31) showed that following activation with IL-33, ILC2s in the gut increased the expression of *AREG*, limited intestinal inflammation, and decreased disease severity in mice treated with dextran sodium sulfate. Moreover, it was reported that the number of ILC2s increased in the respiratory tract after infection influenza virus and that depletion of those cells induced impaired airway remodeling and altered lung epithelial integrity, diminishing lung function. Notably, these defects were restored by administration of AREG (32). On the other hand, TFF1 is a stable secretory protein expressed in gastrointestinal mucosa that stabilize the mucus layer and affect healing of the epithelium. By using TFF1-knockout mice, it was showed that this factor plays a

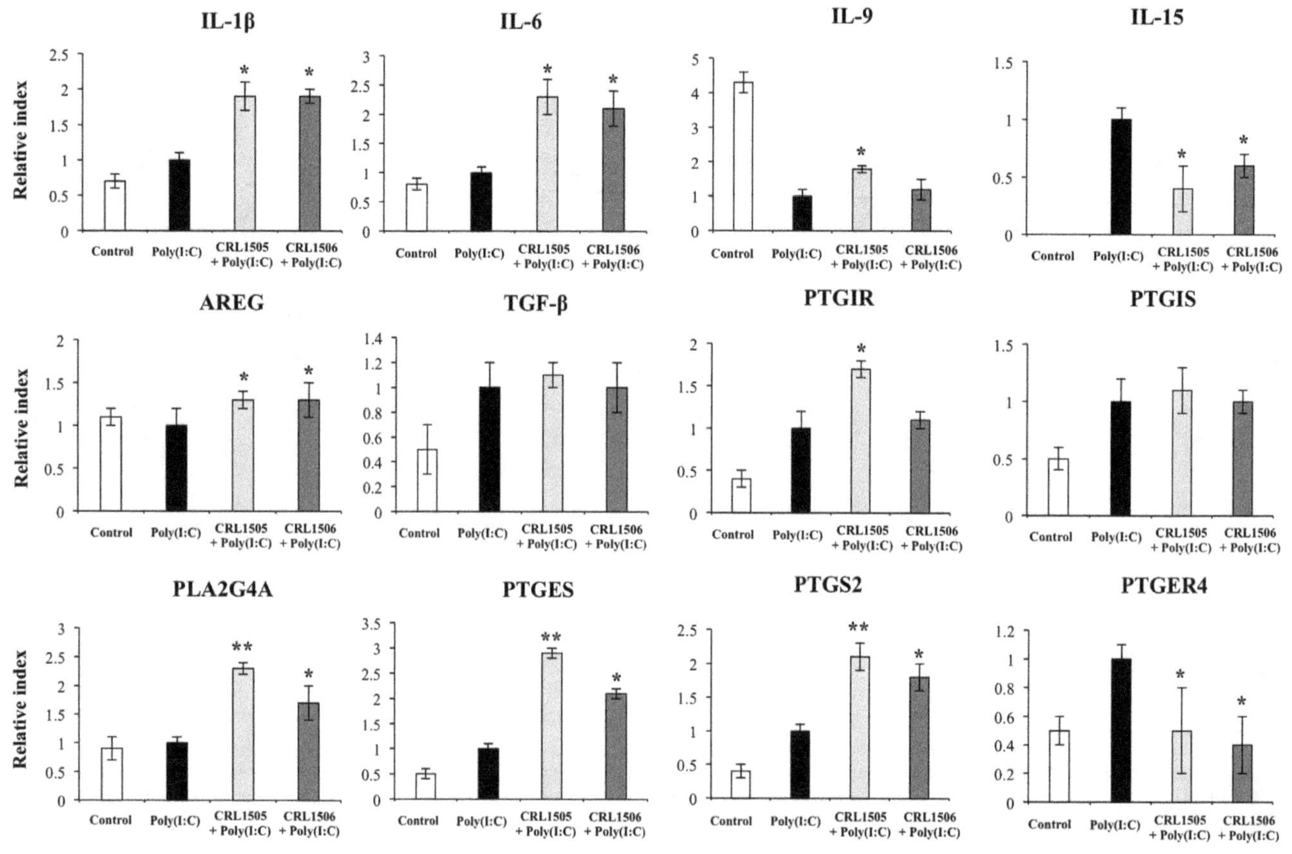

FIGURE 7 | Expression of cytokines and genes involved in prostaglandins biosynthesis in porcine intestinal epithelial (PIE) cells treated with immunobiotic *Lactobacillus rhamnosus* CRL1505 or *Lactobacillus plantarum* CRL1506 and challenged with the viral molecular associated pattern poly(I:C), analyzed by quantitative PCR. Non-lactobacilli-treated PIE cells with or without poly(I:C) challenge were used as controls. The results represent data from three independent experiments. Asterisks indicate significant differences when compared to poly(I:C)-challenged control PIE cells (*$P < 0.05$, **$P < 0.01$).

critical role in maintaining mucosal integrity and regulating the pro-inflammatory response to gastrointestinal pathogens (33). Moreover, a recombinant *Lactococcus lactis* strain, genetically modified to secrete human TFF1, was able to reduce the severity of mucosal damage in an animal model of oral mucositis (34).

We also observed that poly(I:C) stimulation induced transcriptomic changes in several genes involved in the biosynthesis of prostaglandins and that lactobacilli treatments increased the expression of several of those genes including *PLA2G4A*, *PTGES*, and *PTGS2*. Upregulation of *PLA2G4A* and *PTGES* indicates that PIE cells treated with lactobacilli would increase their production of prostaglandin E2 (PGE2). It has been reported that PGE2 regulates immune function in several ways that are able to affect viral pathogenesis. Production of pro-inflammatory cytokines and chemokines by immune cells are inhibited in presence of PGE2, whereas IL-10 is enhanced (35, 36) indicating that PGE2 could have a role in the protective activity of *L. rhamnosus* CRL1505 and *L. plantarum* CRL1506 against inflammatory damage. It was also reported that PGE2 inhibits type I IFN production in epithelial and immune cells, thereby causing an increase in virus replication (37). Interestingly, the expression of PGE2 receptors (*PTGER4* and *PTGER2*) was downregulated in PIE cells treated with the immunobiotic strains indicating that cells were protected from this effect of PGE2.

Whether the capacity of *L. rhamnosus* CRL1505 and *L. plantarum* CRL1506 to differentially modulate AREG, TFF1, and prostaglandins production is involved in their beneficial effects on intestinal or respiratory viral infections *in vivo* is an open question, which we propose to address in the near future.

The zinc-finger protein A20 is capable to terminate TLR signaling, which results in inhibition of NF-κB activation and reduction of inflammatory-induced cytotoxicity (38). Saitoh et al. (39) reported that IRF3 activation is suppressed by A20. The A20 protein is able to induce the suppression of the IFN-mediated immune response and IFN-promoter-dependent transcription following engagement of TLR3 by dsRNA. A20 knock down results in enhanced IRF3-dependent transcription triggered by the stimulation of TLR3 or virus infection. Furthermore, it was reported that A20 was upregulated by different rotavirus strains in IIT29 cells. Interestingly, the same work demonstrated that the knock down of A20 in IECs by siRNA significantly reduced virus titers indicating that A20 is required for rotavirus infection (39). We have reported previously that two immunobiotic bacteria with antiviral capabilities, *Bifidobacterium infantis* MCC12 and

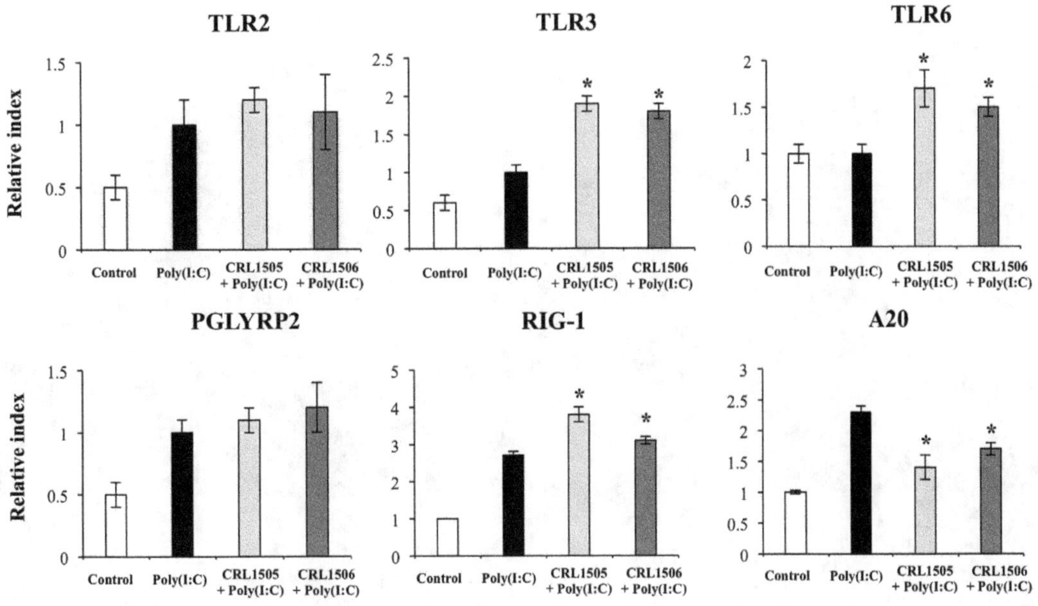

FIGURE 8 | Expression of pattern recognition receptors and A20 genes in porcine intestinal epithelial (PIE) cells treated with immunobiotic *Lactobacillus rhamnosus* CRL1505 or *Lactobacillus plantarum* CRL1506 and challenged with the viral molecular associated pattern poly(I:C), analyzed by quantitative PCR. Non-lactobacilli-treated PIE cells with or without poly(I:C) challenge were used as controls. The results represent data from three independent experiments. Asterisks indicate significant differences when compared to poly(I:C)-challenged control PIE cells (*$P < 0.05$).

Bifidobacterium breve MCC1274, significantly reduced the expression of A20 in rotavirus-infected PIE cells (15), which was in line with the capacity of both strains to improve IRF3 activation and IFN-β production. In line with our findings, MacPherson et al. (23) showed that the stimulation of HT29 cells with poly(I:C) alone increased the expression of A20, but the co-stimulation with poly(I:C) and probiotics significantly reduced A20 expression levels. Although our microarray analysis did not show differences between lactobacilli-treated and control PIE cells when the *A20* (*TNFAIP3*) transcript was evaluated, qPCR analysis showed a significant reduction of A20 expression in immunobiotic-treated cells. Therefore, the reduction of A20 in IECs could be a key effect for the antiviral capabilities of immunobiotics.

Lactobacillus rhamnosus CRL1505 and *L. plantarum* CRL1506 showed quantitative and qualitative differences in their capacities to modulate the innate antiviral immune response in PIE cells. Higher expression levels of the antiviral factors *MX2* and *IFIT2* were found in CRL1505-treated PIE cells when compared to CRL1506-treated cells. Moreover, some antiviral factors were upregulated only with *L. rhamnosus* CRL1505 treatment including *IFIT1*, *IFIT3*, *RIG-1*, *MDA5*, *NLRP3*, and *MSX1*. As mentioned before, *RIG-1*, *MDA5*, and *NLRP3* are important factors in the protection against gastrointestinal virus such as rotavirus. In addition, *MSX1* (also known as *HOX7*) was recently identified as an important modulator of RIG-1-mediated signaling pathway with the ability to induce the activation of the TBK1 kinase and IRF3, increasing the expression of antiviral genes and improving innate antiviral responses (40). Furthermore, *L. rhamnosus* CRL1505 differentially regulated the expression of proinflamamtory and anti-inflammatory factors in poly(I:C)-challenged PIE cells. Higher expression of *CCL4*, *CCL5*, *CCL20*, and *CXCL10* were found in CRL1505-treated PIE cells when compared to CRL1506-treated cells, whereas *CXCL2*, *CXCL5*, and *CXCL11* were upregulated only with *L. rhamnosus* CRL1505 treatment, indicating a higher capacity of this strain to induce recruitment of immune cells. It also seems that the CRL1505 strain would have a higher ability to improve the regulation of the inflammatory response. We observed higher expression of *PLA2G4A* and *PTGES* that would enhance the production of the anti-inflammatory PGE2. Of interest, microarray analysis showed an increase in the expression of IL-27 in *L. rhamnosus* CRL1505 treatment, an effect that was not observed in the other experimental groups. IL-27 is a member of IL-12 family of cytokines that is produced mainly by myeloid cell populations, including macrophages, inflammatory monocytes, and dendritic cells, but its production has been reported in endothelial cells and epithelial cells as well (41). This cytokine has important roles in the early regulation of Th1 differentiation and the suppression of cellular activation and production of proinflammatory cytokines (42). It was demonstrated that IL-27 induces IL-10 production from both mouse and human $CD4^+$ and $CD8^+$ T cells and NK cells (43). Moreover, some recent studies reported a role for this cytokine in restricting virus replication (42). These effects would explain the higher capacity of the CRL1505 strain when compared to CRL1506 to protect against viral infection and inflammatory damage (5, 11, 19).

In conclusion, the genome-wide transcriptional profiling performed in this work allowed us to obtain a global overview of the expression patterns of immune and immune-related genes involved in the response of PIE cells to poly(I:C) stimulation. This study also confirmed that *L. rhamnosus* CRL1505 and *L.*

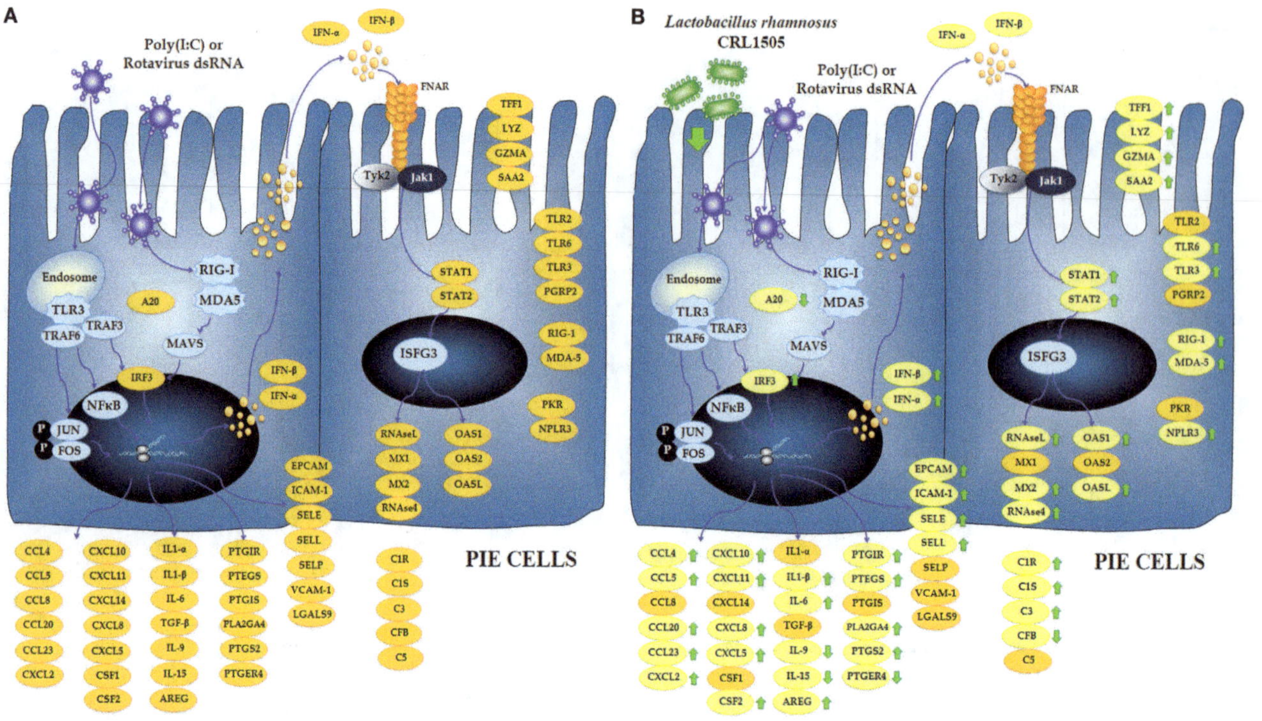

FIGURE 9 | Global overview of the signaling pathways and immune genes differentially regulated in porcine intestinal epithelial (PIE) cells after the challenge with the viral molecular associated pattern poly(I:C) (A). Global overview of the signaling pathways and immune genes differentially regulated in PIE cells treated with *Lactobacillus rhamnosus* CRL1505 and challenged with poly(I:C) **(B)**.

plantarum CRL1506 differently modulate gene expression in poly(I:C)-challenged PIE cells inducing changes that could help to explain the antiviral activities observed in animal models and clinical trials. These results provided clues for the better understanding the mechanism underlying host–immunobiotic interaction.

The main outcome from the study is that our transcriptomic analysis successfully identified a group of genes (*IFN-β*, *RIG1*, *RNASEL*, *MX2*, *A20*, *IL27*, *CXCL5*, *CCL4*, *PTGES*, and *PTGER4*), which can be used as prospective biomarkers for the screening of new antiviral immunobiotics in PIE cells. Classically, the selection of potential immunobiotic strains is performed by studying few biomarkers *in vitro*, and in many cases, the selected strains do not exhibit the same immunomodulatory activity when they are evaluated later in *in vivo* models. Our preliminary studies indicate that the set of biomarkers found in this work allows an efficient *in vitro* selection of new strains with antiviral activity in PIE cells, which present antiviral activity when they are evaluated later in animal models. This efficient selection of immunobiotics could improve the development of novel functional food and feeds, which may help to prevent viral infections.

AUTHOR CONTRIBUTIONS

HA, SA, JV, and HaK designed the study and manuscript writing. LA, HisK, HI, and NS did the laboratory work in the expression and statistical analysis. LA and JV participated in the data analysis of microarray. SS, TN, JV, and HaK contributed to data analysis and interpretation. All the authors read and approved the manuscript.

SUPPLEMENTARY MATERIAL

The Supplementary Material for this article can be found online at http://journal.frontiersin.org/article/10.3389/fimmu.2017.00057/full#supplementary-material.

FIGURE S1 | Expression of adhesion molecules genes in porcine intestinal epithelial (PIE) cells after the challenge with the viral molecular associated pattern poly(I:C), analyzed by quantitative PCR. The results represent data from three independent experiments. Symbols indicate significant differences when compared to unchallenged control PIE cells (time 0 h) (*P < 0.05, **P < 0.01).

FIGURE S2 | Expression of trefoil factor 1, lysozyme, granzyme, and A20 genes in porcine intestinal epithelial (PIE) cells after the challenge with the viral molecular associated pattern poly(I:C), analyzed by quantitative PCR. The results represent data from three independent experiments. Symbols indicate significant differences when compared to unchallenged control PIE cells (time 0 h) (*P < 0.05, **P < 0.01, #P < 0.001).

FIGURE S3 | Heat map analysis of the differentially regulated genes in porcine intestinal epithelial (PIE) cells treated with immunobiotic *Lactobacillus rhamnosus* CRL1505 or *Lactobacillus plantarum* CRL1506 and challenged with the viral molecular associated pattern poly(I:C). Non-lactobacilli-treated PIE cells challenged with poly(I:C) were used as controls.

FIGURE S4 | Expression of trefoil factor 1, lysozyme, granzyme, serum amyloid A2, and complement system factors genes in porcine intestinal epithelial (PIE) cells treated with immunobiotic *Lactobacillus rhamnosus* CRL1505 or *Lactobacillus plantarum* CRL1506 and challenged with the viral molecular associated pattern poly(I:C), analyzed by quantitative PCR. Non-lactobacilli-treated PIE cells with or without poly(I:C) challenge were used as controls. The results represent data from three independent experiments. Asterisks indicate significant differences when compared to poly(I:C)-challenged control PIE cells (*$P < 0.05$).

REFERENCES

1. Basu S, Paul DK, Ganguly S, Chatterjee M, Chandra PK. Efficacy of high-dose *Lactobacillus rhamnosus* GG in controlling acute watery diarrhea in Indian children: a randomized controlled trial. *J Clin Gastroenterol* (2009) 43:208–13. doi:10.1097/MCG.0b013e31815a5780
2. Liu F, Li G, Wen K, Bui T, Cao D, Zhang Y, et al. Porcine small intestinal epithelial cell line (IPEC-J2) of rotavirus infection as a new model for the study of innate immune responses to rotaviruses and probiotics. *Viral Immunol* (2010) 23:135–49. doi:10.1089/vim.2009.0088
3. Maragkoudakis PA, Chingwaru W, Gradisnik L, Tsakalidou E, Cencic A. Lactic acid bacteria efficiently protect human and animal intestinal epithelial and immune cells from enteric virus infection. *Int J Food Microbiol* (2010) 141:S91–7. doi:10.1016/j.ijfoodmicro.2009.12.024
4. Villena J, Salva S, Nuñez M, Corzo J, Tolaba R, Faedda J, et al. Probiotics for everyone! The novel immunobiotic *Lactobacillus rhamnosus* CRL1505 and the beginning of Social Probiotic Programs in Argentina. *Int J Biotechnol Wellness Industries* (2012) 1:189–98. doi:10.6000/1927-3037/2012.01.03.05
5. Villena J, Chiba E, Tomosada Y, Salva S, Marranzino G, Kitazawa H, et al. Orally administered *Lactobacillus rhamnosus* modulates the respiratory immune response triggered by the viral pathogen-associated molecular pattern poly(I:C). *BMC Immunol* (2012) 13:53. doi:10.1186/1471-2172-13-53
6. Chiba E, Tomosada Y, Vizoso-Pinto MG, Salva S, Takahashi T, Tsukida K, et al. Immunobiotic *Lactobacillus rhamnosus* improves resistance of infant mice against respiratory syncytial virus infection. *Int Immunopharmacol* (2013) 17(2):373–82. doi:10.1016/j.intimp.2013.06.024
7. Zelaya H, Tsukida K, Chiba E, Marranzino G, Alvarez S, Kitazawa H, et al. Immunobiotic lactobacilli reduce viral-associated pulmonary damage through the modulation of inflammation–coagulation interactions. *Int Immunopharmacol* (2014) 19:161–73. doi:10.1016/j.intimp.2013.12.020
8. Bardach A, Ciapponi A, Garcia-Marti S, Glujovsky D, Mazzoni A, Fayad A, et al. Epidemiology of acute otitis media in children of Latin America and the Caribbean: a systematic review and meta-analysis. *Int J Pediatr Otorhinolaryngol* (2011) 75:1062–70. doi:10.1016/j.ijporl.2011.05.014
9. Edmond K, Scott S, Korczak V, Ward C, Sanderson C, Theodoratou E, et al. Long term sequelae from childhood pneumonia; systematic review and meta-analysis. *PLoS One* (2012) 7:e31239. doi:10.1371/journal.pone.0031239
10. Gentile A, Bardach A, Ciapponi A, Garcia-Marti S, Aruj P, Glujovsky D, et al. Epidemiology of community-acquired pneumonia in children of Latin America and the Caribbean: a systematic review and meta-analysis. *Int J Infect Dis* (2012) 16:e5–15. doi:10.1016/j.ijid.2011.09.013
11. Tada A, Zelaya H, Clua P, Salva S, Alvarez S, Kitazawa H, et al. Immunobiotic *Lactobacillus* strains reduce small intestinal injury induced by intraepithelial lymphocytes after toll-like receptor 3 activation. *Inflamm Res* (2016) 65:771–83. doi:10.1007/s00011-016-0957-7
12. Parashar UD, Gibson CJ, Bresee JS, Glass RI. Rotavirus and severe childhood diarrhea. *Emerg Infect Dis* (2006) 12:304–6. doi:10.3201/eid1202.050006
13. Greenberg HB, Estes MK. Rotaviruses: from pathogenesis to vaccination. *Gastroenterology* (2009) 136:1939–51. doi:10.1053/j.gastro.2009.02.076
14. Hosoya S, Villena J, Shimazu T, Tohno M, Fujie H, Chiba E, et al. Immunobiotic lactic acid bacteria beneficially regulate immune response triggered by poly(I:C) in porcine intestinal epithelial cells. *Vet Res* (2011) 42:111. doi:10.1186/1297-9716-42-111
15. Ishizuka T, Kanmani P, Kobayashi H, Miyazaki A, Soma J, Suda Y, et al. Immunobiotic Bifidobacteria strains modulate rotavirus immune response in porcine intestinal epitheliocytes via pattern recognition receptor signaling. *PLoS One* (2016) 11:e0152416. doi:10.1371/journal.pone.0152416
16. Moue M, Tohno M, Shimazu T, Kido T, Aso H, Saito T, et al. Toll-like receptor 4 and cytokine expression involved in functional immune response in an originally established porcine intestinal epitheliocyte cell line. *Biochim Biophys Acta* (2008) 1780:134–44. doi:10.1016/j.bbagen.2007.11.006
17. Shimazu T, Villena J, Tohno M, Fujie H, Hosoya S, Shimosato T, et al. Immunobiotic *Lactobacillus jensenii* elicits anti-inflammatory activity in porcine intestinal epithelial cells by modulating negative regulators of the toll-like receptor signaling pathway. *Infect Immun* (2012) 80:276–88. doi:10.1128/IAI.05729-11
18. Tomosada Y, Villena J, Murata K, Chiba E, Shimazu T, Aso H, et al. Immunoregulatory effect of Bifidobacteria strains in porcine intestinal epithelial cells through modulation of ubiquitin-editing enzyme A20 expression. *PLoS One* (2013) 8:e59259. doi:10.1371/journal.pone.0059259
19. Villena J, Chiba E, Vizoso-Pinto MG, Tomosada Y, Takahashi T, Ishizuka T, et al. Immunobiotic *Lactobacillus rhamnosus* strains differentially modulate antiviral immune response in porcine intestinal epithelial and antigen presenting cells. *BMC Microbiol* (2014) 14:126. doi:10.1186/1471-2180-14-126
20. Kobayashi H, Albarracin L, Sato N, Kanmani P, Kober AK, Ikeda-Ohtsubo W, et al. Modulation of porcine intestinal epitheliocytes immunotranscriptome response by *Lactobacillus jensenii* TL2937. *Benef Microbes* (2016) 7(5):769–82. doi:10.3920/BM2016.0095
21. Kitazawa H, Villena J. Modulation of respiratory TLR3-antiviral response by probiotic microorganisms: lessons learned from *Lactobacillus rhamnosus* CRL1505. *Front Immunol* (2014) 5:201. doi:10.3389/fimmu.2014.00201
22. Bagchi P, Nandi S, Chattopadhyay S, Bhowmick R, Halder UC, Nayak MK, et al. Identification of common human host genes involved in pathogenesis of different rotavirus strains: an attempt to recognize probable antiviral targets. *Virus Res* (2012) 169:144–53. doi:10.1016/j.virusres.2012.07.021
23. Macpherson C, Audy J, Mathieu O, Tompkins TA. Multistrain probiotic modulation of intestinal epithelial cells' immune response to a double-stranded RNA ligand, poly(I-C). *Appl Environ Microbiol* (2014) 80:1692–700. doi:10.1128/AEM.03411-13
24. Villena J, Kitazawa H. Modulation of intestinal TLR4-inflammatory signalling pathways by probiotic microorganisms: lessons learned from *Lactobacillus jensenii* TL2937. *Front Immunol* (2014) 4:512. doi:10.3389/fimmu.2013.00512
25. López S, Arias CF. Rotavirus-host cell interactions: an arms race. *Curr Opin Virol* (2012) 2:389–98. doi:10.1016/j.coviro.2012.05.001
26. Sánchez-Tacuba L, Rojas M, Arias CF, López S. Rotavirus controls activation of the 2'-5'-oligoadenylate synthetase/RNase L pathway using at least two distinct mechanisms. *J Virol* (2015) 89:12145–53. doi:10.1128/JVI.01874-15
27. Di Fiore IJ, Holloway G, Coulson BS. Innate immune responses to rotavirus infection in macrophages depend on MAVS but involve neither the NLRP3 inflammasome nor JNK and p38 signaling pathways. *Virus Res* (2015) 208:89–97. doi:10.1016/j.virusres.2015.06.004
28. Zhou R, Wei H, Sun R, Tian Z. Recognition of double-stranded RNA by TLR3 induces severe small intestinal injury in mice. *J Immunol* (2007) 178:4548–56. doi:10.4049/jimmunol.178.7.4548
29. Araya RE, Jury J, Bondar C, Verdu EF, Chirdo FG. Intraluminal administration of poly I:C causes an enteropathy that is exacerbated by administration of oral dietary antigen. *PLoS One* (2014) 9:e99236. doi:10.1371/journal.pone.0099236
30. Zhou R, Wei H, Sun R, Zhang J, Tian Z. NKG2D recognition mediates toll-like receptor 3 signaling-induced breakdown of epithelial homeostasis in the small intestines of mice. *Proc Natl Acad Sci U S A* (2007) 104:7512–5. doi:10.1073/pnas.0700822104
31. Monticelli LA, Osborne LC, Noti M, Tran SV, Zaiss DM, Artis D. IL-33 promotes an innate immune pathway of intestinal tissue protection dependent on amphiregulin-EGFR interactions. *Proc Natl Acad Sci U S A* (2015) 112:10762–7. doi:10.1073/pnas.1509070112
32. Monticelli LA, Sonnenberg GF, Abt MC, Alenghat T, Ziegler CG, Doering TA, et al. Innate lymphoid cells promote lung-tissue homeostasis after infection with influenza virus. *Nat Immunol* (2011) 12:1045–1045. doi:10.1031/ni.2131
33. Soutto M, Chen Z, Katsha AM, Romero-Gallo J, Krishna US, Piazuelo MB, et al. Trefoil factor 1 expression suppresses *Helicobacter pylori*-induced inflammation in gastric carcinogenesis. *Cancer* (2015) 121:4348–58. doi:10.1002/cncr.29644

34. Caluwaerts S, Vandenbroucke K, Steidler L, Neirynck S, Vanhoenacker P, Corveleyn S, et al. AG013, a mouth rinse formulation of *Lactococcus lactis* secreting human Trefoil factor 1, provides a safe and efficacious therapeutic tool for treating oral mucositis. *Oral Oncol* (2010) 46:564–70. doi:10.1016/j.oraloncology.2010.04.008
35. Kunkel SL, Spengler M, May MA, Spengler R, Larrick J, Remick D. Prostaglandin E2 regulates macrophage-derived tumor necrosis factor gene expression. *J Biol Chem* (1988) 263:5380–4.
36. Harizi H, Juzan M, Pitard V, Moreau JF, Gualde N. Cyclooxygenase-2-issued prostaglandin e(2) enhances the production of endogenous IL-10, which down-regulates dendritic cell functions. *J Immunol* (2002) 168:2255–63. doi:10.4049/jimmunol.168.5.2255
37. Coulombe F, Jaworska J, Verway M, Tzelepis F, Massoud A, Gillard J, et al. Targeted prostaglandin E2 inhibition enhances antiviral immunity through induction of type I interferon and apoptosis in macrophages. *Immunity* (2014) 40(4):554–68. doi:10.1016/j.immuni.2014.02.013
38. Ning S, Pagano JS. The A20 deubiquitinase activity negatively regulates LMP1 activation of IRF7. *J Virol* (2010) 84:6130–8. doi:10.1128/JVI.00364-10
39. Saitoh T, Yamamoto M, Miyagishi M, Taira K, Nakanishi M, Fujita T, et al. A20 is a negative regulator of IFN regulatory factor 3 signaling. *J Immunol* (2005) 174:1507–12. doi:10.4049/jimmunol.174.3.1507
40. Chen LT, Hu MM, Xu ZS, Liu Y, Shu HB. MSX1 modulates RLR-mediated innate antiviral signaling by facilitating assembly of TBK1-associated complexes. *J Immunol* (2016) 197:199–207. doi:10.4049/jimmunol.1600039
41. Hall AO, Silver JS, Hunter CA. The immunobiology of IL-27. *Adv Immunol* (2012) 115:1–44. doi:10.1016/B978-0-12-394299-9.00001-1
42. Duan Y, Jia Y, Wang T, Wang Y, Han X, Liu L. Potent therapeutic target of inflammation, virus and tumor: focus on interleukin-27. *Int Immunopharmacol* (2015) 26:139–46. doi:10.1016/j.intimp.2015.03.016
43. Saraiva M, O'Garra A. The regulation of IL-10 production by immune cells. *Nat Rev Immunol* (2010) 10:170–81. doi:10.1038/nri2711

21

Complete Genome Sequence of *Lactobacillus casei* LC5, a Potential Probiotics for Atopic Dermatitis

Jisu Kang[1,2†], Won-Hyong Chung[1†], Tae-Joong Lim[3], Tae Woong Whon[4], Sanghyun Lim[3] and Young-Do Nam[1,2*]*

[1] Research Group of Gut Microbiome, Korea Food Research Institute, Sungnam, South Korea, [2] Department of Food Biotechnology, Korea University of Science and Technology, Daejeon, South Korea, [3] Research and Development Center, Cell Biotech Co. Ltd., Gimpo, South Korea, [4] Department of Biology, Kyung Hee University, Seoul, South Korea

Edited by:
Haruki Kitazawa,
Tohoku University, Japan

Reviewed by:
Margarita Isabel Piazzon,
CONICET, Argentina
Jiu-Yao Wang,
National Cheng Kung University, Taiwan

***Correspondence:**
Sanghyun Lim
shlim@cellbiotech.com;
Young-Do Nam
youngdo98@kfri.re.kr

† These authors have contributed equally to this work.

Keywords: atopic dermatitis, probiotics, *Lactobacillus casei*, genome sequence, PacBio

BACKGROUND

Probiotics are living microorganisms providing health beneficial effect to the host (1). Probiotics have been used for the treatment or prevention of various diseases related to diarrhea (2), cholesterol (3) immune function (4), and inflammatory bowel disease (5). In addition, recent study also presents that probiotic bacteria in the *Bifidobacterium* and *Lactobacillus* genera are able to have therapeutic effects in the patients of psychological disorders, such as depression, anxiety, and memory (6).

Lactobacillus casei is a Gram-positive bacterium that naturally inhabits the human and animal gastrointestinal and mouth organs (7). As its name implies, this heterofermentative microorganism is the dominant species present in ripening cheddar cheese (8). In probiotic aspects, *L. casei* showed beneficial roles in the activation of the gut mucosal immune system (9), treatment of diabetics (10), and chronic constipation (11). In the previous study, we isolated *L. casei* LC5 strain from fermented dairy products, which showed immune regulatory functions, especially, therapeutic effect on atopic dermatitis as a member of complex probiotics (12–14).

In order to gain better insight of the probiotic effect on atopic dermatitis, we analyzed the genome sequence of *L. casei* LC5. According to the report of NCBI Genome,[1] more than two hundreds of *Lactobacillus* organisms are sequenced and their beneficial properties derived from genomic information are used in the food industry. However, the available genomes of *L. casei* strains as members of health promoting probiotics are still insufficient. Furthermore, *L. casei* strains are frequently confused with the closely related strains such as *Lactobacillus paracasei* and *Lactobacillus rhamnosus*. Therefore, comparative study in a whole genome scale is required to clarify taxonomic association of *L. casei* LC5 as well as its functional characteristics. The availability of the genomic information of *L. casei* LC5 will aid as a basis for further in-depth analysis of the probiotic function of *L. casei* strains.

MATERIALS AND METHODS

Bacterial Strains and DNA Preparation

Lactobacillus casei LC5 was isolated from fermented dairy products and commercially used as probiotics in Korea (15). *L. casei* LC5 was cultured aerobically in MRS medium (Difco, USA) at 37°C for 18 h. Genomic DNA from *L. casei* LC5 was extracted and purified using a QIAamp DNA

[1] https://www.ncbi.nlm.nih.gov/genome/?term=Lactobacillus.

Mini Kit (Qiagen, Germany). The concentration of genomic DNA was qualified with NanoDrop 2000 UV–vis spectrophotometer (Thermo Scientific, USA) and Qubit 2.0 fluorometer (Life Technology, USA).

Genome Sequencing, Assembly, and Annotation

Whole genome sequencing of *L. casei* LC5 was carried out by using PacBio RS II platform. A 20 kb DNA library was constructed according to the manufacturer's instruction and sequenced using single molecule real-time (SMRT) sequencing technology with the P6 DNA polymerase and C4 chemistry. A total of 138,180 subreads (1.04 Gb) were obtained with 400-fold coverage. The average length of subreads was 7,550 bp and N50 was 10,940 bp. Genome assembly was performed using HGAP 3.0 (16) with default options. The annotation was carried out with NCBI Prokaryotic Genome Annotation Pipeline (17) through NCBI Genome submission portal (GenomeSubmit at http://ncbi.nlm.nih.gov). The chromosome topology was drawn using DNAPlotter (18). Clusters of orthologous groups (COG) categories were assigned to the coding genes using BLASTP (e-value: 1e−3) against COG database (19).

Phylogenetic Analysis and Comparative Genomic Analysis

For phylogenetic and comparative study, we downloaded 19 genome sequences of *L. casei* group (10 of *L. casei*, 8 of *L. paracasei*, 1 of *Lactobacillus zeae*, and 1 of *L. rhamnosus*) from NCBI genome database.[2] A list of the reference genomes are as follows: *L. casei* Zhang (NC_014334), *L. casei* BL23 (NC_010999), *L. casei* BD-II (NC_017474), *L. casei* LC2W (NC_017473), *L. casei* 12A (NZ_CP006690), *L. casei* W56 (NC_018641), *L. casei* LcY (NZ_CM001848), *L. casei* LcA (NZ_CM001861), *L. casei* LOCK919 (NC_021721), *L. casei* ATCC 393 (NZ_AP012544), *L. paracasei* ATCC 334 (NC_008526), *L. paracasei* 362.5013889 (NC_022112), *L. paracasei* N1115 (NZ_CP007122), *L. paracasei* JCM (NZ_AP012541), *L. paracasei* CAUH35 (NZ_CP012187), *L. paracasei* L9 (NZ_CP012148), *L. paracasei* KL1 (NZ_CP013921), *L. zeae* DSM 20178 (NZ_AZCT01000001), and *L. rhamnosus* GG (NC_013198). The assembly levels of all genomes are "complete genome" or chromosome except *L. zeae* DSM 20178 (includes 55 scaffolds). Because we failed to fetch full-length 16S rRNA gene from the genome of *L. zeae* DSM 20178, we alternatively used a 16S rRNA gene of *L. zeae* RIA 482 (NR_037122), the closest sequence of DSM 20178 (sequence identity = 99.9%), in the phylogenetic analysis.

The evolutionary history was inferred by using the maximum likelihood method based on the Tamura-Nei model (20). All positions containing gaps and missing data were eliminated. There were a total of 1521 positions in the final dataset. Those phylogenetic analyses were conducted in MEGA6 (21). To compute genomic distance, we first computed orthologous average nucleotide identity (OrthoANI) values using orthologous average nucleotide identity tool (22). The OrthoANI values were converted to distance values by following formula: distance = 1 − (OrthoANI/100). The evolutionary distance was computed using the neighbor-joining method of MEGA6 (21). The tree is drawn to scale with branch lengths in the same units as those of the evolutionary distances used to infer the phylogenetic tree. The resulting phylogenetic tree was produced using MEGA6. Pan-genomic study using Panseq (23) was performed to investigate the genomic conservation and finding novel region in the sequenced genome.

RESULTS

Genome Characteristics of *L. casei* LC5

We obtained a complete genome sequence of *L. casei* LC5 using SMRT sequencing. This genome has a chromosome and no organelle sequences. The total size of the genome is 3,132,867 bp and its GC content is 47.9%. A total of 2,925 genes were detected from the genome sequence. The number of coding CDS is 2,817 and pseudogenes is 31. Seventy seven RNAs (15 rRNAs, 59 tRNAs, and 3 non-coding RNAs) were also identified. Repeating region or CRISPR array was not identified. Genomic features of *L. casei* LC5 are shown in **Figure 1A**.

Although *L. casei* LC5 was identified as a strain of *L. casei*, it showed different genomic features compared to the other published *L. casei* strains; According to the summary of 37 *L. casei* genomes deposited in NCBI Assembly, the median length is 3.01993 Mb, the median of coding genes is 2,712, and the median of GC contents is 46.4%. An interesting point is that those genomes can be split into two groups by the difference of GC contents, high-GC group (47.7–47.9%) and low-GC group (46.2–46.6%). Five genomes (ATCC 393, N87, 867_LCAS, Lbs2, JCM 1134) and *L. casei* LC5 belong to the high-GC group and the other genomes belong to the low-GC group (**Table 1**).

Comparative Study of *L. casei* Group

Comparative study of both 16S rRNA genes and whole genome sequences revealed that the closest genome of *L. casei* LC5 was *L. casei* ATCC 393 and second closest one was *L. zeae* DSM 20178. The three genomes which showed distinguishable differences on the comparative study, LC5, ATCC 393, and *L. zeae* DSM 20178, belong to the high-GC group as described in the above section. In contrast to the phylogenetic distances based on 16S rRNA gene among the high-GC group (below 0.001), the distances between the high-GC group and the low-GC group were above 0.003 (**Figure 1C**). It was also supported by the estimation result of the whole genomic comparison. Average nucleotide identity (ANI) values among the high-GC group were above 94% whereas ANI values between two groups were below 80% (**Figure 1D**). All the *L. casei* strains and *L. paracasei* strains belonging to the low-GC group showed the high genomic similarity of 98% or higher.

Functional Classification

Functional classification based on COG assigned the 2,334 CDSs into the 1,309 COG numbers. From the comparison of functional

[2]http://www.ncbi.nlm.nih.gov/genome/.

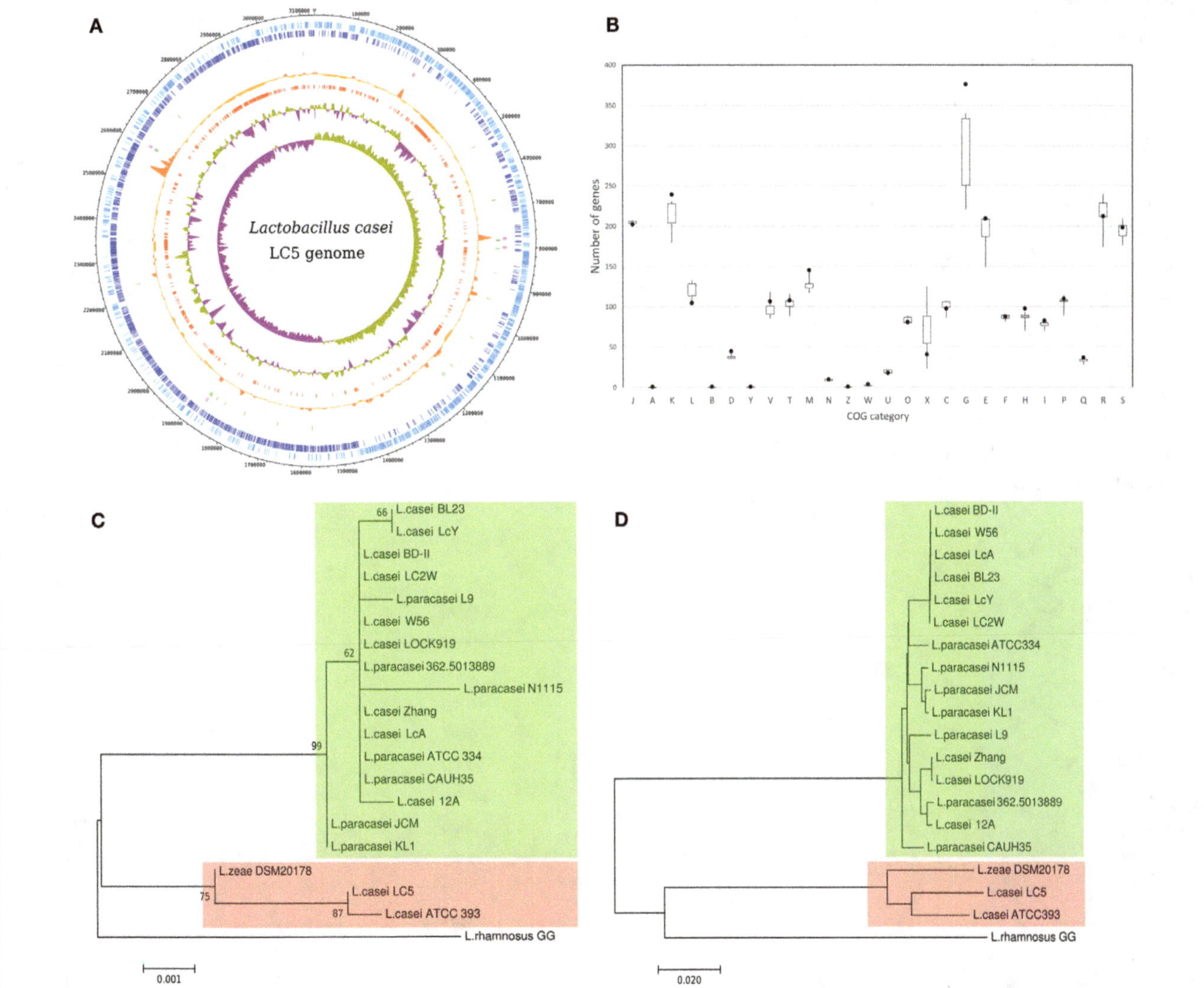

FIGURE 1 | Genome characteristics of *Lactobacillus casei* LC5 genome. (A) Circular map of genomic features; eight tracks were plotted in the map. Track 1 (light blue; outermost), forward-stranded coding CDS; Track 2 (blue), reverse-stranded coding CDS; Track 3 (light purple), rRNA including 5S, 16S, and 23S; Track 4 (green), Trna; Track 5 (orange), peak of pan-genomic conservation; Track 6 (red), novel regions (below 85% similarities with the other genomes); Track 7 (light green and purple), GC content; and Track 8 (light green and purple), GC skew. **(B)** Abundance of clusters of orthologous groups (COG) categories; black point indicates the abundance of LC5 for each category. A box and whisker plot indicates a statistical distribution of the COG categories of 19 *L. casei* genomes. **(C)** Phylogenetic tree of *L. casei* group based on 16S rRNA genes and **(D)** phylogenetic tree of *L. casei* group based on average nucleotide identity. The value 0.02 of the ruler in **(D)** indicates 2% of genomic dissimilarity. Red boxes on the **(C,D)** indicate the genomes associated to the high-GC group and green boxes indicate the genomes associated to the low-GC group.

categories against the 19 *L. casei* group genomes, we found that *L. casei* LC5 contains the high number of proteins which associate with "carbohydrate transport and metabolism (G)" (376 proteins) and "transcription (K)" (239 proteins) excluding two unknown categories, "general function prediction only (R)" and "function unknown (S)" as shown in **Figure 1B**. *L. casei* LC5 has at least 36 more proteins than the other genomes on the category G and has at least 8 more proteins than the other genomes on the category K. The gene expansion of those two functional categories in the LC5 genome is not found on the other members of high-GC group. Although the genomes belonging to high-GC group showed high similarities to each other and the genomes belonging to the high-GC group do not have excessive proteins on the categories, G and K, when compared to those belonging to the low-GC group. Moreover, *L. casei* ATCC 393 which is the most similar genome of LC5 has fewer proteins than the average number of those categories, 223 proteins for the category G and 192 proteins for the category K.

In the previous study, probiotic LC5 strain isolated from Korean fermented dairy product showed great therapeutic effect on atopic dermatitis. Here, we report a genomic overview and distinguishing gene features of LC5 by comparative genomic analysis of 20 related strains. The genomic data presented in this report will broaden our knowledge about roles and mechanisms

TABLE 1 | Genome summary of *Lactobacillus casei* group.

Organism/name	Strain	Clade	Assembly level	Size (Mb)	GC%	GC group
L. casei LC5	LC5	*L. casei*	Complete genome	3.13	47.9	High
*L. case*i str. Zhang	Zhang	*L. casei*	Complete genome	2.90	46.4	Low
L. casei BL23	BL23	*L. casei*	Complete genome	3.08	46.3	Low
L. casei BD-II	BD-II	*L. casei*	complete genome	3.13	46.3	Low
L. casei LC2W	LC2W	*L. casei*	Complete genome	3.08	46.4	Low
L. casei 12A	12A	*L. casei*	Complete genome	2.91	46.4	Low
L. casei W56	W56	*L. casei*	Complete genome	3.13	46.3	Low
L. casei LOCK919	LOCK919	*L. casei*	Complete genome	3.14	46.2	Low
L. casei subsp. casei ATCC 393	ATCC 393	*L. casei*	Complete genome	2.95	47.9	High
L. casei LcY	LcY	*L. casei*	Chromosome	3.10	46.3	Low
L. casei LcA	LcA	*L. casei*	Chromosome	3.13	46.3	Low
L. casei A2-362	A2-362	*L. casei*	Scaffold	3.19	46.2	Low
L. casei	KL1-Liu	*L. casei*	Scaffold	2.85	46.6	Low
L. casei DSM 20011 = JCM 1134	DSM 20011	*L. casei*	Scaffold	2.82	46.5	Low
L. casei 21/1	21/1	*L. casei*	Contig	3.22	46.2	Low
L. casei 32G	32G	*L. casei*	Contig	3.01	46.4	Low
L. casei A2-362	A2-362	*L. casei*	Contig	3.36	46.1	Low
L. casei CRF28	CRF28	*L. casei*	Contig	3.04	46.3	Low
L. casei M36	M36	*L. casei*	Contig	3.15	46.3	Low
L. casei T71499	T71499	*L. casei*	Contig	3.00	46.2	Low
L. casei UCD174	UCD174	*L. casei*	Contig	3.07	46.4	Low
L. casei UW1	UW1	*L. casei*	Contig	2.87	46.4	Low
L. casei UW4	UW4	*L. casei*	Contig	2.76	46.4	Low
L. casei Lc-10	Lc-10	*L. casei*	Contig	2.95	46.4	Low
L. casei Lpc-37	Lpc-37	*L. casei*	Contig	3.08	46.3	Low
L. casei UW4	UW4	*L. casei*	Contig	2.63	46.4	Low
L. casei 12A	12A	*L. casei*	Contig	2.93	46.3	Low
L. casei 5b	5b	*L. casei*	Contig	3.02	46.3	Low
L. casei	N87	*L. casei*	Contig	3.00	47.9	High
L. casei	867_LCAS	*L. casei*	Contig	3.09	47.9	High
L. casei	DPC6800	*L. casei*	Contig	3.05	46.4	Low
L. casei	Lc1542	*L. casei*	Contig	2.92	46.5	Low
L. casei	1316.rep1_LPAR	*L. casei*	Scaffold	2.86	46.5	Low
L. casei	1316.rep2_LPAR	*L. casei*	Scaffold	2.79	46.4	Low
L. casei	844_LCAS	*L. casei*	Scaffold	2.79	46.4	Low
L. casei	BM-LC14617	*L. casei*	Scaffold	3.04	46.3	Low
L. casei	Lbs2	*L. casei*	Scaffold	3.27	47.9	High
L. casei DSM 20011 = JCM 1134	JCM 1134	*L. casei*	Contig	2.78	47.7	High
Lactobacillus paracasei ATCC 334	ATCC 334	*L. paracasei*	Complete genome	2.92	46.6	Low
L. paracasei subsp. *paracasei* 8700:2	8700:2	*L. paracasei*	Complete genome	3.03	46.3	Low
L. paracasei N1115	N1115	*L. paracasei*	Complete genome	3.06	46.5	Low
L. paracasei subsp. paracasei JCM 8130	JCM 8130	*L. paracasei*	Complete genome	3.02	46.6	Low
L. paracasei	CAUH35	*L. paracasei*	Complete genome	2.97	46.3	Low
L. paracasei	L9	*L. paracasei*	Complete genome	3.08	46.3	Low
L. paracasei	KL1	*L. paracasei*	Complete genome	2.92	46.6	Low
Lactobacillus zeae DSM 20178 = KCTC 3804	DSM 20178	*L. zeae*	Scaffold	3.12	47.7	High
Lactobacillus rhamnosus GG	GG (ATCC 53103)	*L. rhamnosus*	Complete genome	3.01	46.7	Low

of microorganisms ameliorating symptoms of immune diseases and help developing functional probiotics for the treatment of immune disorders.

DATA ACCESS

The *L. casei* LC5 genome sequencing project has been deposited at GenBank under the accession number CP017065. The BioProject and BioSample designation for this project is PRJNA340077 and SAMN05631198, respectively. This strain has been deposited in the Korean Collection for Type Cultures (deposit ID: KCTC 12398BP).

AUTHOR CONTRIBUTIONS

Y-DN and SL designed and coordinated all the experiments. T-JL and JK performed cultivation and DNA preparation. JK and W-HC performed genome assembly, gene prediction, gene annotation, and comparative genomic analysis. Y-DN, W-HC, TW, and JK wrote the manuscript. All authors have read the manuscript and approved.

REFERENCES

1. Hill C, Guarner F, Reid G, Gibson GR, Merenstein DJ, Pot B, et al. Expert consensus document: the International Scientific Association for Probiotics and Prebiotics consensus statement on the scope and appropriate use of the term probiotic. *Nat Rev Gastroenterol Hepatol* (2014) 11:506–14. doi:10.1038/nrgastro.2014.66
2. McFarland LV. Meta-analysis of probiotics for the prevention of antibiotic associated diarrhea and the treatment of *Clostridium difficile* disease. *Am J Gastroenterol* (2006) 101:812–22. doi:10.1111/j.1572-0241.2006.00465.x
3. Sanders ME. Considerations for use of probiotic bacteria to modulate human health. *J Nutr* (2000) 130:384S–90S.
4. Reid G, Jass J, Sebulsky MT, Mccormick JK. Potential uses of probiotics in clinical practice. *Clin Microbiol Rev* (2003) 16:658–72. doi:10.1128/CMR.16.4.658-672.2003
5. Saez-Lara MJ, Gomez-Llorente C, Plaza-Diaz J, Gil A. The role of probiotic lactic acid bacteria and bifidobacteria in the prevention and treatment of inflammatory bowel disease and other related diseases: a systematic review of randomized human clinical trials. *Biomed Res Int* (2015) 2015:15. doi:10.1155/2015/505878
6. Wang H, Lee I-S, Braun C, Enck P. Effect of probiotics on central nervous system functions in animals and humans: a systematic review. *J Neurogastroenterol Motil* (2016) 22:589–605. doi:10.5056/jnm16018
7. Cai H, Rodríguez BT, Zhang W, Broadbent JR, Steele JL. Genotypic and phenotypic characterization of *Lactobacillus casei* strains isolated from different ecological niches suggests frequent recombination and niche specificity. *Microbiology* (2007) 153:2655–65. doi:10.1099/mic.0.2007/006452-0
8. Banks JM, Williams A. The role of the nonstarter lactic acid bacteria in Cheddar cheese ripening. *Int J Dairy Technol* (2004) 57:145–52. doi:10.1111/j.1471-0307.2004.00150.x
9. Galdeano CM, Perdigon G. The probiotic bacterium *Lactobacillus casei* induces activation of the gut mucosal immune system through innate immunity. *Clin Vaccine Immunol* (2006) 13:219–26. doi:10.1128/CVI.13.2.219-226.2006
10. Yadav H, Jain S, Sinha PR. Antidiabetic effect of probiotic dahi containing *Lactobacillus acidophilus* and *Lactobacillus casei* in high fructose fed rats. *Nutrition* (2007) 23:62–8. doi:10.1016/j.nut.2006.09.002
11. Koebnick C, Wagner I, Leitzmann P, Stern U, Zunft HF. Probiotic beverage containing *Lactobacillus casei* shirota improves gastrointestinal symptoms in patients with chronic constipation. *Can J Gastroenterol* (2003) 17:655–9. doi:10.1155/2003/654907
12. Hee YJ, Kim DH, Ku JK, Kang Y, Kim M-Y, Kim HO, et al. Therapeutic effects of probiotics in patients with atopic dermatitis. *J Microbiol Biotechnol* (2006) 16:1699–705.
13. Seo J-G, Chung M-J, Lee H-G. Alleviation of atopic dermatitis through probiotic and mixed-probiotic treatments in an atopic dermatitis model. *Korean J Food Sci Animal Resour* (2011) 31:420–7. doi:10.5851/kosfa.2011.31.3.420
14. Yang H-J, Min TK, Lee HW, Pyun BY. Efficacy of probiotic therapy on atopic dermatitis in children: a randomized, double-blind, placebo-controlled trial. *Allergy Asthma Immunol Res* (2014) 6:208–15. doi:10.4168/aair.2014.6.3.208
15. Cha YS, Seo J-G, Chung M-J, Cho CW, Youn HJ. A mixed formulation of lactic acid bacteria inhibits trinitrobenzene-sulfonic-acid-induced inflammatory changes of the colon tissue in mice. *J Microbiol Biotechnol* (2014) 24:1438–44. doi:10.4014/jmb.1403.03064
16. Chin C-S, Alexander DH, Marks P, Klammer AA, Drake J, Heiner C, et al. Nonhybrid, finished microbial genome assemblies from long-read SMRT sequencing data. *Nat Methods* (2013) 10:563–9. doi:10.1038/nmeth.2474
17. Tatusova T, Dicuccio M, Badretdin A, Chetvernin V, Nawrocki EP, Zaslavsky L, et al. NCBI prokaryotic genome annotation pipeline. *Nucleic Acids Res* (2016) 44(14):6614–24. doi:10.1093/nar/gkw569
18. Carver T, Thomson N, Bleasby A, Berriman M, Parkhill J. DNAPlotter: circular and linear interactive genome visualization. *Bioinformatics* (2009) 25:119–20. doi:10.1093/bioinformatics/btn578
19. Galperin MY, Makarova KS, Wolf YI, Koonin EV. Expanded microbial genome coverage and improved protein family annotation in the COG database. *Nucleic Acids Res* (2015) 43:D261–9. doi:10.1093/nar/gku1223
20. Tamura K, Nei M. Estimation of the number of nucleotide substitutions in the control region of mitochondrial DNA in humans and chimpanzees. *Mol Biol Evol* (1993) 10:512–26.
21. Tamura K, Stecher G, Peterson D, Filipski A, Kumar S. MEGA6: molecular evolutionary genetics analysis version 6.0. *Mol Biol Evol* (2013) 30:2725–9. doi:10.1093/molbev/mst197
22. Lee I, Ouk Kim Y, Park S-C, Chun J. OrthoANI: an improved algorithm and software for calculating average nucleotide identity. *Int J Syst Evol Microbiol* (2016) 66:1100–3. doi:10.1099/ijsem.0.000760
23. Laing C, Buchanan C, Taboada EN, Zhang Y, Kropinski A, Villegas A, et al. Pan-genome sequence analysis using Panseq: an online tool for the rapid analysis of core and accessory genomic regions. *BMC Bioinformatics* (2010) 11:1. doi:10.1186/1471-2105-11-461

Permissions

All chapters in this book were first published in IIBMWIS, by Frontiers; hereby published with permission under the Creative Commons Attribution License or equivalent. Every chapter published in this book has been scrutinized by our experts. Their significance has been extensively debated. The topics covered herein carry significant findings which will fuel the growth of the discipline. They may even be implemented as practical applications or may be referred to as a beginning point for another development.

The contributors of this book come from diverse backgrounds, making this book a truly international effort. This book will bring forth new frontiers with its revolutionizing research information and detailed analysis of the nascent developments around the world.

We would like to thank all the contributing authors for lending their expertise to make the book truly unique.

They have played a crucial role in the development of this book. Without their invaluable contributions this book wouldn't have been possible. They have made vital efforts to compile up to date information on the varied aspects of this subject to make this book a valuable addition to the collection of many professionals and students.

This book was conceptualized with the vision of imparting up-to-date information and advanced data in this field. To ensure the same, a matchless editorial board was set up. Every individual on the board went through rigorous rounds of assessment to prove their worth. After which they invested a large part of their time researching and compiling the most relevant data for our readers.

The editorial board has been involved in producing this book since its inception. They have spent rigorous hours researching and exploring the diverse topics which have resulted in the successful publishing of this book. They have passed on their knowledge of decades through this book. To expedite this challenging task, the publisher supported the team at every step. A small team of assistant editors was also appointed to further simplify the editing procedure and attain best results for the readers.

Apart from the editorial board, the designing team has also invested a significant amount of their time in understanding the subject and creating the most relevant covers. They scrutinized every image to scout for the most suitable representation of the subject and create an appropriate cover for the book.

The publishing team has been an ardent support to the editorial, designing and production team. Their endless efforts to recruit the best for this project, has resulted in the accomplishment of this book. They are a veteran in the field of academics and their pool of knowledge is as vast as their experience in printing. Their expertise and guidance has proved useful at every step. Their uncompromising quality standards have made this book an exceptional effort. Their encouragement from time to time has been an inspiration for everyone.

The publisher and the editorial board hope that this book will prove to be a valuable piece of knowledge for researchers, students, practitioners and scholars across the globe.

List of Contributors

Sukumar Kandasamy, Anastasia N. Vlasova, David D. Fischer, Kuldeep S. Chattha, Lulu Shao, Anand Kumar, Stephanie N. Langel, Abdul Rauf, Huang-Chi Huang, Gireesh Rajashekara and Linda J. Saif
Food Animal Health Research Program (FAHRP), Veterinary Preventive Medicine Department, The Ohio Agricultural Research and Development Center, The Ohio State University, Wooster, OH, USA

Krisztian Bene, Zsofia Varga and Eva Rajnavolgyi
Faculty of Medicine, Department of Immunology, University of Debrecen, Debrecen, Hungary

Viktor O. Petrov and Nadiya Boyko
Faculty of Medicine, R&D Centre of Molecular Microbiology and Mucosal Immunology, Uzhhorod National University, Uzhhorod, Ukraine

Takahiro Adachi
Department of Immunology, Medical Research Institute, Tokyo Medical and Dental University, Tokyo, Japan

Shigeru Kakuta
Department of Biomedical Science, Graduate School of Agricultural and Life Sciences, The University of Tokyo, Tokyo, Japan

Yoshiko Aihara
Department of Agrobioscience, Graduate School of Agricultural Science, Kobe University, Kobe, Japan

Tomonori Kamiya, Yohei Watanabe and Noriko M. Tsuji
Biomedical Research Institute, National Institute for Advanced Industrial Science and Technology (AIST), Tsukuba, Japan

Naomi Osakabe and Naoki Hazato
Department of Bio-science and Engineering, Shibaura Institute of Technology, Saitama, Japan

Atsushi Miyawaki
Laboratory for Cell Function and Dynamics, Advanced Technology Development Group, Brain Science Institute, RIKEN, Saitama, Japan

Soichiro Yoshikawa and Hajime Karasuyama
Department of Immune Regulation, Tokyo Medical and Dental University, Tokyo, Japan,

Takako Usami
Laboratory of Recombinant Animals, Medical Research Institute, Tokyo Medical and Dental University, Tokyo, Japan

Hiromi Kimoto-Nira
NARO Institute of Livestock and Grassland Science, National Agriculture and Food Research Organization, Tsukuba, Ibaraki, Japan

Kazuhiro Hirayama
Laboratory of Veterinary Public Health, Graduate School of Agricultural and Life Sciences, The University of Tokyo, Tokyo, Japan

Guanliu Yu, Yao Wang, Tongjie Chai, Yumei Cai and Liangmeng Wei
College of Animal Science and Veterinary Medicine, Shandong Agricultural University, Sino-German Cooperative Research Centre for Zoonosis of Animal Origin Shandong Province, Tai'an, China,

Shouguo Wang and Changmin Duan
Deizhou People's Hospital, Deizhou, China,

Jing Gao
The Central Hospital of Tai'an, Tai'an, China

Zongxin Ling, Li Shao, Yiwen Cheng and Lanjuan Li
Collaborative Innovation Center for Diagnosis and Treatment of Infectious Diseases, State Key Laboratory for Diagnosis and Treatment of Infectious Diseases, The First Affiliated Hospital, College of Medicine, Zhejiang University, Hangzhou, China,

Fengping Liu
Collaborative Innovation Center for Diagnosis and Treatment of Infectious Diseases, State Key Laboratory for Diagnosis and Treatment of Infectious Diseases, The First Affiliated Hospital, College of Medicine, Zhejiang University, Hangzhou, China
Nursing School, Jiangsu Vocational College of Medicine, Yancheng, China

Ting Wan, Yingying Zhao, Fangli Fan, Renjian Hu and Xiuming Jin
Eye Center, Second Affiliated Hospital, School of Medicine, Zhejiang University, Hangzhou, China

Julio Villena
Immunobiotics Research Group, Tucuman, Argentina
Laboratory of Immunobiotechnology, Reference Centre for Lactobacilli (CERELA-CONICET), Tucuman, Argentina
Food and Feed Immunology Group, Laboratory of Animal Products Chemistry, Graduate School of Agricultural Science, Tohoku University, Sendai, Japan

Maria Guadalupe Vizoso-Pinto
Immunobiotics Research Group, Tucuman, Argentina
Faculty of Medicine, INSIBIO (UNT-CONICET), National University of Tucuman, Tucuman, Argentina

Haruki Kitazawa
Laboratory of Immunobiotechnology, Reference Centre for Lactobacilli (CERELA-CONICET), Tucuman, Argentina
Food and Feed Immunology Group, Laboratory of Animal Products Chemistry, Graduate School of Agricultural Science, Tohoku University, Sendai, Japan
Livestock Immunology Unit, International Education and Research Center for Food and Agricultural Immunology (CFAI), Graduate School of Agricultural Science, Tohoku University, Sendai, Japan

Suguru Shigemori
Department of Bioscience and Food Production Science, Interdisciplinary Graduate School of Science and Technology, Shinshu University, Nagano, Japan
Japan Society for the Promotion of Science, Tokyo, Japan

Takeshi Shimosato
Department of Interdisciplinary Genome Sciences and Cell Metabolism, Institute for Biomedical Sciences, Shinshu University, Nagano, Japan
Supramolecular Complexes Unit, Research Center for Fungal and Microbial Dynamism, Shinshu University, Nagano, Japan

René Holst
Research and Innovation, Østfold Hospital Trust, Kalnes, Norway

Stine Indrelid and Morten Jacobsen
Research and Innovation, Østfold Hospital Trust, Kalnes, Norway
Department of Chemistry, Biotechnology and Food Science, Norwegian University of Life Sciences, Aas, Norway

Charlotte Kleiveland and Tor Lea
Department of Chemistry, Biotechnology and Food Science, Norwegian University of Life Sciences, Aas, Norway

Rodrigo D. De Oliveira Carvalho, Fillipe L. R. do Carmo, Alberto de Oliveira Junior, Vasco Azevedo and Marcela S. de Azevedo
Federal University of Minas Gerais - Instituto de Ciências Biológicas, Belo Horizonte, Brazil

Silvia González
Universidad Nacional de Tucumán (UNT), Tucumán, Argentina

Philippe Langella, Jean-Marc Chatel and Luis G. Bermúdez-Humarán
Micalis Institute, Institut National de la Recherche Agronomique, AgroParisTech, Université Paris-Saclay, Jouy-en-Josas, France

Eun Byeol Ko, Sun Kyung Kim and Seung Hyun Han
Department of Oral Microbiology and Immunology, DRI, and BK21 Plus Program, School of Dentistry, Seoul National University, Seoul, South Korea

Ho Seong Seo
Biotechnology Research Division, Korea Atomic Energy Research Institute, Jeongeup, South Korea

Cheol-Heui Yun
Department of Agricultural Biotechnology and Research Institute for Agriculture and Life Sciences, Seoul National University, Seoul, South Korea

Adriaan A. van Beek
Cell Biology and Immunology Group, Wageningen University, Wageningen, Netherlands
Top Institute Food and Nutrition, Wageningen, Netherlands
Gut Health and Food Safety, Institute of Food Research, Norwich, UK

Bruno Sovran and Jerry M. Wells
Top Institute Food and Nutrition, Wageningen, Netherlands
Host Microbe Interactomics, Wageningen University, Wageningen, Netherlands

Floor Hugenholtz and Clara Belzer
Top Institute Food and Nutrition, Wageningen, Netherlands
Laboratory of Microbiology, Wageningen University, Wageningen, Netherlands

Ben Meijer, Joanne A. Hoogerland, Violeta Mihailova and Corine van der Ploeg
Cell Biology and Immunology Group, Wageningen University, Wageningen, Netherlands

Mark V. Boekschoten
Top Institute Food and Nutrition, Wageningen, Netherlands
Human Nutrition, Wageningen University, Wageningen, Netherlands

Susana Salva
Immunobiotechnology Laboratory, CERELA-CONICET, Tucuman, Argentina

Jan H. J. Hoeijmakers
Department of Molecular Genetics, Erasmus University Medical Center, Rotterdam, Netherlands
CECAD Forschungszentrum, Universität zu Köln, Köln, Germany

Wilbert P. Vermeij
Department of Molecular Genetics, Erasmus University Medical Center, Rotterdam, Netherlands

Paul de Vos
Top Institute Food and Nutrition, Wageningen, Netherlands
University of Groningen, Groningen, Netherlands

Pieter J. M. Leenen
Department of Immunology, Erasmus University Medical Center, Rotterdam, Netherlands

Claudio Nicoletti
Gut Health and Food Safety, Institute of Food Research, Norwich, UK
Department of Experimental and Clinical Medicine, University of Florence, Florence, Italy

Rudi W. Hendriks
Department of Pulmonary Medicine, Erasmus University Medical Center, Rotterdam, Netherlands

Huub F. J. Savelkoul
Cell Biology and Immunology Group, Wageningen University, Wageningen, Netherlands
Top Institute Food and Nutrition, Wageningen, Netherlands

Patricia Clua and Susana Salva
Immunobiotics Research Group, Tucuman, Argentina
Laboratory of Immunobiotechnology, Reference Centre for Lactobacilli (CERELA-CONICET), Tucuman, Argentina

Paulraj Kanmani, A. K. M. Humayun Kober and Haruki Kitazawa
Food and Feed Immunology Group, Laboratory of Animal Products Chemistry, Graduate School of Agricultural Science, Tohoku University, Sendai, Japan
4 Livestock Immunology Unit, International Education and Research Center for Food and Agricultural Immunology (CFAI), Graduate School of Agricultural Science, Tohoku University, Sendai, Japan,

Hortensia Zelaya
Immunobiotics Research Group, Tucuman, Argentina
Institute of Applied Biochemistry, National University of Tucumán, Tucuman, Argentina

Asuka Tada
Food and Feed Immunology Group, Laboratory of Animal Products Chemistry, Graduate School of Agricultural Science, Tohoku University, Sendai, Japan

Susana Alvarez
Immunobiotics Research Group, Tucuman, Argentina
Laboratory of Immunobiotechnology, Reference Centre for Lactobacilli (CERELA-CONICET), Tucuman, Argentina
Institute of Applied Biochemistry, National University of Tucumán, Tucuman, Argentina

Julio Villena
Immunobiotics Research Group, Tucuman, Argentina
Laboratory of Immunobiotechnology, Reference Centre for Lactobacilli (CERELA-CONICET), Tucuman, Argentina
Food and Feed Immunology Group, Laboratory of Animal Products Chemistry, Graduate School of Agricultural Science, Tohoku University, Sendai, Japan

Carolina Iraporda, Ana A. Bengoa and Graciela L. Garrote
Centro de Investigación y Desarrollo en Criotecnología de Alimentos (CIDCA, UNLP-CONICET-CIC.PBA), La Plata, Argentina

David E. Romanin, Agustina J. Errea and Martín Rumbo
Instituto de Estudios Inmunológicos y Fisopatológicos (IIFP, UNLP-CONICET), La Plata, Argentina

Delphine Cayet, Benoit Foligné and Jean-Claude Sirard
CNRS, INSERM, CHU Lille, Institut Pasteur de Lille, U1019 - UMR 8204 - CIIL - Center for Infection and Immunity of Lille, University of Lille, Lille, France

Analía G. Abraham
Centro de Investigación y Desarrollo en Criotecnología de Alimentos (CIDCA, UNLP-CONICET-CIC.PBA), La Plata, Argentina
Área Bioquímica y Control de Alimentos, Facultad de Ciencias Exactas, UNLP, La Plata, Argentina

Hortensia Zelaya
Immunobiotics Research Group, Tucuman, Argentina
Institute of Applied Biochemistry, National University of Tucuman, Tucuman, Argentina

Susana Alvarez
Immunobiotics Research Group, Tucuman, Argentina
Institute of Applied Biochemistry, National University of Tucuman, Tucuman, Argentina
Laboratory of Immunobiotechnology, Reference Centre for Lactobacilli (CERELA-CONICET), Tucuman, Argentina

Haruki Kitazawa
Food and Feed Immunology Group, Laboratory of Animal Products Chemistry, Graduate School of Agricultural Science, Tohoku University, Sendai, Japan
Livestock Immunology Unit, International Education and Research Center for Food and Agricultural Immunology (CFAI), Graduate School of Agricultural Science, Tohoku University, Sendai, Japan

Julio Villena
Immunobiotics Research Group, Tucuman, Argentina
Laboratory of Immunobiotechnology, Reference Centre for Lactobacilli (CERELA-CONICET), Tucuman, Argentina
Food and Feed Immunology Group, Laboratory of Animal Products Chemistry, Graduate School of Agricultural Science, Tohoku University, Sendai, Japan

Javier Rodríguez-Carrio, Borja Sánchez, Miguel Gueimonde, Abelardo Margolles and Clara G. de los Reyes-Gavilán
Department of Microbiology and Biochemistry of Dairy Products, Instituto de Productos Lácteos de Asturias (IPLA-CSIC), Villaviciosa, Asturias, Spain

Patricia López and Ana Suárez
Area of Immunology, Department of Functional Biology, University of Oviedo, Oviedo, Asturias, Spain

Sonia González
Area of Physiology, Department of Functional Biology, University of Oviedo, Oviedo, Asturias, Spain

Emanuel Fabersani
Centro de Referencia para Lactobacilos (CERELA) - CONICET, Tucumán, Argentina,

María Claudia Abeijon-Mukdsi and Paola Gauffin-Cano
Centro de Referencia para Lactobacilos (CERELA) - CONICET, Tucumán, Argentina,
Facultad Ciencias de la Salud, Universidad del Norte Santo Tomás de Aquino (UNSTA), Tucumán, Argentina,

Romina Ross
Facultad Ciencias de la Salud, Universidad del Norte Santo Tomás de Aquino (UNSTA), Tucumán, Argentina
Universidad Nacional de Tucumán (UNT), Tucumán, Argentina

Roxana Medina
Centro de Referencia para Lactobacilos (CERELA) - CONICET, Tucumán, Argentina
Universidad Nacional de Tucumán (UNT), Tucumán, Argentina

Tomonori Nochi and Hisashi Aso
Cell Biology Laboratory, Graduate School of Agricultural Science, Tohoku University, Sendai, Japan
Infection Immunology Unit, International Education and Research Center for Food Agricultural Immunology (CFAI), Graduate School of Agricultural Science, Tohoku University, Sendai, Japan

Susana Alvarez
Immunobiotechnology Laboratory, CERELA-CONICET, Tucuman, Argentina
Applied Biochemistry Institute, Universidad Nacional de Tucumán, Tucuman, Argentina

Aline Zazeri Leite, Marina Ignácio Gonzaga, João Luiz Brisotti and Gislane Lelis Vilela de Oliveira
Microbiome Study Group, School of Health Sciences Dr. Paulo Prata (FACISB), Barretos, Brazil

Nathália de Campos Rodrigues and Nadine Aparecida Vicentini Stefanutto
QGene-Solutions and Logistics in Health, Sao Carlos, Brazil

João Carlos Cicogna Paiolo and Carolina Arantes de Souza
Board of Health from Barretos, Barretos, Brazil

Wellington Pine Omori and Daniel Guariz Pinheiro
Department of Technology, School of Agricultural and Veterinarian Sciences, São Paulo State University (UNESP), Sao Paulo, Brazil

Euclides Matheucci Junior
DNA Consult Genetics and Biotechnology, Sao Carlos, Brazil
Biotechnology Department, Sao Carlos Federal University, UFSCAR, Sao Carlos, Brazil

Vânia Sammartino Mariano
Barretos Cancer Hospital (HCB), Barretos, Brazil

Leonardo Albarracin and Julio Villena
Laboratory of Immunobiotechnology, Reference Centre for Lactobacilli (CERELA-CONICET), Tucuman, Argentina
Immunobiotics Research Group, Tucuman, Argentina
Food and Feed Immunology Group, Laboratory of Animal Products Chemistry, Graduate School of Agricultural Science, Tohoku University, Sendai, Japan

Hisakazu Kobayashi, Hikaru Iida, Nana Sato and Haruki Kitazawa
Food and Feed Immunology Group, Laboratory of Animal Products Chemistry, Graduate School of Agricultural Science, Tohoku University, Sendai, Japan
Livestock Immunology Unit, International Education and Research Center for Food Agricultural Immunology (CFAI), Graduate School of Agricultural Science, Tohoku University, Sendai, Japan

Susana Salva and Susana Alvarez
Laboratory of Immunobiotechnology, Reference Centre for Lactobacilli (CERELA-CONICET), Tucuman, Argentina

Immunobiotics Research Group, Tucuman, Argentina

Jisu Kang and Young-Do Nam
Research Group of Gut Microbiome, Korea Food Research Institute, Sungnam, South Korea
Department of Food Biotechnology, Korea University of Science and Technology, Daejeon, South Korea

Won-Hyong Chung
Research Group of Gut Microbiome, Korea Food Research Institute, Sungnam, South Korea

Tae-Joong Lim and Sanghyun Lim
Research and Development Center, Cell Biotech Co. Ltd., Gimpo, South Korea

Tae Woong Whon
Department of Biology, Kyung Hee University, Seoul, South Korea

Index

www.ingramcontent.com/pod-product-compliance
Lightning Source LLC
LaVergne TN
LVHW080947210926
848485LV00004B/794